Essentials of Percutaneous Dialysis Interventions

AF719308

Dheeraj K. Rajan
Editor

Essentials of Percutaneous Dialysis Interventions

Springer

Editor
Dheeraj K. Rajan, MD, FRCPC, FSIR
Head and Associate Professor
Division of Vascular & Interventional Radiology
Department of Medical Imaging
University of Toronto
Toronto, ON, Canada
Dheeraj.Rajan@uhn.on.ca

ISBN 978-1-4419-5656-9 e-ISBN 978-1-4419-5657-6
DOI 10.1007/978-1-4419-5657-6
Springer New York Dordrecht Heidelberg London

Library of Congress Control Number:2011933603

© Springer Science+Business Media, LLC 2011
All rights reserved. This work may not be translated or copied in whole or in part without the written permission of the publisher (Springer Science+Business Media, LLC, 233 Spring Street, New York, NY 10013, USA), except for brief excerpts in connection with reviews or scholarly analysis. Use in connection with any form of information storage and retrieval, electronic adaptation, computer software, or by similar or dissimilar methodology now known or hereafter developed is forbidden.
The use in this publication of trade names, trademarks, service marks, and similar terms, even if they are not identified as such, is not to be taken as an expression of opinion as to whether or not they are subject to proprietary rights.
While the advice and information in this book are believed to be true and accurate at the date of going to press, neither the authors nor the editors nor the publisher can accept any legal responsibility for any errors or omissions that may be made. The publisher makes no warranty, express or implied, with respect to the material contained herein.

Printed on acid-free paper

Springer is part of Springer Science+Business Media (www.springer.com)

Preface

Within the last decade, we have seen a rapid expansion and innovation in dialysis interventions throughout the world and in particular North America. Growth has been fuelled by an aging population, healthcare advances that have prolonged life, and a greater incidence of certain disease states particularly diabetes. These factors have all contributed toward a greater occurrence and prevalence of end-stage renal disease.

The increased need for dialysis and its attendant costs have now moved from a point of obscure interest to one of major concern within medicine. In addition to the increased burden on the medical system, the costs are substantial and growing exponentially. As a result, we have witnessed within a few years a number of new physician groups, organizations, and both medical device and pharmacological companies become involved with all aspects of medical care related to end-stage renal disease.

One particular area, hemodialysis access creation and maintenance, has seen particular focused interest. Prior to 2000, there was little interest in creation and methods to maintain autogenous hemodialysis fistulas, outpatient hemodialysis intervention centers were rare and maintenance interventions were largely performed by Interventional Radiologists. Within the last 10 years, the kidney disease outcomes quality initiative (KDOQI) has been published and revised, within the United States the Fistula First initiative was begun, and the Centers for Medicare and Medicaid Services (CMS) has tied reimbursement to performance measures. In addition, multiple new devices have become available, procedures are now often performed at outpatient centers rather than hospitals, and the profession of Interventional Nephrology has become a major provider of hemodialysis interventions within the United States.

Given all these changes, there is remarkably minimal standardization of education, training, and unbiased independent assessment of technical ability and outcomes for physicians performing percutaneous dialysis interventions. This handbook is a step toward addressing these deficiencies by condensing and simplifying interventions for all medical practitioners who perform these interventions. This handbook also attempts to address all relevant areas associated with percutaneous interventions. The chapters in this book are written by respected experts in their respective areas of specialization. Further, I have endeavored to provide all information in a succinct and practical format for all readers.

This handbook is the first to exclusively focus on percutaneous interventions and is targeted for any medical support personnel, and any physicians who are practicing or in training involved in providing or managing care to dialysis patients.

This project would not have been possible without the unwavering support of my mentors within the United States who have become colleagues and friends, my family, and close personal friends who have tolerated me and my time spent on this book. Finally, I am indebted to the authors for their selfless contributions without which this handbook would not be complete.

Contents

Contributors

Ahmad I. Alomari, MD, FSIR Assistant Professor, Harvard Medical School, Boston, MA, USA

Children's Hospital Boston, Boston, MA, USA

Sandford Altman, MD Open Access Vascular Access Center, Miami, FL, USA

Dirk S. Baumann, MD, FACS Director, Mid Peninsula Wound Care Medical Clinic, Peninsula Surgical Specialists Medical Group, Burlingame, CA 94010, USA

Cynthia Bhola, RN, BN, MN, CNephC Dialysis Vascular Access Coordinator, University Health Network, Toronto, ON, Canada

Jason Blaichman, MDCM Diagnostic Radiology, Department of Medical Imaging, University of Toronto, Toronto, ON, Canada

Micah Chan, MD, MPH, FACP Division of Nephrology, UW Hospitals and Clinics, Madison, WI, USA

Timothy I. Clark, MD, FSIR Associate Professor of Radiology, Director, Interventional Radiology, Department of Radiology, Penn Presbyterian Medical Center, Philadelphia, Pennsylvania, USA

Bairbre Connolly, MB, FRCPC Pediatric Interventional Radiologist, Department of Diagnostic Imaging, The Hospital for Sick Children, Canada; Associate Professor, Earl Glenwood Coulson Chair, Medical Imaging Department, University of Toronto, Toronto, Ontario, Canada

Brian J. Dillon, MD Division of Vascular and Interventional Radiology, Children's Hospital Boston, Harvard Medical School, Boston, MA, USA

Bart Dolmatch, MD, FSIR Professor and Chief of Interventional Radiology, Department of Radiology, UT Southwestern Medical Center, Dallas, TX, USA

Abigail Falk, MD, FSIR American Access Care, Brooklyn, NY, USA

Naveen Goel, MD, FASN American Access Care of Florida, Plantation, FL, USA

Farah G. Irani, MBBS, FRCR, FAMS Consultant, Interventional Radiology Center, Department of Diagnostic Radiology, Singapore General Hospital, Singapore

Shuji Kariya Department of Radiology, Kansai Medical University, Osaka, Japan

Richard Lo, MBBS, MD, FRCR, FAMS Department of Diagnostic Radiology, Interventional Radiology Center, Singapore General Hospital, Singapore

Charmaine E. Lok, MD, FRCPC Associate Professor, Department of Nephrology, Toronto General Hospital and the University of Toronto, Toronto, ON, Canada

David C. Mendelssohn, MD, FRCPC Associate Professor, Department of Nephrology, Nephrolife: Complete Kidney Care Centre, Humber River Regional Hospital and University of Toronto, Toronto, ON, Canada

Joshua G. Mendelssohn University of Western Ontario, London, ON, Canada

Sanjay Misra, MD, FSIR Associate Professor, Department of Radiology, Mayo Clinic School of Medicine, Rochester, MN, USA

Louise Moist, MD, FRCPC Associate Professor of Medicine and Epidemiology, University of Western Ontario, London, ON, Canada

Horacio M. Padua, MD Division of Vascular and Interventional Radiology, Children's Hospital Boston, Harvard Medical School, Boston, MA, USA

William D. Paulson, MD Professor of Medicine, Director, MCG End-Stage Renal Disease Program, Chief of Nephrology, Charlie Norwood VA Medical Center, Medical College of Georgia Augusta, Georgia, USA

Ronald L. Pisoni, PhD, MS Arbor Research Collaborative for Health, Ann Arbor, MI, USA

Robyn A. Pugash, MD, FRCPC Assistant Professor, University of Toronto, Sunnybrook Health Sciences Centre, Toronto, Ontario, Canada

Dheeraj K. Rajan, MD, FRCPC, FSIR Head and Associate Professor, Division of Vascular & Interventional Radiology, Department of Medical Imaging, University of Toronto, Toronto, ON, Canada

John R. Ross, MD Bamberg County Hospital, Bamberg, SC, USA

Theodore F. Saad, MD Nephrology Associates, Newark, DE, USA

Martin E. Simons, MD, FRCPC, FSIR Assistant Professor, Department of Medical Imaging, Toronto Western Hospital, University of Toronto, Toronto, ON, Canada

Bien-Soo Tan, MBBS, FRCR, FAMS Associate Professor, Department of Diagnostic Radiology, Interventional Radiology Center, Singapore General Hospital, Singapore

Manish Taneja, MBBS, MD, FRCR, FAMS Department of Diagnostic Radiology, Interventional Radiology Center, Singapore General Hospital, Singapore

Kiang Hiong Tay, MBBS, FRCR, FAMS Associate Professor, Head and Senior Consultant, Interventional Radiology Center, Department of Diagnostic Radiology, Singapore General Hospital, Singapore

Chapter 1
Introduction

Dheeraj K. Rajan

Globally, there is increasing recognition of the incidence and effects of chronic kidney disease (CKD). Indeed, the scope of CKD appears to be larger than previously believed. The National Kidney Foundation estimates CKD affects 20 million Americans or one in nine adults with the rate of dialysis patients increasing 5–8% per year. Percutaneous interventions are also correspondingly increasing with over 120,000 angioplasties of dialysis access performed every year within the United States and bare metal stent usage has exceeded 12% in all accesses (www.usrds.org). In an effort to regulate and standardize hemodialysis and its method of delivery, the DOQI followed by the K/DOQI guidelines were introduced [1] and subsequently revised in 2006. These documents establish baseline standards to improve patient outcomes within the hemodialysis population. Dialysis access dysfunction contributes significantly to mortality and morbidity with direct costs of dysfunction exceeding one billion dollars annually within the U.S. [2].

D.K. Rajan (✉)
Head and Associate Professor, Division of Vascular & Interventional Radiology, Department of Medical Imaging, University of Toronto, Toronto, Ontario, Canada
e-mail: Dheeraj.Rajan@uhn.on.ca

D.K. Rajan (ed.), *Essentials of Percutaneous Dialysis Interventions*,
DOI 10.1007/978-1-4419-5657-6_1,

© Springer Science+Business Media, LLC 2011

Given the increasing patient population worldwide, a greater proportion of healthcare dollars are being directed to this area of medicine. This has resulted in hemodialysis, an originally forgotten aspect of medicine becoming recognized as a major health issue. Interventions within this area of medicine have become dynamic with many new devices and techniques being developed perpetually. With billions being spent globally, there is significant incentive for policy makers, device and pharmaceutical manufacturers, as well as physicians to become more involved.

Methods for delivery of hemodialysis are via three established methods: (1) catheters, (2) prosthetic grafts, and (3) autogenous fistulas. The hemodialysis fistula is considered the most desired access with dialysis catheters being the least desired. Advantages of autogenous fistulas include longer cumulative patency, lower infection rate, and a lower dysfunction rate, which translates to reduced costs [3–5]. Within this book, percutaneous interventions for management of dysfunctional hemodialysis catheters, grafts, and autogenous fistulas will be discussed. Peritoneal dialysis catheter management is will also be addressed in Chap. 25.

The basis for most percutaneous hemodialysis interventions is the "Seldinger technique." First described by Dr. Seldinger, the basic technique involves puncture of a vessel with a hollow bore trochar needle with passage of a flexible-tipped wire into the vessel. The needle is then removed, and a catheter is advanced into the vessel over the wire, thereby providing maintained access to the vessel [6]. This method has been implemented in many areas of medicine (see Fig. 1.1).

The need for percutaneous intervention should be tempered by clinical findings and a generalized assessment of vascular access requirements in the hemodialysis patient. Every vein segment potentially available for dialysis purposes should be preserved whenever possible, as loss of vein segments directly translates into earlier mortality for many patients. One should intervene with the goal of maintaining current access without loss of future potential access sites. Given the global considerations of the patient and limited healthcare resources, it is important not only to focus on the planned intervention but also to look beyond to future interventions and access needs.

One specific area of concern is placement of peripherally inserted peripheral catheters (PICCs). These devices obliterate veins peripherally in up to 32% of insertions and are the underlying cause of central venous stenosis/occlusion in up to 7% of patients with initial normal

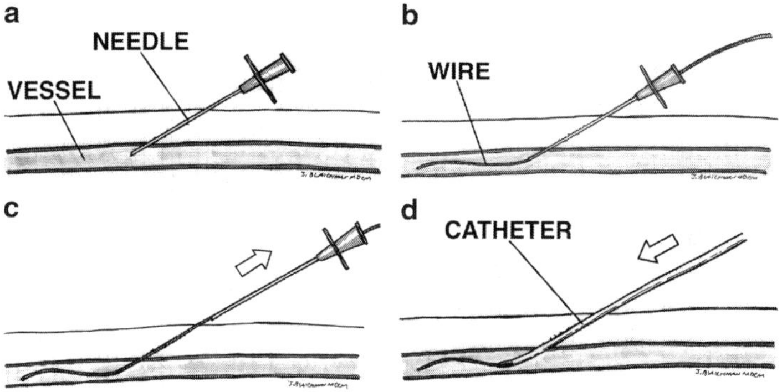

Fig. 1.1 Seldinger technique

venograms [7, 8]. Simply stated, PICC lines destroy future access sites in chronic renal failure patients and should be avoided. Proper management requires a team approach with complementary and coordinated involvement of nephrologists, surgeons, and interventionalists to assure that each patient receives optimal care.

The practicing interventionalist must be diligent in promoting clinical success, outcomes documentation, reliability of service, good clinical practice, and research advances. Some centers have adapted multimodality access conferences to discuss access management issues. Other centers have introduced dialysis access coordinators. Such individuals are highly instrumental in coordinating the care of patients across different clinical services and maintaining proper surveillance of dialysis access. Although initially time consuming, the time saved by patient planning and preprocedure communication far outweighs the small time invested in such a conference. In addition to these strategies, communication and teamwork, development, and adherence to practice guidelines that reflect K/DOQI and local practice patterns are of paramount importance.

This handbook is designed to be a practical "guidebook" for the practicing interventionalist and is structured around the Dialysis Outcome Quality Initiative (K/DOQI) guidelines [9]. K/DOQI can be found at www.kidney.org. Wherever possible, we will attempt to provide several approaches to deal with a specific problem. It is important for the reader to understand that many such approaches will involve the non–FDA-approved off-label use of devices and/or medications within the United States, and by no means is this an exhaustive review of all potential techniques. This is a dynamic field with many new technologies and techniques being developed continuously. Before widely adopting any of these devices or techniques, it is always important to ask if there have been proper review and testing performed. It is always possible to obtain visually good outcomes, but does this translate into clinical benefit for the patient? Finally, it is important to remember that every intervention performed has a permanent effect on the patient, no matter how small or insignificant the intervention is.

References

1. Eknoyan G, Levin NW, Eschbach JW, et al. Continuous quality improvement: DOQI becomes K/DOQI and is updated. National Kidney Foundation's Dialysis Outcomes Quality Initiative. Am J Kidney Dis. 2001;37(1):179–94.
2. Feldman HI, Kobrin S, Wasserstein A. Hemodialysis vascular access morbidity. J Am Soc Nephrol. 1996;7(4):523–35.
3. Hodges TC, Fillinger MF, Zwolak RM, Walsh DB, Bech F, Cronenwett JL. Longitudinal comparison of dialysis access methods: risk factors for failure. J Vasc Surg. 1997;26(6):1009–19.
4. Ifudu O, Mayers JD, Matthew JJ, Fowler A, Friedman EA. Haemodialysis dose is independent of type of surgically-created vascular access. Nephrol Dial Transplant. 1998;13(9):2311–6.
5. Schwab SJ, Oliver MJ, Suhocki P, McCann R. Hemodialysis arteriovenous access: detection of stenosis and response to treatment by vascular access blood flow. Kidney Int. 2001;59(1):358–62.
6. Seldinger SI. Catheter replacement of the needle in percutaneous arteriography; a new technique. Acta Radiol. 1953;39(5):368–76.
7. Gonsalves CF, Eschelman DJ, Sullivan KL, DuBois N, Bonn J. Incidence of central vein stenosis and occlusion following upper extremity PICC and port placement. Cardiovasc Intervent Radiol. 2003;26(2):123–7.
8. Allen AW, Megargell JL, Brown DB, et al. Venous thrombosis associated with the placement of peripherally inserted central catheters. J Vasc Interv Radiol. 2000;11(10):1309–14.
9. National Kidney Foundation Kidney Diseases Outcomes Quality Initiative. Clinical practice guidelines for vascular access: update 2000. Am J Kidney Dis. 2001;37(1 Suppl 1):S137–81.

Chapter 2
Fistula First, K/DOQI and Documentation

Dheeraj K. Rajan

Fistula First represents a collaborative initiative between the Centers of Medicare and Medicaid Services (CMS), ESRD Networks, and relevant members of the renal community within the United States. Its origin is linked to the recognition that within the United States, most patients were not receiving the most optimal form of hemodialysis access, the hemodialysis fistula.

Key principles of the organization are (www.fistulafirst.org):

1. Core strategies and tools that address the fundamental "failure" points in the system that can be adopted easily.
2. Focus on "spreading" successful ideas on a network and national scale.
3. Collaboration – among patients, networks, providers, and key healthcare professionals.

D.K. Rajan (✉)
Head and Associate Professor, Division of Vascular & Interventional Radiology, Department of Medical Imaging, University of Toronto,
Toronto, Ontario, Canada
e-mail: Dheeraj.Rajan@uhn.on.ca

D.K. Rajan (ed.), *Essentials of Percutaneous Dialysis Interventions*,
DOI 10.1007/978-1-4419-5657-6_2,
© Springer Science+Business Media, LLC 2011

4. Leveraging of resources, including Network QI resources and other relevant sources of expertise and support from the Fistula First Breakthrough Initiative (FFBI) Coalition membership.
5. Minimizing burden on dialysis facilities and practitioners.
6. Mission statements and activities.

For the practicing interventionalist, particularly within the United States, this initiative and the resources available through this organization assist in creating a comprehensive program focused on the patient beyond percutaneous interventions. Outside of the United States, the organization provides some resources to enhance practice patterns and quality of care for patients.

Kidney Disease Outcomes Quality Initiative

K/DOQI represents the Kidney Disease Outcomes Quality Initiative. This is an evidence-based clinical practice guideline for providing optimal practices focused on improving the diagnosis and treatment of kidney disease for all stages of chronic kidney disease and patient survival. The document is also a reflection of consensus opinion when evidence is lacking for certain areas of practice. It is imperative for the practicing interventionalists not only to be familiar with guidelines relevant to the interventions they perform but also to understand the limitations of some of these guidelines in select cases where the guideline is based on opinion and/or small retrospective published series.

Updates are determined by conference call when significant findings or results are published. Updated guidelines may be found at www.kidney.org. The latest update occurred in 2006 [1]. Under "Clinical Guidelines for Vascular Access," one can find guidelines and clinical practice recommendations in relation to these guidelines. Key messages focus on improvement in overall nature of hemodialysis vascular access through the primary goals of (1) increasing the placement of AVFs with a lesser dependence on AVGs, (2) detecting AV access dysfunction prior to thrombosis and (3) minimizing long-term dependence on cuffed hemodialysis catheters. The guidelines below do not consider publications after 2006. A synopsis of the relevant points is presented below.

K-DOQI Recommendations Summary

Catheters

1. Short-term catheters should be used for acute dialysis and for a limited duration in hospitalized patients and for less than 1 week. Noncuffed femoral catheters should be used in bedbound patients only.
2. Long-term catheters should not be placed on the same side as a maturing AV access, if possible (i.e., maturing right AVF – place catheter on the left).
3. The preferred insertion site for tunnelled cuffed venous dialysis catheters or port catheter systems is the right internal jugular vein. Subclavian access should be used only when no other upper-extremity or chest-wall options are available.
4. Long-term catheter systems – tunnelled cuffed catheters (TCCs) and tunnelled port catheter systems – should have their tips within the right atrium confirmed by fluoroscopy for optimal flow.
5. For tunnelled cuffed catheters, the recommended target rate of systemic infection is less than 10% at 3 months and less than 50% at 1 year (Opinion).
6. Less than 10% of chronic maintenance hemodialysis patients should be maintained on catheters as their permanent chronic dialysis access. In this context, chronic catheter access is defined as the use of a dialysis catheter for more than 3 months in the absence of a maturing permanent access (Opinion).
7. The primary failure rate of tunnelled cuffed catheters should be no more than 5%. The cumulative incidence of the following insertion complications should not exceed 2% of all catheter placements (Evidence).

    (a) Pneumothorax requiring chest tube insertion.
    (b) Symptomatic air embolism.
    (c) Hemothorax.
    (d) Hemomediastinum.
    (e) Hematoma requiring evacuation [1, 2].

AV Fistulae

1. A fistula with a greater than 50% stenosis in either the venous outflow or arterial inflow, in conjunction with clinical or physiological

abnormalities, should be treated with PTA or surgical revision (Evidence).
2. Stenosis, as well as the clinical parameters used to detect it, should return to within acceptable limits following intervention.
3. Thrombectomy of a fistula should be attempted as early as possible after thrombosis is detected, but can be successful even after several days.

AV Grafts

1. The preferred treatment for central vein stenosis is PTA. Stent placement should be considered in the following situations (Evidence).
   - Acute elastic recoil of the vein (>50% stenosis) after angioplasty.
   - The stenosis recurs within a 3-month period.
2. Stenoses that are associated with AVGs should be treated if the lesion causes a greater than 50% decrease in the luminal diameter and is associated with the following clinical/physiological abnormalities: abnormal physical findings, decreasing intragraft blood flow (<600 mL/min), and elevated static pressure within the graft (Evidence).
3. Angioplasty.
   - The treated lesion should have less than 30% residual stenosis, and the clinical/physiological parameters used to detect the stenosis should return to acceptable limits after the intervention.
   - A primary patency (i.e., time from intervention to next intervention or loss of the graft) of 50% at 6 months (Evidence).
   - If angioplasty of the same lesion is required more than 2 times within a 3-month period, the patient should be considered for surgical revision if the patient is a good surgical candidate.
   - If angioplasty fails, stents may be useful in the following situations: surgically inaccessible lesion, contraindication to surgery. and angioplasty-induced vascular rupture.
4. Outcomes after treatment of AVG thrombosis.
   - Clinical success rate of 85%; clinical success is defined as the ability to use the AVG for at least 1 HD treatment (Evidence/Opinion).

- After percutaneous thrombectomy, primary patency should be 40% at 3 months' patency (Evidence).
- The rate of graft thrombosis should not exceed 0.5 thrombotic episodes per patient year at risk (Evidence/Opinion).
- After adjusting for initial failures (i.e., failures within the first 2 months of fistula use), the rate of thrombosis of AV fistulae should be less than 0.25 episodes per patient year at risk (Opinion).

In Addition

1. The rate of infection should not exceed 1% in primary AV fistulae and should not exceed 10% in dialysis AV grafts, both calculated over the use-life of the access (Opinion).
2. The cumulative patency rate of all dialysis AV grafts should be at least 70% at 1 year, 60% at 2 years, and 50% at 3 years (Evidence/Opinion).
3. Stent placement combined with angioplasty is indicated in elastic central vein stenoses or if a stenosis recurs within a 3-month period (Evidence).

Standards, Documentation and Quality Assurance

Any dialysis interventions practice should take it upon themselves to have a quality assurance program in place that tracks outcomes and complications. We all suffer occasionally from "tunnel vision" in regard to our practices, and a review of outcomes may indicate the need for change in practice for the benefit of patients. An independent unbiased assessment is ideal when possible.

In addition, proper reporting of the intervention performed is highly recommended. A proper report would detail the following elements.

- Patient's access type
- Indication for requested intervention
- Prior relevant history related to the intervention
- Interventions performed and specific devices used with indications for use
- Outcomes of the intervention(s)

- How the puncture site was closed
- An indication if and when additional interventions or change in patient management is required
- Indicating possible dilated outflow veins that may be used for a future access if relevant
- Contrast volume, fluoroscopy time, and medications given

Within the report and for both quality assurance and consistency/uniformity in reporting, it is important for one to follow conventional or consensus reporting terminology. For example, many report a dialysis graft as a fistula. This is incorrect terminology. A consensus document published by Sidawy et al. [3] details proper terminology for hemodialysis accesses. A summary is as follows.

- *Autogenous* is used to describe native vein, whether it is in situ, transposed, or translocated. An *autogenous AV access* is an access created by a connection between an artery and a vein whereby the vein serves as an accessible conduit.
- Nonautogenous AV access is an access created by connecting an artery to a vein with a graft.
- Any man-made material or e-PTFE grafts are called prosthetic grafts.
- *Arterial* inflow site is reported first, followed by a hyphen, and then the *venous* outflow site.
- In instances in which such a descriptor may be ambiguous, the addition of a broader anatomic reference should be included. This is typically reported as the *body region* or *area* where the access procedure is located and where cannulation will occur.
- Configuration reported including if transposed, looped, or straight.

References

1. Vascular Access Work Group. Clinical practice guidelines for vascular access. Am J Kidney Dis. 2006;48 Suppl 1:S176–247.
2. National Kidney Foundation Kidney Diseases Outcomes Quality Initiative. Clinical practice guidelines for vascular access: update 2000. Am J Kidney Dis. 2001;37(1 Suppl 1):S137–81.
3. Sidawy AN, Gray R, Besarab A, et al. Recommended standards for reports dealing with arteriovenous hemodialysis accesses. J Vasc Surg. 2002;35(3): 603–10.

Chapter 3
The Dialysis Outcomes and Practice Pattern Study (DOPPS): Lessons for Interventionalists

Joshua G. Mendelssohn, Ronald L. Pisoni, and David C. Mendelssohn

An Overview of the DOPPS

The Dialysis Outcomes and Practice Patterns Study (DOPPS) is an ongoing prospective, observational study of HD patients and facilities in 12 countries [1]. Vascular access outcomes are among the major study outcomes under investigation. The objective of DOPPS is to determine practice patterns that are associated with better patient outcomes, through the examination of variations in practice patterns around the world. Data collection for the study has been ongoing since 1996 and has yielded information on more than 50,000 patients in over 1,200 dialysis facilities. With over 100 peer reviewed publications, the DOPPS continues to provide numerous important findings that are relevant for patients and practicing clinicians alike. The DOPPS is supported by scientific research grants from Amgen (since 1996), Kyowa Hakko Kirin (since 1999, in Japan), Genzyme (since 2009), and Abbott (since 2009), without restrictions on publications.

D.C. Mendelssohn (✉)
Associate Professor, Department of Nephrology,
Nephrolife: Complete Kidney Care Centre, Humber River Regional Hospital and University of Toronto, Toronto, Ontario, Canada
e-mail: dmendelssohn@hrrh.on.ca

D.K. Rajan (ed.), *Essentials of Percutaneous Dialysis Interventions*,
DOI 10.1007/978-1-4419-5657-6_3,
© Springer Science+Business Media, LLC 2011

DOPPS involves 12 countries: Australia, Belgium, Canada, France, Germany, Italy, Japan, New Zealand, Spain, Sweden, the United Kingdom, and the United States. Briefly, a random sample of dialysis units was selected in each country to be representative of the types of dialysis units and geographic regions of each country. Each unit contributed a random sample of 20–40 prevalent HD patients, and up to 15 incident HD patients. Vascular access data were collected for each patient at study entry, with all access-related events reported throughout study observation. Information collected included type of access, placement location, dates of access creation, removal, first use, infection, and failure, and dates and type of access-related procedures. In addition, the medical director at each participating facility completed a written questionnaire about local practice patterns, including vascular access preferences and practices. Moreover, study patients completed a written questionnaire concerning their feelings about their health, their kidney disease, the effects of kidney disease on their lives, and satisfaction with care. Finally, a vascular access surgery questionnaire was completed by the primary access surgeon at most DOPPS facilities during DOPPS phase II (2002–2004), which assessed vascular access practices, training, and opinions.

Statistical methodology has included applying detailed statistical modeling techniques and model adjustments to allow for comparisons between groups while accounting for measured differences in group characteristics. Facility-level analysis is often performed in addition to patient-level analysis and is a way to partially overcome the treatment by indication bias in patient-level analysis. Because unknown confounders cannot be fully accounted for in an observational study, DOPPS outcomes describe associations only and do not prove causation. Vascular access has been a primary outcome in DOPPS studies and the study has examined surgical practice patterns in detail. However, the DOPPS design has not specifically examined interventional practices per se.

Methods of vascular access. In order to ensure effective and efficient hemodialysis (HD) care, a well-functioning vascular access (VA) is essential. An optimal VA delivers high rates of blood flow to the extracorporeal circuit while minimizing health risks caused by infection, contamination, hemorrhage, and other complications. Native arteriovenous fistulae (AVF), arteriovenous grafts (AVG), and central vein catheters (CVCs) are the three most commonly used methods

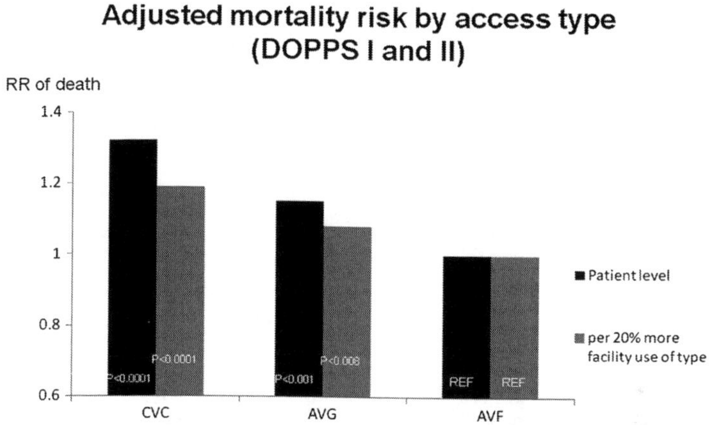

Fig. 3.1 Adjusted mortality risk by access type (DOPPS I and II) [11]

of vascular access. Although catheters avoid needlesticks, catheters are associated with poorer outcomes than either the AVF or AVG options [2]. Catheters result in a high risk of access infection and a relatively shorter period of functional use. Therefore, of the three main VA options, catheters are associated with the highest rates of patient morbidity and mortality [2]. The AVF uses a patient's existing endogenous vasculature to form the fistula. The AVG uses synthetic materials (or rarely, bovine vessels) to form the vascular channel. AVG may be preferred by some practitioners because graft cannulation is easier and maturation times are shorter [3]. However, AV fistulae use requires a significantly smaller number of procedures. Further patient and facility-level research from DOPPS (see Fig. 3.1) and other sources has provided consistent evidence that AV fistulae are associated with significantly lower morbidity and mortality rates [4–7]. Globally, AVF use is considered the preferred method of vascular access [8–10]. AVF use, however, is not ideal for all patients. AVF failure is more common in patients with high levels of comorbidity, women, obese patients, and patients who have previously dialyzed with a catheter [3].

DOPPS and current trends in vascular access. There is large variability in facility-level vascular access practice patterns (see Fig. 3.2) [11]. In Japan, more than 90% of facilities have less than 5% of

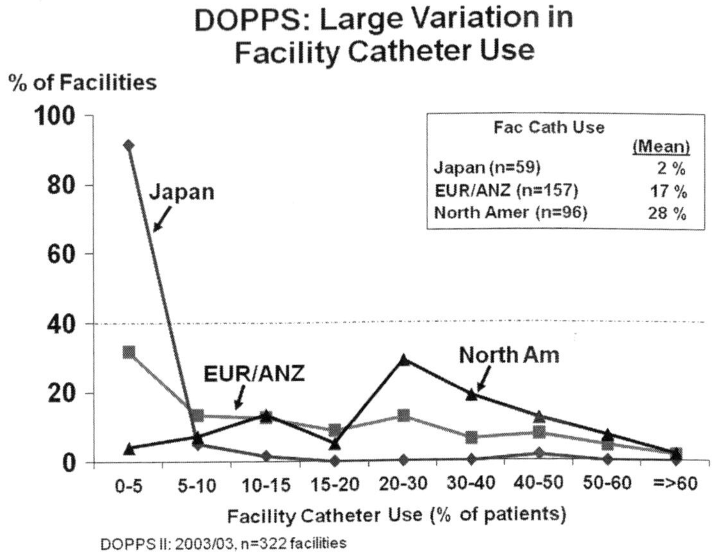

Fig. 3.2 DOPPS: large variation in facility catheter use (DOPPS II: March 2003, $n = 322$ facilities) [11]

patients using CVC, while in North America, facilities with more than 30% CVC utilization are common.

Three longitudinal DOPPS studies (DOPPS I (1996–2001), DOPPS II (2001–2004), and DOPPS 3 (2005–2007)) show significant decreases in AVF use and increases in catheter use over time (see Figs. 3.3 and 3.4) [12]. Although a few countries, such as Japan, have successfully maintained almost universal AVF use, other countries have shown much poorer results [1]. In Japan, 91% of patients dialyzed with an AVF. In France, Germany, the UK, Spain, Belgium, Canada, and the US, catheter use has increased significantly. This increase is most noticeable in Spain where catheter use has increased from 7% of patients at the start of DOPPS I to 21% at the start of DOPPS III. Worse still, in the case of the countries with the highest rates of catheter use (Belgium, Canada, and Sweden), no statistically significant reduction has been observed in recent years. These country trends in the rise in catheter use and decline in AVF use have also been observed in nondiabetic 18–70-year-old HD patients indicating that these patterns are seen even in younger patient populations with lower comorbidity burden.

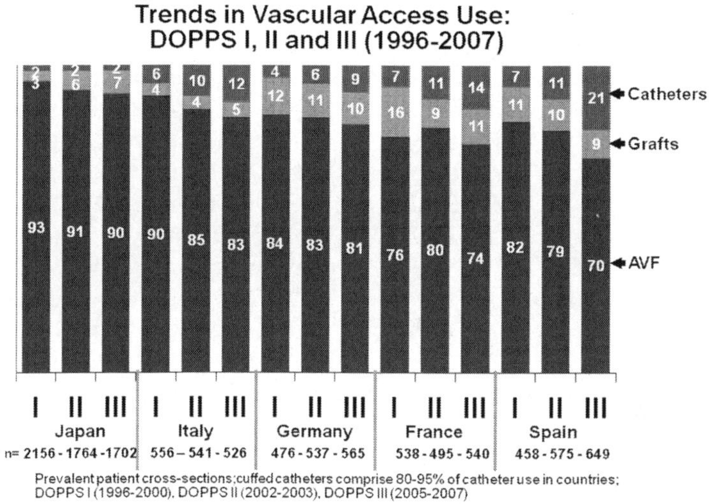

Fig. 3.3 Trends in vascular access use: DOPPS I, II, and III (1996–2007). Prevalent patient cross-sections; cuffed catheters comprise 80–95% of catheter use in countries; DOPPS I (1996–2000), DOPPS II (2002–2003), DOPPS III (2005–2007) [12]

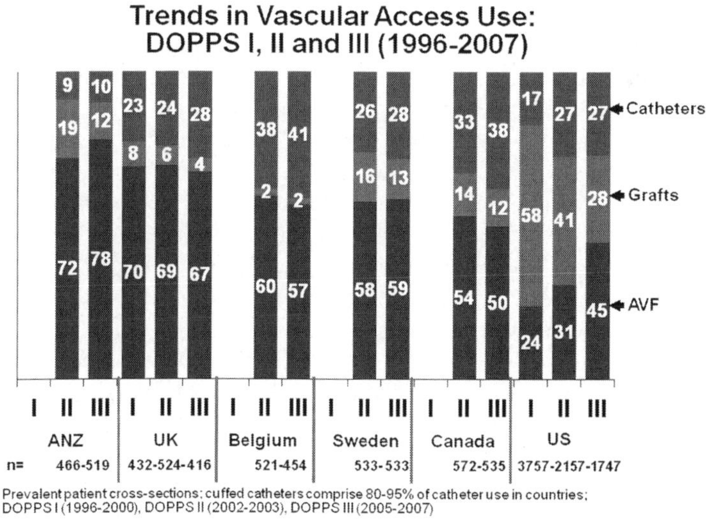

Fig. 3.4 Trends in vascular access use: DOPPS I, II, and III (1996–2007). Prevalent patient cross-sections; cuffed catheters comprise 80–95% of catheter use in countries; DOPPS I (1996–2000), DOPPS II (2002–2003), DOPPS III (2005–2007) [12]

Many countries have initiated programs aimed at increasing AVF use, and these programs have achieved varying degrees of success. In the United States, for example, the successful Fistula First Initiative resulted in a large shift from AVG use to AVF use but did not noticeably reduce the use of catheters. At the onset of DOPPS 1, only 24% of American end-stage renal disease (ESRD) patients were dialyzed with an AVF. The United States remained the only country failing to meet the standard of having >40% of patients dialyzed with an AVF at the start of DOPPS II [12]. However, by the start of DOPPS III, 47% of US HD patients were dialyzed with an AVF. However, catheter use also increased from 17 to 27% in the US from DOPPS I to II (prior to start of the Fistula First Initiative), which is a cause for concern [13]. DOPPS serves to highlight these disturbing international trends in rising catheter use and declining AVF use in many settings, and calls for action from jurisdiction to jurisdiction to reverse them.

Consequences of increasing catheter use. Catheter use is associated with higher rates of patient morbidity and mortality. Patient survival remains the gold standard in measuring the effectiveness of HD treatment. Patients dialyzed with a catheter have consistently lower survival rates than patients dialyzed with either an AVF or an AVG [14]. Catheter use places patients at serious risk of infection. Specifically, catheter use is associated with increased risk of endocarditis, septicemia, and osteomyelitis [14]. According to DOPPS results, a patient dialyzed with an uncuffed catheter is eight times more likely to experience infection than a patient dialyzed with an AV fistula. Infection rates for cuffed, tunneled catheters are still five times higher than native AV fistulae infection rates [14]. Although there is a correlation between catheter use and septicemia, there are significant differences in septicemia rates between countries with similar catheter use. This discrepancy is likely the product of variance in quality of care.

CVCs have a relatively short functional use [2]. As a result, HD patients who initially dialyzed with a CVC must often undergo further surgical procedures to implement a permanent VA (AVG or AVF). In such cases, the patient is exposed to the relatively high risk of infection and surgical complications associated with both initial CVC utilization and the risks of secondary vascular surgery [2]. Furthermore, the high blood flow rates used for delivery of dialysis via AVF or AVG are not feasible with many common catheter designs resulting in lower overall delivered dialysis dose.

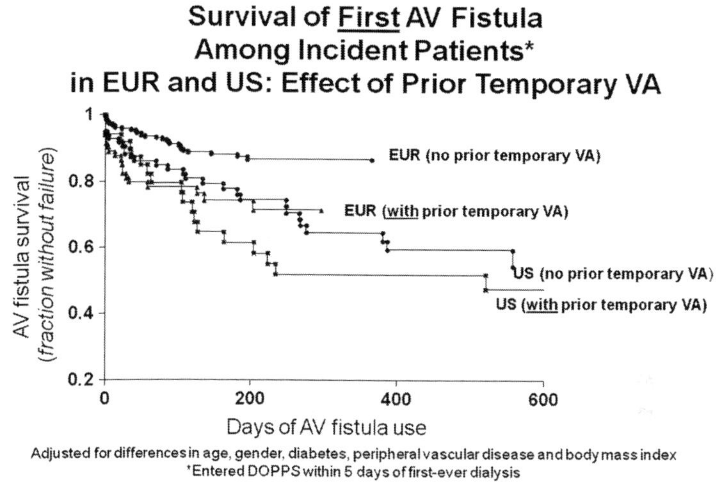

Fig. 3.5 Survival of First AVF in incident patients with or without temporary vascular access [3]

Case-mix-adjusted studies show that facilities with every 20% greater catheter use compared to AVF use have an associated 20% higher mortality risk. Furthermore, patient demographics and comorbidities explain only a small amount of the variance associated with differences in catheter use between facilities. Indeed, facility practice patterns explain more of the variance than patient characteristics. After adjusting for patient-level factors, greater facility-level catheter use is strongly associated with substantially higher rates of patient hospitalization, morbidity, and mortality. In fact, data show a linear increase in mortality risk as facility catheter use increases [11].

CVC use in incident patients has consequences for subsequent AVF/AVG. After controlling for patient characteristics, both AVF and AVG display better survival if used at the initiation of HD, compared to being used after incident patients begin HD with a CVC (see Fig. 3.5) [3]. Avoiding CVC use in incident patients and in patients with problematic AVF/AVG is desirable.

Surgical training. Significant differences in surgical training and access creation exist between countries. In DOPPS II, in Italy, nephrologists performed 85% of vascular access surgeries. By contrast, 92% of vascular access surgeries in Spain are performed by vascular surgeons. In the United States, 61% of VA surgeries are conducted by vascular surgeons while another 31% are conducted by general surgeons [15]. In general, the more surgical training designated to AVF creation in a country, the more likely the prevalent and incident hemodialysis patients in that country are to dialyze with an AVF [14]. Similarly, the more AVGs and catheters created during surgical training in a country, the more likely a hemodialysis patient is to dialyze with an AVG or catheter, respectively. The lowest median number of permanent vascular accesses created during surgical training was seen in the United States ($n=36$). In addition to this, less than 50% of the VA creation in US surgical training was AVF creation. In Germany ($n=426$) and Canada ($n=171$), a significantly larger portion of surgical training was devoted to VA creation. In Germany, Canada, and all other European participants in DOPPS, well over 50% of vascular accesses created during surgical training were AVF [15]. Furthermore, for every doubling of number of AVF created during surgical training, the odds of a patient receiving a fistulae versus a graft in practice increased significantly (AOR=2.17, $P<0.0001$) [15].

One measure of AVF survival is the time from first use until first fistula failure (i.e., primary failure). AVF created by surgeons who created <25 AVF during training were significantly more prone to failure, resulting in a much shorter median survival time [15].

General Recommendations

Minimize incident patient catheter use. When first initiating HD therapy, high rates of catheter use is apparent around the world and in particular in North America [14]. Even in the case of patients who had been seeing a nephrologist for >4 months before HD commencement, catheter use is common [14]. Still, DOPPS data does indicate that in some countries the majority of HD patients initiate HD treatment with a fistula or graft. Analysis of combined data from France, Germany, and Italy shows that 70–80% of new ESRD patients do start treatment with an AVF or AVG. In the United States, however, only 30–40% of patients who have seen a nephrologist >4 months prior to starting HD treatment begin therapy with an AVF or AVG [14]. Furthermore, patients who initiate dialysis using a CVC and are quickly switched to an AVF have a substantially lower risk of mortality than patients who continue with chronic CVC use during the first year of HD therapy [14]. Decreasing the number of patients who begin HD care using a CVC is a key modifiable practice expected to improve patient care and outcomes in the future.

Minimize time between referral and VA creation. There is a large variation in the average time between patient referral and VA creation between countries. According to DOPPS data, the shorter the process time between referral and VA creation, the greater the odds that a patient will dialyze with a permanent VA. Thus, initiatives aimed at reducing process time between referral and VA creation can lead to significant benefits for patients and dialysis facilities.

Optimize time before first AVF cannulation. Two weeks is the minimal maturation time for an AVF. AV fistulae that are cannulated within a relatively short period after creation (2–6 weeks) have, on average, a survival rate that is equivalent to AV fistulae cannulated later (>6 weeks) [14]. In facilities with a larger time period between AVF creation and cannulation, catheter use is generally higher. It is, therefore, ideal to cannulate those AV fistulae that are mature after 2 weeks (earlier than is standard practice in many countries) and to remove CVCs. Such practices would allow dialysis facilities to decrease their dependence on CVCs, greatly improving quality of care.

Recommendations for Interventionalists

While these are based on opinion, we believe the data from DOPPS can be interpreted to support the following approaches.

1. The interventional radiologist or interventionalist is a key player within the vascular access team of a dialysis patient. Over time, more and more secondary procedures on AVF/AVG are performed by interventionalists and more and more catheter insertions and revisions are done by them as well. As a priority, the team should work together to avoid CVCs in incident patients suitable for other permanent forms of AV access, and to convert suitable prevalent patients with a CVC to AVF or AVG.
2. The common practice of inserting a CVC in order to deal with AVF/AVG problems electively the next day or after a weekend may have inadvertent consequences in the long term. Urgent interventions

that salvage an AVF/AVG and completely avoid a temporary CVC are optimal and would be expected to decrease the number of procedures a patient must undergo and ultimately improve the long-term access mix at a facility and longevity of an AVF (since AVF survival is substantially diminished with prior catheter use).

3. There are likely to be significant variations in interventional practice patterns that contribute to patient survival, hospitalization rates, and quality of life. In the future, analyzing these variations with DOPPS methodology may reveal new and important ways to improve patient outcomes on hemodialysis. Furthermore, as was seen in DOPPS with surgical training, it seems likely that increased emphasis on dialysis vascular access procedures during the training of interventionalists would lead to better VA outcomes.

References

1. Young EW, Goodkin DA, Mapes DL, et al. The dialysis outcomes and practice patterns study (DOPPS): an international hemodialysis study. Kidney Int. 2000;57(S74):S74–81.
2. Pisoni RL, Young EW, Mapes DL, Keen ML, Port FK. Vascular access use and outcomes in the U.S., Europe, and Japan: results from the Dialysis Outcomes and Practice Patterns Study. Nephrol News Issues. 2003;17(6):38–43, 7.
3. Pisoni RL, Young EW, Dykstra DM, Greenwood RN, Hecking E, Gillespie B, et al. Vascular access use in Europe and the United States: results from the DOPPS. Kidney Int. 2002;61(1):305–16.
4. Dhingra RK, Young EW, Hulbert-Shearon TE, Leavey SF, Port FK. Type of vascular access and mortality in U.S. hemodialysis patients. Kidney Int. 2001;60(4):1443–51.
5. Xue JL, Dahl D, Ebben JP, Collins AJ. The association of initial hemodialysis access type with mortality outcomes in elderly Medicare ESRD patients. Am J Kidney Dis. 2003;42(5):1013–9.
6. Pastan S, Soucie JM, McClellan WM. Vascular access and increased risk of death among hemodialysis patients. Kidney Int. 2002;62(2):620–6.
7. Woods JD, Turenne MN, Strawderman RL, Young EW, Hirth RA, Port FK, et al. Vascular access survival among incident hemodialysis patients in the United States. Am J Kidney Dis. 1997;30(1):50–7.
8. Jindal K, Chan CT, Deziel C, Hirsch D, Soroka SD, Tonelli M, et al. Chapter 4: vascular access. J Am Soc Nephrol. 2006;17 Suppl 1:S16–23.
9. National Kidney Foundation Kidney Diseases Outcomes Quality Initiative. Clinical practice guidelines for vascular access: update 2000. Am J Kidney Dis. 2001;37(1 Suppl 1):S137–181.
10. Vascular Access Work Group. Clinical practice guidelines for vascular access. Am J Kidney Dis. 2006;48 Suppl 1:S248–73.

11. Pisoni RL, Arrington CJ, Albert JM, Ethier J, Kimata N, Krishnan M, et al. Facility hemodialysis vascular access use and mortality in countries participating in the DOPPS: an instrumental variable analysis. Am J Kidney Dis. 2009; 53(3):475–91.
12. Ethier J, Mendelssohn DC, Elder SJ, Hasegawa T, Akizawa T, Akiba T, et al. Vascular access use and outcomes: an international perspective from the dialysis outcomes and practice patterns study. Nephrol Dial Transplant. 2008;23(10):3219–26.
13. Lok CE. Fistula first initiative: advantages and pitfalls. Clin J Am Soc Nephrol. 2007;2(5):1043–53.
14. Rayner HC, Pisoni RL. The increasing use of hemodialysis catheters: evidence from the DOPPS on its significance and ways to reverse it. Semin Dial. 2010;23(1):6–10.
15. Saran R, Elder SJ, Goodkin DA, Akiba T, Ethier J, Rayner HC, et al. Enhanced training in vascular access creation predicts arteriovenous fistula placement and patency in hemodialysis patients: results from the Dialysis Outcomes and Practice Patterns Study. Ann Surg. 2008;247(5):885–91.

Chapter 4
Controversies in Vascular Access Monitoring and Surveillance

William D. Paulson, Louise Moist, and Charmaine E. Lok

In North America, there are over 350,000 patients receiving hemodialysis for end stage renal disease (ESRD) [1, 2]. Reliable vascular access performance is necessary to ensure adequate dialysis, yet creating and maintaining functional accesses is both challenging and costly. For example, in 2008, ESRD only represented approximately 1% of the Medicare population but accounted for 24 billion dollars or 6–7% of Medicare expenditures. Hemodialysis accounted for 19.4 billion dollars, with access placement and complications estimated to contribute approximately 15% [3]. Of note, the costs of managing access events have increased by up to 17% over the past year [3].

The marked growth in the number of older ESRD patients roughly accounts for the increase in dialysis patients, as they are less likely to be candidates for renal transplantation. Furthermore, an aging ESRD population has greater comorbidity, such as cardiac and vascular disease, that may impact on the successful creation and maintenance of an access. Indeed, the vascular access has been shrouded with so many

W.D. Paulson (✉)
Professor of Medicine, Director, MCG End-Stage Renal Disease Program,
Chief of Nephrology, Charlie Norwood VA Medical Center,
Medical College of Georgia Augusta, Georgia, USA
e-mail: wpaulson@georgiahealth.edu

D.K. Rajan (ed.), *Essentials of Percutaneous Dialysis Interventions*,
DOI 10.1007/978-1-4419-5657-6_4,

© Springer Science+Business Media, LLC 2011

challenges that it has been coined the "Achilles Heel of dialysis" and the certainty of its dysfunction has been equated to death and taxes [4].

Several decades ago, access monitoring (e.g., physical examination) and/or surveillance (e.g., non-physical exam measurements of access function) were introduced in an attempt to reduce access failure rates. The basic premise was that access monitoring and surveillance could detect access dysfunction early so that it could be corrected by preemptive intervention and thereby improve access outcomes. Whether this strategy is effective depends upon many factors, including the cause of dysfunction and the type of intervention.

This chapter focuses on the pathophysiology and hemodynamics of access dysfunction and failure, and how these factors may impact the ability of monitoring and surveillance to improve access outcomes.

Pathophysiology of Arteriovenous Fistula and Graft Failure

Arteriovenous fistulae (AVFs) and arteriovenous synthetic grafts (AV-grafts) are intrinsically different accesses. The AVF is a direct anastomosis between an artery and a vein, created by either an end-to-side or side-to-side connection. An AV-graft requires the interposition of a synthetic vessel, most commonly polytetrafluoroethelyene (PTFE), between the artery and vein. Because of their different natures, it may seem that AVFs and AV-grafts should fail for different reasons. While there are some differences in the pathophysiology of their dysfunction, AVFs and AV-grafts also share common pathologic features. On the other hand, their timing and degree of contributing pathology differs, as reflected by their different clinical courses.

For example, AVFs primarily "fail to mature" early in the post-operative course. Failure of AVF maturation is complex and may include early development of stenosis (neointimal hyperplasia) and thrombosis, inability of the vessels to dilate and remodel because of intrinsic mechanisms (e.g., poor vessel elasticity) or indirect mechanisms (e.g., effect of accessory veins and poor cardiac output). AV-grafts are more likely to be usable for dialysis, but fail later because of stenosis and thrombosis. These processes and interactions are less well understood for AVFs than for AV-grafts (Ashley I. 2008, FAVOURED trial: fish oil and aspirin in vascular access outcomes in renal disease. Personal communication [5–8]).

The pathophysiologies of AVF and AV-graft stenosis are likely to share common features that involve patient factors (e.g., genetic predisposition, integrity of the vessels prior to surgery), surgical factors (e.g., response of the anastomosis and access to surgical stretching and angulations, the specific surgical anastomotic interface between graft and vessel, and the techniques used, such as type of closures or stitches), and dialysis factors (e.g., effect of the uremic environment, inflammatory and coagulation response to repeated needling, turbulent access flow and low and/or oscillatory shear stress on and off dialysis).

The relative contribution and specific interplay of the above factors is undoubtedly unique to the individual and poorly understood. However, the basic process of vascular access stenosis and thrombosis is likely initiated by endothelial dysfunction which encompasses several pathological conditions including dysregulation of vascular tone and remodeling, impaired modulation of vascular growth, and abnormal endothelial and smooth muscle cellular responses to injury, anticoagulation, and inflammation [9]. The cascade of events that lead to access failure begins with access creation, when blood vessels are severed, foreign material is introduced (in the case of AV-grafts), and turbulent flow with low or oscillatory shear stress is initiated [10].

AVFs are more likely to have early failure because arteries and veins may have low elasticity and may not dilate adequately, whereas AV-grafts already have a synthetic vessel of optimal diameter for needling. Low elasticity and poor vessel dilatation promote turbulent flow and low or oscillatory shear stress within the access. These factors interact with endothelial dysfunction to stimulate the development of neointimal hyperplasia and are exacerbated during dialysis, when further fluctuations in flow turbulence, vessel stretch, and shear stress occur. These events lead to the activation of "healing" pathways, such as lipoxygenase and cyclooxygenase pathways, multiple inflammatory cytokines, hemostatic mediators, growth factors, and other molecules [e.g., interleukins, adhesion molecules, platelet activating factor, basic fibroblast growth factor (bFGF), platelet-derived growth factor (PDGF), and metalloproteinases]. These, in turn, lead to abnormalities in vascular tone (increased vasoconstriction and/or impaired relaxation), smooth muscle proliferation, myofibroblast expression and transformation to fibroblasts [11], and altered coagulation. This is evidenced in healed explanted PTFE grafts that have shown large quantities of thrombotic factors such as fibronectin, fibrinogen, and platelet membranes imbedded within the graft material [12].

The vasculature receives further insult with cannulation during dialysis. Each venipuncture results in the formation of a platelet plug, with its attendant expression of cytokines and growth factors, such as PDGF, endothlin-1, and transforming growth factor-beta (TGF-b). These growth factors stimulate smooth muscle cell hyperplasia and are implicated in neointimal hyperplasia, the pathologic lesion in AVF and AV-graft stenosis [13–19]. For example, PDGF is a powerful smooth muscle mitogen and chemotactic agent; it is required for smooth muscle proliferation and migration from the media to intima. The PDGF content of graft tissue anastomosis directly correlates with the degree and development of intimal hyperplasia [20, 21]. TGF-b is also associated with proliferation and repair in AVF neointima and in AV-graft pseudointima [22]. In addition, these mitogens are increased in the presence of oxidative stress in both AVFs and AV-grafts [22].

Oxidative stress, or oxidant-derived tissue injury, takes place when the production of oxidants [intermediate forms or "radicals" of reduced oxygen, also known as reactive oxygen species (ROS)] exceeds local anti-oxidant capacity. Increased oxidative stress results from uremia [23–25], activation of phagocyte metabolism and direct peroxidation of lipids on the dialysis membrane [26, 27], and release of free radicals during dialysis [28]. Thus, the patient's anti-oxidant system becomes overwhelmed [16, 25]. ROS are observed at sites of vascular injury and have been shown to alter the balance in vascular tone and integrity [22, 29]. ROS can promote a procoagulant state [30, 31], inflammatory and growth cytokines [32] resulting in hypertrophy and growth of smooth muscle [22, 33], vessel wall lipid peroxidation and damage [34], and the development of atherosclerosis/vessel restenosis [30, 35]. Some of these adverse effects of ROS can be prevented; in experimental models, vein graft intimal hyperplasia has been limited by administration of anti-oxidants [36]. Clinical study of anti-oxidant use in AV-grafts is ongoing [37]. Finally, other pathophysiologic processes have been proposed [8, 38, 39]. The role of endothelial progenitor cells in promoting neointimal hyperplasia, angiogenesis, and rapid endothelialization may be particularly important in the context of repeated angioplasty and its consequent vascular injury. Novel therapies are under investigation to target these specific processes [8].

To summarize, while AVFs tend to fail because of their inability to dilate and remodel (maturation failure) and AV-grafts are plagued with late stenosis and thrombosis, key common features include endothelial dysfunction, poor vessel elasticity, and development of neointimal hyperplasia. Neointimal hyperplasia involves myointimal proliferation, matrix deposition, infiltration with macrophages, and neovascularization. Active participants in this process include vasoactive, thrombogenic, and mitogenic factors, among which ROS, inflammation, and platelet aggregation are major components. This traditional triad of neointimal hyperplasia, myointimal proliferation, and matrix deposition results in progressive stenosis and thrombosis.

Clinical trials of agents directly targeting these factors have shown little to no effect in combating access failure (see Table 4.1). For example, in a randomized controlled trial, clopidogrel was effective in reducing early AVF thrombosis but did not improve AVF suitability for dialysis [40]. Indeed, approximately 61% of all fistulas created failed to be used for dialysis. However, there was modest improvement in AV-graft cumulative survival in a randomized trial of Aggrenox (dipyridamole/ASA) versus placebo [41]. Lingering questions concerning the longer-term impact on AV-graft patency and cost effectiveness of Aggrenox use remain, particularly with its continued use beyond the first thrombotic episode or after the first radiological or surgical intervention [42]. In addition to currently ongoing clinical trials designed to improve access patency [5, 6, 38], exciting novel therapies are being evaluating with translational research [9]. In the meantime, we are left with the traditional strategy of vascular access monitoring and surveillance with preemptive intervention in an attempt to reduce thrombosis and prolong access survival.

History and Controversies in Access Surveillance

In the first two decades following the introduction of AV-grafts, it was considered a normal part of nephrology practice that patients underwent frequent treatment for AV-graft thrombosis and failure. The cycle of access thrombosis, thrombolysis with correction of stenosis (usually by angioplasty), and recurrent thrombosis was considered the natural order of things. This changed when two paradigm-changing studies [43, 44] reported that surveillance could improve access outcomes. The studies applied dynamic [43] and static (and derived static) [44] dialysis venous pressure (VP) surveillance to AV-grafts and AVFs, and reported large reductions in rates of thrombosis and access replacement. Static VP refers to pressure measured

Table 4.1 Clinical trials of medical prophylaxis of thrombosis

Study	Access type	Drug	*N*	Follow-up	Results
Kaegi et al. [87]	Shunt	Sulfinpyrazone	52	6 months	76% ↓thrombosis
Harter et al. [88]	Shunt	Aspirin	44	5 months	56% ↓thrombosis
Kobayashi et al. [89]	Shunt	Ticlopidine	107	3 months	21% ↓thrombosis
Andrassy et al. [90]	Fistula	Aspirin	92	2 weeks	4 vs. 23% thrombosis
Grontoft et al. [91]	Fistula	Ticlopidine	42	1 month	11 vs. 47% thrombosis
Dember et al. [40]	Fistula	Clopidogrel	877	6 months	12.2 vs. 19.5% thrombosis; however 59.5% and 61.8% in control and clopidogrel groups, respectively, were not suitable for dialysis
Sreedhara et al. [92]	AV-graft	Dipyridamole, Aspirin	84	18 months	Dipyridamole RR 0.35; ASA RR = 1.99
Crowther et al. [93]	AV-graft	Warfarin	107	0–2–3 years	↑Bleeding in warfarin arm; No benefit
Kaufman et al. [94]	AV-graft	Clopidogrel	200	Stopped early	↑Bleeding in warfarin arm; Trend to benefit
Schmitz et al. [95]	AV-graft	Fish oil	24	12 months	Primary patency 75.6% Fish Oil Group and 14.9% control group
Dixon et al. [41]	AV-graft	Dipyridamole, Aspirin	649	12 months	1 year primary unassisted patency 28% in dipyridamole-aspirin group and 23% in control

Clinical trials of $>n=20$

by the venous dialysis needle with the blood pump turned off, whereas derived static VP uses a regression equation to convert VP measurements with the blood pump running (dynamic VP) to static VP. These reports prompted the National Kidney Foundation's (KDOQI) Clinical Practice Guidelines [45] to recommend that AV-grafts and AVFs should undergo routine surveillance with pre-emptive correction of stenosis, and this recommendation has continued in subsequent KDOQI updates [46]. The Guidelines have recommended an intervention referral when AV-graft blood flow (Q) is less than 600 mL/min, or when Q has decreased by more than 25% and falls below 1,000 mL/min. In contrast, they recommend that AVFs be referred when Q is less than 400–500 mL/min because AVFs may remain patent at lower Qs than has been observed in AV-grafts.

The KDOQI Guidelines have reflected a growing trend of applying an organized evidence-based approach to the art of medicine. However, acceptance of these KDOQI Guidelines has been more controversial than originally anticipated. The problem is that clinical practice guidelines depend on clear and reliable answers to these questions: what do we think we know, is this knowledge accurate, and will interventions based upon this knowledge actually improve patient outcomes? It turns out that the answers are not as straightforward as they may seem.

The surveillance recommendation in the KDOQI Guidelines was based upon a critical appraisal of the strength and quality of the evidence. The most recent KDOQI update [46] gave an "A" rating to the surveillance recommendation. However, the paradigm changing studies [43, 44] were not randomized controlled trials (RCTs) nor were they followed by timely RCTs. Rather, the KDOQI recommendation has been based upon studies that used historical or nonconcurrent control groups. Such studies are biased toward finding a treatment benefit [47–49]. Further, claims that surveillance accurately predicts access thrombosis were based upon statistical methods that were not appropriate for evaluating the usefulness of diagnostic tests. For example, the influence of Q on relative risk of thrombosis was used to justify surveillance. Thus, these deficiencies have resulted in persistent controversy [50–55].

When proper statistical methods were applied, such as receiver operating characteristic (ROC) curves, Q and VP surveillance were found to be inaccurate predictors of AV-graft thrombosis [56–60]. For example, Ram et al. [60] studied 176 patients who underwent a total of 1,957 monthly Q measurements over 6 years. They evaluated the accuracy of a single monthly Q measurement, or percentage decrease in Q (ΔQ) computed over 2 months, in predicting thrombosis within the next month. They found that Q predicts thrombosis with a sensitivity of 80% at a false-positive rate of 60%, and ΔQ has a sensitivity of 81% at a false-positive rate of 50%. Areas under the curve were relatively low: 0.698 for Q and 0.713 for ΔQ. Moreover, the majority of thromboses were not preceded by a ΔQ measurement, usually because thrombosis occurred before a second measurement could be taken. Thus, a high sensitivity requires a high false-positive rate that likely yields many unnecessary invasive procedures. Thus, the study did not support the routine application of Q surveillance to predict AV-graft thrombosis. The poor accuracy of surveillance in detecting stenosis and predicting thrombosis follows in large part from our understanding of access hemodynamics.

Access Hemodynamics

A clear understanding of access hemodynamics is important in evaluating the potential effectiveness of surveillance. To this end, mathematical models have been used to analyze AV-graft and AVF hemodynamics [61–64]. These models have provided the important insight that the luminal diameters of vessels in the access circuit control the relation between Q or VP and stenosis (see Fig. 4.1), and this relation impairs the accuracy of surveillance in predicting thrombosis.

These models are based on engineering equations that relate Q to intra-access pressure and other key variables in the access circuit. The models have been validated with data from an in vitro apparatus and have shown a good correlation with clinical data. The AV-graft model [61, 64] includes the inflow artery, arterial and venous anastomoses, AV-graft, stenosis, and outflow vein. It is designed to resemble a loop graft that is anastomosed end to side to the brachial artery and cubital vein for forearm configuration, or brachial artery and basilic or axillary vein for upper arm configuration. The model has applied the luminal diameters of arteries and veins from duplex ultrasound studies of 94 patients. A key characteristic of these diameters was that they varied over a wide range, but the artery was usually narrower than the vein.

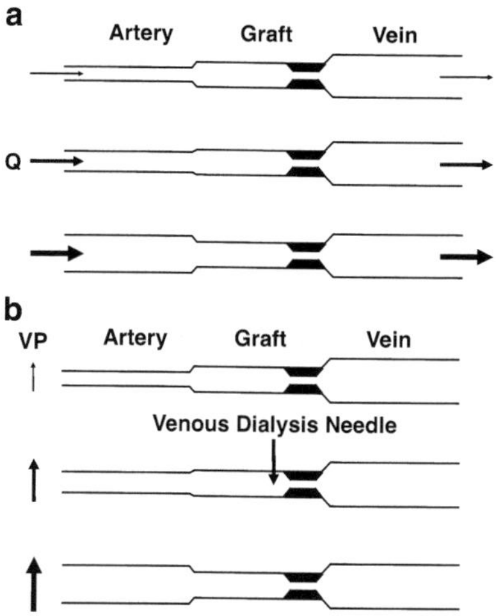

Fig. 4.1 Luminal diameters strongly influence blood flow (Q) and dialysis venous pressure (VP) in a vascular access circuit. In (**a**), an increasing artery luminal diameter reduces overall circuit resistance, so that AV-graft Q increases despite no change in stenosis or other diameters. Similarly, in (**b**), an increasing artery luminal diameter facilitates transmission of vascular pressure to the dialysis needle, so that VP increases. *Thicker arrows* represent larger values for Q and VP, but do not indicate relative numerical values

Figure 4.2 shows predicted pressure (as percentage of initial value) along segments of the AV-graft vascular circuit at different levels of stenosis at the venous anastomosis [61]. The initial pressure is taken to be the pressure in the ascending aorta. Because the inflow artery of a graft is generally narrower than the outflow vein, the ratio of artery/vein luminal diameters is usually less than 1.0. In Fig. 4.2, the artery/vein ratio was set at the median value of the 94 patients (0.77). The model predicts that in the nonstenotic circuit, arterial pressure in the arm falls to 67% of the initial value by the time blood flow reaches the artery-graft anastomosis, and falls by a total of 49% by the time it crosses the anastomosis. Thus, in the absence of stenosis, the blood pressure in the access arm falls approximately 50% by the time flow has entered the graft. The large pressure drop in the nonstenosed circuit occurs because the graft bypasses the arteriolar resistances, resulting in a high-flow shunt. The high flow generates friction with a large dissipation of pressure and energy. Therefore, it is unlike the normal circulation in which pressures in the arm are only

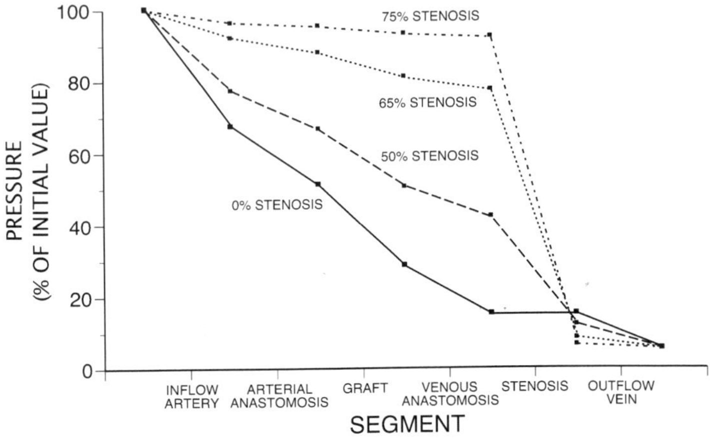

Fig. 4.2 Pressures predicted by mathematical model along segments of AV-graft vascular circuit at different levels of stenosis at the venous anastomosis [61]. For no stenosis, a large pressure drop occurs by the time blood flow enters the AV-graft. In contrast, an arm without an access has an arterial pressure that is only slightly lower than in the ascending aorta. Ratio of artery/vein luminal diameters was set at the median of 94 patients (0.77). Conditions (Figs. 4.2–4.4): initial pressure = mean arterial pressure (MAP) = 93 mmHg, central venous pressure = 5 mmHg, and hematocrit = 36%. MAP of 93 mmHg is equivalent to 120/80 mmHg

slightly lower than in the ascending aorta. Figure 4.2 shows, however, that as stenosis progresses, pressure upstream to the stenosis increases, and the pressure drop across the stenosis eventually accounts for most of the pressure drop in the access circuit. At 75% stenosis, the pressure in the arm is similar to that observed in an arm with no access.

Figure 4.3a shows that the relation between Q and stenosis in AV-grafts is sigmoid: as stenosis progresses, Q initially remains unchanged but then rapidly decreases as critical stenosis (60–80%) is reached [61]. The influence of luminal diameters on Q is evident in the figure. As the artery narrows (lower artery/vein diameter ratio), overall circuit resistance increases (see Fig. 4.1). Thus, Q is reduced and the curve is flattened downward and shifted to the right. This is further illustrated in Fig. 4.3b, which shows Q as a percentage of its initial value. Ratios below the median value shift the curve to the right, so that Q initially remains unchanged as stenosis progresses, but then rapidly falls as critical stenosis is reached. It follows that

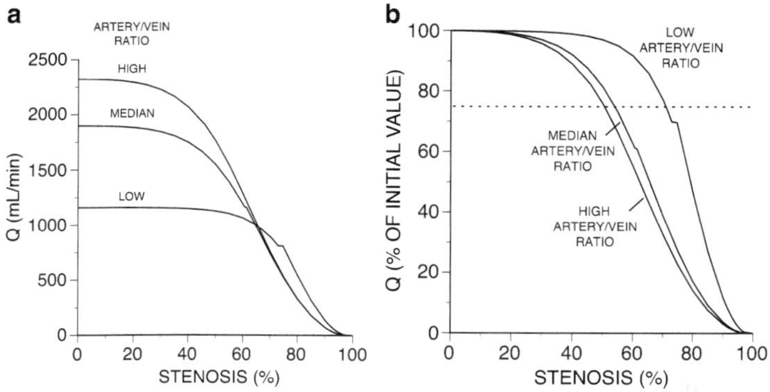

Fig. 4.3 (**a**) Relation between AV-graft blood flow (Q) and stenosis at venous anastomosis [61]. Mathematical model predicts that artery and vein diameters control relation between Q and stenosis [59]. For narrower arteries (lower artery/vein diameter ratios), the sigmoid flow curve is flattened and shifted to the right. High (1.28), median (0.77), and low (0.40) artery/vein ratios derived from 94 patients; low and high ratios enclosed 95% of patients. (**b**) Figure shows same Qs as in Fig. 4.2 except that they are plotted as percentage of initial value [61]. Mathematical model predicts that as an artery becomes narrower (lower artery/vein ratios), the sigmoid curve shifts to the right [61]. This promotes delay and then rapid reduction in Q as stenosis progresses. Q values below *dashed line* represent decrease in Q of greater than 25% (KDOQI referral threshold [46]). Note that by the time Q has fallen by 25%, it is on the rapidly falling part of the curve. Thus, standard monthly Q surveillance fails to detect a decrease in Q before thrombosis

vessel diameters control the relation between Q and stenosis. Because arteries are usually narrower than veins, the artery dominates circuit resistance until stenosis is well advanced. Assuming stenosis progresses at a constant rate, Q may then fall so rapidly that there is insufficient time to detect the decrease before thrombosis. The rapid progression of stenosis in many AV-grafts may further impair the ability to detect stenosis before thrombosis [65]. These results question the viability of standard *monthly* Q surveillance because the frequency of surveillance is unlikely to be adequate given the potential rapidity of Q decline.

Similar results are obtained when considering static VP surveillance (see Chap. 5 for details) [64]. Figure 4.4 shows that the artery/vein ratio controls the relation between static VP and stenosis. In VP surveillance, the VP is normally adjusted for the mean arterial pressure (MAP) because a higher MAP causes VP to increase. The KDOQI recommended threshold for referral for intervention is static

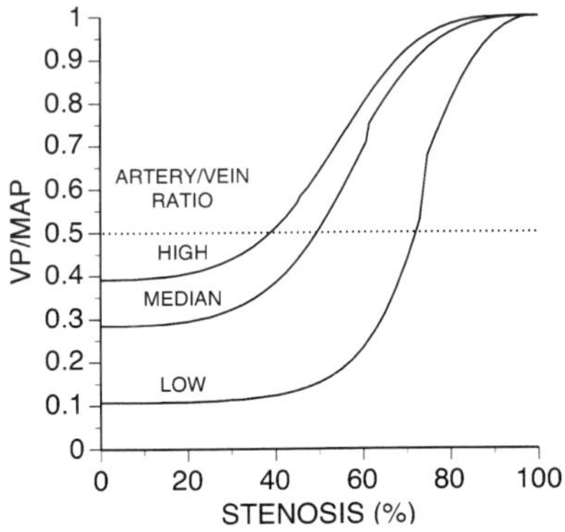

Fig. 4.4 Relation between static venous pressure adjusted for mean arterial pressure (VP/MAP) and AV-graft stenosis varies depending on the artery/vein diameter ratio [64]. At KDOQI referral threshold VP/MAP=0.50 (*dotted line*) [46], the stenosis may range from 38 to 73%. Thus, VP/MAP does not accurately indicate level of stenosis. High (1.28), median (0.77), and low (0.40) artery/vein ratios derived from 94 patients; low and high ratios enclosed 95% of patients

VP/MAP=0.50 (0.55 for derived static VP) [46]. However, Fig. 4.4 shows that 0.50 is not a reliable threshold for detecting significant stenosis. At a high artery/vein diameter ratio, the VP/MAP threshold of 0.50 is reached when stenosis is only 38%. This occurs because at a relatively large arterial diameter, arterial pressure is easily transmitted through the artery and AV-graft to the venous dialysis needle (see Fig. 4.1), yielding a relatively high VP/MAP despite the presence of insignificant stenosis. On the other hand, at a low ratio, the threshold is not reached until stenosis is 73%. This delay occurs because when the artery is relatively narrow, the high arterial resistance causes a large pressure drop, so that by the time flow reaches the needle, the pressure is low (see Fig. 4.1). Because of this delay, VP/MAP will not reach 0.50 until critical stenosis has been reached. Also note that the upward slope of the VP/MAP curve is very steep at the low ratio, so that VP/MAP may then increase so quickly that thrombosis may occur before the next surveillance measurement.

Thus, the artery/vein diameter ratio controls the relation between static VP/MAP and stenosis, and this ratio varies widely between patients. At the median ratio of 0.77, VP/MAP=0.50 at 50% stenosis [46], so that the KDOQI recommended referral threshold is optimal if a single value is to be used. However, the standard referral threshold of 0.50 does not accurately identify significant stenosis.

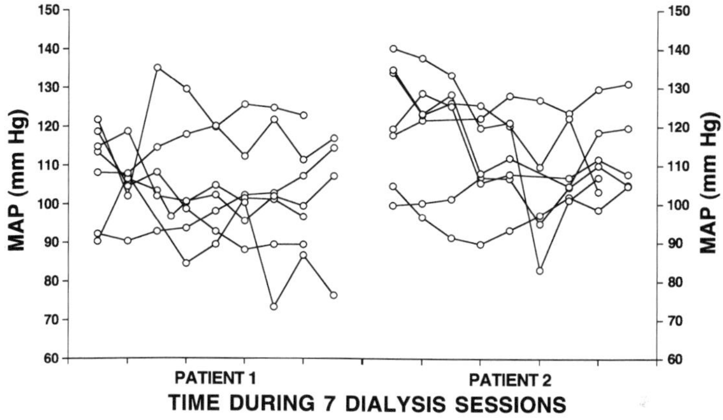

Fig. 4.5 Mean arterial pressures (MAPs) of two representative patients with AV-grafts during seven consecutive dialysis sessions (reprinted with permission of the National Kidney Foundation [66]). Note the very large MAP variations that occurred from the beginning of the sessions. This helps explain why there is no benefit to restricting Q or VP measurements to early in dialysis

Moreover, each AV-graft has its own specific VP/MAP versus stenosis relation, so that an increase in VP/MAP indicates an increase in stenosis. However, the rate at which VP/MAP increases with stenosis may influence surveillance outcomes. Relatively narrow inflow arteries are predicted to delay the stenosis-induced increase until critical stenosis is reached. Assuming stenosis progresses at a constant rate, the delay and then rapid increase in VP/MAP helps explain why standard monthly surveillance often fails to warn of thrombosis [46].

Another practical issue affecting surveillance is that hemodynamic variation is large during dialysis, and this affects surveillance measurements [66, 67]. Consider that Q is determined by MAP, central venous pressure (CVP), and vascular resistance of the access circuit (R) according to the following equation: $Q=(MAP-CVP)/R$ [61]. All three variables rapidly change during dialysis, so that Q is unstable. Figure 4.5 shows the variation in MAP during seven dialysis sessions in two patients whose variations were at the average for a group of 51 dialysis patients [66]. These variations cause large changes in Q, VP, and MAP even during a single dialysis session (Fig. 4.6) [67–70]. Variations may even be larger when compared from session to session [67]. Thus, a change in Q must be >33% to be significant at $p<0.05$.

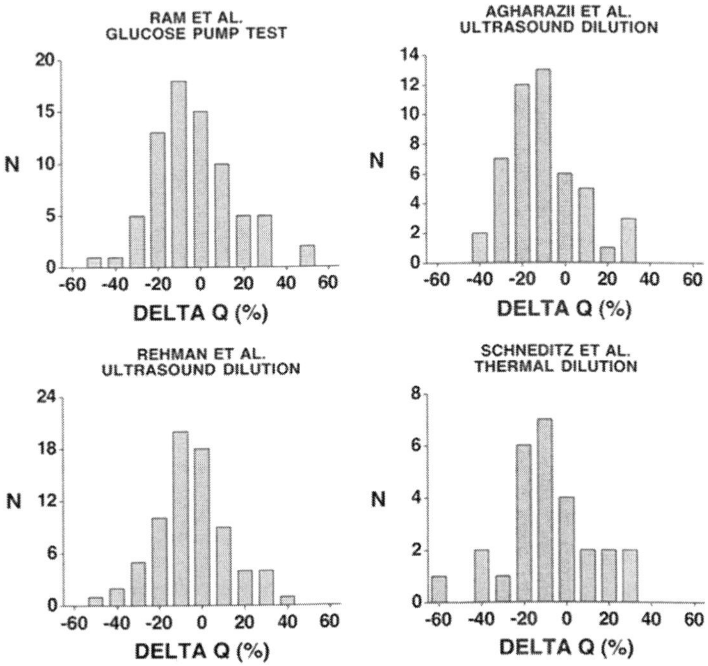

Fig. 4.6 Histograms computed with data from four studies [67–70] show large percentage change in Q (delta Q) in AV-grafts within single dialysis sessions. Changes were measured over periods ranging from 1 to 3 h by three measurement methods. Positive delta Q indicates a decrease in Q; negative delta Q indicates an increase

To minimize these variations, KDOQI recommends that surveillance measurements be taken early in dialysis before hemodynamic changes caused by ultrafiltration occur. However, in reality, published data show that hemodynamic variation is not reduced early in a session, so that this approach is unlikely to be successful [66, 67]. Moreover, higher ultrafiltration volumes increase risk of thrombosis in the period after a dialysis session [71]. Hence, one could argue that measurements should be taken late in a session, which most closely approximates the hemodynamics during the period following the dialysis session, when thrombosis often occurs.

Surveillance might improve outcomes if measurements were taken more frequently. This would allow calculation of average values that may neutralize hemodynamic variation and might make it easier to detect rapid changes in Q or VP before thrombosis. However, Q surveillance measurements take significant time, so it is probably impractical to increase measurement frequency. In contrast, online methods are available that facilitate frequent-derived static VP measurements [72]. Frequent and direct visualization of stenosis by duplex ultrasound might also be successful [73].

Non-vascular Challenges with Access Surveillance

Patient factors such as vessel diameter and configuration are clearly integral to access hemodynamics, and these factors, in turn, predominantly dictate the efficacy of surveillance. However, other factors may also contribute to surveillance efficacy. Consider the ultrasound dilution method, which is widely accepted as the gold standard for measuring Q [74–76] (see Chap. 5). The method involves setting the blood pump to a given flow rate, reversal of the dialysis lines on the dialysis needles, followed by the injection of saline (as a dilution indicator) into the venous side of the dialysis circuit. Reversal of the lines causes access recirculation, so that dialyzed blood reenters the arterial side of the dialysis circuit. The method uses the fact that once percent recirculation is determined by the diluted blood, and the blood pump speed is set, Q can then be determined. Of note, as Q increases, less of the injected saline enters the arterial line, as measured by an ultrasound sensor.

Several key factors may influence the accuracy of the method [76, 77]. Thorough mixing of the saline dilution indicator is required after being injected into the dialysis circuit. Adequacy of mixing is influenced by both the distance between and the orientation of the dialysis needles. For example, the arterial needle must be placed in the direction of the incoming flow. In the AVF, the two needles must be in sequence or series with the arterial needle in the main branch of the AVF. Secondly, cardiopulmonary recirculation (CPR) may cause underestimation of Q. In CPR, blood from the dialysis circuit flows through the heart and pulmonary circulation and then returns to the vascular access where it reenters the dialysis circuit. CPR increases as Q increases (CPR = Q/CO), and return of the saline indicator to the arterial line before systemic mixing causes underestimation of Q. Thirdly, reversal of the blood lines also affects the measurement. Hence, studies have shown that ultrasound dilution underestimates true access flow by an average of 40–60 mL/min [76]. Others have confirmed these both theoretically with hemodynamic calculations and in an in vitro model of hemodialysis [78].

Finally, dialysis blood pump flow (Qb) must be measured accurately as pump readings from the dialysis machine have been shown to overestimate delivered Qb flow by between 10 and 20% because of flow resistance by the dialysis needle [79].

Currently, despite the above issues that may affect ultrasound dilution accuracy, it is probably the most reliable and accurate method of measuring Q. Moreover, the major problems with Q surveillance are not the limitations of the method, but rather that hemodynamics impair the ability of flow surveillance to detect an increase in stenosis before thrombosis, especially when measurements are taken only monthly (the current standard).

Clinical Controversies in Access Surveillance

Recently, Tonelli et al. [80] published a systematic review and meta-analysis of studies that have evaluated Q or duplex ultrasound surveillance in AVFs and AV-grafts (Table 4.2). Only RCTs were included (four studies of AVFs and seven of AV-grafts), and the primary outcome was access thrombosis. They found that AVF surveillance reduced the risk of thrombosis without prolonging AVF life, and AV-graft surveillance showed no benefit at all. However, these RCTs have been criticized for design flaws, such as small sample size, so that they have not resolved the ongoing controversy concerning the benefit and optimal approach to surveillance.

There is also a need to examine additional factors that predict access failure. For example, Ram et al. [60] evaluated the relation between Q and probability of thrombosis, only allowing preemptive angioplasty when there was clinical suspicion of hemodynamically significant stenosis. They found that older AV-grafts were unlikely to thrombose even at low Q or large decreases in Q (Fig. 4.7), suggesting that large decreases in Q in older AV-grafts were likely caused by hemodynamic variation rather than increased stenosis. On the other hand, new AV-grafts were far more likely to thrombose in the next 2–3 months. Thus, AV-graft age should be considered when deciding whether to refer for intervention and referrals should not be based solely upon Q or decrease in Q.

Table 4.2 RCTs in vascular access surveillance

VA type	Author	Sites and population	Surveillance method in treatment group (T)	Comparator method in control group ©	Interventions	Thrombosis	Access survival
AV-graft	Lumsden et al. [96]	Single center; inner city; graft >50% found on AN	PTA + Color flow duplex q 2 months; $N = 32$	No PTA + color flow duplex q 2 months $N = 32$	Average = 1.94/ patient (T)	N/A	6 months patency: 63% (T) vs. 67% (C)
AV-graft	Moist et al. [84]	Multicenter; graft – no clinical or functional abN with Qb >650 mL/min	US dilution + DVP and PE; $N = 59$	DVP + PE; $N = 53$	0.93 PTA/patient-year (T) vs. 0.61 PTA/ patient-year (C)	0.51/patient-year (T) vs. 0.41/ patient-year (C)	No difference $p = 0.89$
AV-graft	Ram et al. [97]	Multicenter	Referral for Ix based on (a) Q <600 mL/min or clinical criteria (Q group); $N = 32$, (b) Stenosis >50% or clinical criteria; $N = 35$	Referral for I× based on clinical criteria only; $N = 34$	0.34/patient-year (Q) vs. 0.65 PTA/ patient-year (Stenosis group) vs. 0.22 PTA/ patient-year (C)	0.91/patient-year (Q) vs. 0.50/ patient-year (Stenosis group) vs. 0.68/patient-year (C)	All patients: Ultrasound dilution (Qa) monthly vs. Duplex US (stenosis detection) q 3 months; it was criteria for intervention that patients were randomized to
AV-graft	Dember et al. [98]	Multicenter; general and VA population	SVP (average of two consecutive sessions) + PTA in response to SVP >0.4; $N = 32$	SVP and no interventions; PTA based on clinical indication only; $N = 32$	3.1/patient-year (T) vs. 1.2/patient-year (C)	0.89/patient-year (T) vs. 1.03/ patient-year (C); 44% (T) vs. 72% (C)	Study stopped at interim analysis due to futility; no difference

(continued)

Table 4.2 (continued)

VA type	Author	Sites and population	Surveillance method in treatment group (T)	Comparator method in control group ©	Interventions	Thrombosis	Access survival
AV-graft	Malik et al. [99]	Multicenter (25 HD units); unselected	Duplex Doppler US q 3 months + standard care; $N=97$	Standard care: DVP, recirculation, blood flow monitoring; $N=92$	2.1/graft (T) vs. 1.8/graft (C)	N/A	Greater cumulative patency in T group vs. C ($p<0.001$)
AV-graft	Robbin et al. [100]	Multi-HD units; prevalent patients with no access intervention in prior month or one planned prior month or one planned	Duplex Doppler US q 4 months + clinical monitoring; $N=65$	Clinical monitoring; $N=61$	1.05 PTA/year (T) vs. 0.64 PTA/year (C) 0.13 surg rev/year (T) vs. 0.16 surg rev/year (C)	0.67/year (T) vs. 0.78/year (C)	Median survival 38 months (T) vs. 37 months (C)
AVF	Tessitore et al. [101]	Multicenter; no history of prior access intervention; subclinical stenosis detected on fistulography	Preemptive PTA within 3 weeks of detection of stenosis; $N=44$	Intervention based on clinical access dysfunction (i.e. inability to sustain dialysis) or thrombosis; $N=39$	N/A	3.7/year at risk (T) vs. 13.9%/year at risk (C)	Greater cumulative patency in the T group vs. C AVF loss rate 5.1%/year at risk (T) vs. 15.6%/year at risk (C)
AVF	Polkinghorne et al. [102]	Single HD units (satellite units); all received US dilution	Referred to angiography based on clinical criteria or Qa by US dilution; $N=69$	Referred to angiography based on clinical criteria only; $N=68$		Overall rate 0.052/patient-years; no difference in groups	

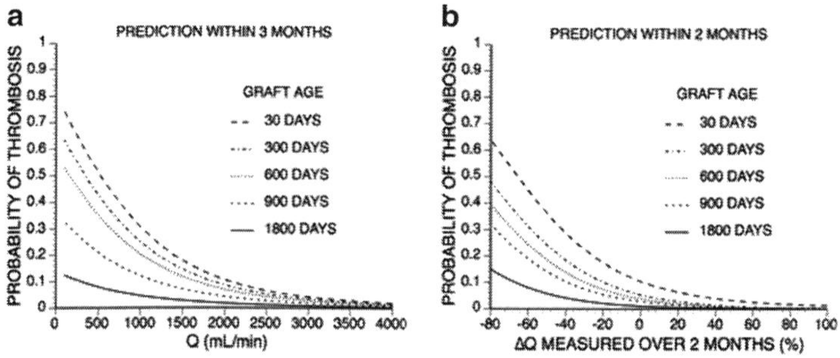

Fig. 4.7 Influence of synthetic AV-graft blood flow (Q), percentage change in flow (ΔQ), and AV-graft age on probability of thrombosis within the next 3 months (**a**) or 2 months (**b**) [60]. Negative ΔQ indicates a decrease in Q. Note that AV-graft age has a strong influence on thrombosis. New grafts are particularly prone to thrombosis, whereas older grafts are unlikely to thrombose even at low Q or large decrease in Q

Finally, another issue is that the usual "corrective" intervention, angioplasty, may itself be harmful [81, 82]. Angioplasty causes endothelial disruption and intimal stretching, thereby stimulating cellular proliferation that may promote neointimal hyperplasia with aggressive restenosis [18, 83]. The potential for a high false-positive rate of referrals with unnecessary angioplasty procedures may, in part, explain the failure of surveillance to prolong access life in RCTs. Thus, the ability to correctly identify those accesses that are likely to fail, and avoid procedures in accesses that are not likely to fail, is of prime importance.

Prolongation of Access Survival

Ideally, the primary goal of access monitoring and surveillance is to preemptively correct stenosis so that thrombosis is reduced and access survival is prolonged. While both Q and static or derived static VP surveillance are recommended to detect access dysfunction and stenosis, there is little evidence that surveillance with angioplasty improves AV-graft survival (see Table 4.2 of RCTs). For example, Moist et al. [84] studied time to AV-graft thrombosis and AV-graft loss, comparing the study treatment group, monthly Q plus standard monitoring (dynamic VP and physical examination) to the control group (standard monitoring). In this blinded RCT of 112 patients, there was no difference in time to AV-graft thrombosis or loss. However, it is not necessary to establish prolonged access survival if there are important benefits. A nonrandomized study [85] found that Q surveillance of AVFs was associated with fewer thromboses and central venous catheters. A secondary analysis of a RCT found that Duplex ultrasound surveillance of stenosis in AV-grafts reduced hospitalizations and cost of care [86]. However, these benefits have generally not been demonstrated in RCTs. This question remains: how can surveillance with preemptive correction be recommended if its benefits have not been established?

Future Directions

The pathophysiology of AVF and AV-graft failure is not fully understood, and this limits us to methods such as surveillance and intervention that do not address the underlying cause of access failure (neointimal hyperplasia, endothelial dysfunction, etc.). Vascular access hemodynamics clearly plays a role in the effectiveness of access surveillance. Standard monthly surveillance has failed to improve outcomes in RCTs. While some have argued that inadequacies of study design accounts for these negative results, it seems more likely that the strategy of standard monthly surveillance with preemptive intervention is a flawed concept. Patients have wide hemodynamic variation during dialysis, so that the reproducibility of measurements from session to session is poor and may falsely suggest increases in stenosis. Q and VP may change so rapidly that there is insufficient time to detect the change before thrombosis. Surveillance might improve outcomes if measurements were taken more frequently so that calculation of average values neutralizes hemodynamic variation, making it easier to detect rapid changes in Q or VP before thrombosis. This increased frequency might be met by on-line monitoring methods [72]. In addition, the current interventional method of angioplasty with possible stenting has the potential to cause more harm than good. The ability to correctly identify those accesses that are likely to fail, and avoid procedures in accesses that are not likely to fail, remains an elusive goal that can only be reached with properly designed studies.

Key Points

- AVFs primarily fail to mature early after creation, whereas AV-grafts are more likely to be usable for dialysis but fail later because of stenosis and thrombosis
- Endothelial dysfunction, poor vessel elasticity, and neointimal hyperplasia are key common features in AVF and AV-graft failure
- Randomized controlled trials have generally not confirmed the claim of nonrandomized trials that access surveillance reduces thrombosis and increases access survival
- An understanding of access hemodynamics helps explain why standard monthly access surveillance has been generally unsuccessful in improving access outcomes
- Surveillance outcomes might be improved if surveillance measurements were taken more frequently

References

1. Canadian Organ Replacement Register. CORR report – treatment of end-stage organ failure in Canada, 1999 to 2008. Ottawa, ON: CORR; 2010.
2. U.S. Renal Data System. USRDS 2009 annual data report: atlas of chronic kidney disease and end-stage renal disease in the United States, National Institutes of Health, Fig. 6.4, Chap. 6. Bethesda, MD: National Institute of Diabetes and Digestive and Kidney Diseases; 2009. p. 273.
3. U.S. Renal Data System. USRDS 2010 annual data report: atlas of chronic kidney disease and end-stage renal disease in the United States, National Institutes of Health. In: Costs of end-stage renal disease, vol. 2. Bethesda, MD: National Institute of Diabetes and Digestive and Kidney Diseases; 2010.
4. Nosher JL. Death, taxes, and vascular access dysfunction. Semin Dial. 1991;4:67–8.
5. NIoHNaTNIoDaDaKD. Identification of factors associated with failure of arteriovenous fistulas to mature in hemodialysis patients (U01). Vol. 2010. Bethesda, MD: National Institute of Diabetes and Digestive and Kidney Diseases; 2007.
6. Lok CE, Allon M, Donnelly S, Dorval M, et al. Design of the fish oil inhibition of stenosis in hemodialysis grafts (FISH) study. Clin Trials. 2007;4:357–67.
7. Conte MS, Nugent HM, Gaccione P, Guleria I, et al. Multicenter phase I/II trial of the safety of allogeneic endothelial cell implants after the creation of arteriovenous access for hemodialysis use: the V-HEALTH study. J Vasc Surg 2009; 50: 1359–1368 e1351.

8. Lee T, Roy-Chaudhury P. Advances and new frontiers in the pathophysiology of venous neointimal hyperplasia and dialysis access stenosis. Adv Chronic Kidney Dis. 2009;16:329–38.
9. Gimbrone Jr MA. Vascular endothelium: an integrator of pathophysiologic stimuli in atherosclerosis. Am J Cardiol. 1995;75:67B–70.
10. Roy-Chaudhury P, Kelly BS, Miller MA, Reaves A, et al. Venous neointimal hyperplasia in polytetrafluoroethylene dialysis grafts. Kidney Int. 2001;59: 2325–34.
11. Roy-Chaudhury P, Wang Y, Krishnamoorthy M, Zhang J, et al. Cellular phenotypes in human stenotic lesions from haemodialysis vascular access. Nephrol Dial Transplant. 2009;24:2786–91.
12. Anderson J, Abbuhl M, Hering T, Johnston K. Immunohistochemical identification of components in the healing response of human vascular grafts. ASAIO J. 1985;8:79–85.
13. Swedberg SH, Brown BG, Sigley R, Wight TN, et al. Intimal fibromuscular hyperplasia at the venous anastomosis of PTFE grafts in hemodialysis patients. Clinical, immunocytochemical, light and electron microscopic assessment. Circulation. 1989;80:1726–36.
14. Hehrlein C. How do AV fistulae lose function? The roles of haemodynamics, vascular remodelling, and intimal hyperplasia. Nephrol Dial Transplant. 1995;10:1287–90.
15. Golden MA, Au YP, Kenagy RD, Clowes AW. Growth factor gene expression by intimal cells in healing polytetrafluoroethylene grafts. J Vasc Surg. 1990;11:580–5.
16. Porter KE, Olojugba DH, Masood I, Pemberton M, et al. Endothelin-B receptors mediate intimal hyperplasia in an organ culture of human saphenous vein. J Vasc Surg. 1998;28:695–701.
17. Roy-Chaudhury P, Arend L, Zhang J, Krishnamoorthy M, et al. Neointimal hyperplasia in early arteriovenous fistula failure. Am J Kidney Dis. 2007;50:782–90.
18. Chang CJ, Ko PJ, Hsu LA, Ko YS, et al. Highly increased cell proliferation activity in the restenotic hemodialysis vascular access after percutaneous transluminal angioplasty: implication in prevention of restenosis. Am J Kidney Dis. 2004;43:74–84.
19. Wang Y, Krishnamoorthy M, Banerjee R, Zhang J, et al. Venous stenosis in a pig arteriovenous fistula model – anatomy, mechanisms and cellular phenotypes. Nephrol Dial Transplant. 2008;23:525–33.
20. Ombrellaro MP, Stevens SL, Schaeffer DO, Freeman MB, et al. The role of platelet-derived growth factor in intraluminal stented graft healing. J Am Coll Surg. 1997;184:49–57.
21. Faries PL, Marin ML, Veith FJ, Ramirez JA, et al. Immunolocalization and temporal distribution of cytokine expression during the development of vein graft intimal hyperplasia in an experimental model. J Vasc Surg. 1996;24:463–71.
22. Weiss MF, Scivittaro V, Anderson JM. Oxidative stress and increased expression of growth factors in lesions of failed hemodialysis access. Am J Kidney Dis. 2001;37:970–80.
23. Roselaar SE, Nazhat NB, Winyard PG, Jones P, et al. Detection of oxidants in uremic plasma by electron spin resonance spectroscopy. Kidney Int. 1995;48:199–206.

24. Witko-Sarsat V, Friedlander M, Capeillere-Blandin C, Nguyen-Khoa T, et al. Advanced oxidation protein products as a novel marker of oxidative stress in uremia. Kidney Int. 1996;49:1304–13.
25. Himmelfarb J, Stenvinkel P, Ikizler TA, Hakim RM. The elephant in uremia: oxidant stress as a unifying concept of cardiovascular disease in uremia. Kidney Int. 2002;62:1524–38.
26. Descamps-Latscha B, Goldfarb B, Nguyen AT, Landais P, et al. Establishing the relationship between complement activation and stimulation of phagocyte oxidative metabolism in hemodialyzed patients: a randomized prospective study. Nephron. 1991;59:279–85.
27. Zima T, Haragsim L, Stipek S, Bartova V, et al. Lipid peroxidation on dialysis membranes. Biochem Mol Biol Int. 1993;29:531–7.
28. Toborek M, Wasik T, Drozdz M, Klin M, et al. Effect of hemodialysis on lipid peroxidation and antioxidant system in patients with chronic renal failure. Metabolism. 1992;41:1229–32.
29. Beckman JS, Koppenol WH. Nitric oxide, superoxide, and peroxynitrite: the good, the bad, and ugly. Am J Physiol. 1996;271:C1424–37.
30. Ruef J, Peter K, Nordt TK, Runge MS, et al. Oxidative stress and atherosclerosis: its relationship to growth factors, thrombus formation and therapeutic approaches. Thromb Haemost. 1999;82 Suppl 1:32–7.
31. Griendling KK, Sorescu D, Ushio-Fukai M. NAD(P)H oxidase: role in cardiovascular biology and disease. Circ Res. 2000;86:494–501.
32. Stracke S, Konner K, Kostlin I, Friedl R, et al. Increased expression of TGF-beta1 and IGF-I in inflammatory stenotic lesions of hemodialysis fistulas. Kidney Int. 2002;61:1011–9.
33. Aviram M. LDL-platelet inteaction under oxidative stress induces macrophage foam cell formation. Thromb Haemost. 1997;74(1):560–4.
34. Fukai T, Folz RJ, Landmesser U, Harrison DG. Extracellular superoxide dismutase and cardiovascular disease. Cardiovasc Res. 2002;55:239–49.
35. Berk BC. Redox signals that regulate the vascular response to injury. Thromb Haemost. 1999;82:810–7.
36. Huynh TT, Davies MG, Trovato MJ, Barber L, et al. Reduction of lipid peroxidation with intraoperative superoxide dismutase treatment decreases intimal hyperplasia in experimental vein grafts. J Surg Res. 1999;84:223–32.
37. Lok CE, Allon A, Donnelly S, Dorval M, Hemmelgarn B, Moist L, et al. Design of the fish oil inhibition of stenosis in hemodialysis (FISH) Graft Study. Clin Trials. 2007;4(4):357–67.
38. Roy-Chaudhury P, Sukhatme VP, Cheung AK. Hemodialysis vascular access dysfunction: a cellular and molecular viewpoint. J Am Soc Nephrol. 2006;17:1112–27.
39. Dixon BS. Why don't fistulas mature? Kidney Int. 2006;70:1413–22.
40. Dember LM, Beck GJ, Allon M, Delmez JA, et al. Effect of clopidogrel on early failure of arteriovenous fistulas for hemodialysis: a randomized controlled trial. JAMA. 2008;299:2164–71.
41. Dixon BS, Beck GJ, Vazquez MA, Greenberg A, et al. The effect of dipyridamole plus aspirin on hemodialysis graft patency. N Engl J Med. 2009;360(21):2191–201.
42. Lok CE. Antiplatelet therapy and vascular-access patency. N Engl J Med. 2009;360:2240–2.

43. Schwab SJ, Raymond JR, Saeed M, Newman GE, et al. Prevention of hemodialysis fistula thrombosis. Early detection of venous stenoses. Kidney Int. 1989;36:707–11.
44. Besarab A, Sullivan KL, Ross RP, Moritz MJ. Utility of intra-access pressure monitoring in detecting and correcting venous outlet stenoses prior to thrombosis. Kidney Int. 1995;47:1364–73.
45. NKF-DOQI. Clinical practice guidelines for vascular access. National Kidney Foundation-Dialysis Outcomes Quality Initiative. Am J Kidney Dis. 1997;30:S150–91.
46. NKF-DOQI. Clinical practice guidelines for vascular access. Am J Kidney Dis. 2006;48:S176–247.
47. Hulley SB, Cummings SR, Browner WS, Grady D, Hearst N, Newman TB, editors. Designing clinical research. 2nd ed. Philadelphia: Lippincott Williams & Wilkins; 2001. p. 143–55.
48. Lok CE, Moist. LM. Challenges for randomized controlled trials in nephrology: illustrations in vascular access science and care. J Nephrol. 2007;20:632–45.
49. Gordis L. Epidemiology. 2nd ed. Philadelphia: W.B. Saunders; 2000. p. 100–9.
50. Besarab A. Access monitoring is worthwhile and valuable. Blood Purif. 2006;24:77–89.
51. Paulson WD, Work J. Controversial vascular access surveillance mandate. Semin Dial. 2010;23:92–4.
52. Abreo K, Allon M, Asif A, Atray N, et al. Which direction is right for vascular access surveillance? A debate. Nephrol News Issues. 2010;24:30, 32, 34.
53. Paulson WD. Access monitoring does not really improve outcomes. Blood Purif. 2005;23:50–6.
54. Sands JJ. Vascular access monitoring improves outcomes. Blood Purif. 2005;23:45–9.
55. White JJ, Bander SJ, Schwab SJ, Churchill DN, et al. Is percutaneous transluminal angioplasty an effective intervention for arteriovenous graft stenosis? Semin Dial. 2005;18:190–202.
56. Dember LM, Holmberg EF, Kaufman JS. Value of static venous pressure for predicting arteriovenous graft thrombosis. Kidney Int. 2002;61:1899–904.
57. McDougal G, Agarwal R. Clinical performance characteristics of hemodialysis graft monitoring. Kidney Int. 2001;60:762–6.
58. Paulson WD, Ram SJ, Birk CG, Work J. Does blood flow accurately predict thrombosis or failure of hemodialysis synthetic grafts? A meta-analysis. Am J Kidney Dis. 1999;34:478–85.
59. Paulson WD, Ram SJ, Birk CG, Zapczynski M, et al. Accuracy of decrease in blood flow in predicting hemodialysis graft thrombosis. Am J Kidney Dis. 2000;35:1089–95.
60. Ram SJ, Nassar R, Work J, Abreo K, et al. Risk of hemodialysis graft thrombosis: analysis of monthly flow surveillance. Am J Kidney Dis. 2008;52:930–8.
61. White JJ, Ram SJ, Jones SA, Schwab SJ, et al. Influence of luminal diameters on flow surveillance of hemodialysis grafts: insights from a mathematical model. Clin J Am Soc Nephrol. 2006;1:972–8.
62. Kheda MF, Brenner LE, Patel MJ, Wynn JJ, et al. Influence of arterial elasticity and vessel dilatation on arteriovenous fistula maturation: a prospective cohort study. Nephrol Dial Transplant. 2010;25:525–31.

63. Paulson WD, Asif A, Salman LH, Jones SA. Mathematical model of artrio-venous fistula (AVF): a powerful method to improve understanding of the hemodynamics of AVF failure (abstract). J Am Soc Nephrol. 2010; 21:248A.
64. White JJ, Jones SA, Ram SJ, Schwab SJ, et al. Mathematical model demonstrates influence of luminal diameters on venous pressure surveillance. Clin J Am Soc Nephrol. 2007;2:681–7.
65. Atray NK, Ram SJ, Work J, Eason JM, et al. A longitudinal study of hemodialysis graft stenosis: role of progressive stenosis in thrombosis (abstract). J Am Soc Nephrol. 2001;12:281A.
66. DeSoto DJ, Ram SJ, Faiyaz R, Birk CG, et al. Hemodynamic reproducibility during blood flow measurements of hemodialysis synthetic grafts. Am J Kidney Dis. 2001;37:790–6.
67. Ram SJ, Nassar R, Sharaf R, Magnasco A, et al. Thresholds for significant decrease in hemodialysis access blood flow. Semin Dial. 2005;18:558–64.
68. Schneditz D, Fan Z, Kaufman A, Levin NW. Stability of access resistance during haemodialysis. Nephrol Dial Transplant. 1998;13:739–44.
69. Rehman SU, Pupim LB, Shyr Y, Hakim R, et al. Intradialytic serial vascular access flow measurements. Am J Kidney Dis. 1999;34:471–7.
70. Agharazii M, Clouatre Y, Nolin L, Leblanc M. Variation of intra-access flow early and late into hemodialysis. ASAIO J. 2000;46:452–5.
71. Paulson WD, Ram SJ, Faiyaz R, Caldito GC, et al. Association between blood pressure, ultrafiltration, and hemodialysis graft thrombosis: a multivariable logistic regression analysis. Am J Kidney Dis. 2002;40:769–76.
72. Zasuwa G, Frinak S, Besarab A, Peterson E, et al. Automated intravascular access pressure surveillance reduces thrombosis rates. Semin Dial. 2010;23:527–35.
73. Dossabhoy NR, Ram SJ, Nassar R, Work J, et al. Stenosis surveillance of hemodialysis grafts by duplex ultrasound reduces hospitalizations and cost of care. Semin Dial. 2005;18:550–7.
74. Depner TA, Krivitski NM. Clinical measurement of blood flow in hemodialysis access fistulae and grafts by ultrasound dilution. ASAIO J. 1995; 41:M745–9.
75. Krivitski NM. Theory and validation of access flow measurement by dilution technique during hemodialysis. Kidney Int. 1995;48:244–50.
76. Krivitski NM, MacGibbon D, Gleed RD, Dobson A. Accuracy of dilution techniques for access flow measurement during hemodialysis. Am J Kidney Dis. 1998;31:502–8.
77. Polkinghorne K. The CARI guidelines. Vascular access surveillance. Nephrology (Carlton). 2008;13 Suppl 2:S1–11.
78. Bos C, Smits JH, Zijistra JJ, Blankestijn PJ, et al. Underestimation of access flow by ultrasound dilution flow measurements. Phys Med Biol. 2002;47:481–9.
79. Sands J, Glidden D, Jacavage W, Jones B. Difference between delivered and prescribed blood flow in hemodialysis. ASAIO J. 1996;42:M717–9.
80. Tonelli M, James M, Wiebe N, Jindal K, et al. Ultrasound monitoring to detect access stenosis in hemodialysis patients: a systematic review. Am J Kidney Dis. 2008;51:630–40.
81. Allon M, Robbin ML. Hemodialysis vascular access monitoring: current concepts. Hemodial Int. 2009;13:153–62.

82. Paulson WD, White JJ. Should arteriovenous fistulas and synthetic grafts undergo surveillance with pre-emptive correction of stenosis? Nat Clin Pract Nephrol. 2008;4:480–1.
83. Levit RD, Cohen RM, Kwak A, Shlansky-Goldberg RD, et al. Asymptomatic central venous stenosis in hemodialysis patients. Radiology. 2006;238:1051–6.
84. Moist LM, Churchill DN, House AA, Millward SF, et al. Regular monitoring of access flow compared with monitoring of venous pressure fails to improve graft survival. J Am Soc Nephrol. 2003;14:2645–53.
85. Tessitore N, Bedogna V, Poli A, Mantovani W, et al. Adding access blood flow surveillance to clinical monitoring reduces thrombosis rates and costs, and improves fistula patency in the short term: a controlled cohort study. Nephrol Dial Transplant. 2008;23:3578–84.
86. Ram SJ, Nassar R, Work J, Eason JM, et al. Stenosis surveillance of hemodialysis grafts by Duplex Ultrasound reduces hospitalizations and cost of care. Semin Dial. 2005;18:550–7.
87. Kaegi A, Pineo GF, Shimizu A, Trivedi H, et al. Arteriovenous-shunt thrombosis. Prevention by sulfinpyrazone. N Engl J Med. 1974;290:304–6.
88. Harter HR, Burch JW, Majerus PW, Stanford N, et al. Prevention of thrombosis in patients on hemodialysis by low-dose aspirin. N Engl J Med. 1979;301:577–9.
89. Kobayashi K, Maeda K, Koshikawa S, Kawaguchi Y, et al. Antithrombotic therapy with ticlopidine in chronic renal failure patients on maintenance hemodialysis – a multicenter collaborative double blind study. Thromb Res. 1980;20:255–61.
90. Andrassy K, Malluche H, Bornefeld H, Comberg M, et al. Prevention of p.o. clotting of av. cimino fistulae with acetylsalicyl acid. Results of a prospective double blind study. Klin Wochenschr. 1974;52:348–9.
91. Grontoft KC, Mulec H, Gutierrez A, Olander R. Thromboprophylactic effect of ticlopidine in arteriovenous fistulas for haemodialysis. Scand J Urol Nephrol. 1985;19:55–7.
92. Sreedhara R, Himmelfarb J, Lazarus JM, Hakim RM. Anti-platelet therapy in graft thrombosis: results of a prospective, randomized, double-blind study. Kidney Int. 1994;45:1477–83.
93. Crowther MA, Clase CM, Margetts PJ, Julian J, et al. Low-intensity warfarin is ineffective for the prevention of PTFE graft failure in patients on hemodialysis: a randomized controlled trial. J Am Soc Nephrol. 2002;13:2331–7.
94. Kaufman JS, O'Connor TZ, Zhang JH, Cronin RE, et al. Randomized controlled trial of clopidogrel plus aspirin to prevent hemodialysis access graft thrombosis. J Am Soc Nephrol. 2003;14:2313–21.
95. Schmitz PG, McCloud LK, Reikes ST, Leonard CL, et al. Prophylaxis of hemodialysis graft thrombosis with fish oil: double-blind, randomized, prospective trial. J Am Soc Nephrol. 2002;13:184–90.
96. Lumsden AB, MacDonald MJ, Kikeri D, Cotsonis GA, et al. Prophylactic balloon angioplasty fails to prolong the patency of expanded polytetrafluoroethylene arteriovenous grafts: results of a prospective randomized study. J Vasc Surg. 1997;26:382–90; discussion 390–382.
97. Ram SJ, Work J, Caldito GC, Eason JM, et al. A randomized controlled trial of blood flow and stenosis surveillance of hemodialysis grafts. Kidney Int. 2003;64:272–80.

98. Dember LM, Holmberg EF, Kaufman JS. Randomized controlled trial of prophylactic repair of hemodialysis arteriovenous graft stenosis. Kidney Int. 2004;66:390–8.
99. Malik J, Slavikova M, Svobodova J, Tuka V. Regular ultrasonographic screening significantly prolongs patency of PTFE grafts. Kidney Int. 2005;67:1554–8.
100. Robbin ML, Oser RF, Lee JY, Heudebert GR, et al. Randomized comparison of ultrasound surveillance and clinical monitoring on arteriovenous graft outcomes. Kidney Int. 2006;69:730–5.
101. Tessitore N, Mansueto G, Bedogna V, Lipari G, et al. A prospective controlled trial on effect of percutaneous transluminal angioplasty on functioning arteriovenous fistulae survival. J Am Soc Nephrol. 2003;14:1623–7.
102. Polkinghorne KR, Lau KK, Saunder A, Atkins RC, et al. Does monthly native arteriovenous fistula blood-flow surveillance detect significant stenosis–a randomized controlled trial. Nephrol Dial Transplant. 2006;21:2498–506.

Chapter 5
Clinical Relevance of Vascular Access Monitoring and Surveillance

Louise Moist, William D. Paulson, and Charmaine E. Lok

In the United States, the National Kidney Foundation Kidney Disease Outcomes Quality Initiative (NKF-KDOQI) have set a goal of 65% functional arteriovenous fistulae (AVF) with <10% central venous catheter (CVC) prevalent use [1]. The Canadian Society of Nephrology has recommended a prevalent AVF rate of 60% [2].The rationale behind these goals is the excellent long-term survival and low complication rates associated with successfully matured and functional AVF and the high morbidity and mortality associated with CVCs. Arteriovenous grafts (AV-grafts) represent a reasonable alternative to AVF. Data comparing the cumulative survival of AVF and AV-grafts demonstrate equivalency when they are compared from the time of creation and include the early fistula failures [3–5]. This equivalency occurs because the natural histories of AVF and AV-grafts differ with their characteristic problems arising at different time intervals. AVF are more likely to have early complications such as its failure to mature, while AV-grafts suffer from late complications such as AV-graft

L. Moist (✉)
Associate Professor of Medicine and Epidemiology,
University of Western Ontario, 800 Commissioners Road,
London, Ontario, Canada
e-mail: louise.moist@lhsc.on.ca

D.K. Rajan (ed.), *Essentials of Percutaneous Dialysis Interventions*,
DOI 10.1007/978-1-4419-5657-6_5,
© Springer Science+Business Media, LLC 2011

stenosis and thrombosis (see Chap. 4). Vascular access (access) monitoring and/or surveillance to detect access problems are some of the first logical step(s) to take in trying to improve outcomes. This chapter will discuss the most common methods of access monitoring and surveillance, and will include illustrations of practical applications.

Vascular Access Monitoring and Surveillance

The basic principle for vascular access monitoring and surveillance is that an access abnormality can be detected and intervened upon with improved outcomes. Vascular access stenoses develop over variable intervals in the great majority of accesses; if they are detected and corrected before thrombosis, complications, and inadequate dialysis can be minimized or avoided, and the rate of thrombosis may be reduced.

Monitoring refers to the examination and evaluation of the access by means of physical examination to detect clinical signs that suggest the presence of dysfunction. These abnormal clinical signs include arm swelling, changes in the access bruit or thrill or prolonged bleeding post dialysis. Dr Gerald Beathard has refined and highlighted specific exam techniques to detect stenosis (below), which have demonstrated excellent accuracy when compared with radiological imaging of the access.

Surveillance refers to the periodic evaluation of the access by using device-based methods of detecting hemodynamically significant stenosis, such as measurement of access blood flow. It is the combination of the monitoring and surveillance that provides the greatest likelihood of detecting a clinically significant access problem requiring intervention [1].

Access Monitoring

Physical Exam

While controversy continues as to whether the use of access surveillance improves outcomes related to stenosis and thrombosis in AVFs and AV-grafts (see Chap. 4), physical examination of the vascular access is a necessary part of the routine care of a hemodialysis access and should be performed at each dialysis session by trained health care providers. While this has practical limitations (e.g., ability of the nephrologist to routinely examine a non-cannulated access), the exam supplements the history to provide information on the integrity of the access, such as signs of trauma, inflammation or infection and/or changes in the access (e.g., changes in size of aneurysms) or complications associated with the access (e.g., signs of vascular steal). The physical exam is in national guidelines [1, 6] with recommendation for it to be incorporated into all monitoring and surveillance programs.

The steps in examining a new AVF have been well described by Dr Gerald Beathard [7]. The approach below has been adapted from a United States initiative on improving vascular access outcomes, the Fistula First Initiative [8].

Establish a Baseline: Examine the Patient Prior to Access Placement

The patient's chest, breast, and upper arms should be evaluated for the presence of swelling or collateral veins. In patients with normal venous pressure, central venous occlusion may not be associated with swelling; however, the presence of collateral veins should alert the examiner to the problem. The presence of pacemakers or scars indicating previous neck or thoracic surgery or trauma should also raise the possibility of a venous anomaly that might affect access creation.

Arterial Evaluation

Two important considerations arise when evaluating the arterial system for access creation and maturation. Firstly, the vessel must be capable of delivering blood flow at a rate to provide adequate dialysis and secondly, access creation must not jeopardize the viability of the extremity, such as may occur with a vascular steal phenomenon. Arterial narrowing and calcification are common in patients with end stage renal disease

(ESRD), especially among those with atherosclerosis, diabetes, and hypertension. Three key physical examination maneuvers can be used to determine the adequacy of arterial inflow: (1) pulse examination, (2) segmental blood pressure measurement, and (3) the Allen Test.

Pulse examination – The presence and strength of the axillary, brachial, radial, and ulnar pulses should be determined in both upper extremities.

Segmental blood pressures – The blood pressures in both arms should be obtained, compared, and graded [9]. A difference of <10 mmHg is considered normal while a difference of 10–20 mmHg is marginal and >20 mmHg is problematic and should trigger further evaluation.

The Allen Test – The Allen Test is used to determine the competence of the palmar arch. It is performed by having the patient clench their fist several times while the radial and ulnar arteries are occluded at the wrist. The patient then extends their fingers, palm up, which should show a "blanched" hand. The pressure on the ulnar artery is then released and the patient's hand is observed for "blushing." If the color of the hand does not return in 5–10 s [10] the Allen test is considered positive, indicating an inadequate collateral circulation. Use of vascular Doppler can increase the effectiveness of the Allen test in predicting collateral arterial perfusion of the hand.

If clinical examination results are clearly satisfactory, no further testing is mandatory. However, if problems are apparent, then noninvasive or even invasive studies should be used for evaluation.

Venous Evaluation

The integrity of the receiving vein is essential for both AVF and AV-graft creation. The patient's vein should be evaluated to determine its potential for distention and to evaluate for outflow obstruction (Fig. 5.1). This is easily done using a blood pressure cuff inflated to a pressure about 5 mmHg above diastolic pressure. This should be left in place for no more than 5 min. A study of three methods to facilitate venous distention demonstrated that hydrostatic pressure combined with warmth generates the greatest venous distensibility in the lower arm in hemodialysis patients in a sitting position [11]. While venous

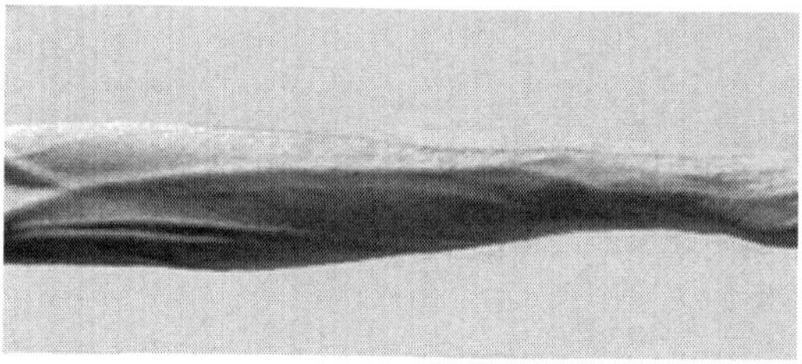

Fig. 5.1 Well-preserved veins in the forearm and upper arm for creating a functional arteriovenous fistula (AVF). Vessel preservation is essential in chronic kidney disease patients (courtesy Tushar J. Vachharajani, *Atlas of Dialysis Vascular Access Fistula First* [8])

evaluation by physical exam provides excellent information in many patients [12, 13], vascular mapping in obese patients may identify surgically feasible vessels for access creation [14].

Critical Evaluation Post Vascular Access Creation

Physical examination is important immediately after surgical creation of a vascular access. The vascular access is a newly created "life-line" that should be evaluated for its integrity, signs of infection and its effect on the surrounding vascular bed and soft tissues. The exam follows an organized manner with a general inspection, palpation and auscultation. On inspection, the arm may be red and swollen for the first few weeks following surgery. It may be warm, possibly with a faint thrill, but there should be an intact pulse. On auscultation, a bruit should be present over the body of the access. The absence of a bruit indicates early thrombosis and necessitates assessment for possible surgical salvage.

After the immediate post operative period, two causes of early access failure include "failure to mature" (when the AVF does not dilate and remodel enough to allow for adequate needle cannulation and blood flow to support dialysis) and thrombosis and stenosis (AV-grafts and AVF) (see Chap. 4). Fistulae fail to mature when the increase in shear stress and pressure (which cause release of nitric oxide) fail to yield adequate vessel dilatation and remodeling; this

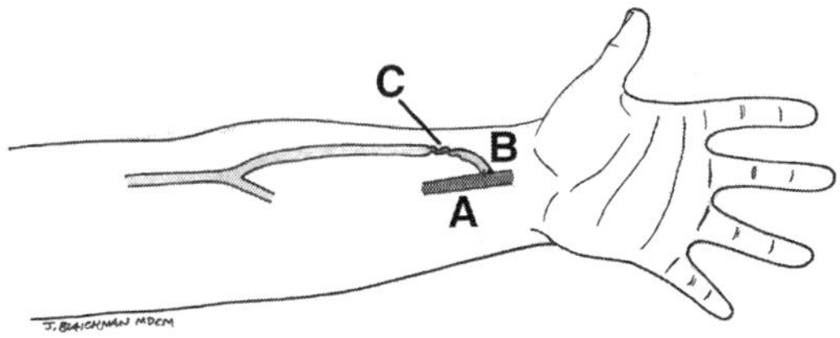

Fig. 5.2 Physical examination of juxta-anastomotic stenosis. (A) Radial artery. A strong pulse and thrill are present at the anastomosis (B). It diminishes or disappears as the examining finger crosses and moves downstream to the stenosis (C)

may be caused by a number of factors, such as poor vessel elasticity, stenosis that limits flow, or the dissipation of flow by accessory veins or collateral veins. The most common type of stenosis is juxta-anastomic [15, 16], a stenosis adjacent to the anastomosis. Accessory vessels are naturally occurring branches of vessels while collateral vessels develop in response to a pathologic, stenotic lesion [7].

Juxta-anastomotic venous stenosis – can be easily diagnosed by palpation of the anastomosis and distal vein (see Fig. 5.2). In the absence of abnormalities, the pulse is soft and easily compressible. With juxta-anastomotic stenosis, a water-hammer pulse is felt at and upstream to the anastomosis. The thrill, which is normally continuous in both systole and diastole, may be present only in systole. As one moves downstream (up the vein towards the heart) from the anastomosis with the palpating finger, the pulse diminishes rather abruptly as the site of stenosis is crossed. After this level, the pulse is very weak and the vein is poorly developed.

Collateral and accessory veins can be easily identified through physical examination (see Fig. 5.3). Frequently, they are visible. If not, then they can be detected by palpating the AVF. Again, palpate the thrill at the anastomosis and simultaneously occlude the AVF downstream (antegrade) with another finger. Normally, the access flow will stop and cause the palpated thrill to disappear. If it does not disappear, an outflow channel (accessory vein) is present upstream to the point of occlusion. Palpation of the fistula upstream to the occlusion will generally reveal the location of the accessory vein by the presence of a thrill over its trunk. As long as the main AVF channel

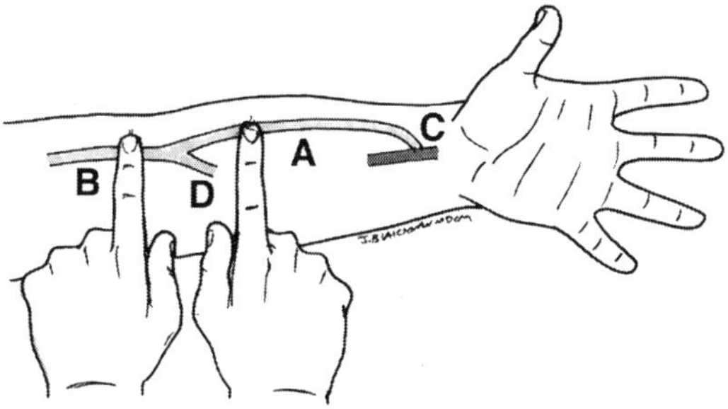

Fig. 5.3 Physical examination of accessory vein. When the fistula is occluded at point A, the thrill will disappear at the anastomosis (C). As the point of occlusion is moved downstream to past the accessory vein (D) to point B, the thrill will continue because flow has an escape route

can be identified for occlusion, its entire length can be evaluated by moving the point of AVF occlusion progressively downstream from the anastomosis.

Maintenance Evaluation of the Vascular Access

After an access is matured and successfully cannulated, the most common cause of failure is stenosis and consequent thrombosis. Vessel stenosis can be detected on routine physical exam of both AVF and AV-grafts (see Fig. 5.4). Normally, the mature AVF and AV-graft have a soft pulse and the entire structure is easily compressed. If stenosis is suspected in an AVF, elevation of the arm will confirm its presence. When the arm is elevated, a normal AVF will have some degree of collapse. When the arm of a stenotic AVF is elevated, that portion of the AVF upstream to the stenosis remains distended, while the downstream portion collapses, thereby allowing easy localization of the stenotic area. In addition, the pulse diminishes abruptly downstream to the stenosis as does the caliber of the vessel.

If stenosis is suspected in AV-grafts, palpation of its thrill and pulse and auscultation of the bruit's pitch will be informative (see Table 5.1). Normally, at the anastomosis, the pulse is compressible and the thrill is continuous (only palpable at the anastomosis). In the presence of a stenosis, the pulse becomes hyperpulsatile or "water-hammer" upstream to the stenosis. Thrill characteristics may be associated with

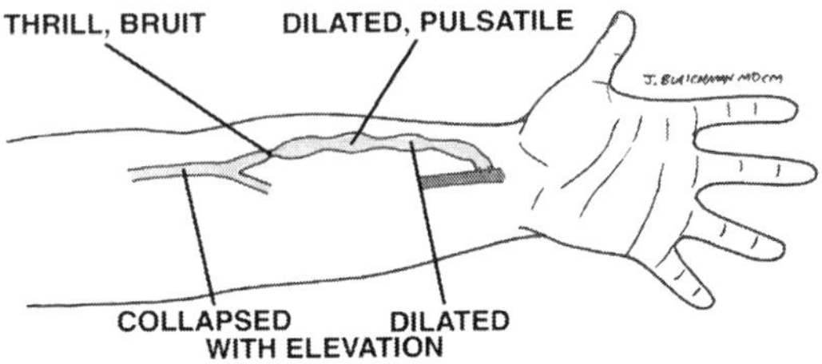

Fig. 5.4 Physical examination of venous stenosis in an arteriovenous fistulae (AVF). Elevation of the arm lowers the pressure in a normal AVF so that there is at least partial collapse of the AVF. In the presence of severe stenosis, the AVF downstream to the stenosis collapses with arm elevation, whereas pressure remains high upstream to the stenosis and there is no collapse

Table 5.1 Description of the characteristics of bruit and thrill after access creation

Clinical sign	Normal	Abnormal
Pulse	Soft, easily compressible	Bounding pulse, difficult to compress (flow is trying to overcome a stenosis) or Low amplitude, hypopulsation (stenosis is limiting blood flow through the access)
Bruit	Low pitch Continuous In diastole and systole	High pitched, "whistling" Discontinuous In systole only
Thrill	Only at the arterial anastomosis for AV-grafts	At site of stenotic lesion

A palpable thrill and audible bruit should be present throughout the body of the access, during systole and diastole, and is expected to be strongest at the anastomosis. The pitch of the bruit should decrease from the arterial to the venous end of the access as pressure decreases. Abnormalities, such as a sudden rise in the bruit's pitch may indicate turbulent blood flow due to an underlying stenotic lesion

AV-graft outcomes [17, 18]; for example, the presence of a thrill in the axilla is correlated with subsequent AV-graft failure [19]. The stenotic narrowing will cause access flow turbulence that is manifested as a thrill over the area of stenosis. The pitch of the bruit will change from a low to high pitch as the stenosis progressively narrows. With the increase in flow resistance, Q may be reduced so much during diastole (when pressure is lowest) that the bruit is no longer heard. The degree of stenosis inversely correlates with the duration of the diastolic component.

Accuracy of the Physical Exam in Detecting Stenosis

How well does physical exam detect stenosis within an AVF or AV-graft? Such an important question can be answered by considering two distinct questions:

1. How does physical exam *compare* to technology in detecting stenosis in the (a) AVF and (b) AV-graft?
2. How does physical exam compare to technology in reducing the rate of and time to (a) AVF and (b) AV-graft thrombosis. These two questions will be addressed below.

How Does Physical Exam Compare to Technology in Detecting Stenosis?

Arteriovenous Fistula

There is no debate that the physical exam plays an essential role in evaluating a newly created AVF. A newly created AVF should be examined by an experienced person at 4–6 weeks after its creation [7]. Physical examination by an experienced person can predict, with 80% accuracy, the ultimate adequacy of the AVF [20] and that physical exam can determine the major cause of early AVF failure [16]. The utility of the physical exam after the initial assessment is given less importance and is often replaced by technology. However, evidence supports a role of physical examination to monitor for access dysfunction. Asif identified 142 dysfunctional AVFs that were referred for angioplasty [21]. A physical exam of the AVF was performed by a blinded interventional nephrologist based on the elements of the physical examination provided by Beathard and others [7, 22–25] as described above. Patients then underwent both upstream and downstream angiography to detect stenosis. Stenosis was defined as luminal narrowing ≥50% compared to the normal vascular segment located closest to the stenosis. The agreement between physical exam and angiography depended on the location of the stenosis. Multiple locations of stenosis were common and 61% of AVFs had an outflow stenosis and 64% had an upstream stenosis.

There was good agreement between the physical examination and angiography in diagnosing downstream stenosis (agreement 89%, κappa (κ)=0.78) with a sensitivity of 92% and a specificity of 86%. The diagnostic elements of the physical examination used in the evaluation of a downstream lesion included the presence of a water-hammer pulse (hyperpulsation), limited systolic bruit, and abnormal arm elevation test [7, 24, 25]. Upstream stenosis had similar results (agreement 83%, κ=0.55; sensitivity of 85% and a specificity of 71%). Central vein stenosis and stenosis within an 8- to 10-cm cannulation segment extending downstream from the juxta-anastomotic area were less common lesions and showed only weak agreement between physical examination and angiography (κ=0.17 and 0.18, respectively). Analysis of the forearm and upper arm AVFs revealed no significant difference in the level of agreement between physical examination and angiography.

This study does not reflect true screening per se, as all the AVF were already diagnosed as dysfunctional. The criteria for defining dysfunction at the time of the referral were not reported and there was no reported comparison of the physical exam to access flow. Additionally, the examining physician was highly trained and without inter-observer bias.

How then does physical examination fare when in the hands of a lesser experienced clinician? Leon addressed this issue by comparing the accuracy of the physical exam performed by nephrology fellows to the angiogram [26]. Fellows were trained in the physical exam using both didactic methods and hands on training as described above. A total of 45 AVF were examined by the renal fellow; agreement was high between the physical exam and angiogram for detection of outflow stenosis (agreement=81% κ=0.63) and for inflow stenosis (agreement=80%, κ=0.56). The fellow had a higher agreement and κ score for the physical exam of the central stenosis than the nephrologist; however, there was poor agreement for both nephrologist and fellow in detecting stenosis within the AVF body. This study strengthens the principle that the physical exam is an important tool in detecting stenosis within the AVF and training of renal fellows should be a priority.

Arteriovenous Grafts

It is important to consider the predictive value of physical exam separately for AVF and AV-grafts due to their different pathophysiologies. Leon again studied 45 AV-grafts with previously identified dysfunction and compared the ability of the physical exam to detect stenosis compared to the gold standard of angiography [27]. The location of the stenosis was key in determining the accuracy of the physical exam. Physical exam for stenosis at the vein graft anastomosis had a sensitivity of 57% and a specificity of 89% with a κ score of=0.52. For inflow and intragraft lesions, the agreement was moderate (K=0.4 and K=0.43, respectively) and lower for the venous outflow stenosis (k=0.23) and central vein stenosis (k=0.18). The detection of stenosis by physical exam was lower in AV-grafts than AVF, and may be related to the lower compliance in the system due to the synthetic nature of the AV-graft material.

How Does Physical Exam Compare to Technology in Reducing the Rate of and Time to Thrombosis?

The answer to this question is currently unavailable. However, to begin to answer such a question, one must also ask at what point does an underlying stenosis manifest a clinical sign or symptom that can be detected by physical exam? Mathematical modeling informs us that in some patients, a stenosis must be much greater than 50% before hemodynamics are affected, whereas in other patients a stenosis well under 50% may have a significant effect (see Chap. 4). Also, it has been argued that not all stenosis >50% are likely to progress and yield thrombosis, especially in the absence of a clinical sign or symptom. Lumsden demonstrated this using color flow duplex scanning to detect >50% stenoses in functioning AV-grafts, without any clinical signs of stenosis. Those who had angiographic stenoses >50% were randomized to balloon angioplasty or observation. There was no difference in 6 and 12 month patency between the two groups [28]. The difficulty is in determining which "clinical signs" indicate that the stenosis is "significant" in the AVF or AVG. Clinical indicators that have been used to predict a clinically significant stenosis include excessive bleeding post needle removal, decreased solute clearance, difficulty with access cannulation, or high venous pressures. In evaluating a vascular access, all the information gathered from physical exam and surveillance measurements may be needed to assist in determining the functionally significant stenosis in which treatment with angioplasty improves outcome without increasing the risk of future thrombosis. Research is needed to determine the outcome of intervention in those with asymptomatic stenosis compared to those with symptomatic stenosis with documentation of the harm as well as the benefit.

Vascular Access Surveillance

Access Flow

Access blood flow (Q) can be measured by a number of different techniques including estimation of flow by Doppler ultrasound, dilution techniques such as ultrasound dilution (UD), differential conductivity, glucose infusion, ionic dialysance, and timed ultrafiltration methods or by magnetic resonance angiography (MRA).

Ultrasound Dilution

Ultrasound dilution is considered the "gold standard" for access flow measurement and detection of stenosis in the vascular access. It is derived from the principles of recirculation (R) (see Fig. 5.5). Recirculation is induced by reversing the arterial and venous dialysis bloodlines, then the blood is diluted, e.g., by saline, in the venous line and then detected in the arterial line. Ultrasonic sensors measure changes in the protein concentration, which yield dilution curves that are used for the calculation of Q. A key relationship between Q, dialysis blood flow rate (Qb) (i.e., blood pump speed), and recirculation within the dialysis vascular access was described and validated as below by Krivitski (see Fig. 5.6a–c). This relationship allows for estimation of Q by means of any method that quantifies access recirculation (also measured when the arterial and venous dialysis tubing is temporarily reversed).

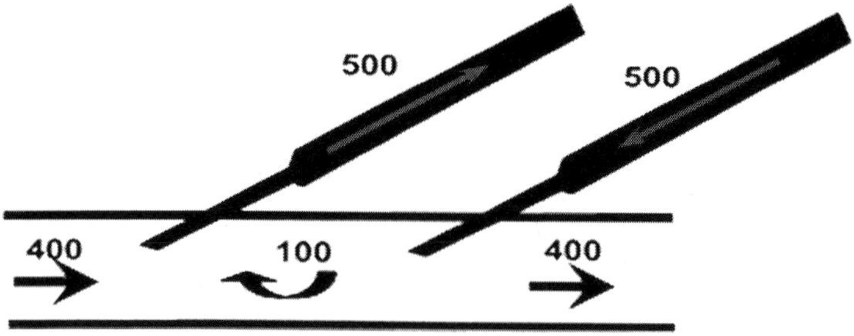

Fig. 5.5 Access recirculation. 100 mL/min of blood is recirculated since the intra-access flow (Q=400 mL/min) is lower than the blood pump speed (500 mL/min)

When Q is measured on a regular schedule, trends of a decreasing Q may indicate an anatomical abnormality (progressive stenosis), particularly when associated with clinical or hemodynamic changes. Single, abnormal measurements are less informative because of the large hemodynamic variations that occur during dialysis (when measurements are taken), described in Chap. 4. Since the patient's hemodynamic state at the time of the test can influence the result [29], NKF-KDOQI recommends measurement in the first 90 min of dialysis, due to the theoretical assumption that hemodynamic stability is greatest before significant ultrafiltration occurs [30, 31]. However, hemodynamic fluctuations usually occur throughout dialysis and variations of flow and arterial blood pressure are not significantly reduced early in a dialysis session (see Chap. 4) [32, 33]. Currently, there is no known published evidence that such a time restriction improves predictive accuracy or surveillance outcomes. Finally, a higher ultrafiltration volume increases the risk of thrombosis during the period after a session [34]. This suggests that measurement late in a session may better approximate hemodynamic conditions associated with thrombosis between sessions (see Chap. 4).

Since the benefit of restricted timing of measurements is not established, and it is not clear when such measurements should be taken, we do not recommend measurements be taken at a particular time in a dialysis session. Confirmed $Q<600$ mL/min in an AV-graft and <400–500 mL/min in an AVF or a decrease in flow of >33% usually indicates hemodynamically significant stenosis [35]. Monthly AV-graft and bi-monthly AVF surveillance by flow studies is recommended by some national guidelines [1, 2]; however, controversy as to its benefit continues [36] (see Chap. 4).

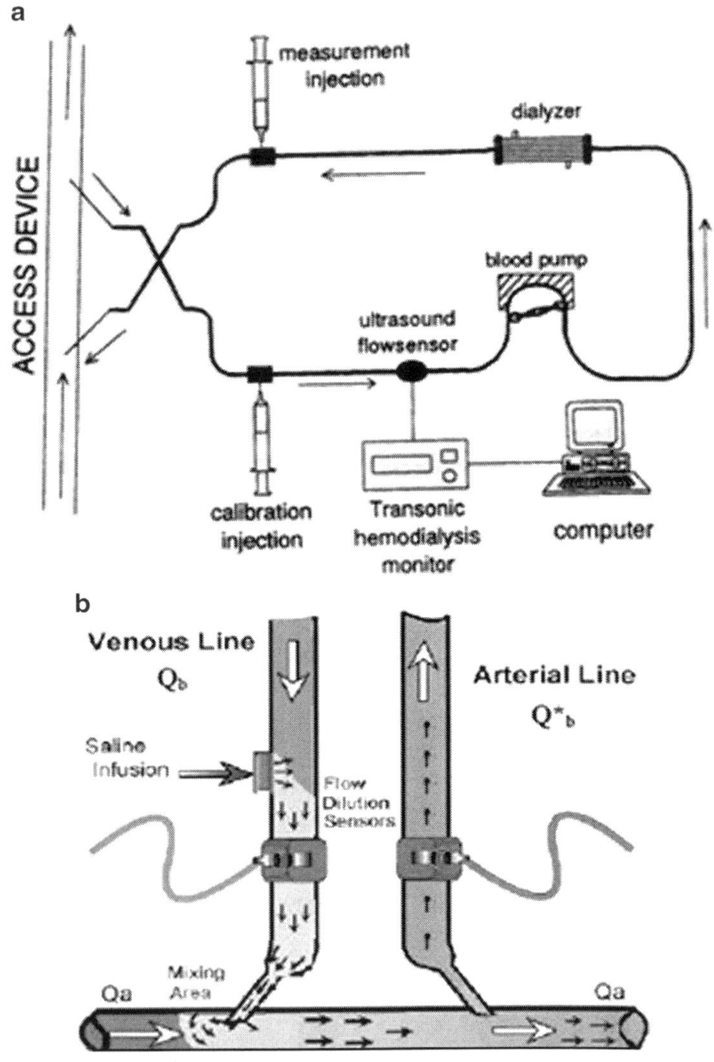

Fig. 5.6 (**a–c**) Key relationship between Q, dialysis blood flow rate (Qb) and recirculation within the dialysis vascular access described and validated by Krivitski. Krivitski elegantly described and validated the application of dilution principles to measure vascular access blood flow (Q) [67, 68]. According to the dilution method, $Q = VS$, where V is the amount of injected indicator that completely mixes in the blood flow stream Q; S is the area under the dilution curve which is equal to the average concentration of indicator in the blood multiplied

c

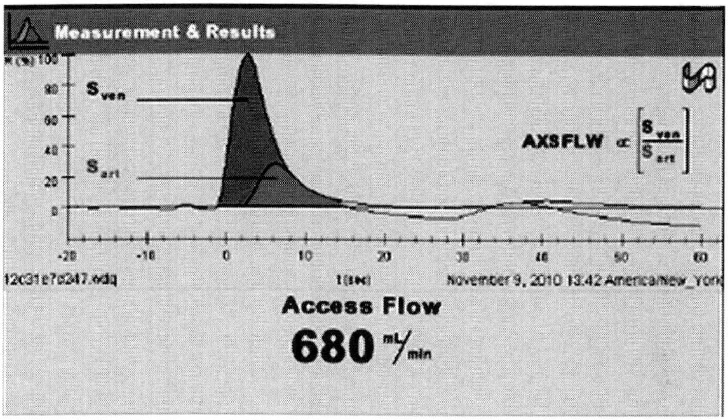

Fig. 5.6 (continued) by the duration of the curve. By reversing the dialysis blood lines (inducing access recirculation) and measuring both the blood flow in the tubing and the changes in velocity of ultrasound transmission induced by a saline bolus (using ultrasound probes attached to the blood line) access blood flow (Q) is equal to: Q=Qb*(SvSa−1) where Qb is the venous line blood flow (blood pump speed) and Sv/Sa is the ratio of areas under the dilution curves recorded by matched arterial (Sa) and venous dilution sensors generated by the saline bolus injection. The above equation can then be rewritten into the now widely recognized form: Qa=Qb*(1R−1) where R is the fractional access recirculation caused by the reversal of the dialysis lines

There are many challenges using saline ultrasound dilution (see Chap. 4). For example, there needs to be at least one available ultrasound dilution machine, a trained technician, a quality assurance and maintenance program, provisions for travel as well as a backup plan if the trained technician becomes unavailable [37]. The need for specialized equipment and trained personnel encouraged others to develop measurement of Q based on different blood properties such as electrical impedance (conductivity) [37–39], optical properties (hematocrit) [40, 41] and temperature[42]. Newly developed techniques include the variable flow Doppler method [43, 44], the transcutaneous flow monitor [45] and the glucose pump test [45].

Online Flow Measurement

Recently, the electrical impedance technology has been incorporated as proprietary integrated modules in Fresenius hemodialysis machine (Fresenius USA, Walnut Creek, CA). Gotch et al. [38] developed an indirect Q measurement method using online (real-time) conductivity dialysance that was validated against direct volumetric flow measurements in vitro and serum urea-based measurements in vivo. Gotch et al. [46] proposed that determining access recirculation by using conductivity dialysance measurements, performed with dialysis tubing reversed, will allow for applying the mathematical relationship between Q and recirculation to estimate Q.

Measurement of Q with the online conductance technique and ultrasound dilution technique has been compared. Studies of online conductance did not accurately measure Q above 2,000 mL/min in one study [39] or above 1,000 mL/min in the other [37] and the ultrasound dilution had flows greater than the online conductance (29 ± SD117) [39] and (135 ± SD229) [37], respectively.

This highlights an important issue when discussing the interpretation of the Q. According to Tonelli et al. [47], a Q<500 mL/min has a strong positive predictive value for stenosis in an AVF. On the contrary, Tessitore [48] reported a Q<700–1,000 mL/min and/or a Q reduction of 25% as best predictors of stenosis (91% efficiency). For AV-grafts, the current recommendation to evaluate the access for stenosis is when Q<600 mL/min [1]. Most of these thresholds were determined using the ultrasound dilution methods. Use of online conductance may reduce these threshold values to <400 mL/min [37]. The guidelines for use of access flow monitoring will have to take into account the measurement tool when recommending threshold targets for intervention.

Doppler Ultrasound

Doppler ultrasound measures blood flow velocity rather than Q directly. In order to determine Q, cross-sectional area of the access is estimated. The estimated Q is subject to operator dependent error in determining the blood velocity, and subject error in estimating the cross sectional error and the Doppler angle [49, 50], and it is labor intensive. Several studies have compared Q determined by ultrasound dilution to that by ultrasound [51–54]. Three compared Q by correlation coefficients only and thus did not assess agreement between the methods. Zanen et al. [54] compared the two methods with the intraclass correlation coefficients (ICC) and Bland and Altman limits of agreement.The investigators used the same ultrasound machine to estimate Q by conventional Doppler and quantitative color velocity index (CVI-Q), which is not as operator dependant and is associated with less error [53, 54]. Compared to ultrasound dilution, conventional Doppler performed very poorly with an ICC of 0.10 and demonstrated significant bias with an increasing difference between the two as the mean Q increased. Access blood flow estimated using CVI-Q faired better with the ICC 0.56 and no systematic bias on the Bland and Altman plot.

The variable flow Doppler method determines Q from the pump speed-induced change in the Doppler signal between the arterial and venous needles [43, 44]. This method had reasonable correlation coefficients for $Q<1{,}000$ mL/min [44]. Access flow can also be measured by MRA. However as this technique is expensive and cannot be performed during dialysis, it is impractical as a screening tool [55].

Static Venous Pressure (VP)

Dialysis venous pressure (VP) refers to the intra-access pressure at the venous dialysis needle and is widely used to evaluate for access dysfunction. Simply, when a stenosis develops, the pressure upstream to the stenosis increases and Q decreases. Dynamic VP is measured by the dialysis machine VP transducer with the blood pump running; it is traditionally measured with 15 gauge needles at a Qb of 200 mL/min. Measurements >125–150 mmHg (different on each brand of hemodialysis machine) on three consecutive treatments have been considered abnormal [56]. Although dynamic VP is relatively simple and inexpensive to perform, it has been discredited as a surveillance strategy and is considered to be *monitoring.* Dynamic VP is confounded by variables such as flow resistance of the dialysis needle, differences in needle size, dialysis machine type, and hematocrit.

Static VP measures intra-access pressure at the venous dialysis needle with the dialysis blood pump turned off. The tubing between the dialyzer and venous drip chamber is clamped. The static VP is then recorded 30 s after the blood pump speed has been turned off. Simultaneous measurements of the mean arterial pressure (MAP) are made with a conventional sphygmomanometer. The height (H) difference between the patient's access and venous pressure transducer is measured and the intra-access pressure (P_{IA}) is calculated with the following equation: $P_{IA}=\text{VP}+(0.35*\Delta H+3.6)$. The ratio of P_{IA} to MAP is then determined as this corrects for the influence of MAP on VP. When P_{IA}/MAP increases to >0.50, the AV-graft is conventionally considered to have a stenosis of >50% with a high risk of thrombosis. Derived static VP, which is a more practical approach to VP surveillance, uses a regression equation to convert VP measurements with the blood pump running (dynamic VP) to static VP. However, mathematical modeling suggests that static VP is not a reliable indicator of significant stenosis (see Chap. 4). Thus, trend analysis appears to be the key to successful VP surveillance whether done with static or derived static VP. On-line methods of VP measurement that allow multiple measurements/month instead of the standard monthly measurement are probably the most effective method of VP surveillance [57], although this awaits confirmation by randomized controlled trials.

VP measurements are less reliable for detecting stenosis in AVFs, due to the development/presence of collateral vessels. Other circumstances whereby static VP may be unreliable (e.g., falsely normal or abnormal) include hemodynamic variation (see Chap. 4), arterial stenosis or stenosis located between the arterial and venous needles.

In the mid to late 1990s, Besarab et al. [58, 59] demonstrated through observational studies that elevated static VP was associated with a sensitivity of 91 and 48% and a specificity of 86 and 100% in AV-grafts and AVF, respectively, for a 50% reduction in access lumen with a SVP/MAP>0.4. This high sensitivity and specificity was questioned by a more recent study by Dember et al. [60] which found that static VP measurement had a poor sensitivity and specificity for predicting AV-graft thrombosis and concluded that VP is not an optimal screening test for identifying AV-graft at risk for thrombosis. A static VP/MAP ≥0.4 would lead to unnecessary interventions in 53% of patients who would not have thrombosed in the next month, yet 27% of patients destined to thrombose would not have had an intervention. Furthermore, static VP in AVF is even less effective in detecting stenosis, as collaterals permit blood-outflow without significant increase in VP. Lastly, stenosis in AVF can occur downstream or upstream of the anastomosis, while the venous needle is usually placed downstream of the stenosis such that there would be no increase in the static VP in the presence of a significant stenosis.

Direct Imaging

Duplex ultrasound incorporates color-flow Doppler with gray scale imaging and has the significant advantage of being noninvasive, providing direct access information on both anatomic and flow characteristics. Early studies showed that AV-graft flows <300–450 mL/min or stenosis >30% were associated with thrombosis and early AV-graft failure [61–63]. Shackleton et. al demonstrated that an AV-graft Q threshold of 450 mL/min showed a sensitivity of 83% and a specificity of 75% for predicting AV-graft thrombosis within 2–6 weeks [64]. Peak systolic velocity (PSV) measurements at stenotic areas have been measured against the PSV immediately upstream to the stenosis. This PSV ratio has a positive predictive value of 80% when it is ≥2.0 for angiographically confirmed stenosis [65]. However, a later randomized controlled trial demonstrated only a trend towards thrombosis reduction with duplex detection of stenosis and no overall improvement in AV-graft survival [66]. Furthermore, duplex ultrasound is highly operator dependent, costly and often inconvenient for patients. MRA can detect stenosis but is rarely used due to its high cost, limited availability, and impracticality (above).

Conclusions and Future Directions

Whether prospective monitoring and surveillance with pre-emptive intervention can prolong access survival currently is unproven (see Chap. 4). However, such a strategy allows for (a) regular assessment of the access including its integrity, evidence of infection, vascular steal and (b) the ability to salvage access sites through planning, coordination of effort, and elective corrective intervention, rather than urgent procedures or replacement. A number of monitoring and surveillance methods are available, such as physical examination and sequential Q or static VP measurements. Physical exam is considered a standard of care and should be incorporated into every monitoring and surveillance program. Recommendations are summarized in the Summary section.

Surveillance by Q or VP might improve outcomes if measurements were taken more frequently. This would allow calculation of average values that neutralize hemodynamic variation, and would make it easier to detect rapid changes in Q or VP before thrombosis. The challenge is that correctly performed Q surveillance takes significant time, so it is probably impractical to increase measurement frequency beyond the standard monthly interval. However, online methods are available that facilitate frequent static VP measurements.

More frequent and direct visualization of stenosis by duplex ultrasound might also be successful (portable devices are available). However, these speculations need to be tested by properly designed and powered prospective studies. Until science can put the surveillance controversy to rest, we rely on the physical examination aspect of monitoring: that cost effective art of medicine that needs to be relearned and re-emphasized again and again.

Terminology

Terminology used in chapter	Upstream[a]	Downstream[a]
Defined	That portion of the vasculature-access circuit leaving the heart to the point of the anastomosis or stenosis	That portion of the vasculature-access circuit traveling towards the heart from the point of the anastomosis or stenosis
Other terminology	Retrograde Proximal to Inflow portion	Antegrade Distal to Outflow portion; access body

[a]Usually in reference to the anastomosis but can also be in reference to the stenosis and will be indicated as such in the text

Summary

Key Signs and Symptoms of Access Dysfunction

- Swelling within the face, chest wall, shoulder, breast or neck may be indicative of high venous pressure suggestive of central stenosis (e.g., superior vena cava or innominate vein). Collateral veins may also be evident on physical exam
- Localized edema is indicative of potential infection or venous outflow impairment e.g., isolated forearm edema suggests a stenosis in the main draining vein
- Palpably increased access pulsation: May be predictive of venous anastomotic stenosis and/or stenosis in the access body
- Palpation may detect fibrotic stenotic lesions, e.g., a "step" can be felt at the anastomosis
- An overly strong (water hammer) pulse may be detected upstream to a stenotic lesion. The access downstream to the stenosis may collapse on arm elevation

- High bruit pitch and/or short diastolic component may indicate stenosis; recall bruit should be heard throughout systole and diastole
- Reduction in bruit intensity following arm elevation is indicative of arterial inflow abnormalities limiting flow
- Prolonged bleeding time after needle withdrawal of >10 min or a change from current baseline with no change in anticoagulation: This should be measured and documented as a potential indicator for AV-graft or AVF stenosis and requires evaluation

Key Points

- Physical exam is an essential part of maintenance of a vascular access and should be performed routinely
- Abnormalities in the access can be determined by feeling, listening and seeing: Palpable changes in the pulse and thrill, auscultatory changes in the duration and pitch of the bruit, and observed bleeding post needle removal are all signs of access dysfunction
- Surveillance of access *Q* or static (or derived) static VP/MAP may be helpful as ancillary tests that should be correlated with physical examination and other data, such as Kt/*V*
- Because hemodynamic variability causes large changes in *Q* and static VP/MAP, it is important to confirm changes in measurements. It is unwise to refer an access for intervention based upon a single monthly measurement
- *Q*<400–500 mL/min in an AVF and <600 mL/min in an AV-graft are usually associated with stenosis.
- Trend analysis is key in using static VP/MAP to detect a significant stenosis. The traditional threshold of VP/MAP>0.50 (or derived static VP/MAP>0.55) on its own is an unreliable indicator of stenosis

References

1. KDOQI. Clinical practice guidelines for vascular access. Am J Kidney Dis. 2006;48:S176–247.
2. Jindal K, Chan CT, Deziel C, Hirsch D, et al. Hemodialysis clinical practice guidelines for the Canadian Society of Nephrology. J Am Soc Nephrol. 2006;17 Suppl 1:S16–23.

3. Allon M, Lockhart ME, Lilly RZ, Gallichio MH, et al. Effect of preoperative sonographic mapping on vascular access outcomes in hemodialysis patients. Kidney Int. 2001;60:2013–20.
4. Allon M, Lok CE. Dialysis fistula or graft: the role for randomized clinical trials. Clin J Am Soc Nephrol. 2010;5(12):2348–54.
5. Allon M, Robbin ML. Increasing arteriovenous fistulas in hemodialysis patients: problems and solutions. Kidney Int. 2002;62:1109–24.
6. Tordoir J, Canaud B, Haage P, Konner K, et al. EBPG on vascular access. Nephrol Dial Transplant. 2007;22 Suppl 2:ii88–117.
7. Beathard GA. An algorithm for the physical examination of early fistula failure. Semin Dial. 2005;18:331–5.
8. Fistula First National Vascular Access Improvements Initiative. 2010. http://www.fistulafirst.org/. Accessed on 17 Nov 2010.
9. Sidawy AN, Gray R, Besarab A, Henry M, et al. Recommended standards for reports dealing with arteriovenous hemodialysis accesses. J Vasc Surg. 2002;35:603–10.
10. Jarvis MA, Jarvis CL, Jones PR, Spyt TJ. Reliability of Allen's test in selection of patients for radial artery harvest. Ann Thorac Surg. 2000; 70:1362–5.
11. Korten E, Spronk S, Hoedt MT, de Jong GM, et al. Distensibility of forearm veins in haemodialysis patients on duplex ultrasound testing using three provocation methods. Eur J Vasc Endovasc Surg. 2009;38:375–80.
12. Wells AC, Fernando B, Butler A, Huguet E, et al. Selective use of ultrasonographic vascular mapping in the assessment of patients before haemodialysis access surgery. Br J Surg. 2005;92:1439–43.
13. Nursal TZ, Oguzkurt L, Tercan F, Torer N, et al. Is routine preoperative ultrasonographic mapping for arteriovenous fistula creation necessary in patients with favorable physical examination findings? Results of a randomized controlled trial. World J Surg. 2006;30:1100–7.
14. Niyyar VD, Wasse H. Vascular mapping: does it help to maximize fistulae placement? Adv Chronic Kidney Dis. 2009;16:316–20.
15. Beathard GA, Settle SM, Shields MW. Salvage of the nonfunctioning arteriovenous fistula. Am J Kidney Dis. 1999;33:910–6.
16. Beathard GA, Arnold P, Jackson J, Litchfield T, et al. Aggressive treatment of early fistula failure. Kidney Int. 2003;64:1487–94.
17. Trerotola SO, Scheel Jr PJ, Powe NR, Prescott C, et al. Screening for dialysis access graft malfunction: comparison of physical examination with US. J Vasc Interv Radiol. 1996;7:15–20.
18. Trerotola SO, Ponce P, Stavropoulos SW, Clark TW, et al. Physical examination versus normalized pressure ratio for predicting outcomes of hemodialysis access interventions. J Vasc Interv Radiol. 2003;14:1387–94.
19. McDougal G, Agarwal R. Clinical performance characteristics of hemodialysis graft monitoring. Kidney Int. 2001;60:762–6.
20. Robbin ML, Chamberlain NE, Lockhart ME, Gallichio MH, et al. Hemodialysis arteriovenous fistula maturity: US evaluation. Radiology. 2002;225:59–64.
21. Asif A, Leon C, Orozco-Vargas LC, Krishnamurthy G, et al. Accuracy of physical examination in the detection of arteriovenous fistula stenosis. Clin J Am Soc Nephrol. 2007;2:1191–4.

22. Mischler R, Schon D, Hubert B, Nissenson AR. Development and usefulness of a physical examination tool to diagnose vascular access dysfunction. J Am Soc Nephrol. 2000;11:190A.
23. Choi JR, Kim Y, Yoon SA, Won YD, Son YS, Son YS, et al. Accuracy of physical examination in detecting arteriovenous fistula dysfunction in hemodialysis patients: comparison with venographic findings. Korean J Nephrol. 2006;25:797–802.
24. Beathard GA. Physical examination: the forgotten tool. In: Gray RJ, Sands JJ, editors. A multidisciplinary approach for hemodialysis access. New York: Lippincott, Williams & Wilkins; 2002. p. 11–118.
25. Beathard GA. Physical examination of the dialysis vascular access. Semin Dial. 1998;11:231–6.
26. Leon C, Asif A. Physical examination of arteriovenous fistulae by a renal fellow: does it compare favorably to an experienced interventionalist? Semin Dial. 2008;21:557–60.
27. Leon C, Orozco-Vargas LC, Krishnamurthy G, Choi KL, et al. Accuracy of physical examination in the detection of arteriovenous graft stenosis. Semin Dial. 2008;21:85–8.
28. Lumsden AB, MacDonald MJ, Kikeri D, Cotsonis GA, et al. Prophylactic balloon angioplasty fails to prolong the patency of expanded polytetrafluoroethylene arteriovenous grafts: results of a prospective randomized study. J Vasc Surg. 1997;26:382–90.
29. Schneditz D, Fan Z, Kaufman A, Levin NW. Stability of access resistance during haemodialysis. Nephrol Dial Transplant. 1998;13:739–44.
30. Neyra NR, Ikizler TA, May RE, Himmelfarb J, et al. Change in access blood flow over time predicts vascular access thrombosis. Kidney Int. 1998;54:1714–9.
31. Bosman PJ, Boereboom FT, Eikelboom BC, Koomans HA, et al. Graft flow as a predictor of thrombosis in hemodialysis grafts. Kidney Int. 1998;54:1726–30.
32. Ram SJ, Nassar R, Sharaf R, Magnasco A, et al. Thresholds for significant decrease in hemodialysis access blood flow. Semin Dial. 2005;18:558–64.
33. DeSoto DJ, Ram SJ, Faiyaz R, Birk CG, et al. Hemodynamic reproducibility during blood flow measurements of hemodialysis synthetic grafts. Am J Kidney Dis. 2001;37:790–6.
34. Paulson WD, Ram SJ, Faiyaz R, Caldito GC, et al. Association between blood pressure, ultrafiltration, and hemodialysis graft thrombosis: a multivariable logistic regression analysis. Am J Kidney Dis. 2002;40:769–76.
35. Ram SJ, Nassar R, Work J, Eason JM, et al. Stenosis surveillance of hemodialysis grafts by duplex ultrasound reduces hospitalizations and cost of care. Semin Dial. 2005;18:550–7.
36. Paulson WD, Work J. Controversial vascular access surveillance mandate. Semin Dial. 2010;23:92–4.
37. Lacson Jr E, Lazarus JM, Panlilio R, Gotch F. Comparison of hemodialysis blood access flow rates using online measurement of conductivity dialysance and ultrasound dilution. Am J Kidney Dis. 2008;51:99–106.
38. Gotch F, Peter H, Panlilo F, et al. On-line measurement of delivered Kt/V during dialysis. J Am Soc Nephrol. 1995;6:600A.

39. Whittier WL, Mansy HA, Rutz DR, Lewis AM, et al. Comparison of hemodialysis access flow measurements using flow dilution and in-line dialysance. ASAIO J. 2009;55:369–72.
40. Lindsay RM, Bradfield E, Rothera C, Kianfar C, et al. A comparison of methods for the measurement of hemodialysis access recirculation and access blood flow rate. ASAIO J. 1998;44:62–7.
41. Yarar D, Cheung AK, Sakiewicz P, Lindsay RM, et al. Ultrafiltration method for measuring vascular access flow rates during hemodialysis. Kidney Int. 1999;56:1129–35.
42. Schneditz D, Fan Z, Kaufman A, Levin NW. Measurement of access flow during hemodialysis using the constant infusion approach. ASAIO J. 1998;44: 74–81.
43. Lin CC, Chang CF, Chiou HJ, Sun YC, et al. Variable pump flow-based Doppler ultrasound method: a novel approach to the measurement of access flow in hemodialysis patients. J Am Soc Nephrol. 2005;16:229–36.
44. Weitzel WF, Rubin JM, Leavey SF, Swartz RD, et al. Analysis of variable flow Doppler hemodialysis access flow measurements and comparison with ultrasound dilution. Am J Kidney Dis. 2001;38:935–40.
45. Steuer RR, Miller DR, Zhang S, Bell DA, et al. Noninvasive transcutaneous determination of access blood flow rate. Kidney Int. 2001;60:284–91.
46. Gotch FA, Buyaki R, Panlilio F, Folden T. Measurement of blood access flow rate during hemodialysis from conductivity dialysance. ASAIO J. 1999;45: 139–46.
47. Tonelli M, Jhangri GS, Hirsch DJ, Marryatt J, et al. Best threshold for diagnosis of stenosis or thrombosis within six months of access flow measurement in arteriovenous fistulae. J Am Soc Nephrol. 2003;14:3264–9.
48. Tessitore N, Bedogna V, Gammaro L, Lipari G, et al. Diagnostic accuracy of ultrasound dilution access blood flow measurement in detecting stenosis and predicting thrombosis in native forearm arteriovenous fistulae for hemodialysis. Am J Kidney Dis. 2003;42:331–41.
49. Gill RW. Measurement of blood flow by ultrasound: accuracy and sources of error. Ultrasound Med Biol. 1985;11:625–41.
50. Oates CP, Williams ED, McHugh MI. The use of a Diasonics DRF400 duplex ultrasound scanner to measure volume flow in arterio-venous fistulae in patients undergoing haemodialysis: an analysis of measurement uncertainties. Ultrasound Med Biol. 1990;16:571–9.
51. May RE, Himmelfarb J, Yenicesu M, Knights S, et al. Predictive measures of vascular access thrombosis: a prospective study. Kidney Int. 1997;52: 1656–62.
52. Depner TA, Krivitski NM. Clinical measurement of blood flow in hemodialysis access fistulae and grafts by ultrasound dilution. ASAIO J. 1995;41: M745–9.
53. Sands J, Glidden D, Miranda C. Hemodialysis access flow measurement. Comparison of ultrasound dilution and duplex ultrasonography. ASAIO J. 1996;42:M899–901.
54. Zanen AL, Toonder IM, Korten E, Wittens CH, et al. Flow measurements in dialysis shunts: lack of agreement between conventional Doppler, CVI-Q, and ultrasound dilution. Nephrol Dial Transplant. 2001;16:395–9.

55. Oudenhoven LF, Pattynama PM, de Roos A, Seeverens HJ, et al. Magnetic resonance, a new method for measuring blood flow in hemodialysis fistulae. Kidney Int. 1994;45:884–9.
56. Schwab SJ, Raymond JR, Saeed M, Newman GE, et al. Prevention of hemodialysis fistula thrombosis. Early detection of venous stenoses. Kidney Int. 1989;36:707–11.
57. Zasuwa G, Frinak S, Besarab A, Peterson E, et al. Automated intravascular access pressure surveillance reduces thrombosis rates. Semin Dial. 2010; 23:527–35.
58. Besarab A, Sullivan KL, Ross RP, Moritz MJ. Utility of intra-access pressure monitoring in detecting and correcting venous outlet stenoses prior to thrombosis. Kidney Int. 1995;47:1364–73.
59. Besarab A, Frinak S, Sherman RA, Goldman J, et al. Simplified measurement of intra-access pressure. J Am Soc Nephrol. 1998;9:284–9.
60. Dember LM, Holmberg EF, Kaufman JS. Value of static venous pressure for predicting arteriovenous graft thrombosis. Kidney Int. 2002;61:1899–904.
61. Rittgers SE, Garcia-Valdez C, McCormick JT, Posner MP. Noninvasive blood flow measurement in expanded polytetrafluoroethylene grafts for hemodialysis access. J Vasc Surg. 1986;3:635–42.
62. Older RA, Gizienski TA, Wilkowski MJ, Angle JF, et al. Hemodialysis access stenosis: early detection with color Doppler US. Radiology. 1998;207:161–4.
63. Passman MA, Criado E, Farber MA, Risley GL, et al. Efficacy of color flow duplex imaging for proximal upper extremity venous outflow obstruction in hemodialysis patients. J Vasc Surg. 1998;28:869–75.
64. Shackleton CR, Taylor DC, Buckley AR, Rowley VA, et al. Predicting failure in polytetrafluoroethylene vascular access grafts for hemodialysis: a pilot study. Can J Surg. 1987;30:442–4.
65. Robbin ML, Oser RF, Lee JY, Heudebert GR, et al. Randomized comparison of ultrasound surveillance and clinical monitoring on arteriovenous graft outcomes. Kidney Int. 2006;69:730–5.
66. Ram SJ, Work J, Caldito GC, Eason JM, et al. A randomized controlled trial of blood flow and stenosis surveillance of hemodialysis grafts. Kidney Int. 2003;64:272–80.
67. Krivitski NM, Depner TA. Development of a method for measuring hemodialysis access flow: from idea to robust technology. Semin Dial. 1998; 11:124–30.
68. Krivitski NM. Theory and validation of access flow measurement by dilution technique during hemodialysis. Kidney Int. 1995;48:244–50.

Chapter 6
Molecular Mechanisms of Hemodialysis Graft Failure

Sanjay Misra

Introduction

Today there are more than 400,000 patients with end-stage renal disease (ESRD) in the United States, and the vast majority of patients use long-term hemodialysis as their mode of renal replacement therapy [1]. This population is expected to double in the next decade. For patients using chronic hemodialysis as their mode of renal replacement therapy, a highly functioning vascular access is their "lifeline" because it ensures adequate reduction of uremic toxins and maintenance of appropriate electrolyte balances. Hemodialysis vascular access dysfunction occurs in patients and is frequently caused by the development of venous stenosis at the vein-to-graft anastomosis site or in the proximal outflow vein [2].

Revision(s) and optimal maintenance of poorly functioning hemodialysis arteriovenous (AV) grafts are costly with estimates of

S. Misra (✉)
Associate Professor, Department of Radiology,
Mayo Clinic School of Medicine,
Rochester, MN, USA
e-mail: misra.sanjay@mayo.edu

D.K. Rajan (ed.), *Essentials of Percutaneous Dialysis Interventions*,
DOI 10.1007/978-1-4419-5657-6_6,
© Springer Science+Business Media, LLC 2011

medical costs exceeding a billion dollars per year. Despite aggressive treatment with invasive vascular procedures, including angioplasty and/or surgical revision, the 1-year patency rates for AV grafts and/or AV fistulas (AVFs) remain disappointingly low averaging 23–50% for polytetrafluoroethylene (PTFE) AV grafts and 65% for AVFs. Typically, venous stenoses are treated with angioplasty and thrombosed grafts are treated with thrombectomy. It is estimated that an average of 1.22 procedures is needed to maintain patency for every hemodialysis graft year: 0.54 angioplasties, 0.51 thrombectomies, and 0.17 surgical revisions [3]. The 6-month patency of angioplasty of venous stenosis is very low which is comparable to restenosis of coronary arteries after angioplasty [4]. Therefore, greater than 200,000 procedures are performed annually in hemodialysis patients with PTFE grafts [3]. Despite these disappointingly low patency rates of AV grafts and fistula, there has been a paucity of understanding of the mechanisms responsible for venous stenosis formation.

In order to develop new therapies aimed at reducing venous neointimal hyperplasia (VNH), the following information is important: (1) Which genes and proteins are responsible for VNH formation? (2) What cells are responsible for the gene/protein production? (3) Where in the vessel wall are these genes/proteins located? (4) When do they need to be inhibited (e.g., at the time of access creation) and for how long? VNH formation is a dynamic and complicated process. The present review will discuss potential mechanisms of VNH formation including hypoxic injury, the role of fibroblast and myofibroblast contributing to VNH formation, role of various angiogenic and matrix regulatory proteins, potential translatable therapies which may limit VNH, and an update on current clinical trials.

Current Theories of Venous Neointimal Hyperplasia Formation in AV PTFE Grafts

VNH formation is a dynamic and complicated process. The mechanisms that can potentially contribute to early venous injury with subsequent initiation of the signaling pathways that promote VNH are multifactorial and felt to include hemodynamic factors such as high and low wall shear stress (WSS) [5–13] as well as local vessel wall hypoxia [14, 15]. Our

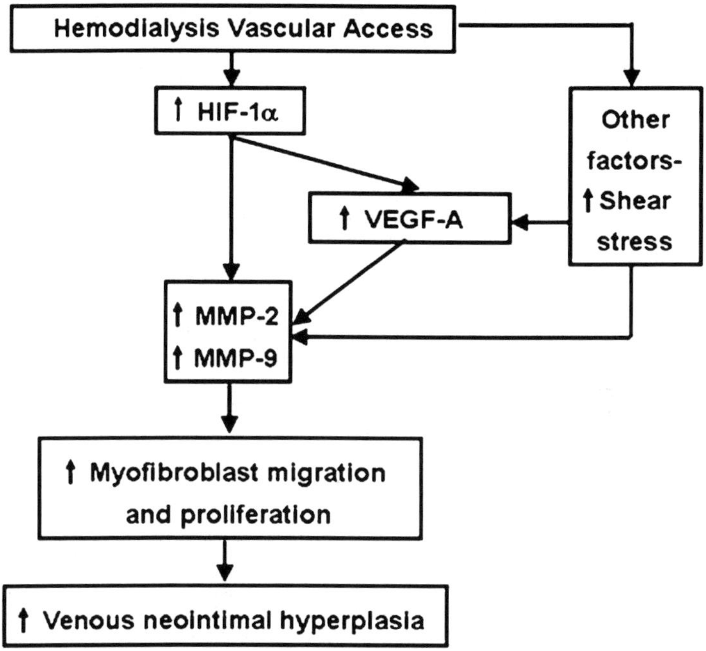

Fig. 6.1 Factors implicated in venous neointimal hyperplasia (VNH)

laboratory has been interested in WSS and has used phase contrast magnetic resonance angiography (MRA) with magnetic resonance imaging (MRI) to determine blood flow and luminal vessel area in order to estimate WSS and have showed that there is increased WSS at the vein-to-graft anastomosis and subsequent VNH formation [16–20].

Recently, we have shown that there is increased hypoxia inducible factor-1α (HIF-1α) associated with VNH formation. Several lines of evidence prompted our investigation of HIF-1α, including increased hypoxia within the vessel wall in regions of intimal hyperplasia in prosthetic vascular grafts used as arterial conduits in experimental animal models and atherosclerosis [21, 22]. Second, at a cellular level, hypoxia increases gene expression of several important matrix regulatory proteins through increased expression of HIF-1α which is known to regulate expression of vascular endothelial growth factor-A (VEGF-A), matrix metalloproteinases (MMPs), tissue inhibitors of matrix metalloproteinases (TIMPs), and others (see Fig. 6.1) [23, 24].

Third, in patients with failed hemodialysis vascular access grafts, increased cellular proliferation with matrix deposition has been shown to occur within the neointima and adventitia [25–28]. Recent studies from our laboratory showed that there was increased expression of HIF-1α in VNH removed from both clinical and experimental samples [14, 15]. These observations suggest that HIF-1α may play an important role in VNH formation in hemodialysis grafts.

Adventitial and Medial Cells Contribute to Venous Stenosis Formation

Adventitial and medial cellular proliferation and migration have been demonstrated in VNH and furthermore can lead to venous stenosis formation in experimental animal models [27, 28]. This is consistent with arterial restenosis and we hypothesize therefore that the early proliferating cells are fibroblasts which have differentiated into myofibroblasts (α-smooth muscle actin (α-SMA) positive cells) [29–31]. Subsequently, many investigators have targeted the adventitia with local delivery of adenoviruses overexpressing proteins or using biodegradable platforms which have been coated with drugs for local drug delivery [26, 32–36]. Because of these reasons, the adventitia is an appealing target for limiting restenosis either at time of access creation or using image guided therapy at the time of venous stenosis formation.

Histologic Features of Hemodialysis Venous Stenoses

Venous injury and subsequent venous stenosis formation are responsible for hemodialysis graft failure. Histologically, the venous stenosis is characterized by a hyperplastic intima with increased cellular proliferation and angiogenesis at the vein-to-graft anastomosis (see Fig. 6.2) [25, 26, 37–39]. There is increased cellular proliferation within the media and adventitia consisting primarily of α-SMA staining cells with a few macrophages and leukocytes being found [37–39].

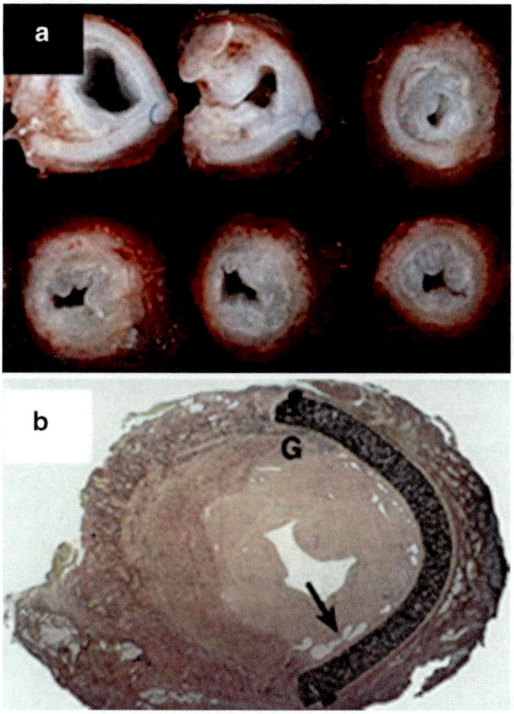

Fig. 6.2 Venous stenosis is characterized by thickened neointima and increased cellular proliferation. (**a**) Gross specimen showing the thickened venous neointima. (**b**) is 10× H and E staining of the venous stenosis at the vein to graft (G) anastomosis (*arrow*)

Proteins Implicated in Venous Stenosis Formation

It is hypothesized that VNH is caused by increased expression of several different matrix regulatory proteins including platelet-derived growth factor (PDGF), basic fibroblast growth factor (B-FGF), vascular endothelial growth factor-A (VEGF-A), and matrix metalloproteinases (MMPs) which have been shown to be increased at the venous stenosis in patients [25, 26, 40]. Because these observations are from clinical specimens that are at the end stage of the venous stenotic and thrombotic process, it is not clear whether the increased VEGF-A contributed to the development of VNH or was a result of the advanced process.

Proteins Implicated in Stenosis Formation After Angioplasty

The mechanisms underlying the formation of stenosis formation after angioplasty are not well understood but probably are similar to those contributing to venous stenosis formation.

Biological and Signaling Activities of Vascular Permeability Factor/Vascular Endothelial Growth Factor

Vascular permeability factor/vascular endothelial growth factor (VPF/VEGF) is a multi-functional cytokine with important roles in cellular proliferation, migration, and angiogenesis [41–47]. It was originally described as a tumor-secreted protein [41, 43, 46] and its activities are mediated primarily by its interaction with two high-affinity receptor tyrosine kinases, VEGFR-2 (KDR in humans, Flk-1 in mice) and VEGFR-1 (Flt-1) that are selectively expressed on vascular endothelium. A number of laboratories including ours have been dissecting the role of VPF/VEGF and its two tyrosine kinase receptors in VNH in hemodialysis grafts. We have recently shown that there is increased expression of VEGF-A in early venous stenosis formation followed by an increase in VEGFR-2 and finally VEGFR-1 in our experimental porcine model [20].

Rationale for VEGF-A

There are several proteins which have been shown to be up regulated in VNH formation. We chose to examine the role of VEGF-A in VNH for several important reasons: (1) It has been shown to be increased in both clinical and experimental specimens of venous stenosis formation; (2) It regulates cellular proliferation and migration with angiogenesis which are the essential hallmarks of VNH; (3) There is cross talk between VEGF-A and MMPs – a second family of proteins which we have observed to be increased in both clinical and experimental venous stenosis specimens; and (4) Finally, there are commercially available inhibitors of both VEGF-A and MMPs which would allow for rapid translation into clinical trials. The role of VEGF-A in restenosis involving the artery remains controversial because of different results by different groups [48, 49]. A clinical trial using adenoviral-VEGF-D delivery to the adventitia of hemodialysis grafts at the time of surgery was planned, however, no results have been published [50].

Matrix Metalloproteinases

Another group of proteins that are thought to play a key role in hemodialysis graft failure are the MMPs and their endogenous inhibitors, TIMPs [15, 27, 51–53]. MMPs are a family of Zn^{2+}-dependent enzymes involved in normal and pathologic states. The three major classes of MMPs are named according to their respective substrate affinity: collagenases, gelatinases, and stromelysins. The gelatinases (MMP-2 and MMP-9) degrade type IV collagen, which is found in basement membranes of blood vessels along with types V, VII, and X collagen fibers. There is strict regulation of the activity of these enzymes by way of transcription of MMP genes, secretion of the latent proenzymes (zymogens) into the extracellular matrix, activation of the zymogens, and inhibition of proteolytic activity by TIMPs. TIMPs are naturally occurring proteins that bind and inactivate MMPs. Vascular smooth muscle cells, monocytes, macrophages, and endothelial cells have all been shown to express MMPs. It has been observed that an imbalance of MMP activity over TIMPs promotes migration and proliferation of smooth muscle cells [54, 55], and that certain MMPs increase the bioavailability of VEGF-A, potentially accelerating the development of intimal hyperplasia [56].

Role of Matrix Metalloproteinases in Hemodialysis Vascular Access Failure

Previous work from our laboratory supports a prominent role for MMPs in hemodialysis graft failure; we reported that PTFE grafts in pigs exhibited early up-regulation of MMP-2 associated with increased cell migration from the adventitia to the media and intima, and subsequent formation of venous stenosis [27]. Furthermore, systemic delivery of a nonspecific broad spectrum MMP-2 and MMP-9 inhibitors reduced the formation of neointima in the same model [53]. One weakness of this study is that the inhibitors used were nonspecific systemic inhibitors thus making it difficult to determine the exact mechanism for the reduction in VNH. A recent study from our laboratory showed in human hemodialysis graft samples that there was significantly increased expression of pro MMP-2, pro MMP-9, and TIMP-1 when compared with control vessels [15]. Recently, we have showed that there is increased expression of pro MMP-9 early in venous stenosis, followed by increased activation of pro and active MMP-2, and finally increased expression of TIMP-1 [20]. Taken collectively, these studies suggest that MMPs (specifically MMP-2 and MMP-9) may play a prominent role in the pathogenesis of VNH of hemodialysis grafts with a potential target being fibroblasts resident in the adventitia.

Rationale for MMPs

Cellular proliferation and migration is a hallmark feature of VNH formation. They have been shown to be regulated and coordinated by activation of MMPs. Increased activity of MMPs has been associated with VNH formation in many different experimental animal models including the mouse, rat, and pig and observed to be significantly elevated in clinical specimens. Certain MMPs can increase the bioavailability of VEGF-A, and thereby possibly accelerating its effect in VNH formation. In this aim, we will investigate the individual role of MMP-2 and MMP-9 using a genetic knockout of each protein in a mouse with an AVF. Successful completion of this aim will provide insight into crucial aspects of VNH pathology: (1) The individual roles both temporal and spatially of MMP-2 or MMP-9, (2) Synergistic roles of MMP-2 and MMP-9, and (3) The simultaneous roles for VEGF-A and MMP-2 or MMP-9 in VNH formation. This information is important as it will allow us to proceed rapidly to a clinical trial aimed at inhibiting VNH using either mono or dual therapy with either VEGF-A and/or MMP compounds as there are multiple commercially available inhibitors of both proteins. Finally, a recent study performed in experimental animal model of atherosclerosis showed that MMPs could be imaged using a novel contrast agent with MRI, thus potentially offering an ability to track MMPs noninvasively [57, 58].

Role of HIF-1α in Protein Expression

Hypoxia mediates gene expression through increased expression of HIF-1α. HIF-1α causes increased expression of VEGF-A, B-FGF, MMPs, and others [23, 24, 59]. Several lines of evidence suggest that hypoxia (HIF-1α) is a key determinant in neointima formation in both arterial and vein graft pathology [14, 15, 21, 22, 60, 61]. Prosthetic vascular grafts used as arterial conduits in experimental animal models have demonstrated increased hypoxia within the vessel wall in regions of intimal hyperplasia [60, 61]. Recently, we demonstrated increased expression of HIF-1α in clinical specimens removed from failed PTFE hemodialysis grafts and our experimental porcine model [14, 15]. Taken collectively, these observations suggest that HIF-1α plays a role in hemodialysis graft failure.

Role of Fibroblasts in VNH

There is substantial evidence that the fibroblasts play a significant role in the response to vascular injury [27, 29, 30, 62–65]. It is well established in experimental animal models of arterial stenosis and interposition of saphenous vein grafts used as arterial conduits that fibroblasts migrating from the adventitia contribute to stenosis formation [65, 66]. Recently, we have shown in the experimental AV graft porcine model that there is migration of adventitial and medial cells contributing to venous stenosis formation [27, 65, 66].

Role of Hypoxia in Transformation of Fibroblasts to Myofibroblasts

It is well known that hypoxia will stimulate fibroblasts from the pulmonary artery to differentiate into myofibroblast, which is hypothesized to cause fibrosis associated with chronic inflammatory lung disease [67–70]. Fibroblasts isolated from different vascular beds have differing abilities to proliferate and migrate [71]. This is felt to be because of subpopulations of fibroblasts which have differing abilities to respond to hypoxia [71]. The role of hypoxia on converting venous fibroblasts to myofibroblasts and subsequent stenosis formation

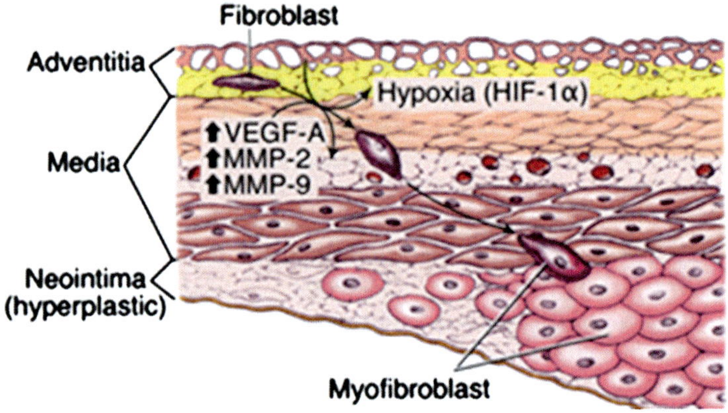

Fig. 6.3 Role of hypoxia via hypoxia inducible factor-1α (HIF-1α) in adventitial migration of fibroblasts

has not been studied. Furthermore, the differentiation process is mediated through an MMP pathway; however, the exact role of MMP-2 and MMP-9 has not been investigated. Understanding the exact role of each MMP has implications in the development of therapeutic options. Preliminary data from our laboratory and others demonstrates that hypoxia will induce the conversion of fibroblasts to differentiate into myofibroblasts through increased production of MMP-2 and MMP-9 (see Fig. 6.3) [67–70].WSS cellular proliferation and migration is a key hallmark feature of VNH formation and have been felt to be secondary to medial smooth muscle cell migration and proliferation. Recently this concept has evolved to include the adventitia as a potential source for cells contributing to stenosis formation involving vascular injury [72]. They have been shown to be regulated and coordinated by activation of multiple different proteins such as PDGF, transforming growth factor β (TGF-β), and recently MMPs [67, 69, 72].

Summary

Vascular access grafts for hemodialysis are a critical necessity for hundreds of thousands of US patients. Unfortunately, these "lifelines" are subject to serious dysfunction due to stenosis at a yearly rate of approximately 50–65%. Understanding the molecular mechanisms could help develop novel new therapies which may inhibit BNH. Such therapies would include drug-coated balloons, stents, and oral medications aimed at reducing proteins increased in VNH formation.

Acknowledgment The project described was supported by Award Number R01HL098967 (SM) from the National Heart, Lung, And Blood Institute and a CR20 grant which is funded by 1UL1RR024150 from the National Center for Research Resources (NCRR), a component of the National Institutes of Health (NIH), and the NIH Roadmap for Medical Research. The content is solely the responsibility of the authors and does not necessarily represent the official views of the National Heart, Lung, And Blood Institute or the National Institutes of Health.

References

1. Collins AJ, Kasiske B, Herzog C, et al. Excerpts from the United States Renal Data System 2003 Annual Data Report: atlas of end-stage renal disease in the United States. Am J Kidney Dis. 2003;42(6 Suppl 5):A5–7.
2. Sullivan KL, Besarab A, Bonn J, Shapiro MJ, Gardiner Jr GA, Moritz MJ. Hemodynamics of failing dialysis grafts. Radiology. 1993;186(3):867–72.
3. Miller PE, Carlton D, Deierhoi MH, Redden DT, Allon M. Natural history of arteriovenous grafts in hemodialysis patients. Am J Kidney Dis. 2000;36(1):68–74.
4. Misra S, Bonan R, Pflederer T, Roy-Chaudhury P. BRAVO I: A pilot study of vascular brachytherapy in polytetrafluoroethylene dialysis access grafts. Kidney Int. 2006;70(11):2006–13.
5. Fillinger M, Reinitz E, Schwartz R, Resetarits D, Paskanik A, Bredenberg C. Beneficial effects of banding on venous intimal-medial hyperplasia in arteriovenous loop grafts. Am J Surg. 1989;158(2):87–94.
6. Fillinger M, Reinitz E, Schwartz R, et al. Graft geometry and venous intimal-medial hyperplasia in arteriovenous loop grafts. J Vasc Surg. 1990;11(4):556–66.
7. Haruguchi H, Teraoka S. Intimal hyperplasia and hemodynamic factors in arterial bypass and arteriovenous grafts: a review. J Artif Organs. 2003;6(4):227–35.
8. Heise M, Schmidt S, Kruger U, et al. Local haemodynamics and shear stress in cuffed and straight PTFE-venous anastomoses: an in-vitro comparison using particle image velocimetry. Eur J Vasc Endovasc Surg. 2003;26(4):367–73.
9. Hofstra L, Bergmans DC, Hoeks AP, Kitslaar PJ, Leunissen KM, Tordoir JH. Mismatch in elastic properties around anastomoses of interposition grafts for hemodialysis access. J Am Soc Nephrol. 1994;5(5):1243–50.
10. Keynton R, Evancho M, Sims R, Rodway N, Gobin A, Rittgers S. Intimal hyperplasia and wall shear in arterial bypass graft distal anastomoses: an in vivo model study. J Biomech Eng. 2001;123(5):464–73.

11. Krueger U, Zanow J, Scholz H. Computational fluid dynamics and vascular access. Artif Organs. 2002;26(7):571–5.
12. Meyerson SL, Skelly CL, Curi MA, et al. The effects of extremely low shear stress on cellular proliferation and neointimal thickening in the failing bypass graft. J Vasc Surg. 2001;34(1):90–7.
13. Van Tricht I, De Wachter D, Tordoir J, Verdonck P. Comparison of the hemodynamics in 6 mm and 4-7 mm hemodialysis grafts by means of CFD. J Biomech. 2006;39(2):226–36.
14. Misra S, Fu A, Pugionni A, et al. Increased expression of hypoxia inducible factor-1a in a porcine model of chronic renal insufficiency with arteriovenous polytetrafluoroethylene grafts. J Vasc Interv Radiol. 2008;19(2):260–5.
15. Misra S, Fu A, Rajan D, et al. Expression of hypoxia inducible factor-1 alpha, macrophage migration inhibition factor, matrix metalloproteinase-2 and -9, and their inhibitors in hemodialysis grafts and arteriovenous fistulas. J Vasc Interv Radiol. 2008;19(2):252–9.
16. Box FMA, van der Grond J, de Craen AJM, et al. Pravastatin decreases wall shear stress and blood velocity in the internal carotid artery without affecting flow volume: results from the PROSPER MRI Study. Stroke. 2007;38(4):1374–6.
17. Marshall I, Zhao S, Papathanasopoulou P, Hoskins P, Xu XY. MRI and CFD studies of pulsatile flow in healthy and stenosed carotid bifurcation models. J Biomech. 2004;37(5):679–87.
18. Misra S, Woodrum D, Homburger J, et al. Assessment of wall shear stress changes in arteries and veins of arteriovenous polytetrafluoroethylene grafts using magnetic resonance imaging. Cardiovasc Intervent Radiol. 2006;29:624–9.
19. Oshinski J, Ku D, Mukundan SJ, Loth F, Pettigrew R. Determination of wall shear stress in the aorta with the use of MR phase velocity mapping. J Magn Reson Imaging. 1995;5(6):640–7.
20. Misra S, Fu AA, Puggioni A, et al. Increased shear stress with up regulation of VEGF-A and its receptors and MMP-2, MMP-9, and TIMP-1 in venous stenosis of hemodialysis grafts. Am J Physiol Heart Circ Physiol. 2008;294(5):H2219–30.
21. Nakata T, Shionoya S. Vascular lesions due to obstruction of the vasa vasorum. Nature. 1966;212:1258–9.
22. Santilli SM, Tretinayak AS, Lee ES. Transarterial wall oxygen gradients at the deployment site of an intra-arterial stent in the rabbit. Am J Physiol Heart Circ Physiol. 2000;279:H1518–25.
23. Koong AC, Denko NC, Hudson KM, et al. Candidate genes for the hypoxic tumor phenotype. Cancer Res. 2000;60(4):883–7.
24. Semenza GL. Targeting HIF-1 for cancer therapy. Nat Rev Cancer. 2003; 3(10):721–32.
25. Roy-Chaudhury P, Kelly BS, Miller MA, et al. Venous neointimal hyperplasia in polytetrafluoroethylene dialysis grafts. Kidney Int. 2001;59(6):2325–34.
26. Roy-Chaudhury P, Sukhatme VP, Cheung AK. Hemodialysis vascular access dysfunction: a cellular and molecular viewpoint. J Am Soc Nephrol. 2006;17(4):1112–27.
27. Misra S, Doherty MG, Woodrum D, et al. Adventitial remodeling with increased matrix metalloproteinase-2 activity in a porcine arteriovenous polytetrafluoroethylene grafts. Kidney Int. 2005;68(6):2890–900.

28. Wang Y, Krishnamoorthy M, Banerjee R, et al. Venous stenosis in a pig arteriovenous fistula model anatomy, mechanisms and cellular phenotypes. Nephrol Dial Transplant. 2007;22(11):3139–46.
29. Shi Y, O'Brien JE, Fard A, Mannion JD, Wang D, Zalewski A. Adventitial myofibroblasts contribute to neointimal formation in injured porcine coronary arteries. Circulation. 1996;94(7):1655–64.
30. Shi Y, Pieniek M, Fard A, O'Brien J, Mannion JD, Zalewski A. Adventitial remodeling after coronary arterial injury. Circulation. 1996;93(2):340–8.
31. Cai WJ, Koltai S, Kocsis E, et al. Remodeling of the adventitia during coronary arteriogenesis. Am J Physiol Heart Circ Physiol. 2003;284(1):H31–40.
32. Nugent HM, Groothuis A, Seifert P, et al. Perivascular endothelial implants inhibit intimal hyperplasia in a model of arteriovenous fistulae: a safety and efficacy study in the pig. J Vasc Res. 2002;39(6):524–33.
33. Kelly B, Melhem M, Zhang J, et al. Perivascular paclitaxel wraps block arteriovenous graft stenosis in a pig model. Nephrol Dial Transplant. 2006;21(9):2425–31.
34. Rotmans JI, Verhagen HJ, Velema E, et al. Local overexpression of C-type natriuretic peptide ameliorates vascular adaptation of porcine hemodialysis grafts. Kidney Int. 2004;65(5):1897–905.
35. Nugent HM, Sjin RT, White D, et al. Adventitial endothelial implants reduce matrix metalloproteinase-2 expression and increase luminal diameter in porcine arteriovenous grafts. J Vasc Surg. 2007;46(3):548–56.
36. Ylä-Herttuala S, Alitalo K. Gene transfer as a tool to induce therapeutic vascular growth. Nat Med. 2003;9(6):694–701.
37. Swedberg SH, Brown BG, Sigley R, Wight TN, Gordon D, Nicholls SC. Intimal fibromuscular hyperplasia at the venous anastomosis of PTFE grafts in hemodialysis patients. Clinical, immunocytochemical, light and electron microscopic assessment. Circulation. 1989;80(6):1726–36.
38. Rekhter M, Nicholls S, Ferguson M, Gordon D. Cell proliferation in human arteriovenous fistulas used for hemodialysis. Arterioscler Thromb. 1993;13(4):609–17.
39. Hofstra L, Tordoir JH, Kitslaar PJ, Hoeks AP, Daemen MJ. Enhanced cellular proliferation in intact stenotic lesions derived from human arteriovenous fistulas and peripheral bypass grafts. Does it correlate with flow parameters? Circulation. 1996;94(6):1283–90.
40. Misra S, Lee N, Fu A, et al. Increased expression of a disintegrin and metalloproteinase thrombospondin-1 (ADAMTS-1) in thrombosed hemodialysis grafts. J Vasc Interv Radiol. 2008;19(1):111–9.
41. Senger DR, Galli SJ, Dvorak AM, Perruzzi CA, Harvey VS, Dvorak HF. Tumor cells secrete a vascular permeability factor that promotes accumulation of ascites fluid. Science. 1983;219(4587):983–5.
42. Dvorak HF, Dvorak AM, Manseau EJ, Wiberg L, Churchill WH. Fibrin gel investment associated with line 1 and line 10 solid tumor growth, angiogenesis, and fibroplasia in guinea pigs. Role of cellular immunity, myofibroblasts, microvascular damage, and infarction in line 1 tumor regression. J Natl Cancer Inst. 1979;62(6):1459–72.
43. Senger DR, Perruzzi CA, Feder J, Dvorak HF. A highly conserved vascular permeability factor secreted by a variety of human and rodent tumor cell lines. Cancer Res. 1986;46(11):5629–32.

44. Koch AE, Harlow LA, Haines GK, et al. Vascular endothelial growth factor. A cytokine modulating endothelial function in rheumatoid arthritis. J Immunol. 1994;152(8):4149–56.
45. Guidi AJ, Abu-Jawdeh G, Berse B, et al. Vascular permeability factor (vascular endothelial growth factor) expression and angiogenesis in cervical neoplasia. J Natl Cancer Inst. 1995;87(16):1237–45.
46. Leung DW, Cachianes G, Kuang WJ, Goeddel DV, Ferrara N. Vascular endothelial growth factor is a secreted angiogenic mitogen. Science. 1989;246(4935):1306–9.
47. Dvorak HF, Sioussat TM, Brown LF, et al. Distribution of vascular permeability factor (vascular endothelial growth factor) in tumors: concentration in tumor blood vessels. J Exp Med. 1991;174(5):1275–8.
48. Bhardwaj S, Roy H, Heikura T, Yla-Herttuala S. VEGF-A, VEGF-D and VEGF-D(DeltaNDeltaC) induced intimal hyperplasia in carotid arteries. Eur J Clin Invest. 2005;35(11):669–76.
49. Khurana R, Zhuang Z, Bhardwaj S, et al. Angiogenesis-dependent and independent phases of intimal hyperplasia. Circulation. 2004;110(16):2436–43.
50. Fuster V, Charlton P, Boyd A. Clinical protocol. A phase IIb, randomized, multicenter, double-blind study of the efficacy and safety of Trinam (EG004) in stenosis prevention at the graft-vein anastomosis site in dialysis patients. Hum Gene Ther. 2001;12(16):2025–7.
51. Chan CY, Chen YS, Ma MC, Chen CF. Remodeling of experimental arteriovenous fistula with increased matrix metalloproteinase expression in rats. J Vasc Surg. 2007;45(4):804–11.
52. Misra S, Fu A, Anderson J, et al. The rat femoral arteriovenous fistula model: Increased expression of MMP-2 and MMP-9 at the venous stenosis. J Vasc Interv Radiol. 2008;19(4):587–94.
53. Rotmans JI, Velema E, Verhagen HJ, et al. Matrix metalloproteinase inhibition reduces intimal hyperplasia in a porcine arteriovenous-graft model. J Vasc Surg. 2004;39(2):432–9.
54. Birkedal-Hansen H, Moore W, Bodden M, et al. Matrix metalloproteinases (MMPs) are a family of nine or more highly homologous Zn(++)-endopeptidases that collectively. Crit Rev Oral Biol Med. 1993;4(2):197–250.
55. Johnson C, Galis ZS. Matrix metalloproteinase-2 and -9 differentially regulate smooth muscle cell migration and cell-mediated collagen organization. Arterioscler Thromb Vasc Biol. 2004;24(1):54–60.
56. Lee S, Jilani SM, Nikolova GV, Carpizo D, Iruela-Arispe ML. Processing of VEGF-A by matrix metalloproteinases regulates bioavailability and vascular patterning in tumors. J Cell Biol. 2005;169(4):681–91.
57. Lancelot E, Amirbekian V, Brigger I, et al. Evaluation of matrix metalloproteinases in atherosclerosis using a novel noninvasive imaging approach. Arterioscler Thromb Vasc Biol. 2008;28(3):425–32.
58. Sanz J, Fayad ZA. Imaging of atherosclerotic cardiovascular disease. Nature. 2008;451(7181):953–7.
59. Pugh CW, Ratcliffe PJ. Regulation of angiogenesis by hypoxia: role of the HIF system. Nat Med. 2003;9(6):677–84.
60. Lee ES, Bauer GE, Caldwell MP, Santilli SM. Association of artery wall hypoxia and cellular proliferation at a vascular anastomosis. J Surg Res. 2000;91(1):32–7.

61. Santilli SM, Wernsing SE, Lee ES. Transarterial wall oxygen gradients at a prosthetic vascular graft to artery anastomosis in the rabbit. J Vasc Surg. 2000;31(6):1229–39.
62. Shi Y, Patel S, Niculescu R, Chung W, Desrochers P, Zalewski A. Role of matrix metalloproteinases and their tissue inhibitors in the regulation of coronary cell migration. Arterioscler Thromb Vasc Biol. 1999;19(5):1150–5.
63. Scott NA, Cipolla GD, Ross CE, et al. Identification of a potential role for the adventitia in vascular lesion formation after balloon overstretch injury of porcine coronary arteries. Circulation. 1996;93(12):2178–87.
64. Zalewski A, Shi Y. Vascular myofibroblasts. Lessons from coronary repair and remodeling. Arterioscler Thromb Vasc Biol. 1997;17(3):417–22.
65. Kalra M, Miller VM. Early remodeling of saphenous vein grafts: proliferation, migration and apoptosis of adventitial and medial cells occur simultaneously with changes in graft diameter and blood flow. J Vasc Res. 2000;37(6):576–84.
66. Shi Y, O'Brien Jr JE, Mannion JD, et al. Remodeling of autologous saphenous vein grafts. The role of perivascular myofibroblasts. Circulation. 1997;95(12):2684–93.
67. Karakiulakis G, Papakonstantinou E, Aletras AJ, Tamm M, Roth M. Cell type-specific effect of hypoxia and platelet-derived growth factor-BB on extracellular matrix turnover and its consequences for lung remodeling. J Biol Chem. 2007;282(2):908–15.
68. Leufgen H, Bihl MP, Rudiger JJ, et al. Collagenase expression and activity is modulated by the interaction of collagen types, hypoxia, and nutrition in human lung cells. J Cell Physiol. 2005;204(1):146–54.
69. Papakonstantinou E, Aletras AJ, Roth M, Tamm M, Karakiulakis G. Hypoxia modulates the effects of transforming growth factor-beta isoforms on matrix-formation by primary human lung fibroblasts. Cytokine. 2003;24(1–2):25–35.
70. Short M, Nemenoff RA, Zawada WM, Stenmark KR, Das M. Hypoxia induces differentiation of pulmonary artery adventitial fibroblasts into myofibroblasts. Am J Physiol Cell Physiol. 2004;286(2):C416–25.
71. Das M, Dempsey EC, Reeves JT, Stenmark KR. Selective expansion of fibroblast subpopulations from pulmonary artery adventitia in response to hypoxia. Am J Physiol Lung Cell Mol Physiol. 2002;282(5):L976–86.
72. Stenmark KR, Gerasimovskaya E, Nemenoff RA, Das M. Hypoxic activation of adventitial fibroblasts: role in vascular remodeling. Chest. 2002;122 (6 Suppl):326S–34.

Chapter 7
The Vascular Access Coordinator

Cynthia Bhola

Arteriovenous (AV) access-related complications result in considerable morbidity and are associated with millions of health care dollars being spent each year. With a dedicated access team that includes a nephrologist, an access surgeon, an interventionalist, and a dialysis nurse with expertise in vascular access, a hemodialysis (HD) program can develop and maintain skills that lead to better patient care, better long-term outcomes, and efficient use of resources. The role of the vascular access coordinator (VAC) is pivotal to the success of this program.

Setting up the Vascular Access Coordinator Position

The introduction of VAC role to many of the HD programs differs greatly, depending on the resources and the needs of the specific programs. The first challenge facing a VAC is to understand the

C. Bhola (✉)
Dialysis Vascular Access Coordinator, University Health Network,
Toronto, Ontario, Canada
e-mail: Cynthia.bhola@uhn.on.ca

D.K. Rajan (ed.), *Essentials of Percutaneous Dialysis Interventions*,
DOI 10.1007/978-1-4419-5657-6_7,
© Springer Science+Business Media, LLC 2011

institution's organizational structure and develop an appreciation for the unique patient population that he or she will be responsible for. The VAC will need to adapt the role to meet these needs.

For those setting up the role of a VAC for the first time they will need to be resourceful, networking with other institutions that have an established VAC role, and take advantage of the many online resources (see below). The VAC will need to set realistic goals and develop vital relationships with those who will ultimately form a vascular access team (VAT). These members should include nephrologists, interventionalists including interventional radiologists and nephrologists, vascular surgeons, and the VAC. Often the relationship between the key players of the VAT was previously competitive or nonexistent. Building this relationship is time consuming, but necessary. The VAC is the bridge between the divisions. Ideally, the VAC should be a nurse with AV access cannulation experience.

For programs that have very large patient populations or have multiple satellite centers, the role of the VAC may require two or more people. For programs that are small, it is best to combine hemodialysis and peritoneal vascular access management for one VAC, rather than have a part-time position that risks having the VAC assigned to other duties. For a vascular access program to be successful, the VAC needs to be dedicated to that role and only that role due to the unpredictable or episodic nature of vascular access dysfunction. At minimum, a VAC should establish and maintain a VA surveillance program, provide vascular access-related education to patients and caregivers, and coordinate his or her care by liaising with referring physicians, nephrologists, radiologists, and surgeons.

Scope of Practice

The VAC role varies greatly among hemodialysis programs. The VAC should be the key resource responsible for coordinating and overseeing vascular access information and care for the nephrology program, with a focus on maintaining optimal access function and longevity. The role of the VAC is to provide "seamless" patient care with respect to vascular access. The following highlights the practical but important aspects of developing a VAC role that promotes a successful vascular access program.

Establish a Vascular Access Clinic

Weekly Vascular Access Clinic

- The access surgeon and the VAC assess the patient together, to provide continuity of care. The VAC provides a detailed access history including prior interventions for the surgeon and clearly articulates the vascular access issue that the patient is referred for.
- The VA Clinic should see patients for new access creation, problems with established access, and follow-up of newly created access.
- Referrals can come from the predialysis clinics, nephrologists, and primary dialysis nurses (for those patients who have initiated HD).
- First goal of the vascular access clinic: Facilitate early access placement with emphasis on fistula placement and reduce admissions for vascular access surgery.
- Patient-focused clinic that provides preoperative and postoperative surgical management.
- VAC provides vascular access teaching on access creation and its care, preop and postop teaching. The VAC has many opportunities to provide patient education and stress early vein preservation.
- VAC will arrange anesthesia consults and endocrine consults as appropriate.
- The VAC will organize vein mapping, venograms, specific interventional radiology tests, and consults deemed appropriate by the vascular surgeon (e.g., dermatology). Should the patient have a contrast allergy, orders will be obtained for premedication prior to the patient's intervention.
- The VAC will experience a high degree of autonomy within this role.

Ongoing Surveillance and Managing Vascular Access Complications

The VAC is Responsible for all Access Issues

- Provide ongoing patient support and education related to AV Access.
- For a VAC to be abreast of vascular access issues, it is best to coordinate and arrange *ALL* procedures – a daunting task, but it

provides the VAC with the ability to prioritize patient procedures in an institution that has limited resources. The VAC is the only person who knows the complete vascular access history for the patient. If the VACs give up the opportunity to arrange all their own AV access procedures, they miss the opportunity to prioritize AV access procedures and allow others not familiar with the HD patient's status to do the arranging. Valuable time slots in the OR could potentially be given to a patient who is elective while an urgent access case waits for their procedure.

- Access surveillance is critical to the success of a vascular access program with "preservation of a functioning access" a vital goal.
- VACs intervene on vascular access issues based on their critical assessment skills and the surveillance information tracked (e.g., transonic monitoring, Doppler's, prior interventions). Surveillance leads to improved outcomes and a decrease in thrombosis rates of AV fistulae and grafts by identifying potential stenosis and arranging appropriate percutaneous and occasional surgical interventions.
- VAC reviews all diagnostic screening tests including ongoing interventional procedures arranged to maintain vascular access patency.

Setting up and Maintaining a Vascular Access Database

A prospective data collection mechanism is vital for the success of a VA program and as such, the VAC needs to oversee the database "management." Without accurate data, the program has no idea how it is doing and if the program is reaching the national target guidelines. The VAC will require resources to setup a database and to input data so that he or she is free to fulfill the nursing aspects of his or her role. The database can provide many opportunities for continuous quality improvement (CQI) and research endeavors by the VAT. Even though initially the management of the database can be costly, it will pay for itself with potential cost savings to a HD program with CQI initiatives. The information that is important to track needs to be decided by the VAT and may be determined in some programs by the resources available to a VAC. Ideally, the database should include the following (see Fig. 7.1):

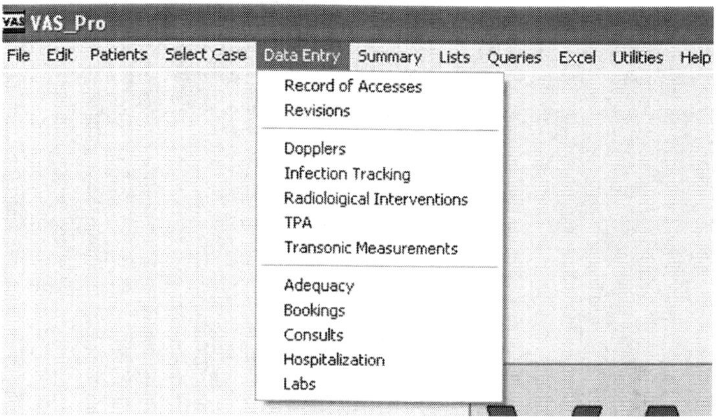

Fig. 7.1 Sample database. Data entry pull down tab with some of the representative input data fields

- A detailed access history for all patients
- Access type and site by surgeon
- Access monitoring and surveillance data such as transonic flows and Doppler results
- Track laboratory results associated with dialysis adequacy measurements such as urea reduction rates and Kt/V
- Monitor waiting times from time of referral to access creation
- Dialysis adequacy according to access type (linking access data with lab data)
- Track overall patency rates by following the number and type of dysfunction events
- Number and type of interventions with outcomes and complications
- Incident access placement should be monitored and compared to prevalent access use. Follow fistula maturation rate
- Infection rates and consequences
- VA-related Hospitalizations

Education of Patient/Staff/Resource Personnel

The VAC should educate the newly hired HD nurses on vascular access and keep all staff updated on new vascular access technology such as catheters, cannulation needles, and stent grafts. VAC should be a participant in the predialysis clinic, providing patient education on vascular access to those patients who have chosen HD as their modality and to those who have not but have an eGFR <25 mL/min. Specific points are as follows:

- The VAC should educate nurses on reporting and managing access problems and provide diagramming of new accesses, communicating specific issues with an access.
- The VAC needs to be involved in the development of vascular access policy and procedures.
- The VAC should be visible in the HD units remaining approachable to staff and patients. Being visible in the HD unit doing access rounds helps establish a trusting relationship with patients and provides opportunities for educating the patient and staff.
- The VAC should remain readily accessible for consultation on all access-related issues, and it is essential to foster excellent working relationships with all those who are involved in the coordination of AV access procedures including the secretaries and technical staff. *The Staff Nurses are Your Eyes and Ears* when you are not in the unit; treat them with respect.
- All patients should have a secondary vascular access plan in place even when the current access is functioning well.
- All patients and their families should be educated on the care of their vascular access and how to preserve their veins for potential future vascular access options.

Monthly Meeting with VAT Leader

To be successful as a VAC, a nurse must have the full support and collaboration of his/her VAT. A nephrologist is usually the leader of the VAT and sets the standard for the expectations of what a VAT hopes to achieve for their program. It is important to keep the channels of communication open between all members of the team, and it is the VAC who is the liaison between the members.

- The VAT leader and the VAC should be in close communication and work diligently on new quality initiatives for VA.
- The VAT leader and the VAC should lead a multidisciplinary approach to infection control management for vascular access and

meet at least monthly to review the HD infections to promote adherence to infection control policies.
- A VAC is part of the optimal team for Nephrology and should be a member of quality assurance and accreditation committees.

CQI Role

The VAC role is based on the premise of CQI of patient vascular access care and outcomes. For example, CQI initiatives should use the PDSA (Plan-Do-Study-Act) model of improvement. The cycle begins with identifying a problem and developing an improvement plan and ends with actions based on the learning gained from the Plan, Do, and Study phases. Once a Plan is determined, the VA program implements the plan in the Do phase. The Study, or analysis, phase not only evaluates whether the change was an improvement but also acknowledges, synthesizes, and considers new knowledge gained. The results of this evaluation will determine changes to be made in the Act phase, completing the cycle. Specific examples of successes using this PDSA model are described below. Outcomes are documented by use of a prospective VA database and communicated to patients, radiologists, and surgeons involved. This raises the awareness and commitment to vascular access of all parties involved and quantifies the effectiveness of VA initiatives. Collecting prospective data allows program to review day-to-day clinical data, as well as the intended and unintended consequences of any CQI initiatives. Benchmarking of VA practices and outcomes is essential in the CQI process.

Multidisciplinary Rounds

The VAC should organize and manage monthly vascular access rounds with the surgeons, interventionalists and nephrologists to review the difficult access cases. A future plan of care can be decided at this time for each patient based on the findings. The VAC is responsible for communicating this to the primary nephrologist and the dialysis unit.

- The VAC should point out trends and events that predict access dysfunction and obtain the expert opinions of the VAT to identify the cause for the events and how they should be managed.

- The VAT has the opportunity to evaluate interventions and their outcomes set goals to improve outcomes.
- The VAT should review current literature for vascular access–associated research and recommendations and seek opportunities to lead their own research. Meeting monthly stimulates the interest and commitment of all members of the VAT to vascular access.
- The concept of the VAT was included in the DOQI guidelines as a prerequisite for best practices and better outcomes through a CQI process in 2006.

Other Expectations of the VAC Role Include

- To assist and participate in vascular access research with authorship of papers and presentations when opportunities present themselves.
- Being "the" contact person and resource for all vascular access issues is critical to the success of a VAC role.
- The VAC is the central person for all the disciplines that deal with vascular access creation, care, use, and ongoing maintenance. The VAC is a strong patient advocate.
- The VAC is the contact person for vascular access sales representatives.
- The VAC must be proficient in vascular access care and management and constantly is required to problem solve.
- Promote patient-centered care and provide emotional support. A vascular access is a patient's lifeline, and any dysfunction or loss of this access causes the patient considerable stress and anxiety. They need compassion.
- Must be able to troubleshoot vascular access problems and know whom to call and when. Must be accountable for their actions.
- VAC often acts as a consultant to other hospital and agencies, especially to those who have limited vascular access resources.
- Routinely monitors dialysis treatment sheets and monthly adequacy labs that pertain to access function.
- Collaborates with dialysis staff in developing and recommending strategies to prevent complications and improve the function of existing access.

- Become a member of a professional VA network and keep up to date on best practices and national guidelines. There is considerable variability in nursing practices among the dialysis units often related to the resources available to the VAC and the organizational structure of the institution one practices.
- Attend conferences and other educational events to remain current in advances in patient management.

Impact of the Role

The major benefit of the VAC role is the management and continuity of care through one contact person. With coordination of vascular access care through one person, there is a decrease in vascular access–related hospitalizations. There is a focused increase in AV fistula placement and close follow-up for the potential for failure to mature. Vascular access dysfunction is captured quickly with ongoing surveillance. The VAC will be relentless in getting patients to appointments. The VAC is committed to patient-centered care and constantly advocates for the patient. The VAC is in continuous search for innovative solutions to access dysfunction. Due to the unpredictability of access dysfunction, it is difficult to have all the experts in place when an emergency occurs, such as vascular access thrombosis. Quick communication and organization with various departments is required to deal with this issue, highlighting the need for a single dedicated individual, the VAC, to coordinate and solve the problem, thereby avoiding fragmented care.

Recommended Reading

1. http://www.fistulafirst.org/HealthcareProfessionals/FFBIChangeConcepts/ChangeConcept1.aspx.
2. http://www.bcrenalagency.ca/professionals/VascularAccess/ProvGuide.htm.
3. Clinical Educators Network. Clinical educators network nursing recommendations for management of vascular access hemodialysis patients. CANNT J. 2006;16 Suppl 1:e1–20.
4. Dinwiddie LC. Investing in the lifeline: the value of a vascular access coordinator. Nephrol News Issues. 2003;17(49):52–3.

5. Dinwiddie LC. Overview of the role of a vascular access nurse coordinator in the optimisation of access care for patients requiring haemodialysis. Hong Kong J Nephrol. 2007;9(2):99–103.
6. Mermel LA, Allon M, Bouza E, Craven DE, Flynn P, O'Grady NP, et al. Clinical practice guidelines for the diagnosis and management of intravascular catheter-related infection: 2009 update by the Infectious Diseases Society of America. Clin Infect Dis. 2009;49:1–45.

Chapter 8
The Procedure Room, Equipment and Radiation Safety

Dheeraj K. Rajan

When performing dialysis interventions, it is important to have optimal imaging equipment to assist in maximizing outcomes for patients. Although many consider basic imaging equipment to be sufficient for such "basic procedures," high imaging quality does translate into improved outcomes and fewer complications. Considerations for the procedure room and equipment include sterility, functionality, practicality and safety. The ideal suite would promote operative aseptic practices (Chap. 11) and contain single-use disposables for the cases to be performed, an ultrasound machine, and the fluoroscopic imaging equipment.

Disposables including wires, access needles, access sheaths, balloons, stents, and medications are ideally available within the procedure room to reduce the risk of introducing microorganisms into the sterile environment and to provide greater efficiency in performing procedures and managing potential complications.

D.K. Rajan (✉)
Head and Associate Professor, Division of Vascular & Interventional Radiology, Department of Medical Imaging, University of Toronto, Toronto, Ontario, Canada
e-mail: Dheeraj.Rajan@uhn.on.ca

D.K. Rajan (ed.), *Essentials of Percutaneous Dialysis Interventions*, DOI 10.1007/978-1-4419-5657-6_8,
© Springer Science+Business Media, LLC 2011

Common Disposable Equipment for Interventions

1. Needle sizes are expressed in gauge with increasing gauge size representing smaller needle size. Stent and balloon sizes (diameter and length) are expressed in millimeters. Wires and wire lumen sizes are expressed in inches. Sheath, catheter, and overall device size or diameter is expressed using the French scale where 1 French (Fr) = 0.33 mm.
2. Access needles: 19-gauge single-wall puncture needles and 18-gauge IV angiocatheters. These have the advantage of allowing access for imaging of the access and also are large enough to pass a 0.035 in. wire. A micropuncture set (see Fig. 8.1) contains a 21-gauge needle through which a 0.018 in. wire is passed. The set is considered less traumatic by many and is used commonly for jugular punctures. The set produced by many manufacturers allows transition to a 0.035 in. wire delivery via two catheters passed as a unit with the inner removable catheter tapered to 0.018 in. and the outer catheter tapered to 0.035 in. It is also useful for brachial/radial artery punctures and complicated venous punctures as the inner cannula is 3 Fr and can be used to image the access circuit with minimal trauma.
3. Wires: The standard diameter is 0.035 in. At least one hydrophilic angled glidewire with a length of 150 cm should be stocked. This wire assists in crossing difficult lesions, and the tip is directable. Nonhydrophilic wires are used for initial access and interventions. Wires should be of sufficient length to allow for exchange of devices without losing access across the lesion being treated. Typical lengths are 145 cm, 180 cm, and occasionally 260 cm lengths of varying stiffness. Stiffer wires are preferred for delivery of stents or stent grafts. At least one wire stocked should have a floppy straight tip to aid in access and occasionally cross or push through thrombus. Depending on advanced devices stocked, additional wire diameters and lengths may be needed.
4. Angioplasty balloons. For dialysis grafts, the most common size used is 8 mm diameter × 40 mm length. For fistulas, the common range is 4–10 × 40 mm lengths. Shorter lengths often lead to migration or slipping of the balloon off the stenosis. For

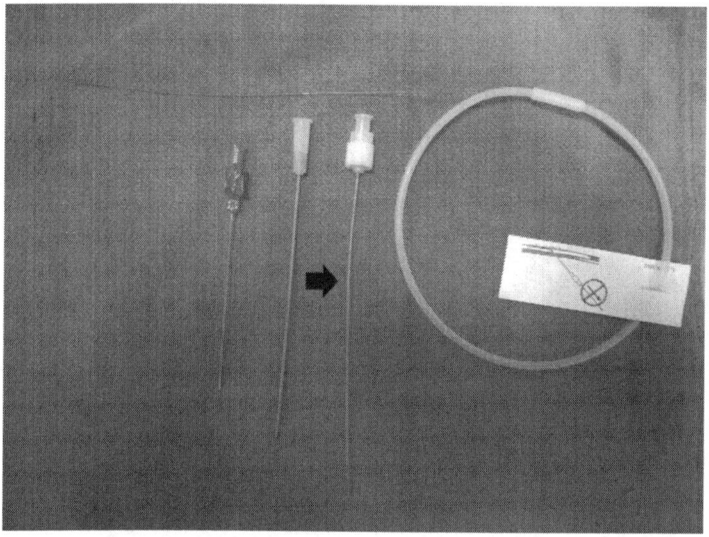

Fig. 8.1 Micropuncture set. Includes 21-gauge puncture needle, 0.018-in. wire and a transition catheter set which allows transition from a 0.018-in. wire to a 0.035-in. wire. The inner catheter (arrow) is 3 Fr and can be used for diagnostic arterial punctures where minimal size is preferred

central lesions, 12–16 mm balloons are needed. Stocked balloons <12 mm should be able to reach inflation pressures up to 18 atm. A small collection of balloons for peripheral interventions which are able to exceed these pressures is recommended as up to 30% of stenoses require inflation pressures exceeding 20 atm.

5. Balloon inflators. Devices that inflate beyond 20 atm are recommended. A cost-effective alternative described by Foering et al. [1] is use of 1-cc polycarbonate syringes to inflate balloons where >40 atm of pressure is possible.
6. Stents. As there is no routine indication for stent usage, a minimal number on hand are required for bailout situations. Nitinol self-expanding stents are recommended (Chap. 15), and common sizes used peripherally are 8 mm diameter × 40 mm length. For central lesions, 12–16 mm diameter stents are most commonly used.

7. Stent grafts. With the exception of the FLAIR stent graft, no others have been investigated sufficiently to advocate for routine use. However, as with stents, 8 and 12 mm × 40 mm devices are suggested in minimal numbers as basic stock. These devices can act as bailout devices for catastrophic vein or access ruptures peripherally and centrally and can potentially save a patient's life.
8. Snares. These come as a simple snare commonly the Amplatz Gooseneck Snare (EV3) and a three loop snare called the Ensnare (Merit Medical). Device size used is determined by the device to be retrieved and vessel size where the device resides. Some prefer the Ensnare as its shape gives better cross sectional coverage.
9. Sharp object disposable containers.
10. Sutures. 2–0 and 3–0 monofilament sutures are most commonly used which are on cutting needles which are indicated for skin use only. Tapered needles on sutures are for nonskin use.
11. Other devices. These are specific to the challenges of one's practice and are not common required equipment but are discussed throughout this book.

Ultrasound

A portable ultrasound machine is often sufficient for dialysis interventions. The machine should have a 12-MHz or similar linear probe available to allow for venipuncture, for line insertions and basic interrogation of AVFs and AVGs, as well as for aiding punctures of these accesses when required. Ultrasound is useful in identifying open veins, length and location of thrombus and/or stenoses within dialysis accesses and collateral veins compared to the normal outflow tract for fistulas. Color Doppler images and velocity measurement capabilities are added features that are desirable but not absolutely required for interventions. Ideally, the machine should be on a mobile platform, have minimal boot-up or start-up time, be easily moveable, and have a small footprint within the room to allow for maximum flexibility. Although larger machines provide diagnostic quality imaging, their usefulness is diminished by their weight, large size, cost, poor mobility, and poor positioning flexibility (see Fig. 8.2).

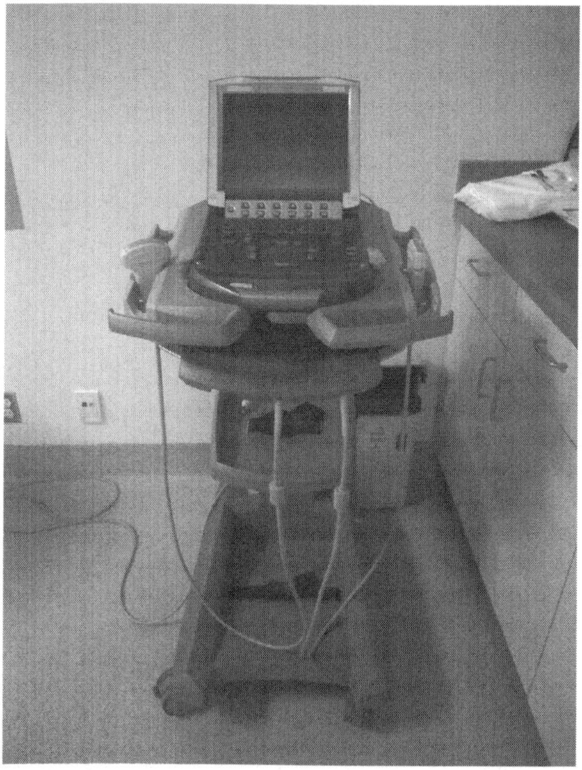

Fig. 8.2 Portable ultrasound machine

Imaging Equipment

When choosing what digital angiography system is appropriate, one should consider the uses for the equipment both present and future, compatibility issues with current and future equipment acquisitions, digital storage solutions, and soon-to-be-required documentation of radiation doses per examination. Cost of the equipment and the servicing contract are very important as well as the expected service life of the equipment.

The ideal system specifically for dialysis interventions would allow for flexible access to the patient for imaging both arms and neck with access to the groin. The imaging field should be of sufficient size to image large parts of the access circuit rather than small areas that are obtained with cardiac-specific imaging units. When the imaging field is restricted, potential pathology can be missed, complications can occur, and overall there is a greater dose of radiation delivered due to more imaging time required to compensate for the narrow field of view. Recommended image intensifier size is a minimum of 12 in. Our image intensifiers are 12×16 in. (rectangular and rotational) which provides greater imaging flexibility for dialysis interventions. Imaging quality should be sufficient to detect subtle differences in contrast density that may indicate areas of vessel narrowing. The imaging equipment should be repositionable with the aid of the imaging table to allow imaging from the fingertips of the patient to the heart. The image intensifier which is responsible for generation of the image (or the C-arm containing the radiation source and the intensifier) should be able to rotate to different obliquities to obtain different planes of imaging. The table that supports the patient must be radiolucent and designed for imaging purposes. At least two monitors are recommended, one for viewing the active image and one for displaying a static image, of a previous fistulogram, previous study etc. with a minimum resolution of 1,000×1,000 matrix.

Adjustable shielding or cones within the intensifier that reduce the field of view and thereby reduce radiation exposure and scatter should also be available and operator adjustable on the unit. Additionally, shielding between the operator and the ionizing radiation source that is both table mounted and ceiling mounted are desired but not absolutely required. The patient table itself should be made of low radiation adsorption material and should be capable of being raised, lowered, and rotated so that in conjunction with tube rotation, imaging from the center of the patient to the fingertips is easily possible. A portable focal bright light source is also of benefit to illuminate areas of intervention.

Digital subtraction imaging (an initial noncontrast image is electronically subtracted from subsequent images) is a must and data archiving in the form of DICOM images (Digital Imaging and Communications in Medicine) which is the standard for handling, storing, printing, and transmitting information in medical imaging. Within North America, there will be future requirement to document radiation doses per examination. This is another consideration when choosing equipment.

Radiation Safety

For every interventionalist, radiation exposure is a primary concern, and the risk to oneself and the patient cannot be ignored or understated. Although ionizing radiation doses and radiation safety is core teaching for radiologists, this is not necessarily so for other practitioners. There is an increasing concern within regulatory bodies in North America regarding this issue as more imaging studies and interventions are performed with little safety oversight or understanding.

For the interventionalist, there are basic steps that can be undertaken to reduce ionizing radiation dose. Radiation safety glasses reduce the dose to the corneas where cumulative radiation dose leads to cataracts. Wearing glasses reduces dose significantly and also protects against splash injury. Radiation shielding in the form of table-mounted lead curtains below the table reduces radiation scatter to the legs and body (from 25 to 80%). Reducing the air gap between the area imaged and the image intensifier as well as coning out areas that don't need imaging (see Fig. 8.3) reduces dose and scatter. Further dose reduction can be obtained by increasing the distance between the x-ray tube and the patient. The simple concept of "if you are not looking at the

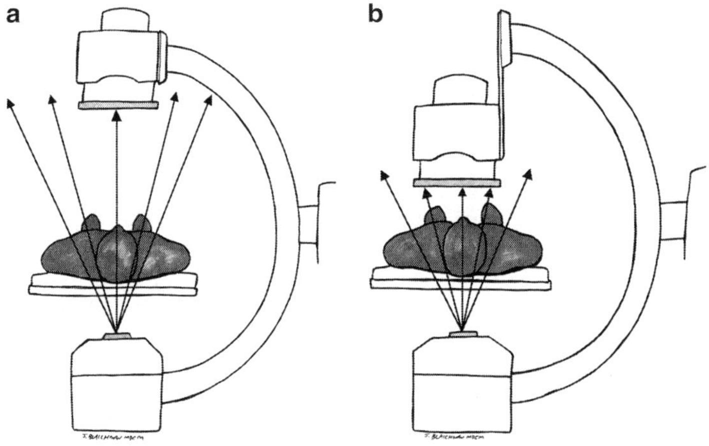

Fig. 8.3 (**a**) If the image intensifier is far from the patient and the air gap is large, more radiation scatter occurs. (**b**) When the air gap is reduced, scatter is reduced

screen, your foot should not be on the pedal" reduces radiation dose for obvious reasons. Filming digital subtraction runs or sequences at two frames per second is sufficient for most interventions. With the exception of carbon dioxide imaging (Chap. 12), rates above this are unnecessary. Many imaging machines also offer the option of pulsed fluoroscopy. Pulsed fluoroscopy (the rate at which images are created) is an important tool for dose reduction in fluoroscopic procedures. Rates can be reduced to 15 frames per second yet retain effective image information.

Radiation safety gowns are integral to significantly reducing dose to an interventionalist. The gown should be well fitting with minimal gaps to the body. If working with others, a full-body gown is preferred compared to a 1/2 body gown. There is no protection if your backside is exposed to the radiation source with the 1/2 gown. A thyroid protection collar is also worn to reduce the risk of radiation-induced thyroid cancer. The gowns themselves are rated in terms of exposure based on reduction of scattered radiation exposure. Within Canada the minimum standard is 0.5 mm lead equivalency up to 130 kVp, and within the United States, for some states, it is a minimum of 0.5 mm lead equivalency at 80 kVp for 95% reduction in scatter whereas others only state equivalency to 0.5 mm lead. One should seek proper required standards from the appropriate government organization that regulates radiation safety within their state/country.

Although many refer to the gowns as lead gowns, many are now available in much lighter materials with similar lead attenuation equivalency. Regardless of the material, proper storage of the gowns is important to prevent the protective material within them from cracking or tearing. Cracks and tears allow ionizing radiation in. The gowns should be properly stored or hung when not in use rather than laid somewhere. In addition, a proper quality assurance program for radiation safety should be in place to assess the gowns routinely for damage, and monitoring of body dose to the interventionist should be done with body dosimeters and ring dosimeters on a monthly basis. This service is available through multiple organizations.

For the patient, the aforementioned measures also reduce ionizing radiation dose. For interventional procedures, the tissue of concern is the skin. At a minimum, it is important to report or record fluoroscopy times. Fluoroscopy times greater than 30 min should impart caution on behalf of the operator. The skin at the site where radiation enters the body receives the highest radiation dose, and beyond a threshold dose, injury becomes more severe with increasing dose.

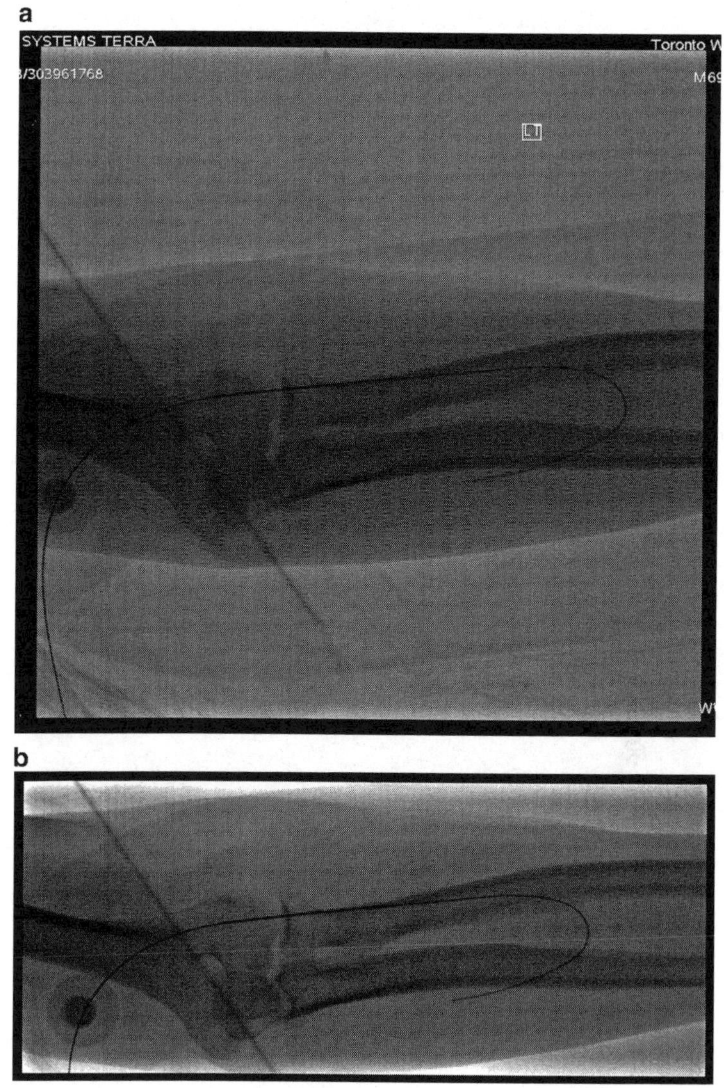

Fig. 8.4 (**a**) Unconned image leads to greater radiation exposure to the patient and the operator. (**b**) Properly conned field of view

Radiation injury often manifests itself weeks to months after the procedure with only exceedingly high doses manifesting within 24 h [2]. Scatter contributes greatly to body dose absorption. Reducing the rate of pulsed fluoroscopy, the source to image receptor distance should be maximized, reducing the air gap between the patient and imaging receptor, and coning out areas or collimating that are not of interest reduces scatter and radiation dose (see Fig. 8.4). Avoid the magnification or "zoom" feature as this also increases radiation dose. Also, for young patients, a radiation shield can be placed under the pelvis of the patient to reduce dose to the gonads. Also, radiation risk is higher for patients who weigh <10 or >135 kg. If the patient is exposed to large amounts of radiation, the area irradiated should be pointed out to the patient and he or she should be warned about possible rash or skin irritation. If this occurs, a referral to a dermatologist or plastic surgeon familiar with radiation skin damage is highly recommended.

An important concept taught in Radiology is ALARA which represents "as low as reasonably achievable." It means making every reasonable effort to maintain exposures to ionizing radiation as far below the dose limits as practical. This concept should be followed by anyone performing fluoroscopic imaging. Ionizing radiation is dangerous. It is not something you can see, feel, or smell. However, the damage it can cause is permanent and potentially fatal. Using fluoroscopy i.e., ionizing radiation requires respect for its utility and also its harmful properties.

Key Points

- Ionizing radiation in imaging studies is dangerous. Proper practices and quality assurance procedures should be in place to protect both the patient and the interventionist.
- Record fluoroscopy times and only equipment that at a minimum display fluoroscopy times should be used so that the operator is roughly aware of radiation exposure.
- Fluoroscopy time greater than 60 min is not a dose value but is an indirect indicator of significant radiation dose.
- Keep in mind the concept of "as low as reasonably achievable" or "ALARA" when subjecting the patient to ionizing radiation.
- If you are not looking at the screen, your foot should not be on the fluoroscopy pedal.
- An ultrasound machine available within the procedure room is a valuable tool for diagnosis and treatment.
- Fluoroscopy equipment should be flexible enough to adapt to your needs, not the other way around.

References

1. Foering K, Chittams JL, Trerotola SO. Percutaneous transluminal angioplasty balloon inflation with syringes: who needs an inflator? J Vasc Interv Radiol. 2009;20(5):629–33; quiz 571.
2. Stecker MS, Balter S, Towbin RB, et al. Guidelines for patient radiation dose management. J Vasc Interv Radiol. 2009;20(7 Suppl):S263–73.

Chapter 9
Patient Considerations and Preparation

Dheeraj K. Rajan

The key to delivering good care to any patient remains a proper history and physical examination. This is no different for dialysis patients despite the short nature of interventions and relative low-risk of complications. A proper history and physical helps guide short- and long-term therapy. Below is an outline of major points to be considered.

History and Physical

Besides knowing the patient's basic medical history, it is important to know multiple specific aspects related to their access. These include:

1. Allergies – IV contrast and heparin in particular.
   (a) If allergic to contrast, alternative agents can be considered or the procedure can be rebooked with premedication.

D.K. Rajan (✉)
Head and Associate Professor, Division of Vascular & Interventional Radiology, Department of Medical Imaging, University of Toronto,
Toronto, Ontario, Canada
e-mail: Dheeraj.Rajan@uhn.on.ca

D.K. Rajan (ed.), *Essentials of Percutaneous Dialysis Interventions*,
DOI 10.1007/978-1-4419-5657-6_9,

© Springer Science+Business Media, LLC 2011

   (b) Heparin induced thrombocytopenia (HITT) is a serious condition which is an immune-mediated response leading to thromboses. Alternative medications include lepirudin and argatroban.

2. What medications are they taking?
   (a) See further.
3. What type of access do they have?
   (a) Fistula vs. graft, upper vs. lower arm.
   (b) Which side is arterial? Often the patient can tell you which side of the graft loop access is arterial and which is venous. Simply ask.
4. When was it placed?
   (a) Age of access helps determine how extensive intervention should be.
5. How long has it been functional?
   (a) If it has not been functional long, there may be an underlying technical issue that is not correctable percutaneously.
6. What problems are they having related to the access?
   (a) If they are having problems with recirculation, accessing the access, or aspirating blood clots, then stenosis is more strongly suspected. If no flows are obtained, then thrombosis.
   (b) Have recent flow measurements or noninvasive testing (Duplex ultrasound) been performed, and if so what are the results?
7. When and what was the last intervention? How many interventions have been performed?
   (a) Knowing how many times an access has been intervened on helps determine if POBA will be sufficient or if another intervention is required.
8. What other accesses and/or catheters have been placed and where?
   (a) If the current access is the last access available for the patient, one should be more committed to doing whatever preserves the access long term. Prior catheter insertions may indicate the presence of central venous stenoses or occlusions.

9. Are they being considered for transplantation and when?

    (a) If the patient is potentially getting a transplant within less than a year, one may consider doing more to preserve an access that would normally be abandoned.

10. Any recent echocardiogram?

    (a) Does the patient have a patent foramen ovale? If they do, air and clot on the venous side can pass to the arterial side causing cardiac, brain, or visceral artery ischemia/infarction.

Physical examination can reveal many key findings that are relevant to planned and future interventions. This should be part of the workup prior to any intervention on the patient (also see Chap. 5). Relevant physical findings include:

1. Where and what type of access does the patient have?

    (a) Is the access upper or lower arm and is it a fistula or graft. Type of access is associated with potential location of stenoses.
    (b) What are the arterial inflow and venous outflow vessels?

2. What does the access look like?

    (a) Are there areas of bulging that are aneurysms in fistulas and points of graft material breakdown forming pseudoaneurysms in grafts? Do any of these bulging areas have a shiny overlying skin with or without a scab? This may indicate a site of pending rupture.
    (b) If a fistula, is the access superficial or deep? If deep, the access may be difficult to puncture and inappropriately considered to be immature or have poor flows.
    (c) Is there a portion that is dilated and an area that is not? This may be a point of stenosis.
    (d) Are there multiple dilated collateral veins? These could either indicate an outflow stenosis/occlusion or represent a cause for the fistula to have delayed maturation.

3. How does the access feel?

    (a) Is there a thrill or pulsatility? No thrill or pulsatility indicates either an inflow lesion or thrombosis. If thrombosed, the fistula or graft will not be compressible.
    (b) Is there a point where pulsatility disappears? Is there a point along the access that feels focally hard? These may be points

of stenosis. A continuous thrill in a graft reliably indicates acceptable flow rates (>450 mL/min: 100% sensitivity) and is useful in determining an endpoint of an interventional procedure. Conversely, a pulse in the graft suggests unacceptable flow rates (<450 mL/min: 75% sensitivity, 77% specificity) [1, 2].

(c) Is the fistula warm to touch, red, and feels like a rope or cord-like? Is there no thrill or compressibility? The fistula is likely thrombosed.

(d) Is the fistula very easy to palpate and puncture? This may indicate an outflow stenosis.

(e) If the patient has a graft, if there is redness and tenderness with or without some fluctuance, graft infection should be suspected and excluded prior to any intervention.

4. Are there scars to indicate prior accesses and catheter insertions?

   (a) These findings may tip off the interventionalist to sites of stenosis.

5. Does the patient have a swollen arm, neck, or face?

   (a) This indicates a central venous stenosis or occlusion. If the whole face, neck and arms are swollen, then the patient either has or is at risk of developing SVC syndrome which is a medical emergency.

6. Are there dilated subcutaneous veins on the chest wall?

   (a) This is an indicator of central venous stenosis/occlusion.

7. Location of needle punctures and scars along the dysfunctional access.

   (a) If the fistula is flat, the needle marks give you an indication of the course of the fistula. Surgical scars indicate the location of the anastomosis and can give you an idea of the access type present. For example, if the patient has a long scar along the upper arm, they likely have a transposed brachiobasilic fistula.

8. Brachial, radial, and ulnar pulses?

   (a) If pulses are diminished, the patient may have a subclavian artery origin stenosis. They may also have a stenosed inflow artery problem. For instance, if the radial artery is not palpable, it may be occluded and flow to a radiocephalic fistula may be via retrograde flow through the palmar arch of the hand from the ulnar artery.

(b) If the hand is cold, numb, pale, and/or painful, arterial ischemia is present and related to "steal syndrome."

9. With a fistula, what happens when you raise the arm?

(a) If the fistula flattens out, then the patient has an inflow stenosis.

Patient Preparation

Most interventions can be performed on an outpatient basis. In preparation, patients should not eat solid food 8 h and liquids 4 h prior to intervention. Rather than providing variable instructions, it is less confusing to state to the patient that they should take nothing orally with the exception of clear liquids and necessary medications after midnight. With the exception of anticoagulants, injected insulin, and oral hypoglycemics, all other medications including antihypertensive medications should be taken with sips of water in the morning.

In most cases, intravenous access is not necessary as medications can be given via the indwelling dialysis catheter or access to the AVF or AVG. If dealing with a thrombosed access or complicated intervention, establishing peripheral venous access is highly recommended. For infusion, D5 1/2NS or 2/3 and 1/3 (0.3 NaCl with 3.3% dextrose) is recommended in volumes of less than 100 mL/min.

Hypoglycemics and Insulin

As the patients will have low blood sugar related to no oral intake, if they are taking injectable insulin, half the dose should be taken the morning of the procedure. Patients can continue to take their usual dose of Lantus Insulin (insulin glargine) the night before the procedure, as this covers their basal requirements. If they are taking oral hypoglycemics, we ask the patient not to take their morning dose.

Anticoagulants

Anticoagulation prior to interventions is more dependent on operator preference rather than any proven indication [3]. Antiplatelet agents, such as aspirin or Plavix should be continued through the procedure, as limiting platelet deposition in the area of the intervention may lessen later intimal hyperplasia. The risk of bleeding from antiplatelet agents when performing percutaneous interventions is minimal. If desired, aspirin and/or antiplatelet agents should be discontinued for a minimum of 5–7 days, and more commonly 10 days for their effects to diminish. Subcutaneous heparin is also not usually withheld. Simple interventions can be performed while patients are on Coumadin with minimal bleeding risk. Puncture site closure should be secure, as described in Chap. 23. However, if a major intervention is planned or expected, such as a thrombectomy, recanalization of occluded vein segments, complex dilation of central veins, or tunneled catheter insertion/exchange, the patient should have normal clotting parameters including a normal PTT and INR. In general, Coumadin needs to be withheld for a minimum of 3 days before a patient's coagulation factors begin to normalize. If the patient requires continued anticoagulation, they can be switched over to full dose subcutaneous or intravenous heparin or low-molecular weight heparin several days prior to the procedure and continued on it until the INR reaches therapeutic levels when Coumadin is restarted. After interventions, Coumadin can be restarted the same or the next day. For patients on dabigatran (Pradaxa, Boehringer Ingelheim Pharmaceuticals, Inc.) requiring cessation of anticoagulation prior to a major intervention, dabigatran should be stopped 3–5 days before the intervention in these patients with renal dysfunction. If bleeding is controlled, it can be restarted 6–12 h after the procedure.

Although many interventionalists administer heparin prior to any dialysis interventions, there is no evidence of benefit during routine angioplasty and/or stenting in dialysis grafts and fistulas. However, heparin, either intravenous or intra-access should always be administered during declotting procedures because it may inhibit serotonin-mediated bronchospasm related to pulmonary emboli, as well as prevent rethrombosis during the procedure.

Coagulation Parameters and Management

Normal coagulation parameters are international normalized ratio of 0.9–1.1. INR has replaced prothrombin time (PT) as a measure of anticoagulation. Normal activated partial thromboplastin time (PTT) is 25–35 s. There are no defined appropriate ranges that have been investigated and most threshold values are based on consensus. *For most dialysis interventions, an INR <1.5, platelets >50,000/μL and a PTT <1.5 times normal are sufficient.* An elevated INR can be reversed over 12–24 h for some time with vitamin K that can be given orally/SC/IM or IV. IV administration is faster acting but carries a significant risk of anaphylactic like reaction, even when given diluted and slowly. Prothrombin complex concentrate can be used in the setting for Coumadin anticoagulation and ongoing bleeding. Fresh frozen plasma (FFP) should be avoided in dialysis patients as the high volume needed to correct Coumadin anticoagulation is contraindicated. Low platelet counts can be corrected for procedures generally with 5–10 units. Dialysis patients are often uremic which causes platelet dysfunction. Desmopressin (1-deamino-8-D-arginine vasopressin (DDAVP) is a synthetic analogue of antidiuretic hormone. DDAVP acts through an unclear mechanism to enhance the plasma levels of factor VIII and von Willebrand factor. Dosing is of 0.3 μg/kg IV diluted in 100 mL of normal saline and infused over 20–30 min.

Dye Allergy

For patients with an intravenous dye allergy, depending on the severity of the allergy, the patient can be premedicated or an alternative contrast agent can be used (Chap. 12). If the allergy is non-anaphylactic, the patient can be premedicated with oral corticosteroids. Although many protocols exist, we use Prednisone 50 mg p.o. 13 h and 1 h pre-examination and diphenyl hydramine (Benadryl®) 50 mg p.o. 1 h pre-examination. If the procedure is urgent, then hydrocortisone 200 mg is intravenously administered immediately, and every 4 h until the procedure is completed (steroids must be given at minimum of 6 h prior to contrast) and diphenhydramine (Benadryl®) 50 mg intravenously 1 h before contrast media injection.

Sickle Cell Disease

If the patient has sickle cell disease, prophylactic measures are undertaken to prevent precipitation of sickle cell crises. These include adequate pain control, proper hydration, and provision of oxygen during the procedure to ensure high levels of blood oxygen saturation.

Antibiotics

Prophylactic antibiotics are not necessary for routine interventions if standard sterile technique (Chap. 11) is used. However, with more stent-grafts being placed within dialysis accesses, given the permanent placement of a foreign body, prophylactic antibiotics are highly recommended. The most concerning organisms are skin flora predominantly *Staphylococcus aureus*. Cefazolin, 1 g given intravenously is recommended an hour prior to intervention to reach peak serum concentration. For patients with suspected allergic reactions to penicillin or cephalosporin derivatives, vancomycin 1 g intravenously can be given. Some use prophylactic antibiotics before thrombectomy while others do not. Although there is no proof that prophylactic antibiotics are helpful in this setting, fatal septic events have been reported following dialysis graft thrombectomy and up to 62% of clinically uninfected thrombosed grafts are colonized with bacteria [4].

Key Points

- A specific history and physical related to the access and access dysfunction is invaluable in determining treatment plan and potential outcomes.
- Almost all percutaneous interventions can be performed on an outpatient basis.
- Routine use of prophylactic antibiotics is not required.

References

1. Trerotola SO, Scheel Jr PJ, Powe NR, et al. Screening for dialysis access graft malfunction: comparison of physical examination with US. J Vasc Interv Radiol. 1996;7(1):15–20.
2. Trerotola SO, Ponce P, Stavropoulos SW, et al. Physical examination versus normalized pressure ratio for predicting outcomes of hemodialysis access interventions. J Vasc Interv Radiol. 2003;14(11):1387–94.
3. Malloy PC, Grassi CJ, Kundu S, et al. Consensus guidelines for periprocedural management of coagulation status and hemostasis risk in percutaneous image-guided interventions. J Vasc Interv Radiol. 2009;20(7 Suppl):S240–9.
4. Ayus JC, Sheikh-Hamad D. Silent infection in clotted hemodialysis access grafts. J Am Soc Nephrol. 1998;9(7):1314–7.

Chapter 10
Patient Monitoring, Sedation and Post-Procedure Care

Dheeraj K. Rajan

Monitoring and Sedation

Prior to sedation, local anaesthetic to the site(s) to be punctured should be used. The preferred agent is lidocaine 1% without epinephrine. Lidocaine with epinephrine should be avoided as inadvertent intravascular injection may lead to tachycardia and elevated blood pressure and rarely death. Maximum recommended dose is 3–5 mg/kg. The concentration in 1% lidocaine is 10 mg/mL and 2% lidocaine is 20 mg/mL. Some interventionalists infiltrate the perivascular area to be dilated with lidocaine. Although not studied, some feel this reduces the pain from balloon dilation. For patients with an allergy to lidocaine, bupivacaine is an alternative agent that may be used.

Most percutaneous procedures performed on dialysis patients require minimal sedation which can be provided within the interventional suite. Moderate IV sedation in the form of a sedative (benzodiazepines e.g. Midazolam 0.5–2 mg IV q30–60 min) and opioid

D.K. Rajan (✉)
Head and Associate Professor, Division of Vascular & Interventional Radiology, Department of Medical Imaging, University of Toronto,
Toronto, Ontario, Canada
e-mail: Dheeraj.Rajan@uhn.on.ca

D.K. Rajan (ed.), *Essentials of Percutaneous Dialysis Interventions*,
DOI 10.1007/978-1-4419-5657-6_10,
© Springer Science+Business Media, LLC 2011

analgesics (Fentanyl 25–75 μg IV q 15–60 min or Morphine 1–5 mg IV every 30–60 min) can be administered. Midazolam and fentanyl are most commonly used. Midazolam is a short acting sedative with amnestic properties and fentanyl sulphate is an opiate pain killer that beyond short-term pain coverage provides synergistic effects with midazolam. Both are short acting and can be titrated upwards for effect. The most common initial dosage to use is 1 mg of versed and 50 μg of fentanyl intravenously. When accesses are not clotted, I routinely deliver medications via the access to avoid placing an intravenous line. Almost all patients experience pain with angioplasty and thrombectomy procedures and adequate sedation should be provided prior to the intervention when required.

Prior to providing conscious sedation, it is necessary to have the appropriate personnel, equipment and medications available. In addition, there should be someone accompanying the patient home following the procedure. At least one person other than the physician should be trained in providing conscious sedation and monitoring the patient. Prior to administration of sedation, baseline vitals should be obtained including blood pressure, oxygen saturation and cardiac monitoring via continual electrocardiography (ECG). ECG monitoring and oxygen saturation should be continually monitored and blood pressure intermittently up to every 10 min. The most common side effect of sedation is respiratory depression. This will be detected with oxygen monitoring. All patients should have oxygen available prophylactically or as necessary. For interventions, blood pressure and ECG monitoring may point to or indicate potential complications. Vitals should be checked every 15 min in stable situations and more frequently with changes in the patient condition. Premature ventricular complexes (PVC's) are often noted when a wire is within the right ventricle and is a precursor to potentially fatal arrhythmias when six or more PVC's occur in succession. Repositioning of the wire is required. If the patient develops a sudden drop in pressure and tachycardia depending on the intervention a significant pulmonary or air embolism may have occurred, the patient may have developed pericardial tamponade or may be bleeding. For syncopal episodes, conservative supportive measures are sufficient. Rarely, in the event of persistent bradycardia, atropine 0.5–1.0 mg can be given IV every 5 min as needed to a maximum total dose of 3.0 mg.

Medications to reverse the effects of sedation should be present which include naloxone to reverse opiate intoxication. In children, a dose of 0.1 mg/kg is recommended and given IM or IV. In adults, an initial naloxone dose of 0.4–2 mg is recommended, with the selection of dose determined by the patient's respiratory status and likelihood of precipitating opiate withdrawal. This dose may be repeated every 2–3 min until full reversal is achieved or to a maximum of 10 mg. This can be delivered intravenously. For benzodiazepine reversal, flumazenil can be given IV. In adults 0.2 mg is given IV initially over 15 s with repeated doses of 0.2 mg given every 60 s as necessary up to a maximum of 5 mg. In children, the dose is 0.01 mg/kg to a maximum of 0.05 mg/kg. For reversal of heparin, 1 mg of protamine sulphate per 100 units of heparin can be delivered. This dose is dependent on the time of heparin administration and should be scaled back in correlation with the half life of heparin which is 60 min. Maximum dose is 50 mg. An infusion rate of a 10 mg/mL solution should not exceed 5 mg/min. Hypersensitivity reactions to protamine sulphate may occur in patients with known hypersensitivity reactions to fish or those previously exposed to protamine therapy or protamine-containing insulin. Reactions include symptoms associated with histamine release, bradycardia, dyspnea and pulmonary hypertension.

Post-Procedure Care

Following completion of interventions, assuming no complications, the patient can resume all medications at their scheduled times. Observation/recovery time is dependent on the interventions performed and medications given. In general, an observation time of 1 h is sufficient for most interventions and to recover from any moderate sedation provided and to monitor for potentially late occurring complications. This monitoring time also allows for heparin effect to wear off rather than reversing it for removal of access sheaths or devices. If unusual amounts of sedation or heparinization were given or there is a concern of complications following the procedure, a greater length of observation time is suggested. The patient should be placed in a monitored environment and be monitored by a person sufficiently trained in conscious sedation and in the recognition of changes in vitals and ECG monitoring. Heparin half life is approximately 60 min but is prolonged in renal failure patients. Continuous patient oxygen saturation and ECG monitoring with intermittent blood pressure should be conducted until the patient is able to tolerate oral intake, is oriented and is freely ambulatory (if possible prior to procedure) with stable vital signs. To date, no medication has been found that can be administered to a patient that confers longer durability of any dialysis interventions performed. At the time of discharge, appropriate written instructions should be given to the patient.

A procedural report should be sent to the dialysis center and managing nephrologist to inform them of the findings and any interventions performed. Possible failure modes for this access should also be documented to direct future monitoring. Close follow-up clinical evaluation, dialysis access pressure measurements, dialysis adequacy determination, and flow rate (if performed) are necessary to verify the effectiveness of the intervention. Additionally, if suboptimal results are obtained percutaneously, personal coordination with the dialysis access coordinator will improve outcomes by allowing better information transfer. Finally, recommendations regarding future access sites and considerations should be detailed to help other physicians in the future care of the patient.

Key Points

- If administering IV sedation, keep reversal medications close at hand.
- Have appropriate equipment/medication on hand to acutely resuscitate patients.
- A proper report is integral to patient care.

Chapter 11
Sterile Technique

Dheeraj K. Rajan

Although percutaneous interventions due to their inherent nature of being minimally invasive have lower infection rates than "open" procedures, proper sterile technique should be followed at all times as an infection of the dialysis access is potentially devastating for a dialysis dependent patient. Patients with dialysis grafts are more prone to infection than dialysis fistulas. However, the risk is minimized with proper sterile technique and prophylactic antibiotics are not necessary. With stent grafts now being placed, for such interventions, antibiotics are recommended (Chaps. 15, 16, 17, 19, 20).

Prevention of nosocomial infections within the interventional suite is of paramount importance. This begins with basic hand sanitation which simply involves washing your hands after seeing each patient. Evolution of this simple process has now evolved to "universal body and blood precautions." Personal protective equipment is part of the overall process as is proper training. This includes sterile gloves, protective eyewear, facemask, gown, shoe covers to protect against

D.K. Rajan (✉)
Head and Associate Professor, Division of Vascular & Interventional Radiology, Department of Medical Imaging, University of Toronto, Toronto, Ontario, Canada
e-mail: Dheeraj.Rajan@uhn.on.ca

D.K. Rajan (ed.), *Essentials of Percutaneous Dialysis Interventions*, DOI 10.1007/978-1-4419-5657-6_11,
© Springer Science+Business Media, LLC 2011

splashes and transmission of infection to the patient, and proper infection control training for all staff. All people who come in contact with blood products should be immunized against hepatitis B. There are specific published guidelines for infection control in healthcare professions by the Centers for Disease Control and Prevention by the U.S. Government [1].

In regards to interventions to be performed, there are a number of steps to obtain maximal sterility of the operating field. They can be broken down into equipment, the operators, and the patient:

1. For equipment, the ideal procedure room would be separated by at least one antechamber from personnel and patients not properly dressed for sterile procedures. Washing stations should be present outside the procedure room. The procedure room itself should ideally be a positive-pressure room with a minimum of six air exchanges per minute.
2. For the operators, proper hand washing techniques prior to each case is required. This should be done with a germicidal and virucidal before each case. Proper barrier precautions of sterile gloves (proper gloving technique), facemask, eye splash protection, a cap to prevent hair from falling into the sterile field, sterile gown, and shoe covers are mandatory. Proper freshly laundered surgical attire (scrubs) should be worn in the procedure room, not be worn in public, and changed daily. Street cloths are not permissible. After completion of each case, the room should be cleaned with washing of the floors with an antiseptic solution and all items that come into patient contact wiped down with antibacterial/antiviral wipes or solutions with changing of any linens on the table.
3. For the patient, they should be changed to a gown with removal of street clothing and footwear. The area of interest where procedures are to be performed should be appropriately prepared. Hair in the area of intervention should be trimmed rather than shaved as shaving causing microabrasions in the skin leading to higher bacterial colonization and therefore a higher risk of infection. If the area of intervention needs to be shaved to trimmed, this should be done immediately prior to sterile preparation to reduce the time for bacterial colonization. The area of intervention should be prepped 2% aqueous chlorhexidine solutions or higher concentrations. This solution has been found to reduce bloodstream infections more than 10% povidone iodine or 70% alcohol

although these solutions may also be used. The preparation solution should be allowed to air dry prior to breaking the skin barrier. Povidone iodine should remain on the skin for at least 2 min before puncture of the skin. The area prepped should widely exceed the area of intervention with large drapes placed (see Fig. 11.1). A few towels around the area to be punctured are not sufficient.

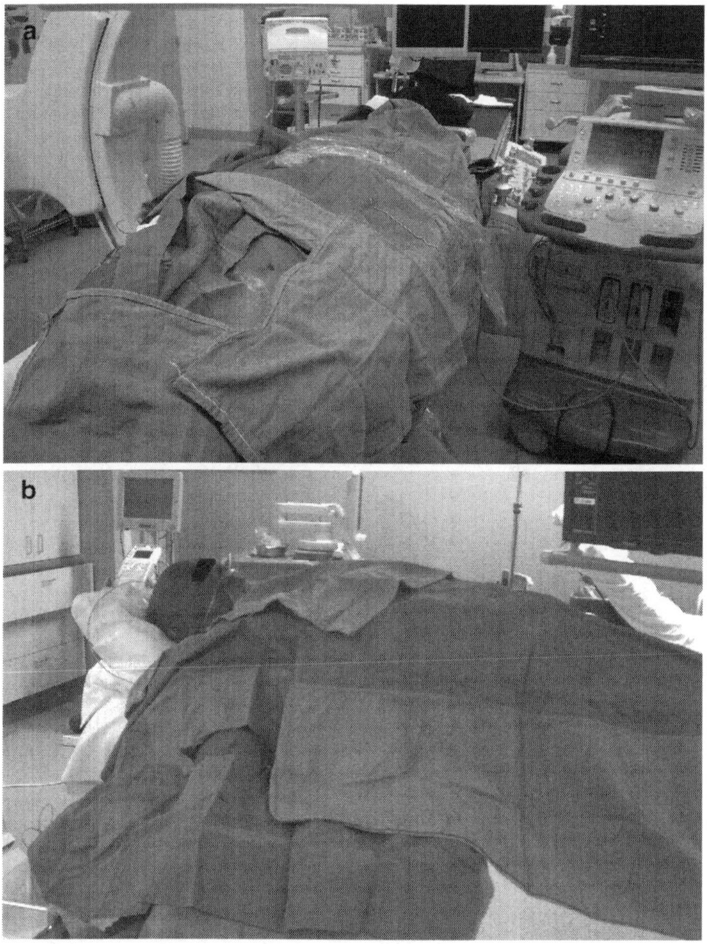

Fig. 11.1 (**a**) Sterile field for jugular catheter insertion. (**b**) Sterile field for arm interventions

At the end of the day, a final cleaning of all surfaces and equipment must be performed.

When working on the patient, basic principals that should be followed include:

1. Proper hand washing before, after and between patients is required.
2. The scrubbed operators function only within the sterile field.
   (a) Sterile operators work on the patient with non-sterile personnel in the periphery.
   (b) The sterile field on the operator is limited to the gown portions directly viewed by the scrubbed person. These sterile areas include the gown front, from chest to the sterile field level, and the sleeves from 5 cm above the elbow to the cuff.
3. Sterile drapes create a sterile area of operation.
   (a) Sterile drapes should cover the patient and exposed equipment with only the area where the punctures are to be performed exposed.
   (b) The drapes should be fluid resistant to prevent soaking through to the patient and therefore preventing a transmission route for bacteria.
4. Only sterile items should be used in the sterile field.
5. All items introduced into the sterile field should be done in a manner to maintain sterility of the items.
   (a) Most packaging of items used for dialysis interventions allow for sterile transfer by allowing the other protective packaging to be peeled back away from the item to be used.
6. All personnel should be aware of the sterile field and move in ways to maintain the field.
7. All sterile items to be used or have been used should remain within the sterile field.
   (a) Transient bacteremia is the most common problem encountered with percutaneous interventions and is often the result of poor wire management from contamination of the distal end of the wire when it leaves the sterile field.
8. If using ultrasound, the probe must also be contained within a sterile protective barrier.

Dialysis dependent patients have limited venous access and are more prone to infections than the general population. It is imperative to do what is possible to prevent infections in these patients as this directly translates into an accelerated rate of mortality through loss of accesses. Aseptic technique prevents the transfer of microorganisms and plays an important role in reduction of puncture site infections. All members involved in interventions should be aware of and knowledgeable of aseptic practices to provide an important component to patient care.

Key Points

- A sterile environment for interventions is created by considering the patient, the operator, and the operating environment.
- All persons interacting within the sterile environment should be properly instructed on sterile technique and sterile environment.
- The back end of the wire straying out of the sterile field is the most common cause of break in sterile technique.

Reference

1. Bolyard EA, Tablan OC, Williams WW, Pearson ML, Shapiro CN, Deitchmann SD. Guideline for infection control in healthcare personnel, 1998. Hospital Infection Control Practices Advisory Committee. Infect Control Hosp Epidemiol. 1998;19(6):407–63.

Chapter 12
Contrast Agents

Dheeraj K. Rajan

Standard Agents

Intravascular use approved iodinated contrast agents should be used unless the patient has a known severe contrast allergy or still retains compromised renal function. An allergy to shellfish does not indicate a risk for an allergic reaction to IV dye and premedication is not necessary. Modern intravenous contrast agents are typically based on iodine. The more iodine, the denser the radiographic image where contrast is present and the contrast is more viscous. For use in dialysis interventions, an iodine concentration around 300 mg/mL is sufficient. There are a variety of manufacturers that supply this product in varying forms and concentrations. In reality, for applications mentioned within this publication, there is little difference. Intravenous contrast may be bound either in an organic nonionic (low osmolarity) compound or an ionic compound (high osmolarity). Although the

D.K. Rajan (✉)
Head and Associate Professor, Division of Vascular & Interventional Radiology, Department of Medical Imaging, University of Toronto,
Toronto, Ontario, Canada
e-mail: Dheeraj.Rajan@uhn.on.ca

D.K. Rajan (ed.), *Essentials of Percutaneous Dialysis Interventions*,
DOI 10.1007/978-1-4419-5657-6_12,
© Springer Science+Business Media, LLC 2011

cost is lower for ionic agents, one should endeavor to use nonionic opposed to ionic contrast when possible. It is associated with a lower incidence of heat sensation, pain, produces fewer cardiovascular changes, allergic reactions, and nephrotoxicity but has not shown a reduction in neurotoxicity or definite life-threatening reactions. The risk of severe life-threatening contrast reaction is lower than 1:10,000 with direct related mortality 10 times lower than this (1:100,000).

For chronic renal failure patients, contrast nephropathy is typically not a concern as there is no residual renal function. However, all attempts should still be made to limit amount of contrast delivered to the patient. The volume delivered should be enough to provide diagnostic images and digital subtraction imaging should be utilized as well. If the patient has residual renal function, depending on how much function is left and the exam to be performed, a choice can be made to use standard contrast agents alone in very limited volumes (as renal damage is dose dependent). Iodixanol (Visipaque, GE Healthcare) is associated with a lower risk of contrast induced nephropathy. Contrast agents can also be used with hydration (0.9% $NaHCO_3$ 1–2 mg/kg/h 3–6 h before the procedure with at least 300–500 mL given before the procedure), and renal protective medications such as fenoldopam (0.1 μg/kg/min initiated 2 h prior to the procedure and continued at a rate of 0.4 μg/kg/min for 4 h during and after the procedure) and/or *N*-acetylcysteine (1,200 mg orally bid, given day before and day of contrast administration) or alternative contrast agents that are not nephrotoxic. There is a substantial amount of evidence that indicates preprocedure hydration is as effective as and potentially more effective than fenoldopam and/or *N*-acetylcysteine.

Alternative Agents

If the patient presents with an IV contrast allergy beyond correction with steroid premedication or retains minimal renal function (Chap. 9), two alternative contrast agents that could be used were gadolinium and carbon dioxide gas. However, within the last couple of years, *nephrogenic systemic fibrosis* (*NSF*) or nephrogenic fibrosing dermopathy has been identified as a distinct potential serious complication of gadolinium injection particularly in renal compromised patients. NSF is a syndrome causing fibrous plaques and nodules to form in the skin, joints, eyes, and internal organs including the heart. Flexion contractures can occur. The Food and Drug Administration has issued warnings regarding its use and guidelines for use of gadolinium-based contrast agents that have been published by the American College of Radiology [1]. Gadolinium should be *absolutely avoided* in any renal compromised patient undergoing percutaneous dialysis interventions.

The remaining alternative is carbon dioxide gas. There are certain characteristics that one needs to know before using the agent. It is naturally occurring and therefore readily available. CO_2 is not associated with any nephrotoxicity or allergic reactions. It is roughly 20 times more soluble than oxygen. Since it is a gas, it has minimal viscosity (>400 times less viscous than iodinated contrast) and therefore flows very rapidly. It also expands in more open spaces and rises to the least dependent position. Gas is a negative contrast agent and will show up as a radiolucent or white area on imaging. Also, outline of the graft or fistula is obtained by displacement of blood. Carbon dioxide as an imaging agent does not mix with blood. Hence, larger volumes are required for imaging. Also, given its low viscosity, it travels very rapidly through the area being imaged and breaks up rather than diluting with blood. Hence, a higher imaging rate is required (at least four frames per second) and images may have be stacked or summated to visualize the access circuit segment being imaged.

Carbon dioxide may be used but should not be refluxed across the arterial anastomosis due to risk of neurological events and death. It should also not be used in patients with a patent foramen ovale. Particular care should be used when refluxing it across the arterial anastomosis as it can very easily reflux back to the aortic arch with potential devastating complications such as a stroke. Also note that CO_2 may overestimate the degree of stenosis [2]. *No carbon dioxide should be directly injected into the arterial system above the diaphragm.* There is associated neurotoxicity. The maximum volume injected should be under 200 cc over a 2–3 min period as carbon dioxide is excreted through the lungs and may build up in the blood system causing hypercapnia. It takes 2–3 min to completely dissolve in blood. Lower volumes and greater caution should be used in patients with chronic obstructive pulmonary disease as their ability to excrete CO_2 is reduced.

Since CO_2 is odorless and colorless, care must be taken to avoid air contamination which may cause potentially serious complications. The CO_2 canister should contain laboratory grade 99.99%

CO_2. The canister should never be directly connected to the imaging catheter or sheath as this can deliver an excessive amount of CO_2. Hand injections via a syringe should be performed. A closed system should be used that allows for purging the syringe at least 3 times to remove air contamination. Our preference is a connection tubing connected to the canister which has a controlled flow valve and at the other end connecting a three-way stopcock. A one-way stopcock is connected to a 20 or 50 cc syringe and connected to the three-way stopcock and both are opened to the canister (see Fig. 12.1). Flow is turned up to the point of filling the syringe at a satisfactory rate. After the syringe fills, the stopcock between the syringe stopcock and canister is turned off to the canister and opened to air to purge the syringe. The stopcock is then turned closed to air to allow refilling of the syringe with CO_2. This process is performed at least 3

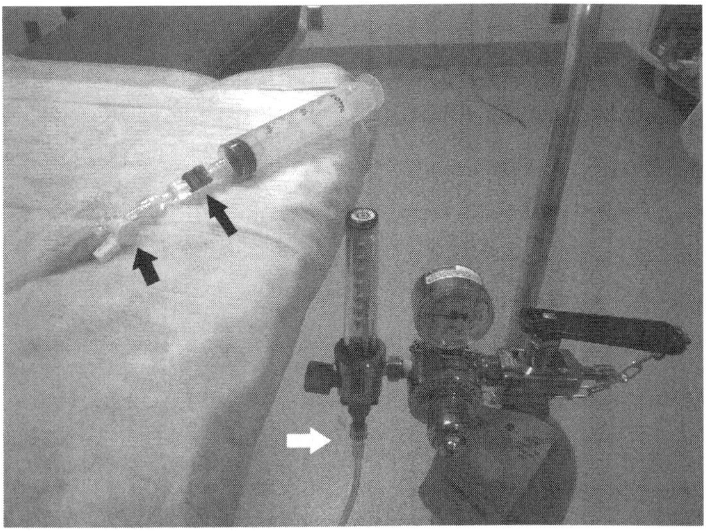

Fig. 12.1 Carbon dioxide system. Flow regulator to control volume and flow rate (*white arrow*). A microfilter can be attached at this level. A 20 cc syringe with a one-way stopcock is connected to the three-way stopcock (*black arrows*) connected via connection tubing to the flow regulator. The system is closed to room air and the three-way stopcock allows for purging of the system to remove air contamination. The one-way stopcock in the closed position after proper filling and purging allows for transfer of the CO_2 filled syringe and connection to the catheter with no air contamination

times to purge air contamination from the system. When completed, the one-way stopcock on the syringe is closed and the filled syringe with the one-way stopcock is removed from the three-way stopcock. One should make sure the three-way stopcock is turned to close off flow from the canister. The syringe is then attached to the imaging catheter or sheath, the one-way stopcock is opened and the CO_2 is injected. Volume and rate of delivery are dependent on the size and flow rate of the territory being imaged where a faster injection rate is required in a high flow state. Commercial systems are not available for delivering CO_2 for imaging purposes at this time but are under development with a potential device available from Merit Medical shortly.

In the dialysis patient, if the systolic blood pressure drops by 10–20 mmHG from baseline, one should suspect air contamination. Since gas rises, it is not uncommon for CO_2 to pool in the upper portion of pseudoaneurysms and aneurysms. No other agents are approved for intravascular imaging use.

Key Points

- CO_2 creates an image of the vascular structure by displacing blood, not mixing with it. Hence, a sufficient volume is needed to displace blood in the structure to be visualized.
- CO_2 should not be used in the arterial system above the diaphragm. Be very careful using it as even a gentle injection within the access can result in reflux back through the arterial system to the brain.
- The degree of stenosis is overestimated with CO_2.
- Do *not* use gadolinium products.
- Nonionic contrast is preferred but not absolutely necessary.

References

1. http://www.acr.org/SecondaryMainMenuCategories/quality_safety/contrast_manual/NephrogenicSystemicFibrosis.aspx.
2. Ehrman KO, Taber TE, Gaylord GM, Brown PB, Hage JP. Comparison of diagnostic accuracy with carbon dioxide versus iodinated contrast material in the imaging of hemodialysis access fistulas. J Vasc Interv Radiol. 1994;5(5):771–75.

Chapter 13
Dialysis Catheters

Sandford Altman and Dheeraj K. Rajan

Dialysis catheters represent a necessary evil for those on dialysis. Referred to as "the great white tube of death" by some, this potentially high risk means of access can be a life saver for others. The DOQI guidelines recommend that no more than 10% of permanent access be in the form of catheters. Despite these recommendations, at many centers the percentage of patients dependent on catheters is significantly higher with rates approaching 40%. Although catheters are associated with poor patency (less than 60% at 6 months), high infection rates (1–5/1,000 catheter days), high overall costs relative to functionality, and central vein destruction, they are required in many situations. These include acute renal failure, emergent presentation of chronic renal failure, bridging device for fistula or graft maturation, temporizing measure related to graft or fistula infiltration, infection or surgical revision, permanent access for those without fistula or graft options or those suffering from labile pressure, and severe hypotension.

S. Altman (✉)
Open Access Vascular Access Center,
Miami, Florida, USA
e-mail: saltman@oavac.com

D.K. Rajan (ed.), *Essentials of Percutaneous Dialysis Interventions*,
DOI 10.1007/978-1-4419-5657-6_13,
© Springer Science+Business Media, LLC 2011

In the past, temporary catheter placement was the norm for patients presenting with a clotted graft or fistula awaiting an elective surgical declotting procedure. Over the last decade there has been a paradigm shift, treating the clotted or dysfunctional access emergently, obviating the need for these temporary catheters. Although this has led to a decline in the use of temporary catheters, permanent catheters still play a role in hemodialysis. As discussed above, temporary catheters often serve as a bridging device for graft or fistula creation and maturation. In some instance, patient preference with regards to access type still plays a role in catheter access. For the ill informed, the idea of having a painless means to connect ones vascular system to the dialysis machine is appealing. Although despite the fact that patient education on the perils of catheter access still occasionally lands on deaf ears, once educated, the majority of patients opt for a fistula or graft. Over the last 5 years in the United States, with an increase in fistula incidence and prevalence as championed by the Fistula First initiative, there had also been a rise in the number of dialysis catheters. The most recent USRDS (United States Renal Data System) data, however, has documented a downward trend with catheter rates now estimated at 19%.

If a dialysis catheter is required, it should be well thought out prior to its placement understanding the long term vascular access needs of the patient. Although for a select few, a tunneled catheter may be the only access option remaining, for the majority, better access options exist. For each and every patient a vascular access plan should be formulated with the goal of creating the best access that will function the longest with the fewest complications. For the majority, a tunneled catheter is not that access. It may be a bridge to that access, but given its patency, morbidity, and mortality, it is less than ideal.

Types of Hemodialysis Catheters

Simplistically, there are two basic types of catheters used for hemodialysis, those with cuffs and those without. Non-cuffed catheters, better known as "temporary" catheters, carry a higher rate of infection than cuffed, tunneled "permanent" catheters. As such, temporary catheters should be reserved for short term use, typically less than 1 week duration. Temporary catheters are often used for emergent dialysis needs. Unless one is absolutely certain that the need of the catheter is less than a week, if a catheter is required it should be a cuffed tunneled catheter. The greatest risk during catheter placement occurs when access to the vascular system is obtained. Creation of the subcutaneous tunnel carries a relatively low risk to the patient, as compared to the benefit the tunnel provides through infection prevention. Although there are a great number of catheter designs; from single lumen to dual lumen to step tip to staggered tip to split tip to reverse flow, none have proven to be truly superior over the other. In fact, a catheter that functions ideally for one individual may perform suboptimally for another. In addition to varying tip designs, there are different hub assemblies, often related to whether the catheter is tunneled antegrade or retrograde. These two insertion techniques each have their unique advantages some of which are dependent upon the site of insertion and whether the catheter is a new placement or an exchange. Over the last several years, surface coatings have fostered interest, however, as of yet, no clear advantage, at least with regards to tunneled catheters, has been demonstrated.

When and What to Place

Vascular catheters, as previously mentioned are typically placed when immediate access is required. Whether it's a patient presenting with acute renal failure that needs dialysis urgently, or a patient with a mature fistula that had a significant infiltration preventing fistula cannulation, the common thread is the immediate need for a conduit to the vascular system to provide hemodialysis.

If a catheter is going to be required for greater than a week, a cuffed tunneled catheter should be placed. If a catheter is required for a single treatment, or for less than a week a temporary, non-cuffed catheter can be used. These catheters are typically dual lumen catheters. Many are straight, but pre-curved or bendable temporary catheters are often preferred because when these catheters are placed in the jugular veins the hubs of the pre-curved catheters can be positioned over the patient's chest rather than taped high in the neck abutting the face. Temporary femoral catheters are typical used either for a single dialysis treatment or for bed-bound patients. Care must be taken to use a temporary femoral catheter having adequate length so that the tip of the catheter can reach the IVC. In temporary catheters, surface coatings, such as silver, have been proven to reduce the short term risk of infection. Care should be taken to appropriately secure temporary catheters in place as the lack of the cuff and tunnel tract increase the easy of dislodgement. Temporary catheters are often placed at the bed side where it may be more difficult to place a tunneled catheter. Whether the catheter being placed is temporary or tunneled, proper sterile technique is essential. For patients who are septic or have positive blood cultures and are in need of a catheter, temporary catheters can be placed as a bridge until the infection has resolved and a tunneled catheter can be inserted.

Cuffed tunneled hemodialysis catheters are the catheter of choice when a catheter is required for longer than a week. The main advantages of tunneled catheters over temporary catheters are their lower infection rates and the tissue in-growth to the cuff securing the catheter to the body. The tunnel serves as a protective barrier for infection, likely related to the distance it creates from the exit site where bacteria reside to the entrance site where the catheter passes into the sterile vascular system. As such the skin and subcutaneous tissues of the tunnel tract serve as a protective barrier that temporary catheters do not have. Another advantage that tunneled catheters provide in infection prevention is with regard to maintenance of hygiene. Maintenance of hygiene, a necessity for those living with catheters, is typically easier and thus more effective with tunneled catheters as compared to temporary catheters. The exit site of a jugular or subclavian tunneled catheter is typically on the anterior superior chest. Maintenance of hygiene for catheters residing in this location is typically easier and thus superior to temporary catheters that often reside on the neck. The other advantage afforded by the cuff of tunneled catheters as mentioned above is the tissue in-growth which secures the catheter in place. These cuffs, typically made from Dacron, allow for tissue in-growth. Once this has occurred, usually by 3 weeks, the catheters are typically secure in place and do not easily fall out. In fact, removal of these catheters often requires a minor surgical procedure to release the cuff from the tissue in-growth. Some also believe that the cuff provides an additional barrier to infection. Although not proven this is plausible. These cuffed tunneled catheters are often referred to as permanent catheters; however, this is or at least should be a misconception. Although in some patients these catheters function for years, for the majority, by 6 months, these catheters fail. Additionally, for the ill informed patient, referring to any catheter as permanent access probably creates unneeded confusion. Many patients like the idea of a catheter. No needles and no disfiguring appearances on your extremities. Telling patients you are going to place a permanent catheter is sending them the wrong message. For the vast majority of patients, all catheters should be perceived as a temporary bridging device to a superior access.

Sites of Placement

The preferred site for dialysis catheter placement is the right internal jugular vein (IJV). This site is associated with the fewest technical failures, and longest catheter patency. Additionally, the straight descending course of the right IJV into the right brachiocephalic vein (BCV) and SVC typically results in less, long term catheter related, central venous damage than that seen with catheters placed from a left sided approach. Given the anatomy of the left IJV, left BCV, and SVC, catheters living in this tortuous environment serve as a constant irritant to walls of the vessels. It is not unusual to see stenosis or occlusion of the left BCV in someone who previously had a left sided chest catheter. In descending order of catheter entrance preferences (see Fig. 13.1) after the right IJV, one should consider the left IJV, the right external jugular vein (EJV), left EJV, the right subclavian vein, the left subclavian vein, and the right and left femoral veins. Some prefer placing external jugular venous catheters prior to placing subclavian venous catheters. Given the high association between subclavian vein catheterization and occlusion, the subclavian vein should preferably not be catheterized until it has been determined that the contralateral extremity cannot support a graft or fistula.

Femoral venous catheters are typically utilized when the central venous anatomy has been compromised in the chest, or when there is only one dominant central vein in the chest being preserved for fistula or graft creation or maturation. Given the higher rates of bacterial skin colonization in the groin as compared to the chest, femoral catheters carry a higher risk of infection. Patients should be instructed of such and encouraged to pay close attention to their personal hygiene. Additionally, femoral venous catheters should be long enough to have their tip positioned either in the IVC or right atrium. Although no

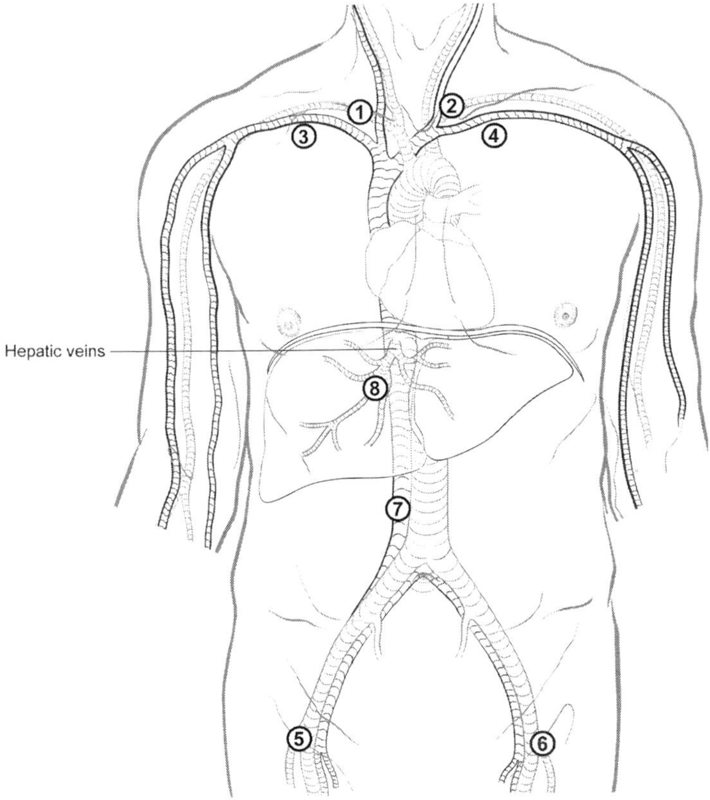

Fig. 13.1 Tunneled catheter insertion sites. (1) Right internal jugular vein. (2) Left internal jugular vein. (3) Right subclavian vein. (4) Left subclavian vein. (5) Right femoral vein. (6) Left femoral vein. (7) Inferior vena cava. (8) Right/middle hepatic veins

studies have conclusively proven whether the IVC or right atrium is the optimal site for femoral catheter tip positioning, if the catheter is too short, resulting in tip placement in the iliac vein, flow will often be sub-optimal. A minimal length of 19 cm should be used to minimize recirculation.

Once the jugular, subclavian, and femoral routes of access have been exhausted, additional sites to gain entrance to the central venous system include the IVC, cervical, thoracic, abdominal, and femoral collateral veins and the hepatic veins. These sites, as one would imagine, often are associated with poorer patency rates. This is usually not related to the site of entrance but the rather the concomitant vascular disease that led to these sites being required. Often, if one takes the time to look for patent vessels utilizing appropriate imaging including ultrasound, CT, MRI, and selective venography, an entrance vessel can usually be obtained. Central venous stenoses or occlusions can often be treated with percutaneous interventions such as angioplasty and stenting to provide a conduit for central venous catheter placement (Chap. 20). Dual access from both cephalad (chest or neck) and caudad (femoral) directions may be required to obtain a route for catheter placement. One should always be aware of anatomic variations which can affect catheter placement such as a duplicated and left sided SVCs and IVCs. In SVC and or IVC occlusion, the tip of the catheter should be placed in the largest draining vein when possible if right atrial positioning is not possible.

In conclusion, catheter placement should be based on the specific needs of the individual patient. The goal is to place the best catheter for the patient that will allow for adequate dialysis with the fewest complications. As catheters are often damaging to the veins in which they live, the choice of the vein utilized for catheter placement should in part be based on the future permanent access (fistula or graft) plans for the patient. When possible it is always best not to place a tunneled catheter on the side of a maturing access.

Placement

There is extensive literature supporting the benefits of image guided catheter placement. Ultrasound guidance for vein cannulation significantly reduces the risks of catheter placement complications such as inadvertent arterial puncture and pneumothorax. Unless the situation calls for emergent placement when image guidance is not available, catheter placement should be performed with imaging. Ultrasound allows for improved venous cannulation while fluoroscopy aids in determining appropriate catheter lengths, guidewire manipulation, and catheter tip positioning. Cardiac monitoring is considered essential by most given the excitability of the atrial-ventricular region and right ventricle which can result in ventricular tachycardia or fibrillation. As outlined in the Center's for Disease Control Guidelines for the Prevention of Catheter infection, appropriate sterile technique including appropriate skin preparation and barriers are essential [1].

Nonimage Guided Placement: Non-Tunneled Catheters

Again, nonimage guided catheter placement should only be performed in emergent conditions to meet the medical needs of the patient. Prior to placing any catheter a detailed history and physical should be performed to determine if prior catheters have been placed in the area you are planning to place the catheter. Prior catheter placement places the patient at greater risk of having an unsuccessful catheter placement. If image guidance is not available, this history is essential. Whether or not image guidance is utilized, take care in insuring that the appropriate skin prep and drape is utilized with full barrier techniques to decrease the incidence of infection. With temporary catheter kits, 18 gauge needles are typically supplied for vein cannulation. Micro access sets (i.e., 22 gauge needle with a 3–5 Fr catheter) may be used instead of 18 gauge needles decreasing the complications associated with inadvertent arterial punctures.

Nonimage Guided IJV Placement (See Fig. 13.2)

1. In the supine position, have the patient turn their head in the opposite direction.
2. Anesthetize the region of anticipated catheter placement.
3. Using the 18 gauge needle (largest needle in the kit) and a small syringe, enter the skin at the top of the jugular triangle. In obese patients where the landmarks are not discernable, a reasonable rule of thumb is to go three finger breadths lateral from the tracheal midline, and three finger breadths up from the clavicle.
4. Palpate for the carotid pulse and make sure you are lateral to this vessel.
5. Insert the needle at 30° and aim for the ipsilateral nipple.
6. Gradually advance the needle, while pulling back on the plunger as you progress; do not apply significant negative pressure on the syringe as it may collapse the vein preventing an intravascular position from being realized. A flash and easy withdrawal of dark blood indicates entrance into the vein. If the blood is pulsating or appears bright red, carotid artery puncture has occurred. Remove

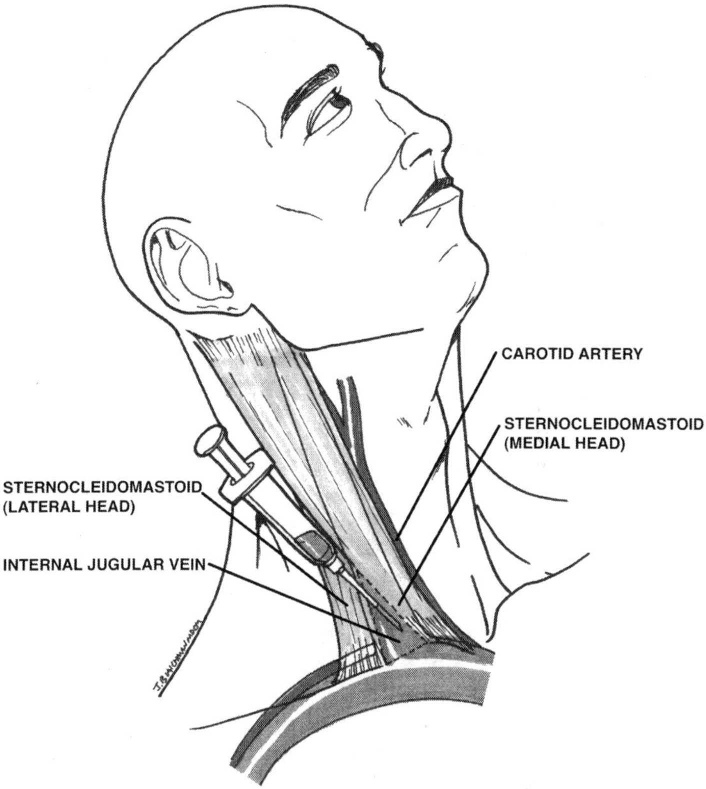

Fig. 13.2 Nonimage guided internal jugular vein (IJV) puncture

the needle, hold pressure for 5–10 min, until bleeding has stopped and there are no signs of hematoma formation and try again.

7. The needle should not need to be advanced more than 2–3 cm in patients with normal body habitus.
8. If more than half the needle has been advanced without blood return, gradually withdraw; you may still get into the vein as you may have collapsed it on the way in.
9. When the vein is entered, venous blood flashback into the syringe will be seen (provided the vein segment is patent). A wire can then be passed through the needle and the temporary dialysis catheter advanced utilizing Seldinger technique.
10. Catheter length is a minimum of 15 cm from the right and 19 cm from the left.

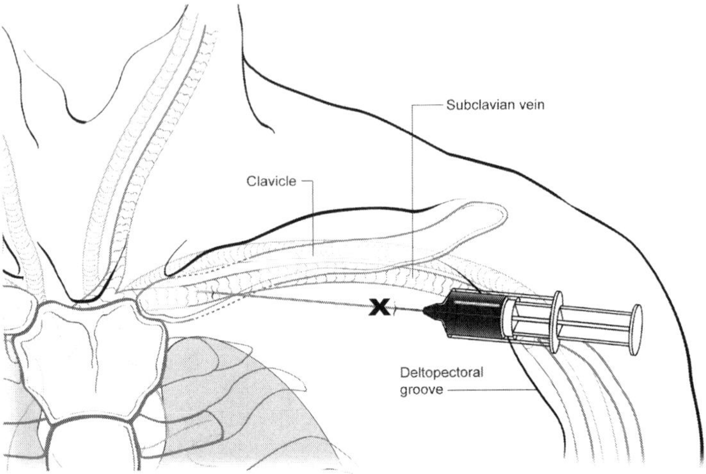

Fig. 13.3 Nonimage guided subclavian vein puncture

Nonimage-Guided Subclavian Vein Puncture (Subclavian Vein Catheters Are Not Recommended Unless Absolutely Necessary as They Place the Greatest Risk on the Patient Including Subclavian Vein Occlusion and Pneumothorax) (See Fig. 13.3)

1. A rolled up towel is placed vertically between the shoulder blades to drop the shoulders back.
2. Prep, drape, and anesthetize as described above.
3. In the supine position, your entrance site should be located two finger widths medial to the deltopectoral groove and two finger widths below the clavicle.
4. Direct the 18 gauge needle medially towards the suprasternal or manubrial notch passing under the clavicle.
5. A shallow angle of passage is important to enter just under the clavicle and avoid piercing the pleura.
6. While advancing the needle, gentle aspiration should be applied until venous blood is aspirated or the needle has passed beyond the clavicle. If the subclavian artery is punctured (located posterosuperior to the vein), the needle should be withdrawn, pressure applied for 5–10 min until bleeding stops and there are no signs of hematoma formation and the angle of cannulation changed slightly.

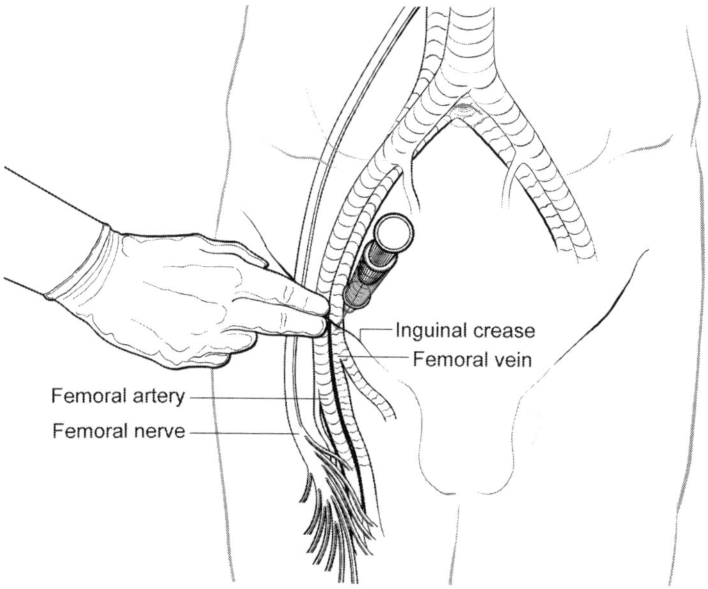

Fig. 13.4 Nonimage guided femoral vein puncture

7. When the vein is entered, venous blood flashback into the syringe will be seen (provided the vein segment is patent). A wire can then be passed through the needle and the temporary dialysis catheter advanced utilizing Seldinger technique.
8. Catheter length is a minimum of 15 cm from the right and 19 cm from the left as with jugular punctures.

Nonimage-Guided Femoral Catheter Placement (Given the High Infection Rate Seen with Femoral Catheters, Their Use Should Be Reserved for Patients Who Cannot Have an IJV or EJV Catheter Placed) (See Fig. 13.4)

1. Prep, drape, and anesthetize the patient.
2. The femoral vein is best cannulated over the medial third of the mid femoral head. In thin patients this is usually at the inguinal crease, however, for heavier patients with a large pannus, the external anatomic landmarks may be obscured.

3. The neurovascular bundle as it exits the inguinal canal is NAVel (Nerve, Artery, Vein) to the navel from lateral to medial. Palpate the femoral artery over the femoral head. Securing the pulsating artery with one hand, puncture the vein with the 18 gauge needle or micro access needle medial to the artery with the other. The femoral vein tracks in most cases immediately adjacent to the artery. Aspirate on your way down and if no venous return is noted, aspirate on the way back. When aspirating do not apply pressure to the femoral artery as this can inadvertently compress the femoral vein preventing venous return.
4. When the vein is entered, venous blood flashback into the syringe will be seen (provided the vein segment is patent). A wire can then be passed through the needle and the temporary dialysis catheter advanced utilizing Seldinger technique.

A simple trick to reduce potential complications for nonimage guided punctures is to find the vein using a much smaller gauge needle, e.g., 22 gauge to aid in localization. All nonimage guided catheter insertions should have a chest X-ray post insertion prior to use to verify catheter tip position and exclude complications. All catheters should be secured with appropriate sutures. Sterile dressing should be applied at the entrance site to decrease the risk of infection.

Image Guided Insertion

There are many studies documenting the benefits of image guided over nonimage guided catheter placement. The main advantages include a lower complication rate, an improved technical success and improved catheter patency. Image guidance typically includes ultrasound imaging for cannulation of the vein and fluoroscopic imaging for guidewire manipulation and catheter tip positioning.

After a focused history and physical has been performed and the anticipated vein for catheter placement has been chosen, an ultrasound should be performed to confirm its patency. Typically, a 7–12 MHz linear ultrasound probe is used. This should be done prior to prepping and draping the patient in order to prevent any potential problems related to unknown central venous occlusion. Sonographically, the vein to be punctured should have a thin wall, be compressible, have flow within it and not be pulsatile. Color Doppler imaging can provide further visual information for the operator with regards to the course of the vessel and its proximity to the neighboring artery. For those not familiar with color Doppler, the color display (i.e., blue or red) is assigned by the operator and is indicative of flow direction, not artery or vein. If one is unsure as to whether they are imaging an artery or vein, wave form analysis and compressibility are good sonographic indicators. Arteries are noncompressible, pulsatile vessels with a high resistance arterial waveform. Veins are compressible, non-pulsatile vessels with a low resistance waveform having respiratory variation.

Once the patient has been examined, and the preferred vessel to be used has been chosen based on current and future permanent access needs of the patients and sonographic confirmation of vessel patency, the patient should be appropriately positioned prepped and draped. A sterile sleeve should be placed on the ultrasound probe to maintain sterility. Additionally sterile ultrasound gel should be utilized. As previously mentioned, one of the main benefits of ultrasound guidance is the lower complication rate. Following this same logic, micro access systems, typically using 21 or 22 gauge needles, are safer than 18 gauge needles and should be considered for vessel cannulation. Scored echogenic needles may also be used to aide in visualization of the needle during ultrasound guidance. After the skin has been anesthetized, the micropuncture needle can be advanced under ultrasound guidance. Once the needle is noted to be abutting the wall of the vein a quick 1–3 mm stab may be useful in allowing passage of the needle through the complaint venous wall. In experienced hands the needle can be visualized cannulating through the wall of the vein, preventing a back wall puncture. Occasionally, the needle will pass through both the front and back walls of the vein. If this occurs, pull the needle back slowly while aspirating until brisk blood is back aspirated through the needle into the syringe. It is preferred to have a 10 cc or smaller syringe on the end of the needle filled with a small amount of saline for aspiration purposes. This also helps to prevent entry of air into the venous system that could occur through an open ended needle.

After entry into the vein, an appropriate wire (typically 0.018 in., included in most catheter sets) is passed into the vein under fluoroscopic visualization. This helps to verify a venous rather than arterial side cannulation. For upper body venous access, whenever possible, the wire should be advanced into the IVC to decrease the incidence of cardiac arrhythmias. Following advancement of the wire the needle can be removed over the wire for introduction of the micro-access catheter. Prior to removal of the 0.018 in. wire, it can be used as a measuring tool to determine the appropriate size catheter to be placed. This measurement is performed by positioning the tip of the wire at the desired future catheter tip location, then bending the end of the wire at the catheter hub, pulling the wire back to the vein entrance site and then bending the wire again at the catheter hub. The distance between the two bends represents the distance from the desired catheter tip position to the vein entrance site. If one then measures the desired length of the tunnel tract, adds that length to the length determined from the guidewire bends and subtracts 1–2 cm for the cuff position in the tunnel tract, the correct cuff to tip length catheter can be determined. Another method is by laying the catheter over the patient's chest wall and positioning the tip and catheter course on the chest wall with fluoroscopy where you want it to end up intravascularily. Then from the exit site, determine how much of the catheter from this point to the hub will be subcutaneous. Based on this length, the location of your exit site will be determined. If this method is employed, care should be taken to compensate for a patient having a large chest which introduces parallax. The catheter length will be longer than what is actually needed (see Fig. 13.5). Catheters are typically made in 19, 23, 27, 31, and 50 cm *tip to cuff* lengths. Most skilled in ultrasound guidance develop their own technique for imaging the vein during cannulation. Many image the vein in its transverse projection (cross section) although some prefer to image it in its longitudinal projection. Scanning the vein with one hand, while cannulating the vein with the other, is a skill that requires time to perfect.

For ultrasound guided IJV punctures the vein should be cannulated along its anterolateral or lateral walls (see Fig. 13.6). A more lateral wall puncture typically allows for a less acute angle from the vein entrance site to the tunnel tract decreasing the incidence of catheter kinking. Care should be taken not to pierce the musculature (i.e., sternocleidomastoid) as this can result in long term catheter pain whenever the patient moves their neck. A low jugular vein puncture is preferable, ideally less than 2 cm above the clavicular head. Higher jugular punctures can cause patient discomfort when moving the neck and are prone to kinking. For ultrasound guided femoral vein punctures, the common femoral vein is punctured anteriorly. For ultrasound guided subclavian vein punctures, the subclavian vein may be difficult to visualize but often can imaged around the lateral

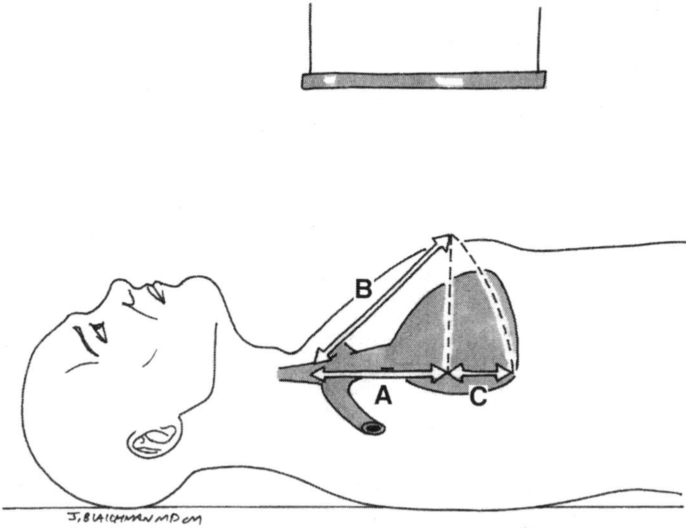

Fig. 13.5 Measurement of catheter length with fluoroscopy. (A) Ideal length of catheter from puncture site to proximal right atrium. (B) If the patient has a sloped or has a barrel chest, AP fluoroscopic imaging would falsely suggest proper length (B). However, when the catheter is inserted, the extra length translates into too long a length (A+C)

a

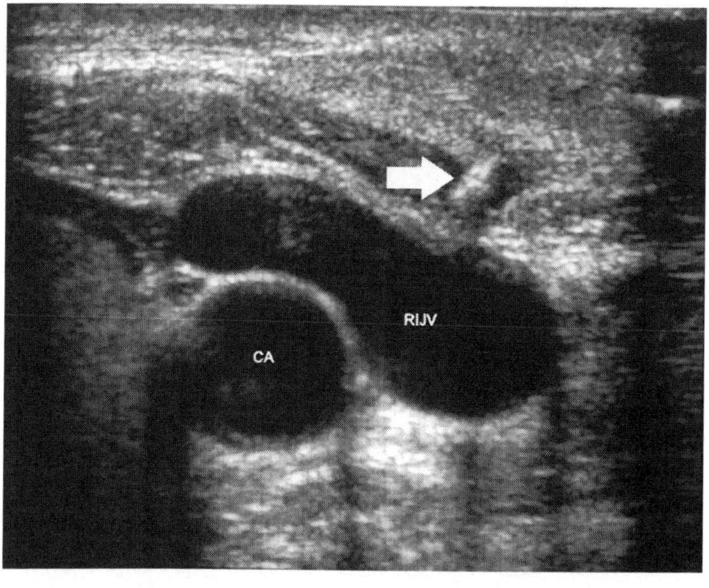

Fig. 13.6 (**a**) Anterolateral puncture of the right internal jugular vein. The needle tip appears as a bright or echogenic line with ultrasound (*arrow*)

b

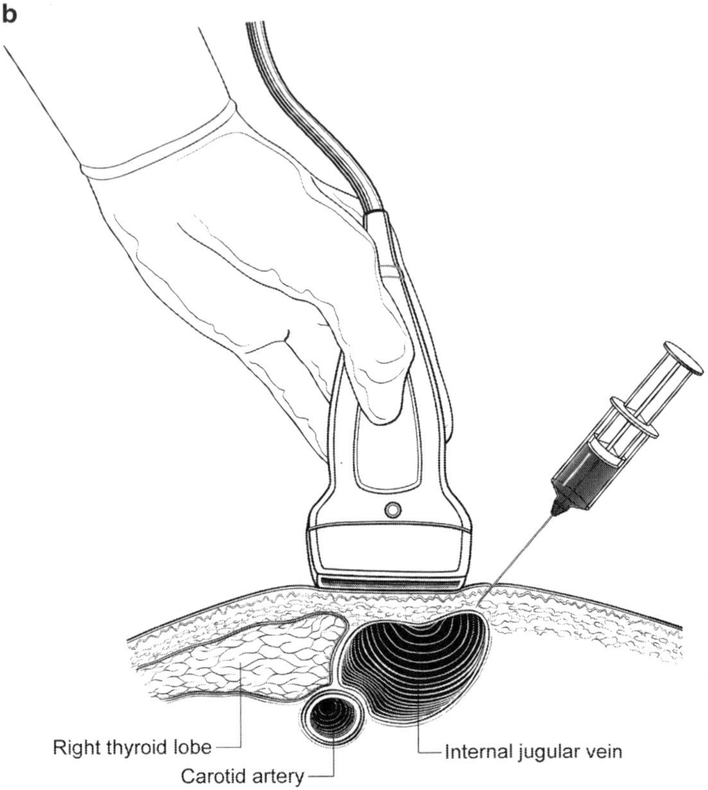

c

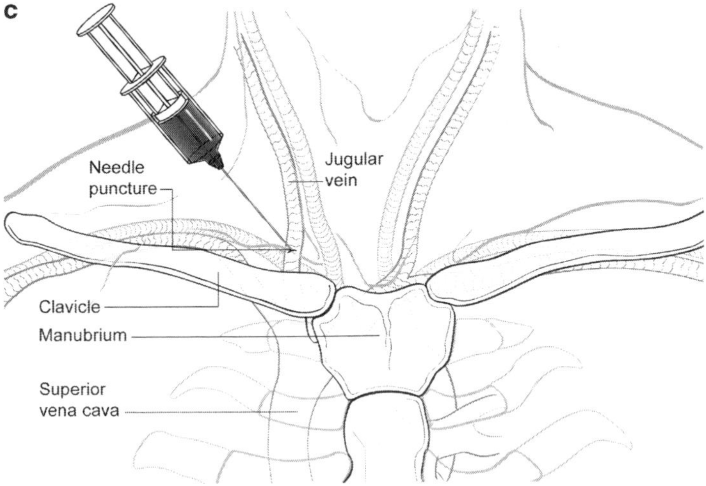

Fig. 13.6 (continued) (*RIJV* right internal jugular vein; *CA* carotid artery). (**b**) Illustration of RIJV puncture location in the axial and (**c**) the coronal plane

third of the clavicle. The puncture is made directly into the antero-inferior aspect of the vein.

If there is any concern that arterial puncture has occurred multiple options exist to verify location. One can pass the wire forward and note the course. The wire should pass to the right of the spine as it passes into the heart (assuming no congenital variations). If the wire crosses to or stays on the left, one should suspect arterial puncture. Another method is to advance a small catheter over the wire and inject contrast to verify intravenous location. If one is using a micro-puncture access set, the inner 3 Fr catheter can be used. One can also transduce the small catheter and determine if arterial or venous pressures are obtained.

Cuffed Tunneled Catheter Placement: Most catheters kits include the appropriate tools required for insertion of the catheters (unless the catheters are ordered specifically without them). The length of catheter to be inserted is dependent on the desired tip and cuff locations. Catheter tips are typically positioned either in the right atrium, caval-atrial junction, SVC, or IVC. Ideal tip positioning may be catheter dependent. No definite studies have proven the ideal location for a catheter tip although the proximal right atrium is considered ideal. The catheter cuff should be situated within 2 cm of the catheter exit site. This allows for easy release of the cuff at time of catheter exchange or removal. Once the desired tip and cuff positions have been determined, the appropriate sized catheter can be chosen.

Internal/External Jugular Vein Insertion (See Fig. 13.7)

Although as previously discussed the veins should be visualized prior to prepping the patient to avoid problems, it is wise when possible to prep both sides of the chest and neck. Occasionally, even though the more superficial veins may appear patent sonographically, unrecognized proximal vein occlusions may prevent successful catheter placement from the intended approach. In this situation, if the contralateral side has already been prepped, the procedure need not be interrupted. After appropriately prepping and draping the area, local anesthesia is administered subcutaneously and subdermally typically using a 25 gauge needle. The micro access needle is then advanced through the skin and puncture of the jugular vein is performed as described above using ultrasound guidance. The catheter length is

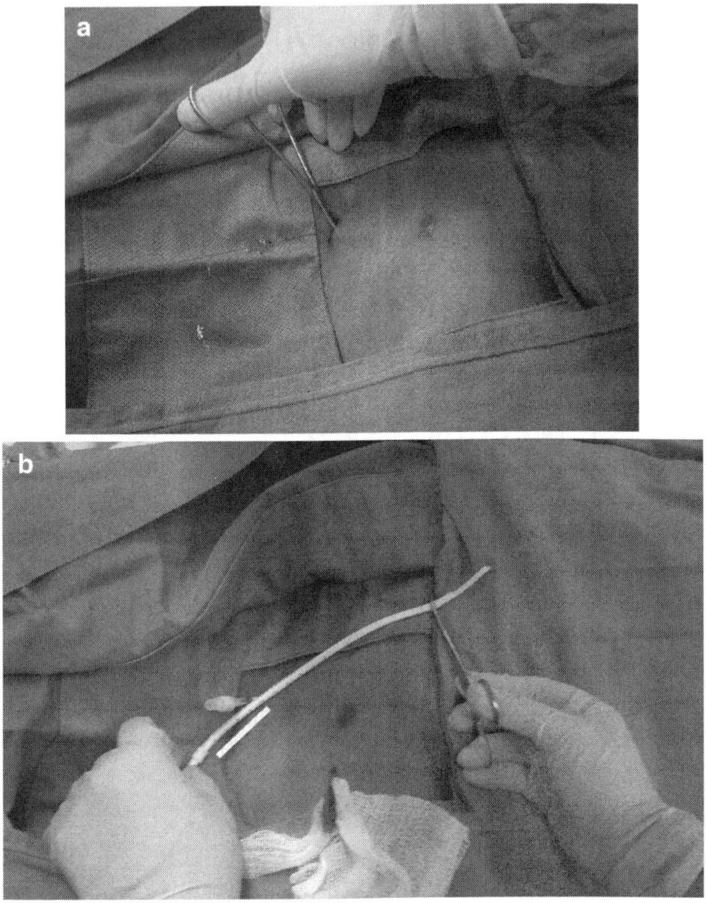

Fig. 13.7 Right internal jugular vein tunneled catheter insertion. After puncture of the vein and insertion of a wire into the SVC or IVC (**A**) a small incision is made by the needle and using small snaps a small pocket is created in the subcutaneous tissues laterally to prevent kinking of the catheter. (**b**, **c**) Intravascular length of the catheter is estimated with fluoroscopy. (**d**) Chest skin incision is made and the catheter is tunneled from the chest incision to the neck incision. (**e**, **f**) Peel away sheath is advanced into the vein with continuous fluoroscopic visualization. (**g**) After removal of peel-away sheath, a small portion of the catheter is knuckled through the incision and this is massaged down with a finger into the vein. (**h**) Catheter now placed with the tip (**i**) in the expected location of the proximal right atrium with arterial lumen pointed away from the atrial wall. (**j**) The skin incision site is stitched to close the gap and a hanging stitch from the exit site secures the catheter

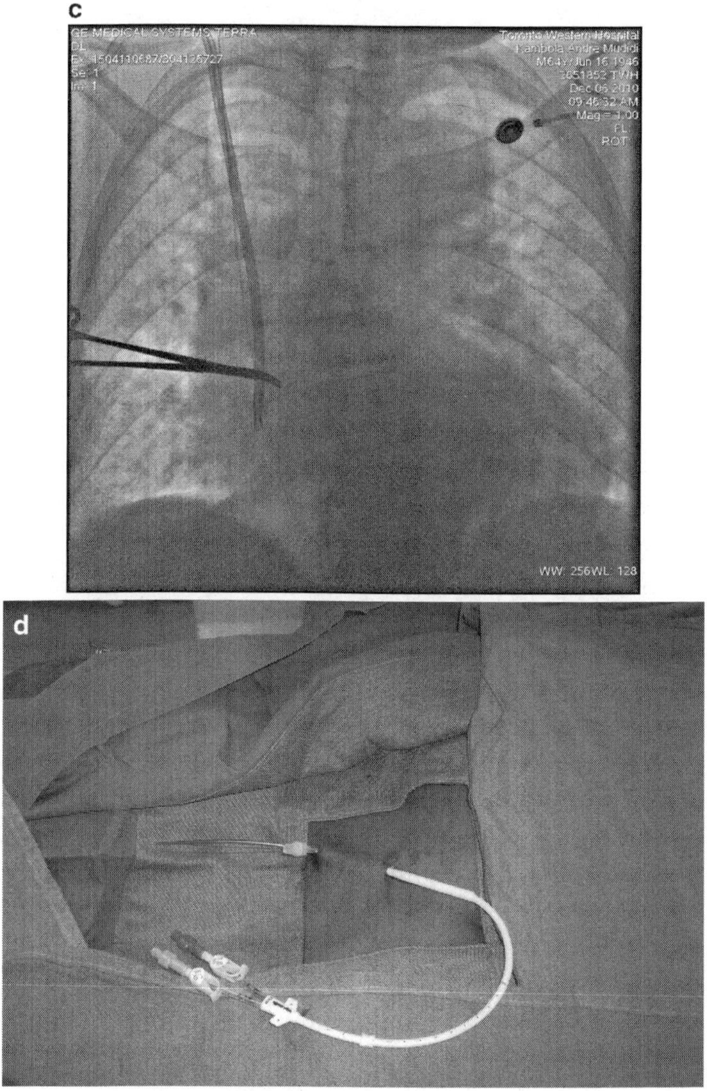

Fig. 13.7 (continued)

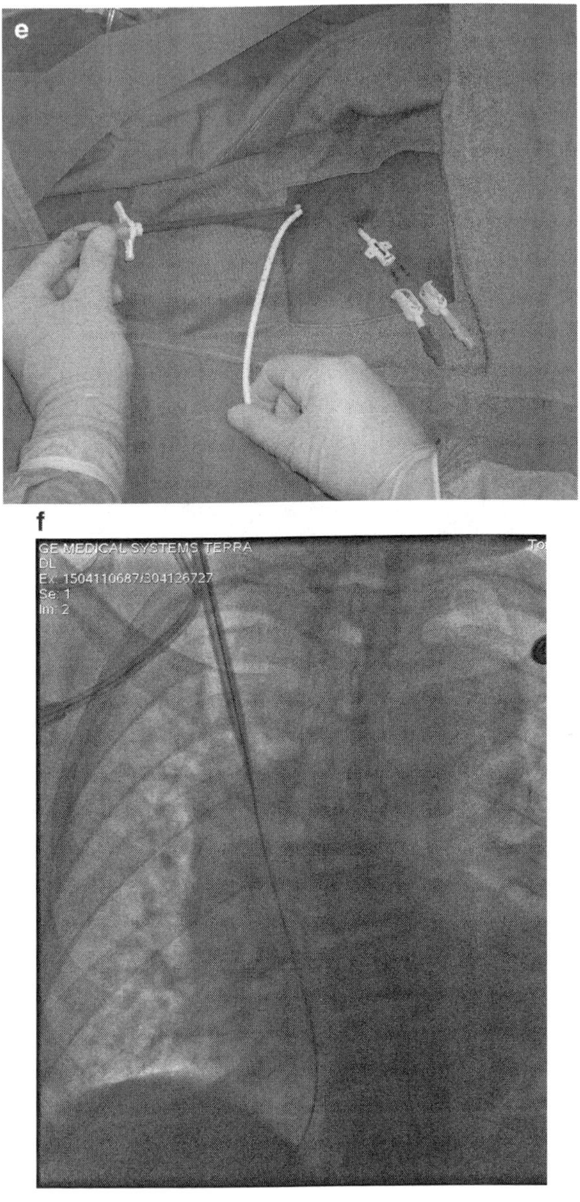

Fig. 13.7 (continued)

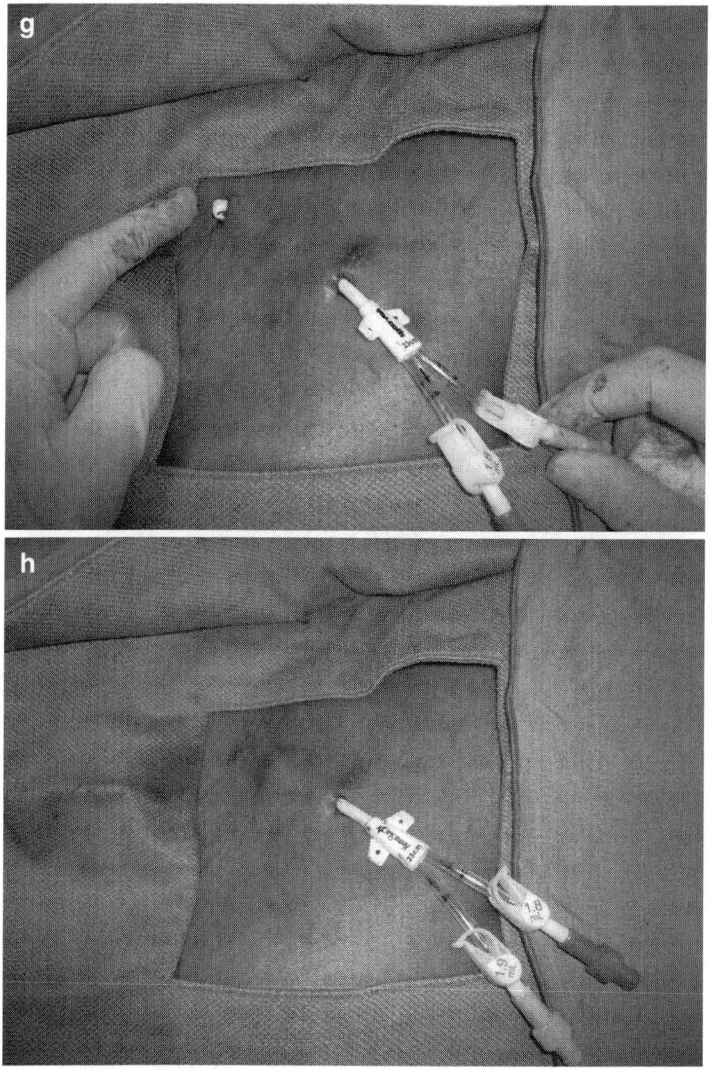

Fig. 13.7 (continued)

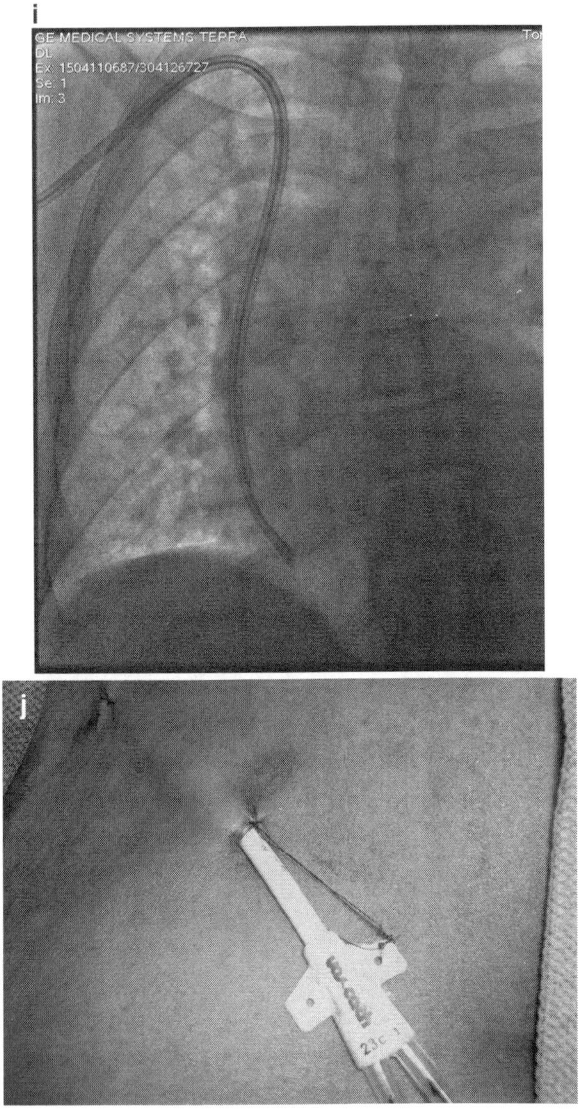

Fig. 13.7 (continued)

determined and the catheter is chosen. As previously mentioned there are many different types of catheters none of which work ideally for every patient. For patients with known "small veins" or central venous stenosis, a smaller diameter catheter may be preferable (14.5 Fr instead of 15.5 Fr) as it may decrease the risk of the patient developing a catheter related SVC syndrome. For small right atria or caval atrial issues, reverse flow catheters may be preferred. Left sided placements may be felt by some to be easier using a retrograde tunneled catheter. As such, the choice of the catheter may be multifactorial. Typically, right sided catheters lengths are *19–23 cm tip to cuff* while left sided catheters lengths are *27–31 cm tip to cuff*. Once the length of the catheter has been determined as described above, the 0.018 in. wire has been removed and the micro access catheter should be remaining in the jugular vein. Next:

1. A small 5–10 mm incision is made using a #11 blade beside the micro-access catheter parallel to the skin folds of the neck extending the size of the access entrance.
2. Using a small angled snap or mosquito forceps, blunt dissection should be performed enlarging the catheter entrance site to accommodate the catheter or peel away sheath (see Fig. 13.7a).
3. The tunneled tract should then be created typically inferolateral to the entrance site, allowing for a gentle angle between the entrance site and the tunnel tract. Prior to creating the tunnel the desired area should be anesthetized appropriately (i.e., 1% lidocaine with or without epinephrine). Most tunnel tracts range from 4 to 8 cm in length. If too short or positioned to far laterally approaching the axilla, there is a higher risk of infection. Care should also be taken to keep the exit site away from the clavicle as catheter related clavicular osteomyelitis has been reported. For antegrade tunneled catheters, the exit site is then created using a #11 blade. A 1–2 cm incision is made with the goal of having a tight fit between the catheter and exit site. Blunt dissection can be performed using long straight hemostats from the exit site to the vein entrance site. For retrograde tunneled catheters, the tunnel isn't created until the dialysis catheter has been placed into the vascular system and its tip positioned accordingly. The remainder of the catheter can then be draped over the skin where the tunnel tract is desired. At this time the tunnel tract exit site can be chosen with the knowledge that the cuff and the tip will be located where desired. The tunnel tract is then created as described above (see Fig. 13.7b).

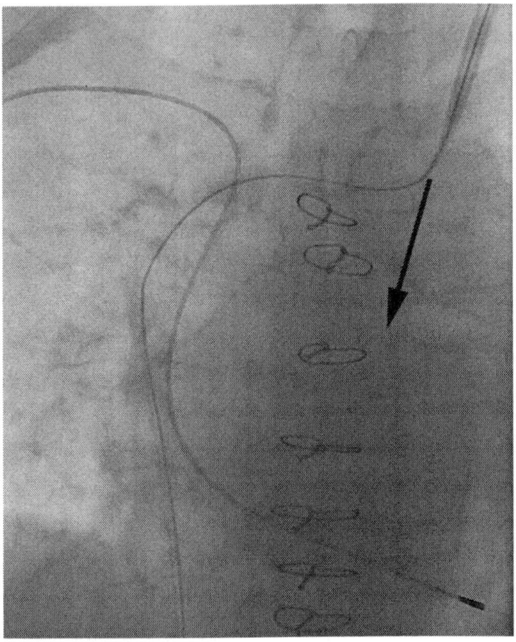

Fig. 13.8 The peel-away sheath introduction vector of travel (*arrow*) is into the mediastinum. If not monitored with fluoroscopy, laceration of the vein is possible. Dilators and peel-away sheaths should be introduced under fluoroscopic visualization

4. Once the tunnel tract has been created the catheter is connected to the tunneling device and pulled through the tunnel. The cuff is pulled into the tunnel tract. If not pulled in at this time it is difficult to do so once the catheter has been inserted in its entirety (see Fig. 13.7d).
5. The vein entrance site micro catheter is then removed over a 0.035 in. guidewire the tip of which should be positioned in the IVC. The entrance site is then dilated up for sheathless placement of the catheter over a wire or for introduction a peel away sheath (see Fig. 13.7e). Dilator advancement often requires a twisting motion and should be performed using fluoroscopic guidance (see Fig. 13.7f) to ensure the dilator is advancing over the wire and not with a kinked wire into an unplanned location (i.e., mediastinum, pleural space, artery) (see Fig. 13.8). Finger compression to the venotomy site should be applied between dilatations to prevent

significant back bleeding and air embolism. Most kits now come with a peel away sheath that has a valve to prevent bleeding and air embolism. Regardless of whether or not a valve is present it is wise to pinch the peel away sheath until the dialysis catheter has been introduced and the peel away sheath removed. For kits that do not have these sheaths there are multiple techniques to prevent air embolism. After the peel-away sheath is advanced the following maneuvers can be performed to introduce the catheter with a low risk of air embolism:

(a) Just before the wire and inner dilator are pulled out, have the patient take a deep breath in and hold it. The wire/dilator are then pulled out and exchanged for the catheter which should be advanced through the peel-away sheath rapidly.
(b) Have the patient continuously hum during the dilator/catheter exchange. With humming the patient is in a constant state of expiration preventing air embolism. Again, don't forget to pinch the sheath.
(c) Pull out the dilator/wire and clamp the peel-away sheath 1–2 cm below the hub thereby closing off the inner lumen. Then advance the catheter through the hub and release the clamp allowing passage of the catheter.
(d) Pinch the sheath with your fingers. Always remember to pinch the peel away sheath below the hub until the catheter resides within the sheath. Remember to always instruct the patient not to take any deep breaths during this maneuver.

If one believes that an air embolism has occurred, the patient should immediately be placed left side down (left lateral decubitus and Trendelenburg), administered oxygen (100% rebreather if possible) and your EMS system should be activated if the patient is symptomatic. Some have reported that air can be aspirated through the catheter that was placed as a means of reducing the amount of air that may be present in the right side of the heart.

6. After the catheter is advanced, the peel-away sheath is peeled away with the peel point outside the vein to prevent tearing of the vein puncture site. In other words, as you advance the catheter, pull the peel-away sheath back a bit and then peel in steps rather than peeling it off down into the vein. Once the peel away sheath has been removed and the catheter introduced there is usually a small portion catheter sticking out through the

entrance site (see Fig. 13.7g). This can usually be gently massaged down below the skin into the tunnel tract and/or entrance site.

7. Now that the catheter has been placed, the tip position should be confirmed fluoroscopically. The ideal position of most catheter tips is in the proximal right atrium. The shorter lumen of the catheter (arterial or red lumen) is ideally pointed towards the tricuspid valve (see Fig. 13.7i). If the catheter tips are not felt to be in the correct position the catheter can be manipulated at this time. If the tips are too far down into the right atrium, IVC, or right ventricle, the catheter can be pulled back as long as the cuff isn't pulled out of the exit site. If the catheter is felt to be positioned to high in the right atrium or SVC, the catheter can be advanced over a stiff 0.035 guidewire. At this time fluoroscopy should also be performed to look for catheter kinks or twists. Occasionally, blunt dissection is required to release bands or tissue that can be causing a kink. Twisting of a catheter may cause a first use phenomenon, most frequently seen with retrograde tunneled catheters. As such, twist should be looked for fluoroscopically and corrected with guidewires manipulation. As most dual lumen catheters have a septum dividing the two lumens a twist can be appreciated when the septum or lack thereof is not visualized throughout the course of the catheter.
8. Functionality of the catheter should be checked for with a 10 cc syringe. Brisk aspiration and forward flushing should be possible. A 10 cc syringe should fill in less than 3 s suggestive of flow rates of greater than 200 cc/min. If the catheter doesn't perform well on the surgical table, don't assume it will work better at dialysis. It is the implanter's responsibility to ensure that the catheter is functioning properly before the patient is removed from the OR table.
9. Once the catheter has been verified to flow freely on aspiration and flushing with a 10 cc syringe, the catheter should be flushed with saline and packed with a locking solution. Typically, most catheters are locked with heparin 1,000–5,000 U/cc with the appropriate volume as marked on each catheter lumen. There are other locking solutions described; however, heparin is still the most commonly used. Most now use 1,000 U/cc as no difference has been reported in patency, and if the heparin is inadvertently flushed into the patient, 1,000 U/cc bolus likely caries less risk to

the patient that a 5,000 U/cc bolus. Care should be taken to avoid over injecting the locking volume as this could lead to systemic heparinization particularly if 5,000 U/cc is being used. This can result in bleeding from the tissues around the catheter after insertion. Sodium citrate (4%) can also be used as an alternative to heparin.

10. The entrance and exit site wounds should be sutured to close the wounds and secure the catheter in place. Most close the entrance site (i.e., neck incision) with either absorbable suture or monofilament. For the catheter exit site (i.e., chest incision) most prefer monofilament to secure the catheter in place until tissue in growth has occurred at the cuff. Often a purse string suture is applied around the exit site securing the catheter in place. This suture can also be twisted around the catheter and sutures. Some suture the wings in place as well. In a responsible patient with a tight exit site and tunnel tract, the wings need not be sutured if the purse string suture is wrapped around the catheter. For many patients suturing of the wing of the catheter to the chest serves as a constant irritant. To avoid this constant irritation, some place a "hanging" knot at the level of the suture wing and then tie the suture wing to the hanging knot to anchor the catheter (see Fig. 13.7j). Sutures should be removed when no longer needed. For the entrance site stitch, if nonabsorbable, the suture should be removed at 7–10 days as the wound should be healed at that time. For the exit site and wing, the sutures can be removed at 3–5 weeks. By this time tissue in growth to the cuff should have occurred. This can be confirmed by tugging on the catheter. If the catheter is secure, the exit site and wing sutures can be removed.
11. Sterile dressings should be placed to protect the new surgical sites. Breathable dressings, typically gauze and tape are preferable as occlusive dressing can promote infection. Patients should also be instructed on how to care for their catheters at home prior to discharge. Although the dialysis center is responsible for changing the dressings during the dialysis treatment, patients need to be instructed on how to care for their catheter when not at dialysis. The CDC guidelines for the Prevention of Catheter Infections states that patients must maintain their hygiene as poor hygiene is associated with an increased risk of catheter infections [1]. When maintaining their hygiene during showering or bathing, these guidelines state that patients must use an impermeable

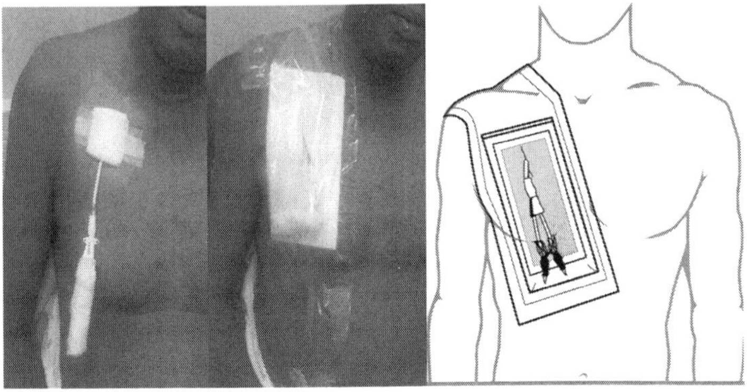

Fig. 13.9 Standard nonocclusive dressing vs. CD-1000 specialized catheter occlusive dressing for showering and bathing associated with reduced infection rate

dressing as water is implicated in catheter infections. This in part is likely related to water mobilizing the normal skin flora allowing it to travel along the catheter into the otherwise sterile subcutaneous tunnel tract and vascular system. One study has shown that dialysis catheter patients who use an impermeable dressing during showering or bathing have a 75% reduction in their incidence of developing a catheter infection (see Fig. 13.9) [2]. Additionally, patients should be instructed that if their daily catheter dressing ever gets moist or wet, it should be immediately changed for a dry breathable dressing (i.e., gauze and tape). These simple instructions can help patients to care for themselves and lower their risk of developing a potentially life threatening catheter related infection.

12. If the patient is going for dialysis immediately after catheter placement, instruct the dialysis nurse not to heparinize the dialyzer or to go "light" on the heparin. If too much heparin is used during the dialysis session, bleeding from the newly placed catheter entrance and exit sites can occur.
13. Sheathless systems now exist and involve insertion of the catheter over a wire without the use of a peel-away sheath. The main advantage is reduction in the risk of air embolism.
14. If twin (i.e., Tesio) dialysis catheters are to be inserted, the above steps are followed twice.

Subclavian Vein Insertion

The insertion technique for a subclavian catheter is essentially the same as that described above. Given the infraclavicular entrance, there may been less room for a long tunnel tract. Care should be taken to make sure that the tunnel is at least 3 cm in length. The lengths of catheters from *tip to cuff* is 19–23 cm from the right and 27 cm from the left.

Femoral Vein Insertion

Femoral venous catheters are typically associated with higher infection rates and poorer patency. The steps for placement are similar to those described in the IJV/EJV section with a few exceptions:

1. The puncture is made into the common femoral vein.
2. The subcutaneous tunnel should extend to the lateral upper thigh and be at least 5 cm in length.
3. The catheter tip should reside either in the IVC or right atrium. The catheter tip should not be positioned in the iliac vein. Furthermore, one should ensure the catheter tip has not advanced into the ascending lumbar vein. Attempted dialysis results in rupture of the vein and potentially life threatening retroperitoneal hemorrhage. No definitive studies have shown improved patency with tip positioning in the IVC vs. the RA. Some believe that if one starts with the tip in the distal IVC, the more proximal IVC and right atrium have been preserved for future access needs. Typical catheter lengths from this approach are 31–50 cm cuff to tip.

Collateral Vein Insertion

In an attempt to stay within the upper body and avoid the subclavian veins when the IJVs are occluded, one can try to find a reasonably sized collateral vein within the neck or upper chest using ultrasound guidance. Collaterals tend to be highly variable in size and course. It is recommended to puncture these vein using ultrasound guidance and a micro-access system. If the wire doesn't freely pass into the region of the right atrium and there is concern about location or patency of the vessel entered, it is best to advance the 3 Fr inner catheter of the micro-access system over the 0.018 wire. Contrast venography can then be performed to evaluate the course and patency of the collateral vein as well as their path to the SVC and/or RA. Stenoses and occlusions can be crossed at this time and dilated if need be. Occasionally, simultaneous use of a femoral approach may help to cross high grade stenoses or functional occlusions. Once a path has been created, hopefully to the right atrium, standard tunneled catheter placement techniques as described above can be employed.

Proper Location of the Catheter Tip

For catheters inserted via the jugular, collateral or SCVs, there is persistent debate about the ideal location of the catheter tip. Many hospital protocols and instructions for use (IFUs) indicate that no part of the catheter should enter the heart. This position is based on a limited number of early case reports of pericardial tamponade and arrhythmias. Many prefer to position the catheter tip within the *proximal right atrium*. This location results in improved flows, less recirculation, less acute failures and better catheter patency. The complications noted previously have not occurred with any consistency. This may be the result of different catheter materials and better technical placements with the use of image guidance. Occasionally, a shallow right atrium or narrow caval atrial junction may prevent tip positioning in the right atrium or caval atrial region as adequate flows may be difficult to obtain from the arterial lumen of the catheter. This can be corrected by using either a shorter catheter an positioning both tips in the SVC, using the planned catheter and re-positioning one tip in the RA and one tip either in the SVC or IVC or by using a reverse flow catheter where the arterial tip would be positioned in the center of the right atrium while the venous tip is positioned in the SVC.

The location of the right atrium tends to be lower than the landmark of 2 cm below the right mainstem bronchus and the tip can extend 2–3 cm beyond this point before reaching the proximal right atrium (see Fig. 13.10). Further reading regarding this debate can be found in summary paper written by Dr. Thomas Vesely [3].

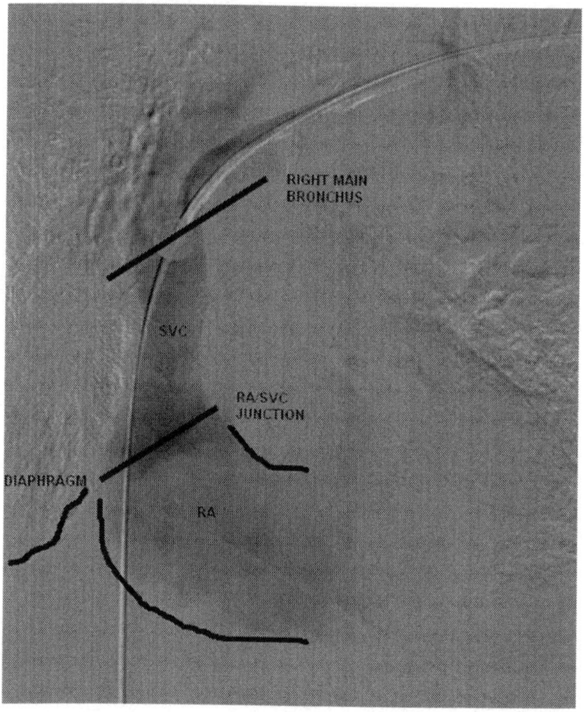

Fig. 13.10 Cavogram demonstrating the cavoatrial junction and right atrium positions relative to the mainstem bronchus (*SVC* superior vena cava; *RA* right atrium)

Complications of Catheter Insertion

These are well described and with image guidance should occur in less than 1% of placements. Complications include:

Pneumothorax, hemothorax, chylothorax
Arterial injury
Arteriovenous fistula
Rupture and/or thromboses of vein segments
Malposition of catheter
Kinking of catheter
Infection
Nerve damage

Pericardial tamponade – the interventionalist should always be aware of this possibility
Cardiac arrhythmias
Cardiac valvular damage
Air embolism
Hematoma formation
Lost wire
Death (although very rare) as a result of a complication

Catheter Problems

I just placed the catheter and it is not working. What could be wrong and what should I do?

1. The first thing that should be done is to inspect the catheter externally to ensure that it is not twisted or that the lumens weren't clamped during testing.
2. The catheter itself should then be investigated fluoroscopically for any kinks or twists. These can be subtle and different projections and magnification views may be necessary (see Fig. 13.11). Kinks are often the result of high jugular punctures or an acute angle between the vein entrance site and tunnel tract. Options include rotating the catheter, exchanging the catheter for a stiffer catheter or a pre-curved catheter, or creation of a new tunnel with a less acute angle.
3. The stitch around the catheter could be to tight "kinking" the catheter. If this is the case simply remove the stitch and replace it with a looser stitch if needed.
4. The catheter lumens have clotted. If this is suspected, attempts should be made to aspirate the clot out with a 20 cc syringe or larger (larger syringes generate larger vacuum pressures). If this fails, clot volume on average is less than 2.5 cc and can be dissolved with thrombolytic agents. If inadvertently flushed out, the clot embolism is usually not large enough to cause a clinically significant pulmonary embolism if the patient has normal lung perfusion and capacity.
5. The catheter tip is resting or sucking up against the venous wall. In such cases, the tip can be repositioned forward or backward until appropriate function is obtained. If it cannot, the catheter may need to be exchanged for a longer or shorter catheter or a catheter with a different tip design (see Fig. 13.11).
6. The SVC is severely narrowed and the tip is within the SVC. In such cases, the catheter needs to be advanced beyond the stenosis.

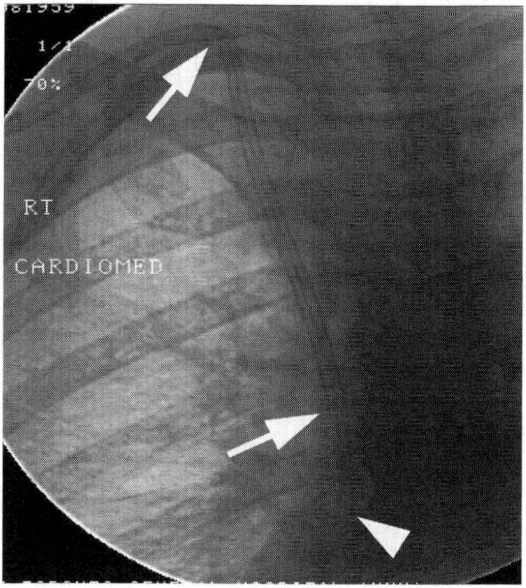

Fig. 13.11 One day after IJV catheter insertion, no flows were obtained. Three problems exist. The catheter is kinked at the vein entry site (*arrow superiorly*), the arterial lumen is facing laterally rather than medially (*lower arrow*) and the catheter tip terminates at the SVC/RA junction (*arrowhead*)

Dilating the SVC can be performed but often these stenoses are elastic and recur causing delayed catheter problems. Stenting of the SVC may be another option with the appropriate sized stent deployed by the appropriately trained individual. Reverse flow catheter may work well in this situation.

7. The catheter tip is in a collateral vein or the azygous vein (see Fig. 13.12). This problem can be determined by injecting a small amount of contrast and/or examining the catheter in the lateral projection. If this has happened, the catheter needs to be pulled back, a guidewire advanced through it and then repositioned in the desired location.
8. From the left side, although the desired length of the catheter may have been measured with a wire, the wire may have underestimated the required length. This occurs in tortuous vasculature (SVC-innominate-jugular veins) where the wire temporarily straightens out the tortuous vasculature which returns back to its configuration once the wire is removed. The net result is the measured catheter length with the wire is actually to short (see Fig. 13.13). For this

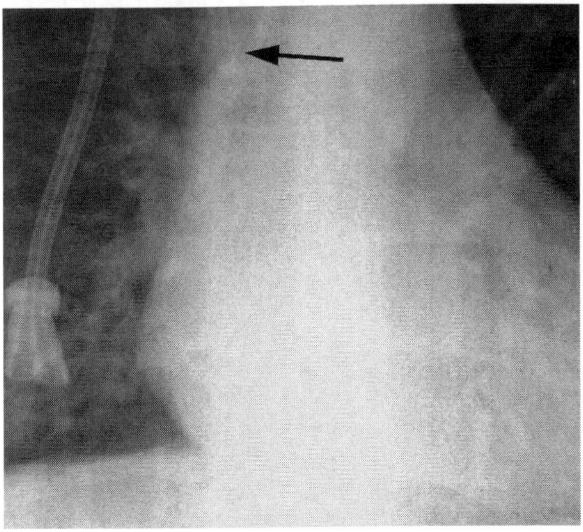

Fig. 13.12 Catheter failed to work after placement. Radiograph demonstrates step tip to catheter (*arrow*) not present. Lateral radiograph later demonstrated the tip angled backwards into the azygous vein

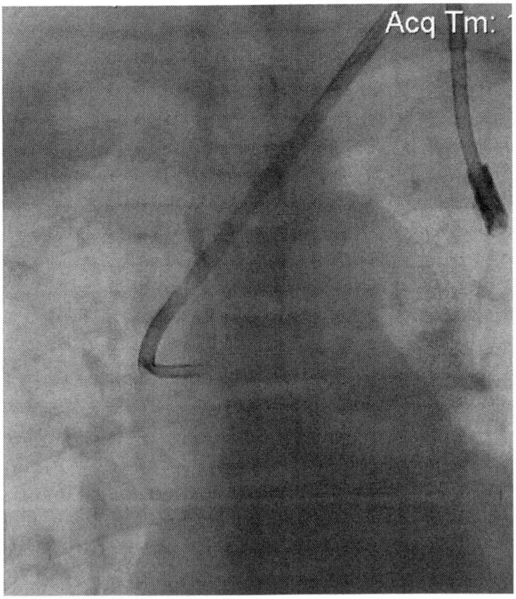

Fig. 13.13 LIJV catheter placement. The catheter tip has retracted up to the innominate vein/superior vena cava junction

problem, the catheter needs to either be exchanged for a longer catheter or advanced further into the tunnel tract. This, however, will result in the cuff being further up the tunnel tract as well.

9. The new catheter may have entered a previously formed fibrin sheath. Disruption techniques are discussed below.
10. First use phenomenon. This was previously eluded too when discussing retrograde tunneled catheters. This phenomenon is most commonly seen with retrograde tunneled catheters. For some poorly described reason, the first time these catheters are used they do not function well. High arterial or venous side pressures may be seen with clotting of the dialyzer. If these catheters are flushed and re-packed with their locking solution (i.e., heparin) they typically work perfectly at their next treatment and beyond. There are many theories about why this occurs, however, it is the authors believe that it is related to unrecognized twisting of the catheter during the retrograde tunneling. After 24–48 h the catheter likely untwists, thus, allowing the catheter to function well.
11. Rarely the catheter is not intravascular but passes perivascular or extravascular. This can occur if fluoroscopy is not used during each of the described steps for catheter insertion. A small amount of contrast may be injected to verify intravascular or extravascular positioning of the catheter.

Late Catheter Dysfunction

Catheter dysfunction is to be expected as catheters have a mean functional patency of less than 6 months. The most common presentation of a dysfunctional catheter is poor catheter flow, either occurring gradually over weeks or abruptly over days. This is usually the result of either catheter thrombosis or fibrin sheath formation. Other less common causes of catheter dysfunction include venous stenosis, thrombosis and occlusion, catheter material breakdown and catheter migration.

Catheter Thrombosis

Catheter thrombosis is a common complication seen with hemodialysis catheters. Varying techniques to rid the catheter of thrombus can be employed. Some dialysis centers pack the catheter with Open-cath (urokinase) for either a timed interval (30 min to 2 h) or an overnight dwell. Others refer clotted catheters directly for treatment. Management with thrombolytic therapy via the catheter or via an adjacent infusion catheter is dependent on the extent and degree of catheter thrombus present. Although most studies treating thrombosed catheters with thrombolytics were performed using urokinase, alteplase and reteplase have been administered in dose equivalents to urokinase for this indication. Results of multiple small studies evaluating catheter declotting techniques have documented success rates ranging from 55 to 97%. Success was defined as restoration to satisfactory flow for at least one dialysis session [4–8]. Approximately half of the catheters treated in these studies demonstrated an uninterrupted primary patency at 30–45 days. Doses used are mentioned in section "Thrombolytic Management." As part of a catheter declotting procedure, after the thrombolytic has been allowed to dwell and subsequently removed, if the flow is still felt to be suboptimal when aspirating or flushing with a syringe, some clean the inner lumen of the catheter with a brush or stiff guidewire. If flow problems persist after these techniques, other abnormalities such as fibrin sheath likely account for the catheter dysfunction. If the thrombosed catheter is associated with a suspected catheter infection, the catheter must be exchanged or removed.

Fibrin Sheath

Fibrin sheath will form around most dialysis catheters given enough time. The fibrin sheath or "biofilm" is initially composed of platelets and typically begins forming within 24 h of catheter insertion. Over time, fibroblasts and other cellular elements form a matrix around the catheter and this sheath, when it reaches the tip of the catheter, disrupts catheter flow. Typically, the arterial lumen is encroached by the fibrin sheath before the venous lumen likely related to the high pressure venous return, which occurs 3 times a week, cleansing the distal venous lumen of the catheter. When infection occurs in can become incorporated into the biofilm and difficult to treat with antibiotics alone. In these cases, many believe that fibrin sheath disruption is required along with catheter exchange and antibiotic therapy to effectively treat the infection. Hemodialysis catheter dysfunction due to fibrin sheath formation has been reported in 13–57% of patients undergoing catheter dialysis. A variety of novel catheter coatings and catheter designs have been developed to address fibrin sheath formation, however, to date there is no clear winner.

There are a variety of methods to address catheter dysfunction related to fibrin sheath formation. Management techniques include:

1. New catheter placement
2. Catheter exchange over a guidewire
3. Balloon PTA disruption of the fibrin sheath during catheter exchange
4. Percutaneous fibrin sheath stripping
5. Thrombolytic infusion

Success and failure has been document with each of these treatment regimens. Although fibrin sheath stripping was the procedure of choice in years past today most treat this problem with balloon disruption using traditional angioplasty balloons. Angioplasty balloon disruption of the sheath has proven to deliver similar if not superior results without the patient having to undergo a femoral venous catheterization.

To identify the presence of a fibrin sheath, after prepping and draping the patient, one must release the catheter cuff and pull the catheter back repositioning the tips closer to the vein entrance site. Prior to pulling back the catheter, a guidewire can be introduced through one of the two catheter lumens with imaging performed through the other lumen. Care should be taken not to inject forcefully as a hole can occur in the sheath filling the cava or vessel being imaged preventing visualization of the sheath. Rates of contrast injection are 2–5 cc/s for 2–3 s filmed at 2 frames/s.

Catheter Exchange for Treatment of Fibrin Sheath

Although catheter exchange has been described as a treatment for fibrin sheath, if the fibrin sheath isn't dislodged with the catheter removal and exchange, and the sheath remains after catheter exchange, flow problems will likely persist.

As with all catheter procedures the patient must be appropriately prepped and draped. Prior to performing a catheter exchange make sure that there are no signs of exit site or tunnel tract infection. Fluoroscopic imaging should be performed to evaluate the location of the catheter tips and to determine the type and size of catheter to be used.

Next, anesthetize the skin and subcutaneous tissue around the exit site and tunnel tract to the catheter cuff. If the cuff is situated within a few centimeters of the exit site blunt dissection can be performed to release the tissue from the cuff. Occasionally blunt dissection will help to mobilize the cuff through the exit site where sharp dissection can be performed to release the tissue from the catheter/cuff. Once this is performed a guidewire should be introduced through one of the two catheter lumens positioning the tip of the wire in the IVC. Many prefer to use stiff nitinol (i.e., glidewire) wires as they will not kink. Once the desired catheter has been chosen, the old catheter can be removed over the wire and the new catheter subsequently introduced over the wire. For staggered tip catheters, the guidewire can be advanced up the distal end of the catheter (typically venous) and out the catheter hub for over the wire introduction. For split tip catheters the wire is usually introduced through the distal most lumen of the catheter then out a side hole and back into the more proximal (arterial) lumen and out the hub for over the wire introduction. If a smaller diameter catheter is being exchanged for a larger diameter catheter, the tract may need to be dilated to accept the larger diameter catheter. Most dilators that come with catheters can be gently curved to aid in tract dilatation. If the dilator is going to be advanced into the vein over the wire this should be performed with fluoroscopic guidance. Occasionally, if a very small diameter catheter (i.e., Tesio 12 Fr) is going to be exchanged for a larger dual lumen catheter (i.e., 15 Fr), the tract may need to be dilated with a PTA balloon. 5 or 6 mm diameter high pressure balloons have been used by some for this purpose.

If the exit site or tunnel tract is felt to be infected but the proximal tract and entrance site are thought to be free of infection and a catheter exchange is required, a cut down at the catheter apex can be performed for a catheter exchange and new tunnel tract creation. After the area has been prepped, draped and anesthetized accordingly, an incision is created using a #11 blade at the catheter apex near its entrance sight into the vein. A guidewire should be advanced through the catheter positioning the tip of the wire in the IVC. The catheter cuff should be released as described in section "Removal of the Cuffed Tunneled Dialysis Catheter." After the incision (i.e., 2–4 cm) has been created, blunt dissection should be performed. Once the catheter is visualized it should be mobilized to the surface. This can be performed with hemostats, Alice clamps or other surgical instruments. Once mobilized, the catheter can be removed. This can performed one of two ways. The first way would be like any other over the wire catheter removal. Once the catheter is removed over the wire, the distal end of the wire can be pulled through the old tunnel tract up and out the new entrance site keeping the tip of the guidewire in the IVC. The down side of this maneuver is that the wire has been pulled through an infected tunnel tract or exit site. The other way to remove the catheter would be to place clamps on both sides of the catheter that had been mobilized up into the new entrance site. Next, cut the catheter in two around the guidewire. Then pull the distal part of the wire through the proximal piece of the catheter so the wire is now exiting the new entrance site. The wire has not passed through the old infected tunnel tract by performing this maneuver. If this is performed take caution that the proximal end of the catheter does not slip into the patient. It should stay clamped until it can be removed over the wire. A new tunnel tract can then be created using either antegrade or retrograde approach. In this situation, a retrograde tunnel is preferred by some as the new catheter can immediately be introduced over the wire prior to creating the tunnel tract. Either way a new catheter is introduced, either over the wire and or through a sheath. Then the new entrance site and exit site are sutured closed as previously described. When a new tunnel tract is created try and keep the exit site away from the old infected catheter exit site to prevent the new site from becoming infected. Also, it is wise to use separate surgical instruments to prevent spread of infection.

Once the catheter has been exchanged check to make sure the tips are in the proper position and the catheter is performing as expected. If the flow is not adequate further intervention will be required.

PTA Balloon Disruption of Fibrin Sheath (See Fig. 13.14)

As described above, once the patient has been prepped, draped and anesthetized, the cuff released, the catheter pulled back and imaging performed documenting the presence of fibrin sheath, balloon disruption of the sheath is a viable option. This is performed by removing the catheter over a guidewire, the tip of which has been positioned in the IVC. Most use standard PTA balloons, ranging from 10 to 14 mm diameters. Some use occlusion balloons for this purpose, however, given the characteristics of these compliant balloons, standard PTA

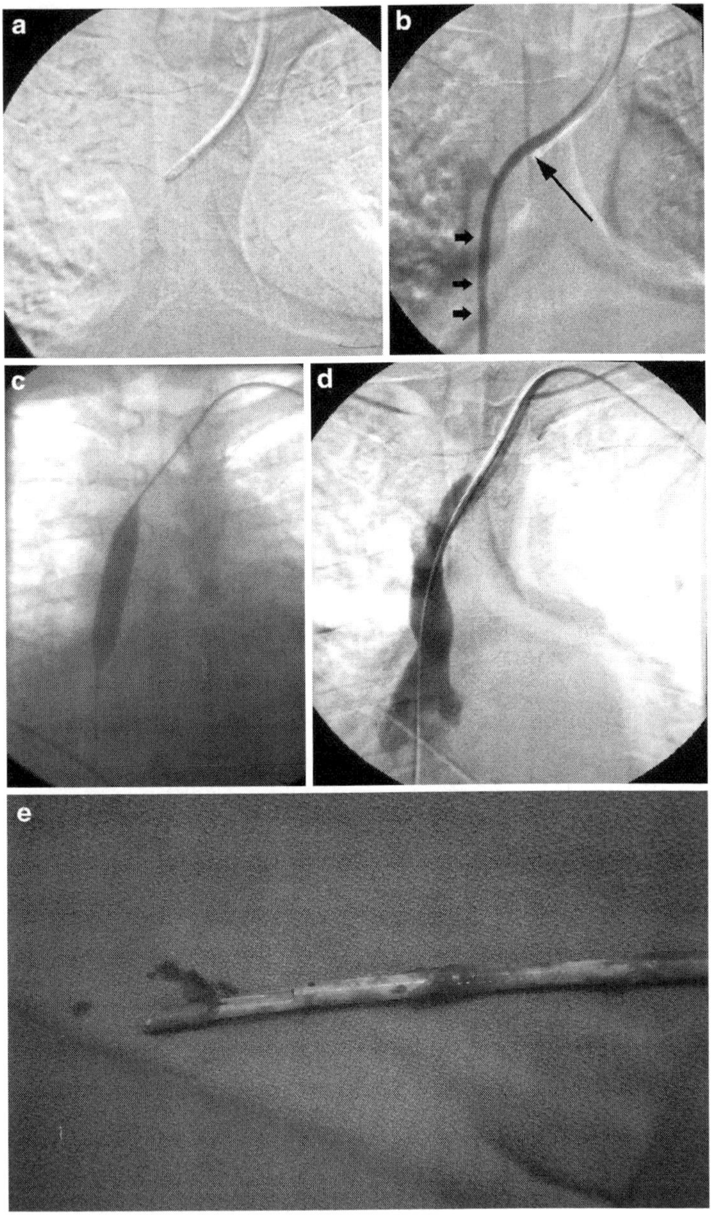

Fig. 13.14 (**a**) Dialysis catheter has been pulled back with tip in the innominate vein. (**b**) After contrast injection a static image demonstrates contrast retained within the fibrin sheath (*arrows*) which extends from the venotomy site to the right atrium. (**c**) Balloon disruption with a 12 mm balloon. (**d**) Repeat central venogram shows complete disruption of the fibrin sheath. (**e**) Soft tissue adherent to the removed catheter is remnants of the fibrin sheath

balloons are felt to be safer by some. With the wire tip in the IVC advance the catheter into the caval-atrial region where the tip of the fibrin sheath ends. Gently inflate and deflate the balloon, pulling it back and repeating inflations. With many fibrin sheaths, if the balloon is being inflated by hand, the operator will feel a popping sensation as the sheath is being disrupted. Once the operator believes that the fibrin sheath has been successfully disrupted, the balloon catheter can be removed over the wire for introduction of the dialysis catheter over the wire. Once the catheter tip is intravascular, as visualized fluoroscopically, venography can be performed through the lumen of the catheter the guidewire is not residing in. On the venogram, if the sheath has been successfully disrupted brisk outflow (i.e., SVC) will be visualized. When this is seen, the remainder of the catheter can be introduced until the tips are in their desired position. Remove the guidewire and check for adequate catheter flow with a 10 cc syringe as previously described. Occasionally, the balloon size chosen is suboptimal at disrupting the fibrin sheath and larger balloon sizes will be required. Occasionally balloon dilatation is not successful and other techniques may be required.

Also, the balloon should not extend up beyond the lower clavicle margin as one is now dilating the venotomy site which cause sustained poorly controlled bleeding back along the tract. If inflation pressures >5 atm are required to dilate and rupture the sheath, underlying venous stenosis rather than a fibrin sheath should be suspected.

Thrombolytic Management

Management with thrombolytic agents for fibrin sheath formation has documented success [4, 5]. Some institutions prefer a protocol involving an initial "lock" of thrombolytic agent for a variable dwell time. Others prefer a short 3-h infusion. Alteplase has been utilized in doses of 1–2.5 mg/h/lumen for a 2–3-h infusion or 2 mg/lumen for dwell times of 1–4 h. A typical protocol is 2.5 mg of reconstituted Alteplase (1 mg/1 mL) mixed with 47.5 mL of normal saline (0.05 mg/mL) and infused into each catheter lumen at 20 mL/h (1.0 mg/h) for 2.5 h (total dose per lumen = 3 mg). For urokinase, instilling 5,000 U/mL/lumen to fill the lumen and allow to dwell for a minimum of 1 h. This can be repeated up to 3 times or 30,000–60,000 U can be infused/

lumen/h for 4 h. Although this method is helpful for intraluminal thrombus buildup for organized fibrin sheath many believe it has limited value. In a soon to be published randomized study, locking the catheter with tPA once a week is associated with a decreased incidence of catheter malfunction and bacteremia.

Fibrin Sheath Stripping

This procedure typically involves a transfemoral venous catheterization, for placement of a sheath to accommodate a snare. Varying size snares are available based on operator preference. Fibrin sheath stripping can be attempted either with the dialysis catheter in place snaring the sheath over the existing catheter or pulling the dialysis catheter back and snaring the sheath prior to exchanging the catheter. Stripping over the existing catheter runs the risk of fracturing the catheter and embolizing catheter fragments to the heart or lungs. Since imaging is typically performed to verify the presence of the fibrin sheath, most perform fibrin sheath stripping with the catheter pulled back.

Prior to advancing the snare, release the dialysis catheter cuff and pulled back the catheter over a 0.035 in. wire positioning the tip of the wire in the IVC. Perform a central venogram through the dialysis catheter to confirm the presence of the suspected fibrin sheath. The loop snare can then be advanced from the femoral approach. Some find it easiest to snare the 0.035 wire that was advanced through the dialysis catheter and advance the snare up the wire and then over the dialysis catheter. The dialysis catheter should be pulled back as far as possible, and the snare should be tightened up against the wire abutting the tip of the catheter. Once the snare is taught, a hemostat can be applied on the snare abutting the hub of the snare catheter allowing for constant pressure by the snare on the sheath. Making sure the guidewire from the catheter approach is freely mobile, pull the snare briskly. Imaging can then be performed through the lumen of the dialysis catheter not occupying the guidewire. If the sheath is gone the snare can be removed and the catheter exchanged for a new catheter. If the sheath is still present repeat the snare procedure. Sometimes the wire through the catheter that the snare is around prevents adequate snaring of the sheath. If this is felt to be the case, place an additional wire through the other lumen of the catheter and remove the wire that the snare was advanced over and repeat the snaring procedure. Occasionally, the fibrin sheath will be adherent to the wall of the SVC. This can be dealt with by placing a pigtail catheter around the hemodialysis catheter thereby lifting the adherent dialysis catheter free from the SVC wall. Thirty-day patency rates with fibrin sheath stripping have been reported in the literature at 30–50%. Given these poor patency rates as well as the added risk of the transfemoral cannulation to the patient, this procedure has been abandoned by most as a routine method for treatment of fibrin sheath and is typically used as a last resort.

Infection

According to the USRDS, the average dialysis catheter develops over 1.4 catheter infections/year (http://www.usrds.org). These infections carry a high morbidity and mortality. A study from Duke University documented a 19% mortality rate at 12 weeks of a dialysis patient being admitted to the hospital with a catheter infection [9]. As such, all efforts should be made at preventing these infections, and when they occur, caring for them timely and appropriately.

Traditionally, catheter infections have been reported per 1,000 catheter days [10, 11]. Dialysis catheters have some of the highest reported infections rates in the medical literature ranging from 1 to over 8 infections/1,000 catheter days. Temporary catheters have even higher rates of infection than tunneled catheters. The KDOQI guidelines recommend establishing protocols to reduce catheter infections rates below 1/1,000 catheter days.

Catheter related infections run the gamut of localized exit site infections, to tunnel track infections, to bacteremia/septicemia and death. Treatments range from local exit site care, to antibiotic therapy, to catheter exchange or removal. Once a catheter infection is suspect it should be dealt with timely given the associated morbidity and mortality. For localized exit site or tunnel tract infections the catheter will need to either be exchanged for a new catheter with a new tunnel tract or removed with a new catheter placed in a different location. This is typically determined by the extent of the tunnel tract infection and whether the proximal tunnel-vein entrance site is felt to be involved. If the proximal tunnel/vein entrance site appears to be uninvolved a catheter exchange with new tunnel tract creation can be performed preserving the current access to the vascular system. For a suspected "catheter infection" which presents typically with fever and chills while on dialysis, or with documented positive blood cultures, the catheter will need to be exchanged or removed completely. Over the wire exchanges with disruption of the biofilm has been proven to be a viable treatment for these infections preserving the central venous access. Most believe that the bacteria don't typically incorporate into the catheter material itself; rather the bacteria enclose themselves in a polymeric matrix, the biofilm, that facilitates bacteria metabolic cooperatively and growth. In fact, it is estimated that the biofilm is responsible for greater than half of the bacterial infections that occur in humans. As such if an exchange is performed without disruption of the biofilm fibrin sheath the infection will likely persist even though the "infected catheter" has been removed. Conversely, if the sheath is disrupted and the exchange performed and appropriate antibiotics utilized, the infection is usually successfully treated.

The most common organisms found in catheter infections are those that colonize the skin including; *Staphylococcus epidermidis*, *S. aureus*, and *Enterococcus*. Up to one third of catheter infections are, however, from gram negative organisms likely related to poor personal hygiene.

Catheter Exit Site and Tunnel Tract Infections

Catheter exit site infection is characterized by exudate at the exit site with or without erythema, crusting, warmth or tenderness. Exit site infections do not present with systemic signs, and blood cultures are negative. Appropriate treatments include topical and or systemic antibiotics and appropriate local exit site care.

Tunnel tract infections occur within the tissue tract between the cuff and vein entrance site. The tract itself is often warm to touch, tender and fluctuant with or without drainage from the exit site. Patients may or may not also present with systemic symptoms. Because tunnel tract infections occur within a closed space without adequate drainage, conservative treatment is often ineffective. Although parenteral antibiotic therapy may on occasion be effective for mild tunnel tract infections, for warm, hot purulent infections, catheter removal with new catheter placement is usually the best treatment option for the patient.

For patients requiring catheter removal due to an infected tunnel tract, two options exist. The first is removal of the catheter with placement of a new catheter in a new location. The second is removal of the infected catheter maintaining the entrance site and creation of a new tunnel tract. This is performed as described above performing a cut down near the vein entrance site and mobilizing the catheter. The old catheter can be removed and a new tunnel tract created. The new tunnel tract should be created away from the infected site, with the exit site cephalad to the old exit site, when possible, to prevent dependent drainage of the infected site on the new exit site. Appropriate wound care and antibiotic therapy should be administered.

Catheter-Related Bacteremia

Catheter-related bacteremia typically presents with a history of fever and chills while on dialysis. The diagnosis is often based on clinical presentation supported by positive blood cultures. IV antibiotic therapy should be initiated once suspected, and modified as needed following blood culture results. Common antibiotics used include vancomycin, gentamicin and cephazolin. As previously mentioned, up to one third of these infections will be from gram negative organisms, and as such broad spectrum coverage should be provided until culture results are obtained. In stable patients without evidence of concomitant exit site or tunnel tract infection, over-the-wire catheter exchange with balloon disruption of the biofilm fibrin sheath is often effective along with accompanying antibiotic therapy. This treatment preserves the central venous real-estate for future access needs. This is a vast improvement when compared to the old dictum of removing the catheter, placing a temporary catheter, waiting for negative blood cultures for 36 h after the patient is asymptomatic, and the placing yet another catheter. This old approach destroyed precious central venous real-estate and as such has been abandoned by most access specialists. The literature supports the over-the-wire exchange technique showing only minimal increased risk of infection when compared to a new catheter placement in a noninfected patient. Typically, antibiotics are administered for 2–3 weeks at dialysis after catheter exchange for catheter related bacteremia. Following cessation of antibiotic therapy, blood cultures should be negative.

Removal of the Cuffed Tunneled Dialysis Catheter

The patient should be prepped and draped accordingly. If the catheter was properly placed, the cuff should be within 1–2 cm of the catheter exit site. The cuff is often palpable and should be located prior to catheter removal. Local anesthesia (i.e., lidocaine) should be injected liberally into the subcutaneous tissue from the exit site to the cuff. The lidocaine not only anesthetizes the area, it helps to spread the tissue surrounding the cuff facilitating removal. From the exit site, forceps can be introduced spreading the tissue around the catheter and catheter cuff. This should be performed with gentle traction being placed on the catheter. Usually, the cuff is mobilized with this type of blunt dissection and can be pulled back through the exit site. If tissue is still adherent to the cuff, it can be cut away using scissors to release the tissue allowing the catheter to be pulled back freely. If the cuff is located far from the exit site (i.e., >6 cm), an incision over the cuff may be required, with subsequent dissection, to release the cuff from the surrounding tissue. Once the cuff has been released the catheter should be able to be removed through the exit site. If this is not possible, the catheter can be removed from the incision site. This can be performed by cutting the catheter proximal to the cuff. This allows the cuff and distal portion of the catheter to be removed from the vein and subsequently the proximal part of the catheter to be removed freely from the exit site. Remember, once you cut the catheter do not release the distal end until it is removed. If care is not taken the distal end of the catheter could migrate into the patient causing concern for both the patient and the operator. The incision can usually be closed with a single interrupted suture. If a deep dissection was required, one or more absorbable sutures placed in the subcutaneous tissues, in addition to the superficial sutures may be required.

Prior to removing the catheter some interventionalists prefer to image the central veins with contrast venography to insure that venous damage such as venous stenosis, thrombosis, or fibrin sheath formation hasn't occurred. If present, some believe that intervention is helpful to maintain patency of this valuable central venous real-estate for the future access needs of the patient. Angioplasty for central vein stenosis or fibrin sheath disruption, performed over the guidewire that was inserted through the catheter prior to its removal, can be a quick and effective way to treat this problem.

After removal of the catheter, the exit site can be closed with a single interrupted monofilament sutures along with compression of the tract and exit site for a several minutes to achieve hemostasis. Conversely, manual pressure alone, without placement of a suture can be performed. In this situation, when the exit site is left unsutured to close on its own, closure typically occurs over 48–72 h. The potential advantage to this is if there is an unrecognized infection at the exit site or in the tunnel tract, the infection can drain freely until healed. If there is an infection present and the exit site is sutured, a large abscess cavity can form. If the exit site is allowed to close unsutured, patients should be instructed on how to compress the exit site if bleeding were to occur at home. Patients should also be instructed not to perform any heavy lifting or valsalva type maneuvers for the first 24–48 h.

Occasionally, only a portion of the cuff comes out when the catheter is removed. If the remainder of the cuff cannot be removed, the cuff can be left behind with no consequence if the exit site is not infected. It is always preferable, however, to remove any foreign body (i.e., cuff) when possible [12].

During attempted catheter removal it is always best to perform the catheter removal over a safety guidewire. Occasionally, during the attempted removal when traction is being placed on the catheter, the catheter can break in two. This usually occurs near the catheter cuff when the cuff has not been completely released and excessive traction is placed on the catheter. Care should also be noted with silicone based catheters (i.e., some Tesio catheters) as these catheters are sometimes easier to break with traction. If this occurs and a safety wire is through the catheter, the fear of distal catheter fragment migration is lessened. If the fractured fragment cannot be reached from the catheter exit site, a cut down should be performed over the end of the fractured catheter. This can be performed with the use of fluoroscopic guidance. Once the distal catheter fragment has been grasped with a forceps or like surgical instrument and the catheter wire combination clamped decreasing the risk of bleeding or air embolism, the proximal end of the catheter should be removed over the wire. Once this is accomplished, the end of the wire exiting the tunnel tract exit site can be pulled back through the surgical cut down site and the clamped distal end of the catheter can then be removed over the wire and the wire subsequently removed. If the distal catheter fragment accidentally migrated back into the vascular system, a snaring procedure may need to be performed. This is usually performed from a femoral approach as described in the fibrin sheath stripping section. The snare is advanced through a femorally positioned sheath and advanced to the level of the catheter (i.e., SVC, RA). Once snared, the snare should be cinched down on the catheter and then clamped against the hub of the snare catheter. Once secure the catheter fragment and snare should be pulled to the sheath. Usually, the snared catheter cannot be pulled into the sheath, but once tightly up against the sheath, the snare sheath combination can be pulled out as a unit. Prior to performing this maneuver, a safety wire may want to be placed through the sheath incase rapid access needs to be regained into the venous system. Also it is advisable to use the largest sheath possible (16 Fr) to remove the snared catheter fragment. Once it has been verified that the catheter has been removed in total, the safety wire can be removed.

Occasionally, a portion of the catheter which has been in place for years becomes incorporated within the tunnel tract and or blood vessel wall and can't be removed by traditional means. This is seen most commonly with silicone based catheters. The catheters become pours and friable and break apart easily. If one is persistent, often requiring one or more incisions over the tunnel tract, the catheter pieces can slowly be removed. Always remember to keep a safety wire through the catheter pieces. An incision will likely be required by the vein entrance site to remove the intravascular portion of the catheter. This portion of the catheter is usually easily removable even though the portion of the catheter in the tunnel tract is friable. If the intravascular portion of the catheter became incorporate into the wall of the vessel, however, its removal may become challenging. For catheters that have become incorporated into the wall of the vessel surgical consultation is prudent as surgical intervention may be required. Percutaneous options that can be attempted WITH some risk are:

1. Cutdown on to the catheter above the cuff, dividing the catheter and then trying to pass a peel-away sheath over the catheter. When attempting this technique, control of the catheter fragment is absolutely required and the fragment should be closed off to prevent bleeding and air embolism. A simple way to accomplish both is to place and tightly tie a braided suture around the end of the catheter that does not easily break (e.g., Tevdek). A hemostat may also be used for this same purpose when technically feasible. The peel-away sheath may force surrounding fibrous tissue off the catheter allowing the catheter to be removed.

2. Either free the cuff from the underlying subcutaneous tissues as discussed above or cutdown above the catheter cuff and divide the catheter. Then with gentle traction on the catheter with guidewire through the catheter, continuously twist the catheter. This may rotate the catheter free of its fibrous attachments.
3. Seek the assistance of a cardiologist and cardiac surgeon for potential laser extraction. Some cardiology centers have laser cardiac lead extraction catheters that may be used to attempt removal of the catheter.
4. If the tunnel tract portion has been removed and a portion of the intravascular catheter is adherent to the wall of the vessel, a snare can also be attempted.

If the catheter has been divided and still can't be removed, tie off the fragment end, close the skin over the cutdown site and seek further surgical consultation. Occasionally, 90% or more of the catheter will be removed with a small intravascular portion remaining. What to do with this portion of the catheter that has likely been incorporated into the wall of the vessel (i.e., SVC, RA) for months to years causing no clinical problems, has been the topic of conversation of experts in years past with no best answer.

Catheter Exchange

A tunneled cuffed catheter may require exchange for infection, poor function, fibrin sheath formation, an exposed cuff, or the catheter is broken. As described above in catheter exchange for fibrin sheath, the catheter and exit site should be prepped and draped and anesthetized accordingly. A guidewire should be advanced through one of the catheter lumens positioning the tip of the wire in the IVC. The catheter cuff should be released and the catheter pulled back. Contrast venography can then be performed through the other catheter lumen to evaluate the vasculature (i.e., SVC and RA). If a fibrin sheath is present and felt to be significant, fibrin sheath PTA may be indicated. As there is typically a well formed tunnel tract, the patient may bleed from the exit site once the catheter has been removed over the wire. This can usually be managed with manual compressions of the tract. Another option (see Fig. 13.15) is to place a purse string suture at the catheter exit site, which can be tightened or loosened during catheter exchanges to prevent significant bleeding and air embolism. The

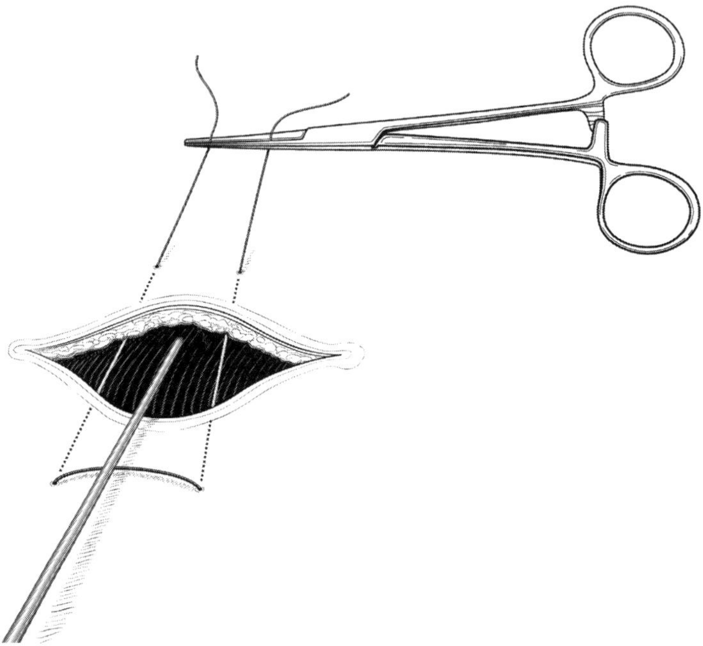

Fig. 13.15 Pursestring stitch placed during catheter exchange

suture can also be used to secure the catheter in place once the final catheter position has been achieved.

The appropriate size and type of catheter should be chosen keeping in mind the desired tip design and position as well as the desired cuff position. If the diameter of the new catheter is larger than that removed, the tract may need to be dilated. The dilator of the peel away sheath can be gently curved to facilitate passage of the sheath. If the peel away sheath can be introduced, the catheter can then be advanced over the wire through the peel away sheath and the sheath subsequently removed. If the peel away sheath cannot be introduced and the catheter cannot be advanced over the wire, the tract and vein entrance site can be dilated with a PTA balloon (i.e., 5 mm) facilitating introduction of the catheter. If there still is a problem with advancing the catheter, a different catheter with a different tip design may be required. Using a stiff guidewire through each lumen may also help. The catheter can then be introduced over the wire and sutured in place as previously described. Another later considered option is to cutdown on the venotomy site and under fluoroscopy, puncture down onto but not into the catheter at the site where the catheter enters the vein. Then pass a wire into the vein. Remove the old catheter and continue as though placing a new catheter but through the old tract with preservation of the vein access from the previous catheter. A variation is to cutdown on the catheter, divide it at the venotomy site and pass a wire through it and then remove the two fragments and then carry on as though it is a fresh catheter insertion.

The Bleeding Exit Site

On occasion, significant oozing of blood can occur from the exit site. This typically is seen more often with catheter exchanges than new catheter placements. The bleeding arises from either the tract itself, or from back bleeding from the venotomy site. Another cause may be heparin. If the patient had a catheter placed or exchanged and immediately proceeded to dialysis, and if the dialysis nurse heparinized the patient which is customary for most patients on dialysis, the heparin used for the dialysis treatment may have caused the bleeding to occur. In addition, many dialysis patients have some form of platelet dysfunction which could contribute to bleeding. With time, all bleeding stops; however, it is best to treat this problem timely. Removing the catheter is almost never the answer. There are a few steps beyond compression to the site which may abate the bleeding:

1. An additional purse string suture at the exit site is often the best and easiest option. This along with a pressure dressing usually is effective at stopping the bleeding.
2. Reversal of anticoagulation. If the patient was heparinized, protamine sulfate may have to be administered. The standard dose is 1 mg/100 U of heparin for reversal. Not more than 50 mg should be given in a 10 min period and it should be administered slowly as rapid infusion has been associated with histamine release, bradycardia, dyspnea, and pulmonary hypertension.
3. Exchange of the catheter. There may be a pinhole in the catheter from suturing. If there is a hole in the catheter this is usually noted by aspirating air from the catheter.
4. Avitene or microfibrillar collagen can be injected up into the tract.
5. Topical thrombin may be injected up into the tract.

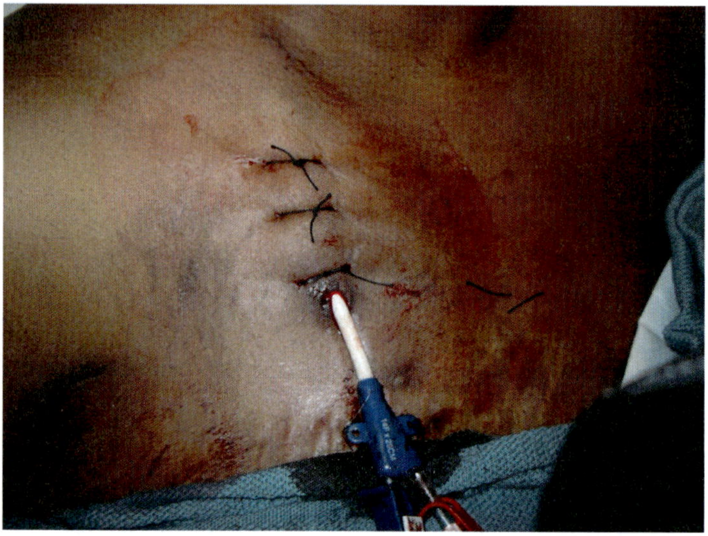

Fig. 13.16 Multiple sutures placed along subcutaneous tract with attention to not passing through the catheter to control bleeding from the tract following catheter exchange

6. DDAVP to improve platelet function.
7. Exchange of the catheter for a larger French sized dialysis catheter if one is available.
8. Place sutures through the skin, around the catheter, back through the skin again and tie a knot. This can be done along the course of the subcutaneous tract multiple times in an effort to compress or close off the subcutaneous tract (see Fig. 13.16).
9. Any combination of the above.

Conversion of a Temporary Catheter to a Tunneled Cuffed Catheter

Although there is an increased risk of infection when converting a temporary dialysis catheter into a tunneled cuffed catheter, the risk is minimal compared to the risk of losing a central vein for future access needs. One study has examined the infectious risks associated with such procedures and found no significant difference in infectious risk [13]. If conversion is to be performed, this should ideally be done within 7 days of temporary catheter placement to reduce the risk of tunneled catheter infection. Prior to attempting a conversion, the catheter exit site must be inspected to rule out infection.

For conversion of low jugular catheters, one can simply create a tunnel tract to the current puncture site and convert the temporary catheter to a tunneled catheter. Some like using retrograde tunneled catheters in the situation. The temporary catheter can be exchanged over the wire for the retrograde catheter. The tips of the catheter can be ideally positioned and the remainder of the catheter can be laid out over the anticipated tunnel tract. The desired cuff position can then be determined, the tunnel tract can be created and the catheter pulled through the tunnel and secured in place. Antegrade tunneled catheters can also be used when converting a temporary catheter to a tunneled catheter. In this situation, the tunnel tract will need to be created first then the catheter introduced either over the wire or through a peel away sheath and positioned accordingly.

Conversion of temporary IJV catheters to tunneled catheters works reasonably well if the puncture is low down on the neck. However, most punctures for temporary catheters are done without image guidance and are frequently higher in the neck. Placing a tunneled catheter through a high puncture increases the risk of catheter kinking significantly. As such many prefer to re-puncture the vein below the original puncture site either with ultrasound or fluoroscopic guidance. Using the temporary catheter as a guide, the vein can be cannulated. Sometimes the vein has collapsed around the catheter making cannulation more difficult. If this is the case one can pull back the temporary catheter over a guidewire increasing the internal luminal diameter of the vein available for the new vein puncture. Once the vein has been cannulated, the temporary catheter can be removed, hemostasis achieved and the new catheter placed using standard techniques. When converting a temporary catheter to a tunneled catheter, the old exit site of the temporary catheter may need to be surgically debrided to allow for clean margins to promote appropriate wound closure. For femoral and subclavian access sites, similar maneuvers can be performed.

Clot Formation at the Tip of the Catheter

With more patients having long term catheters in place and more cardiac imaging being performed, it is not uncommon to find patients with clot hanging off the tip of their catheters. This is now more commonly discovered and depending on the clot burden, this finding can be distressing. Treatment is somewhat subjective as there are no defined algorithms or clinical studies in support of one form of treatment over another. The options below reflect individual's opinions and live under assumption that the patient does not have a right to left intra-cardiac shunt.

If the clot burden is considered to be low (<5 cc) options include:

1. Do nothing
2. Exchange the catheter to prevent further thrombus formation
3. Short course of infusion lytic therapy through the catheter to dissolve or shrink the clot
4. Short course of systemic anticoagulation in an attempt to dissolve or shrink the clot
5. Forceps or basket retrieval of the clot

If the clot burden is larger than 5 cc, options 3–5 are considered as well as surgical extraction of the clot. Option #3, however, is considered with caution as if the clot is pedunculated off the tip of the catheter; the thrombolytic may dissolve the stalk and cause the bulk of the thrombus to embolize.

Catheter Fell Out

In this situation, the patient typically presents with their catheter in their hand saying "I don't know what happened." Usually there is no bleeding as tunnel tracts easily clot once the catheter is removed. If there are no signs of infection, and patient doesn't report any symptoms consistent with infection, a new catheter can usually be replaced through the same tunnel tract. The patient should be prepped and draped accordingly. Using a glide wire, gently advance the wire into the tunnel tract. With gentle pressure the wire can usually be freely introduce back into the central venous system. Rarely, a catheter will be required to aid in this process. If so, try using a 4 Fr Kumpe catheter with a 5 cc syringe of contrast. Under fluoroscopic visualization, with small puffs of contrast the tract is highlighted and the catheter is steered forward along the tract. Using a wire sometimes causes formation of false passages [14]. Once the wire has been introduced into the patient, a diagnostic catheter should be introduced over the wire for contrast venography. If fibrin sheath is present it may need to be treated with balloon disruption. The distance from the desired tip position to the desired cuff location can be measured and the appropriate catheter chose and introduced over the wire. The catheter should then be sutured in place. Broad spectrum prophylactic antibiotics are recommended in this situation.

Key Points

- If the upper body veins are collapsed, having the patient perform a valsalva maneuver or placing them in Trendelenburg position may cause the vein to dilate. Another option, although often well tolerated in dialysis patients is to bolus the patient with 1 L of normal saline to increase the intravascular volume.
- If the vein is noncompressible and appears round then a more central venous obstruction should be considered.
- Follow the course of your anesthetic (lidocaine) needle with ultrasound to give you an idea of the course you are directing your needle.
- The angle of the needle and puncture should roughly approximate the angle of the ultrasound probe.
- Allow the wire to pass to IVC during catheter insertions and exchanges. If the wire passes into the right ventricle, arrhythmias may occur, the tricuspid valve can be damaged, and very rarely cardiac perforation with subsequent pericardial tamponade can occur.
- If unsure of vein access or the vein is small or easily collapsible, use a micropuncture set.
- Always make sure you know where your wire tip is and always maintain control of your wire.
- Think of the right atrium as composed of tissue paper. Any mild trauma can damage it and all actions within it should respect the delicacy of this cardiac chamber.
- The wires included in insertion kits are occasionally short or too floppy. In obese patients, using a longer stiffer wire not included in the kit mitigates future problems.
- In patients with a large body habitus or pendulous breasts, the catheter tip can migrate up to 5 cm when the patient sits

up. For such patients, we deliberately place the catheter tip within the mid right atrium at placement as it will pull up to the proximal right atrium or atrial caval junction when they sit up. This can be verified by pulling down the soft tissue on the patient's chest and seeing the degree of catheter tip retraction on fluoroscopy.

- If a patient's dialysis catheter has fallen out, the tract may be mature enough to negotiate back through it into the central veins.
- For catheter exchange related to infection, a fibrin sheath should be looked for and disrupted if present.

References

1. O'Grady NP, Alexander M, Dellinger EP, et al. Guidelines for the prevention of intravascular catheter-related infections. Centers for Disease Control and Prevention. MMWR Recomm Rep. 2002;51(RR-10):1–29.
2. Altman SD, Ross JJ, Work J. Reducing catheter infections through use of the CD-1000: a retrospective review of a unique catheter specific composite dressing. J Vasc Access. 2008;9(4):236–40.
3. Vesely TM. Central venous catheter tip position: a continuing controversy. J Vasc Interv Radiol. 2003;14(5):527–34.
4. Savader SJ, Haikal LC, Ehrman KO, Porter DJ, Oteham AC. Hemodialysis catheter-associated fibrin sheaths: treatment with a low-dose rt-PA infusion. J Vasc Interv Radiol. 2000;11(9):1131–6.
5. Gray RJ, Levitin A, Buck D, et al. Percutaneous fibrin sheath stripping versus transcatheter urokinase infusion for malfunctioning well-positioned tunneled central venous dialysis catheters: a prospective, randomized trial. J Vasc Interv Radiol. 2000;11(9):1121–9.
6. Janne d'Othee B, Tham JC, Sheiman RG. Restoration of patency in failing tunneled hemodialysis catheters: a comparison of catheter exchange, exchange and balloon disruption of the fibrin sheath, and femoral stripping. J Vasc Interv Radiol. 2006;17(6):1011–5.
7. Hyman G, England M, Kibede S, Lee P, Willets G. The efficacy and safety of reteplase for thrombolysis of hemodialysis catheters at a community and academic regional medical center. Nephron Clin Pract. 2004;96(2):c39–42.
8. Dowling K, Sansivero G, Stainken B, et al. The use of tissue plasminogen activator infusion to re-establish function of tunneled hemodialysis catheters. Nephrol Nurs J. 2004;31(2):199–200.
9. Engemann JJ, Friedman JY, Reed SD, et al. Clinical outcomes and costs due to *Staphylococcus aureus* bacteremia among patients receiving long-term hemodialysis. Infect Control Hosp Epidemiol. 2005;26(6):534–9.

10. Maki DG, Kluger DM, Crnich CJ. The risk of bloodstream infection in adults with different intravascular devices: a systematic review of 200 published prospective studies. Mayo Clin Proc. 2006;81(9):1159–71.
11. Mermel LA. Prevention of intravascular catheter-related infections. Ann Intern Med. 2000;132(5):391–402.
12. Kohli MD, Trerotola SO, Namyslowski J, et al. Outcome of polyester cuff retention following traction removal of tunneled central venous catheters. Radiology. 2001;219(3):651–4.
13. Van Ha TG, Fimmen D, Han L, Funaki BS, Santeler S, Lorenz J. Conversion of non-tunneled to tunneled hemodialysis catheters. Cardiovasc Intervent Radiol. 2007;30(2):222–5.
14. Saad NE, Saad WE, Davies MG, Waldman DL. Replacement of inadvertently discontinued tunneled jugular high-flow central catheters with tract recannulation: technical results and outcome. J Vasc Interv Radiol. 2008;19(6):890–6.

Chapter 14
Dialysis Grafts Versus Fistulas

Dirk S. Baumann and Dheeraj K. Rajan

The type of hemodialysis access and the management of this access greatly influences the survival and quality of life for patients undergoing hemodialysis. The revised Kidney Dialysis Outcome Quality Initiative guidelines recommend primary placement of native or autogenous hemodialysis fistulas over synthetic vascular grafts and central venous catheters, since this form of access has been proven to have longer durability [1, 2]. This durability is well recognized and accepted within Asia, Europe, and Canada. Recent studies have shown that thrombosis occurs roughly ten times more frequently in dialysis grafts compared with autogenous fistulas [3, 4]. Another study reported mean secondary patency rates ranging from 3.6 to 7.2 years for autogenous fistulas compared with 1 year for grafts [5]. With the introduction of these guidelines and the introduction of the Fistula First Initiative, there has been a shift in clinical practice within the United States.

Although autogenous hemodialysis fistulas represent optimal access for hemodialysis, they, like hemodialysis synthetic grafts, are prone to eventual dysfunction and failure. In addition, there is now

---

D.S. Baumann (✉)
Director, Mid Peninsula Wound Care Medical Clinic, Peninsula Surgical Specialists Medical Group, Burlingame, CA 94010, USA
e-mail: dbaumann@pssmg.com

D.K. Rajan (ed.), *Essentials of Percutaneous Dialysis Interventions*,
DOI 10.1007/978-1-4419-5657-6_14,

© Springer Science+Business Media, LLC 2011

some question as to how much better fistulas are given the high initial failure rate to mature compared with grafts, and overall graft survival is now widely suspected to be higher than previously reported.

The Hemodialysis Graft

When an autogenous hemodialysis fistula cannot be created, synthetic grafts constructed of polytetrafluoroethylene (PTFE) or woven Dacron tubes with a diameter of 6–8 mm can be constructed. Synthetic grafts are typically placed in the upper extremities preferably as distal as possible initially. Configurations are straight and looped grafts. Usually grafts in the forearm are looped and grafts in the upper arm are straight. A sufficient length of synthetic conduit is placed to allow for insertion of dialysis needles and to primarily allow for reduced mixing of blood between the two needles.

The forearm loop graft is typically created between the brachial artery and either the antecubital vein or basilic vein (see Fig. 14.1a). A pretapered graft is most commonly used with the arterial anastomotic portion of the graft having a diameter of 4 mm and the venous end of the graft having a diameter of 6 mm. The arterial anastomosis is located medial to the venous anastomosis just below the elbow. Occasionally the venous anastomosis may also be to the cephalic vein. A straight configuration in the forearm can be used where the arterial anastomosis is the radial artery (see Fig. 14.1b). Within the upper arm, the most common configuration is the straight graft between the brachial artery and basilic vein or the axillary vein (see Fig. 14.1c). The size of the graft is 6 mm. When the upper extremities are exhausted, thigh grafts are placed. A loop configuration within the thigh is used with the arterial anastomosis to the common femoral artery and the venous anastomosis to the common femoral vein (see Fig. 14.1d). The size of the grafts is commonly 6 mm at the arterial anastomosis and 6 mm at the venous anastomosis. Unrevised grafts often have a length of 30–40 cm, whereas revised grafts can be up to 60 cm in length. Length and size of all grafts are also slightly variable based on arterial/venous vessel sizes and patient's anthropological characteristics.

There are many variations to the aforementioned standard configurations and as dialysis patients live longer and exhaust traditional access types, variations are performed. One such configuration is called the necklace graft which is connected from the axillary artery across the chest to the axillary vein on the contralateral side (see Fig. 14.1e).

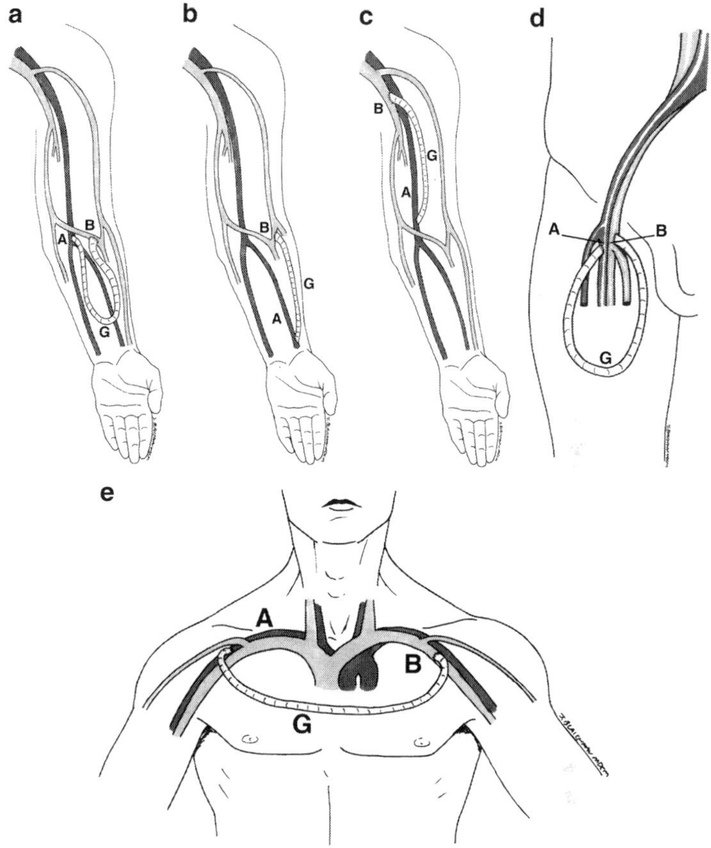

Fig. 14.1 Arteriovenous grafts. A – arterial anastomosis, B – venous anastomosis, G – PTGE graft (**a**) Forearm loop graft. A – brachial artery, B – antecubital vein. (**b**) Forearm straight graft. A – radial artery, B – antecubital vein or cephalic vein. (**c**) Upper arm graft. A – Brachial artery, B – axillary vein. (**d**) Thigh loop graft. A – superficial femoral artery. B – common femoral vein. (**e**) Necklace upper chest graft. A – axillary artery. B – axillary vein

PTFE is considered the material of choice as the microscopic configuration of the material allows for multiple needle punctures over a prolonged period of time. The material is considered "self healing"; however, a rind or layer of perigraft scar tissue forms within months around the graft. This allows for fixation of the graft within the subcutaneous tissues and also facilitates hemostasis after needle punctures for dialysis as well as for percutaneous interventions.

Advantages of grafts include high clinical success rate following placement, limited need for a segment of sufficient vein to act as a venous conduit, short maturation time of 2–3 weeks with some newer graft material allowing puncture within days of insertion, and greater initial durability. Patients who are not candidates for fistulas are often candidates for grafts.

Native Dialysis Fistula

The autogenous hemodialysis fistula represents a native vessel conduit to provide access for hemodialysis. The most recognized conduit is the Brescia Cimino fistula first described in 1966 (see Fig. 14.2a). This hemodialysis conduit was a side to side surgically created anastomosis between the radial artery and the cephalic vein. Arterial pressure resulted in dilation of the cephalic vein as well as wall thickening or so called "arterialization" of the cephalic vein within the forearm. The length of the cephalic vein within the forearm is sufficient to allow for adequate distance between the dialysis needles to prevent recirculation. Compared to AVGs, the AVF has multiple advantages and some disadvantages. Advantages include better cumulative patency, low infection rates, low thrombosis rates, and reduced costs overall compared with grafts. Disadvantages include a failure to mature in up to 30% of placements and some patients not having suitable veins to attempt fistula placement.

Fistulas can fail to mature for a number of reasons. These include: (1) failure for the vein to "arterialize," (2) large and/or multiple venous collaterals reducing flow through the cephalic vein, (3) insufficient size of the cephalic vein, and (4) technical factors at the time of surgery. Methods to intervene to promote maturation are discussed in Chap. 18.

Today, the most common fistula placed is the radiocephalic fistula (see Fig. 14.2b). This like the Brescia Cimino fistula is created between the radial artery and the cephalic vein near the wrist. This is most commonly an end-to-side anastomosis with the cephalic vein cut at the wrist with the end toward the hand ligated and the portion going up the forearm anastomosed to the side of the radial artery. The next most common is the upper arm brachiocephalic fistula, which is typically created just above the elbow, and is an end-to-side anastomosis between the cephalic vein and brachial artery (see Fig. 14.2c).

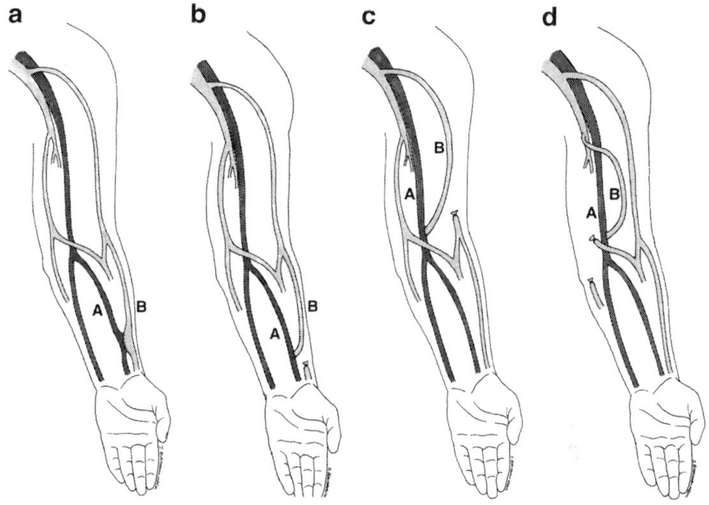

Fig. 14.2 Autogenous hemodialysis fistulas. (**a**) Brescia Cimino fistula with side-to-side anastomosis between the radial artery (A) and the cephalic vein (B). (**b**) Radiocephalic fistula with radial artery (A) side-to-end (B) cephalic vein anastomosis. (**c**) Brachiocephalic fistula (A) brachial artery (B) cephalic vein. (**d**) Transposed brachiobasilic fistula (A) brachial artery (B) basilic vein

The cephalic vein is transected just above the elbow with the portion passing to the forearm ligated and the upper portion mobilized, rotated down, and anastomosed to the side of the brachial artery. Occasionally a side-to-side anastomosis is performed without ligating the other end of the cephalic vein. The third most common fistula is the brachiobasilic fistula which is created between the brachial artery and basilic vein within the upper arm (see Fig. 14.2d). Since the basilic vein is deep within the upper arm, the vein has to be surgically mobilized to a subcutaneous location.

With the drive to place more fistulas within the United States due to the Fistula First Initiative, many unique fistula types have been created. They include fistulas created between the posterior tibial artery at the ankle and the saphenous vein, ulnar cephalic fistulas, and ulnar basilic fistulas within the forearm. The basilic vein in the forearm originates on the medial (ulnar) side of the dorsal venous network of the hand and it travels up the base of the forearm and arm along the dorsal aspect. Other unique forms have been created and are limited in description to case reports.

Combination of Graft and Fistula

When fistulas begin to fail, either due to aneurysm formation or multiple stenosis along the access circuit, rather than abandoning the access, an interposition graft may be placed surgically across the problem area(s) or bypassing them. In most cases, this is done from the artery to the nondiseased venous outflow of the original fistula. In addition, problem areas can be resected with placement of graft across the area removed.

Surgical Considerations for Fistula Versus Graft Construction

Generally, arteriovenous fistulas (AVF) are the preferred primary access for hemodialysis, offering several advantages over arteriovenous nonautogenous grafts (AVG) and tunneled central venous catheters. Overall, AVFs are associated with fewer revisions, lower costs for maintenance, fewer complications, and lower mortality than AVGs and catheters. However, recent reports emphasize that up to 50–60% of fistulas fail to mature sufficiently to provide adequate hemodialysis access [6–8] and that nearly 90% require additional intervention [8]. Therefore, AVGs may be superior alternatives to AVFs and especially catheters in some situations.

Forearm AVGs have several advantages over construction of upper arm AVFs in patients with poor quality forearm vasculature. Forearm loop AVGs have been shown to have improved primary, assisted primary, and secondary patency over radial cephalic AVFs in patients with compromised forearm vessels (radial artery 1–2 mm and/or cephalic vein <1.6 mm) [9]. In patients with an inadequate radial artery but ample cephalic vein, brachial artery to distal forearm cephalic vein AVGs have similar patency to transposed forearm brachial artery to cephalic vein loop AVFs. Yet, these AVGs allow for dialysis access avoiding a catheter during fistula maturation. Finally, while patency rates of forearm loop AVGs may not be as good as upper arm AVFs [10], they allow for maturation of the upper arm veins without the need for a catheter. If done distal to the antecubital fossa, the outflow veins can be later converted to AVFs. Thus, there are several situations that forearm AVGs should be considered prior to upper arm AVF construction.

In patients with multiple factors associated with fistula failure, an AVG may also be acceptable alternative to an AVF. Patients, who are female, are older, have diabetes or have small veins, have poorer overall outcomes from AVFs, with lower maturation rates and higher failure rates. AVGs offer acceptable alternatives in these patients to avoid long-term catheters required for fistula maturation and revision. Poor clinical condition may dictate AVG placement rather than a more complicated transposition AVF. Patients with obese arms, loose tissue, or coagulopathies are often better candidates for AVGs than AVFs. Finally, lower extremity AVGs to the larger femoral vein have satisfactory patency rates, while the saphenous vein AVF tends to have lower patency than arm AVFs. It is important to consider risks of catheter placement and usage, timing of need for dialysis initiation, and factors involved in fistula maturation in order to offer optimal access selection. AVGs offer a preferential option either prior to or instead of AVFs in select circumstances.

Summary

When assessing the patient for what type of access they have, the simplest way to determine this is to ask the patient. Otherwise, physical examination of the arm, based on location of the access, the location and lengths of surgical scars, and the "feel" of the access itself should indicate what type of access you are dealing with.

Key Points

- One should be familiar with the type configuration of accesses placed prior to intervening and for grafts, the size of the graft itself.
- The simplest way to ascertain what type of access the patient has and which side is arterial versus venous is to ask the patient.

References

1. Eknoyan G, Levin NW, Eschbach JW, et al. Continuous quality improvement: DOQI becomes K/DOQI and is updated. National Kidney Foundation's Dialysis Outcomes Quality Initiative. Am J Kidney Dis. 2001;37(1):179–94.
2. Zaleski GX, Funaki B, Kenney S, Lorenz JM, Garofalo R. Angioplasty and bolus urokinase infusion for the restoration of function in thrombosed Brescia-Cimino dialysis fistulas [see comments]. J Vasc Interv Radiol. 1999;10(2 Pt 1): 129–36.
3. Schwab SJ, Oliver MJ, Suhocki P, McCann R. Hemodialysis arteriovenous access: detection of stenosis and response to treatment by vascular access blood flow. Kidney Int. 2001;59(1):358–62.
4. Sands JJ, Kapsick B, Brinckman M. Assessment of hemodialysis access performance by color-flow Doppler ultrasound. J Biomater Appl. 1999;13(3): 224–37.
5. Rodriguez JA, Armadans L, Ferrer E, et al. The function of permanent vascular access. Nephrol Dial Transplant. 2000;15(3):402–8.
6. Miller PE, Tolwani A, Luscy CP, et al. Predictors of adequacy of arteriovenous fistulas in hemodialysis patients [see comments]. Kidney Int. 1999; 56(1):275–80.
7. Dember LM, Beck GJ, Allon M, et al. Effect of clopidogrel on early failure of arteriovenous fistulas for hemodialysis: a randomized controlled trial. JAMA. 2008;299(18):2164–71.
8. Biuckians A, Scott EC, Meier GH, Panneton JM, Glickman MH. The natural history of autologous fistulas as first-time dialysis access in the KDOQI era. J Vasc Surg. 2008;47(2):415–21; discussion 420–21.
9. Rooijens PP, Burgmans JP, Yo TI, et al. Autogenous radial-cephalic or prosthetic brachial-antecubital forearm loop AVF in patients with compromised vessels? A randomized, multicenter study of the patency of primary hemodialysis access. J Vasc Surg. 2005;42(3):481–6; discussions 487.
10. Keuter XH, De Smet AA, Kessels AG, van der Sande FM, Welten RJ, Tordoir JH. A randomized multicenter study of the outcome of brachial-basilic arteriovenous fistula and prosthetic brachial-antecubital forearm loop as vascular access for hemodialysis. J Vasc Surg. 2008;47(2):395–401.

Chapter 15
Commonality of Interventions in AV Accesses

Dheeraj K. Rajan and Dirk S. Baumann

Although dialysis grafts and dialysis fistulas are fundamentally different in many ways, the interventions performed within them and the methods employed are the same. Indications for interventions and endpoints of interventions are also relatively similar. What constitutes success of the intervention performed? There are immediate anatomic, clinical, and hemodynamic endpoints for every case, while one can use anatomic and clinical endpoints only and reserve hemodynamic endpoints for equivocal cases. Hemodynamic endpoints can be determined by measuring intraprocedural blood flow using a Transonic catheter or flow measuring catheter. The clinical endpoint may be as simple as reestablishing a thrill within the access.

D.K. Rajan (✉)
Head and Associate Professor, Division of Vascular & Interventional Radiology, Department of Medical Imaging, University of Toronto, Toronto, Ontario, Canada
e-mail: Dheeraj.Rajan@uhn.on.ca

D.K. Rajan (ed.), *Essentials of Percutaneous Dialysis Interventions*,
DOI 10.1007/978-1-4419-5657-6_15,

© Springer Science+Business Media, LLC 2011

Indications for Intervention

Beyond thrombosis of the accesses discussed in their respective sections, the most common indication for intervention is >50% venous stenosis with angiographic assessment. This indication alone should not be considered absolute or in isolation for reasons discussed in future chapters as angioplasty without proper indication can be harmful in certain situations. Beyond angiographic criteria, there should be at least one other hemodynamic, functional, or clinical indicator of access dysfunction. Clinical indicators would include prolonged bleeding from puncture sites, painful cannulation, and difficult cannulation, clots coming out of the access, swollen extremity, abrupt changes in palpable flow along the access, and no flow or pulsatility through the entire access. Hemodynamic criteria are discussed in Chap. 5 more extensively, but briefly include abnormal pump pressures, high recirculation, poor urea clearance, and poor measured access flow rates/velocities (<600 mL/min). The reason for treatment of venous stenosis is that its presence is strongly associated with an increased risk of access thrombosis which translates into poorer cumulative access patency.

Endpoints of Intervention

The endpoints below are readily achieved in any angiographic suite and are used because they allow an immediate assessment. Obviously, the most important outcome is resumption of normal dialysis with resolution of the abnormal screen or thrombosis that led to the diagnostic fistulogram or thrombectomy procedure. As per K/DOQI, a successful dialysis intervention is defined as anatomic success with resolution of at least one clinical or hemodynamic variable.

Anatomic endpoint: All stenoses should have a maximal *posttreatment anatomic residual stenosis of no greater than 30% relative to the normal adjacent vein*, and preferably less. Recent invasive hemodialysis flow studies suggest there is lack of sensitivity for this anatomic endpoint and point to future trends of assessing endpoints with direct hemodynamic flow measurements.

Clinical endpoint: *A palpable continuous thrill without significant pulsatility* indicates a satisfactory clinical endpoint. Although this has been examined in dialysis grafts [1], this observation is also observed with dialysis fistulas.

Hemodynamic endpoint: Measurement of the *intragraft venous limb pressure to cuff brachial systolic pressure ratio should be less than 33%* [2]. For autologous fistulae, no localized drop in systolic pressure greater than 30% should be accepted, except through the anastomosis where it can be greater than 50%. Lilly et al. report pressures to be the best predictor of patency [3], but Trerotola et al. found the physical exam to be superior to pressures [1].

One can also measure translesional pressures with an intraluminal standard angiography catheter. If there is a >10 mmHg translesional gradient in systolic pressure across a stenotic area, this is considered hemodynamically significant. This method can also be used to evaluate vessel segments for occult stenosis not detected with fistulography.

What is Adequate Angioplasty?

Adequate angioplasty is a matter of debate for many. What is an adequate inflation pressure and for how long? Both questions have never been properly answered. However, adequate inflation pressure by consensus is the point where the angioplasty balloon completely effaces the stenosis and no residual indentation is seen fluoroscopically along the balloon. The length of time the balloon is inflated is another issue. There is no consensus regarding an adequate time of inflation, although most prefer >45 s of inflation time for each lesion treated. In a recently published study comparing 1–3 min inflation times for angioplasty in fistulas and grafts, improved technical success was observed. However, this observation did not translate into improved intervention patency at 6 months [4]. There is some evidence that smooth muscle relaxes after 30 s of ischemic time.

Noncompliant balloons are preferred as the pressure introduced within the balloon is equally distributed along the length of the balloon with no expansion beyond predetermined sizes. With compliant balloons, pressure is not equally distributed and moves to the point of least resistance along the balloon potentially leading to incomplete dilation of the lesion. *In general, the balloon diameter should be equal to or 1 mm larger than the diameter of the immediately adjacent normal vessel* (see Fig. 15.1), although in select cases such as calcified

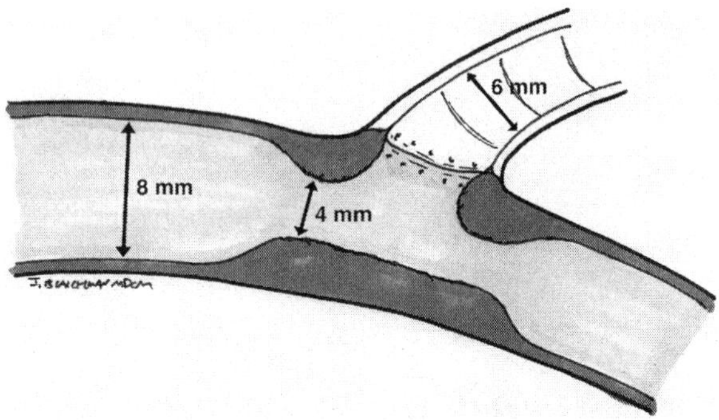

Fig. 15.1 Sizing of balloon catheter. Adjacent normal vessel diameter is 8 mm. An 8 mm angioplasty balloon is chosen

inflow arteries or arterial anastomoses one may undersize the balloon depending on the clinical situation. The balloons should not be inflated beyond the manufacturer-specified rated burst pressure as potential complications can occur. Some interventionalists have been advocating deliberate rupture of the vein segment that is stenosed using larger diameter balloons to obtain better outcomes. There is no evidence to support this practice and it is not recommended.

When not to Intervene

Infection of the vascular access is an absolute contraindication to a percutaneous thrombectomy procedure and a major contraindication to angioplasty. This includes sepsis or bacteremia related to the access. Overlying cellulitis is a relative contraindication as puncture through the skin can seed a graft with bacteria, whereas this is less likely with an autogenous fistula. No implantable devices should be placed in the access. Recurring thrombosis in the absence of an identifiable anatomic lesion or hemodynamic abnormality should raise the suspicion of an occult infection. Severe uncorrectable coagulopathy is also considered by many as an absolute contraindication for fear of hemorrhagic complications.

Relative contraindications to percutaneous thrombectomy techniques include:

- Pulmonary hypertension
- Severe lung disease
- Right heart failure
- Known right to left shunts
- Contrast allergy

Death related to stroke from paradoxical emboli has occurred with percutaneous thrombectomy and deaths from pulmonary emboli have been reported with both mechanical and chemical techniques. Mechanical thrombectomy techniques may offer a lower risk than pharmacologic methods, while surgical thrombectomy offers the lowest risk, due to reversal of flow in the vein during thrombectomy. If a right to left shunt is present (e.g., patent foramen ovale (PFO)), it is preferable to defer percutaneous thrombectomy to surgery for better control against emboli during declotting. Nevertheless, the risk associated with surgery is probably also not zero.

Recent access site creation is considered a relative contraindication to angioplasty and/or pharmaco- or mechanical thrombolysis due to concerns of leak or disruption of the suture line. Although most interventionalists would not intervene within 6 weeks of the access being created, some have successfully done so within 2 weeks. However, surgical correction of technical errors is often necessary in cases of acute access thrombosis. Therefore, consultation with the operative surgeon should be obtained prior to percutaneous intervention in this setting. Early attempts at thrombectomy may be indicated to "define" the anatomy and potential cause of graft failure. Standard contraindications to thrombolysis should be considered for patients in whom thrombolysis is anticipated.

Complications specific to angioplasty are relatively low (<5%) and include:

1. Flow limiting dissection.
2. Vessel spasm.
3. Vessel rupture.
4. Intramural hematoma.
5. Vessel thrombosis.
6. Creation or worsening of arterial steal.
7. Loss of the access related to 1–5.
8. Although not considered a complication, intimal injury leading to or triggering cellular-mediated mechanisms that result in intimal hyperplasia.

Angioplasty Technique

- Although a sheath within the access is recommended to pass the balloon catheter, this is not absolutely required. A sheath allows for easy multiple exchanges and causes less trauma to the access site.
- When advancing the wire, it is important to see where the tip of the wire is going and the wire tip should be followed fluoroscopically to ensure it does not end up in an incorrect or possibly damaging location.
- It is important to have a wire traversing the lesion to be dilated and that the wire is of sufficient length to allow delivery of the balloon catheter without losing wire access across the lesion. Ideally, the wire should be passed into the IVC to prevent intraprocedural arrhythmias from passage of the wire into the right ventricle.
- Many interventionalists use a hydrophilic wire to cross areas to be dilated. It is recommended that the balloon catheter be advanced over a nonhydrophilic wire as the wire is less likely to be displaced.
- The balloon catheter is then advanced up to and across the lesion with the inflatable portion of the catheter (radiopaque markers) centered across the lesion.
- The balloon catheter is then inflated with an inflator after removing any air within the balloon. This is called priming the balloon and can be done by aspirating back on the inflation port with a balloon inflation device or a syringe full of saline. When the air comes out with backward suction, it is replaced by saline. The purpose of this is twofold.

  1. To prevent air embolism from a potentially ruptured balloon.
  2. To apply greater dilation force with fluid than can be applied with air.

- Within the balloon inflator, a 1:1 concentration of saline and contrast should be used. This allows for visualization of the balloon and easy evacuation or deflation of the balloon.
- The balloon catheter is then inflated and gentle traction is maintained on the shaft of the catheter to keep it from slipping off the lesion.
- Inflation is continued until the lesion is effaced completely or the rated burst pressure of the balloon catheter is reached. There is no advantage to inflating the balloon beyond the point where the lesion is effaced completely. Most lesions will efface by 10 atm; however, pressures above 20 atm are not uncommon.

- In general, one can exceed the manufacturer rated burst pressure by 20%, but this is off label practice and not recommended.
- Once dilation has been performed, the balloon should be fully evacuated prior to retrieval/removal. A 20-cc syringe helps evacuate the balloon quicker than common insufflation devices.
- If angioplasty is being performed to dilate a stent/stent graft, the balloon should be fully deflated prior to removal and removal should be visualized with fluoroscopy to ensure the stent/stent graft is not being displaced by the balloon.

Stent Deployment

As with balloon angioplasty, stent or stent graft size is determined by the diameter of the normal adjacent vein segment and is generally *sized 1 mm larger* than the nonstenosed vessel. Centrally, devices 2 mm larger in diameter are used to prevent inadvertent migration. Care must be taken to avoid traversing veins that can be used for future access. For example, stenting from the subclavian vein to the innominate vein thereby blocking the internal jugular vein. Also, if one is going to err in location of the stent, it is best to err on the side of the access rather than on the other side of the lesion. The shortest possible length should be used. Also, recent increased usage of stents has demonstrated another problem/consideration of stent fracture with bare stents. This occurs at points of compression and articulation including the shoulder, elbow, and the subclavian vein. Points of fracture result in accelerated intimal hyperplasia (see Fig. 16.4, Chap. 16).

Premounted Balloon Expandable Stents (the Manufacturers Instructions for Use (IFU) Should be Followed)

Balloon expandable stents have greater outward radial strength when dilated and can be overdilated. These stents change anatomy rather than conforming to it. Also, if crushed or compressed, they will not return to their originally deployed shape. Hence, there is little use for these stents in dialysis patients.

- With balloon expandable stents, deployment is similar to balloon inflation with some minor additional steps.

- Most balloon expandable stents now come premounted on balloons and are shrink wrapped on. Inadvertent partial inflation of the balloon will lead to partial expansion of the stent which may cause it to slip off the balloon and be lost in the patient.
- When advancing the balloon stent combination through the sheath, gentle grip should be maintained on the stent as it is advanced through the diaphragm of the sheath to prevent it from being dislodged.
- The stent should be centered on the lesion prior to expansion and additional verification angiographic runs should be obtained to verify position.
- All attempts should be made to deploy the device with the deployment system in a straight line. Any bends or curves will cause the system to migrate forward.
- Predilation of the lesion is not required and the balloon should be fully deflated prior to withdrawal to prevent dislodgement of the stent.

Self-Expanding Stents/Stent Grafts

Most self-expanding stents are composed of nitinol which is a combination of nickel and titanium. It has unique shapeable characteristics where it has different shapes at different temperatures. Also, these stents are laser cut from single nitinol tubes and have no weld points. This stent type conforms to vessel walls and always tries to reach its designed diameter. If an 8 mm stent is deployed in a 5 mm vessel, the stent will continuously try to reach its predetermined 8 mm diameter. However, if overdilated, it will retract back to its predetermined diameter. Another characteristic is that they have an open cell structure, which implies fewer connection points between the cells or adjacent rings. This feature allows for greater flexibility, conformability, and predictability for how long the stent will be. This allows the stent to be bent, crushed, and twisted within the body yet it will return to its original shape. However, these characteristics also allow the stent to be compressed or elongated when deployed. Both situations lead to improper stress on the stent which leads to fracturing and stent failure. Fracture points are focal points of accelerated intimal hyperplasia. In addition, some say nitinol stents are prone to "jumping" forward. Furthermore, the open cell structure prevents repositioning or recapturing of the stent. The statement "you only get one chance to place a permanently implantable device in a patient once" should always be in one's mind. It is therefore important to have good technique when deploying these stents to avoid misplacement and future fractures. In addition, the nitinol material is not very radiopaque. To compensate for "lack of visibility," many manufacturers have added markers at the ends of the stents to make them more visible. It is recommended to use stents with markers embedded within them to aid in proper deployment. This is not as important in the arm, where stents are better visualized, but is particularly important in the chest or abdomen where visualization can be limited.

The other form of self-expanding stent is the Wallstent by Boston Scientific. This is composed of 16 strands of woven Elgiloy, which is primarily a mixture of nickel, cobalt, and chromium. This stent is now not commonly used in North America and Europe, but is still in use within Asia. The stent is a closed cell structure which allows it to be recaptured and repositioned. However, due to the design, it is difficult to predict where the back end of the stent will end up as the stent shortens considerably from predeployment length to deployed length. The degree of foreshortening is also dependent on diameter of the stent used and the diameter of the vessel into which it is placed. This is in contrast to nitinol stents where length of the stent is not variable. In addition, due to the design of the stent, eccentric external loading of the stent can cause it to migrate or slip away from the lesion. This effect has been called the "water melon seed effect."

Complications specific to stent/stent graft insertion include:

1. Perforation of vessel by the device (<1%).
2. Migration (operator-dependent).
3. Infection (operator- and patient factor-dependent).
4. Hypersensitivity reaction to the metal (<0.1%).
5. Accelerated intimal hyperplasia and in stent stenosis with uncovered stents (100% by 1 year).

Wallstent Deployment (the Manufacturers Instructions for Use (IFU) Should be Followed)

– There are four markers on the delivery system. One is the outer sheath ring that indicates how far the outer restraining sheath for the stent has been withdrawn. The other three markers are on the inner shaft of the delivery system. The marker at the tip indicates where the stent end more centrally will be deployed. The second marker indicates the point where the stent cannot be retrieved or the point of no return. The final marker indicates the end of the stent on the delivery system. In general, when fully deployed, the distal end or end of the stent closest to the operator will end up roughly equidistant between the last two markers.

- The appropriate diameter and length device is chosen based on the lesion to be treated and the proximity of adjacent structures.
- The delivery system is a basic "pin and pull" system. The inner cannula and flush port are flushed with sterile normal saline.
- The system is then delivered over a wire, preferably nonhydrophilic, and centered so that the first or more central marker is located where the beginning part of the stent is to be deployed and the 1/2 way point between the distal two markers is roughly indicative of where the back end of the stent will deploy.
- All attempts should be made to deploy the device with the deployment system in a straight line. Any bends or curves will cause the system to migrate forward.
- The inner portion is stabilized with one hand so that it does not move. This hand and inner cannula of the system can be stabilized against the patient, the procedure table, or oneself by holding the hand tight to the body.
- The other hand is then used to pull the outer sheath back over the inner cannula, keeping the inner cannula perfectly fixed in position. This is the "pin and pull" technique (see Fig. 15.2).
- The deployment must be performed under continuous fluoroscopic visualization.
- Once the outer catheter is pulled back beyond the third inner marker, the stent is fully deployed.
- If recapturing and repositioning is required, the outer sheath can be pushed back over the stent provided the outer sheath ring has not passed the inner shaft second marker.
- Following deployment, the stent should be seated or pushed into the vessel wall by dilating it with an appropriately sized angioplasty balloon (in most cases, the same diameter as the stent if matched to adjacent vessel diameter).
- Following angioplasty, ensure the balloon is fully deflated prior to removal to prevent the balloon from catching on the stent or the stent migrating.

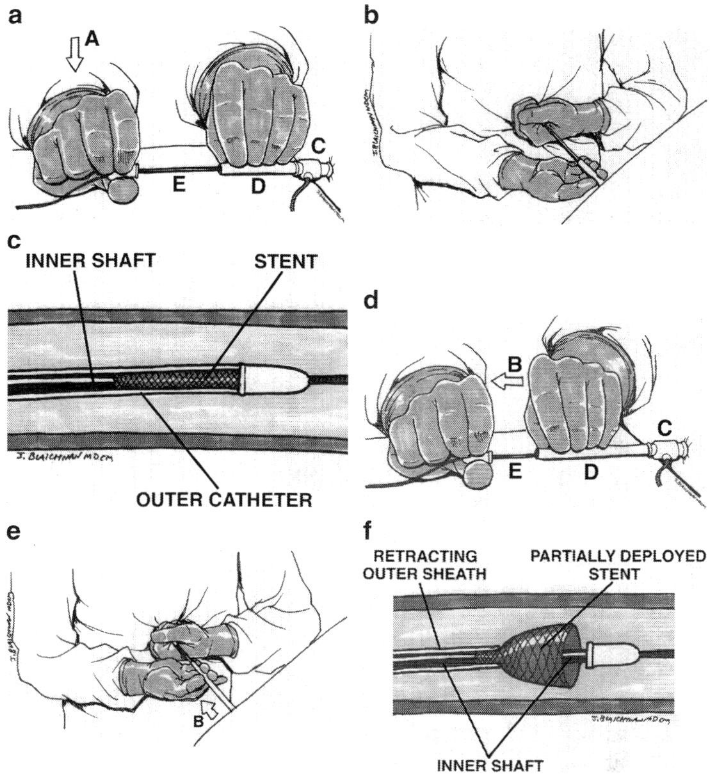

Fig. 15.2 Pin and pull technique. (**a**) The back hand (A) secures the inner metal cannula (E) and stays fixed in place (*arrow*). The outer sheath of the stent system (D) is pulled back along (E) to expose the stent. The vascular sheath (C) should not pull back or out of the vessel/access during deployment. (**b**) Suggested position for deploying the stent. (**c**) Before deployment, with fluoroscopy, one should determine which structure represents the inner shaft, the stent, and the outer constraining sleeve or sheath. These often have radiopaque markers on them and the manufacturer IFU should be reviewed. (**d**) During deployment, the hand on the outer sheath (B) pulls back the sheath (D) along the inner metal cannula (E) towards (*arrow*) the fixed back hand. (**e**) Hand on outer sheath pulling back. (**f**) As the outer sleeve or sheath is pulled back, the stent begins to deploy

Nitinol Stent Deployment (the manufacturers Instructions for Use (IFU) Should be Followed)

- Deployment is essentially the same as with Wallstents and is performed using the "pin and pull" technique described above.
- Differences are that the stents cannot be retrieved and there are typically three markers. One is on the outer delivery sheath to indicate progress of deployment and two inner shaft markers that indicate the front and back end of the stent when deployed. There is no back-end variability as with the Wallstent and the back marker accurately depicts where the back end of the stent will terminate.
- As these stents can be stretched or compressed during deployment, it is very important to prevent the inner cannula of the delivery system from moving during deployment. This is best accomplished by observing the back marker and preventing its movement during deployment.
- Also, given nitinol's characteristic of dilating to predetermined size when heated, the devices tend to migrate forward or try to pull off the delivery shaft. To avoid this problem, all attempts should be made to have the deployment system placed in a straight line. A small amount of back tension on the inner cannula will take out slack from the system and reduce forward motion. Additionally, allowing the initial portion of the stent to enlarge to size and engage the vein wall will limit later forward movement during the remainder of the deployment.

Stent Graft Deployment (the Manufacturers Instructions for Use (IFU) Should be Followed)

- Deployment is again essentially the "pin and pull" technique for most devices with exception of the Gore Viabahn device.
- There is no shortening of the devices.
- Given their increased size, they have increased frictional loads within the catheter and are, therefore, more prone to move forward during deployment. To compensate for this, some operators deploy the device 1 cm further than needed and then pull back the whole system to the point where they want to deploy the device. This maneuver removes slack from the system and reduces forward

motion of the device. This is also possible as the covering material creates little friction with the vein wall and allows the device to be pulled back, but *not* pushed forward (into the patient).

- All attempts should be made to deploy the device with the deployment system in a straight line. Any bends or curves will cause the system to migrate forward.
- As stent grafts have minimal ability to engage the vessel wall, extra care should be taken to seat these devices with postdeployment angioplasty and to ensure the balloon catheter does not dislodge the stent graft.
- For the Gore Viabahn stent graft, the device is deployed by pulling a string or "rip cord" at the hub. This results in peeling away of the outer restraining sheath.

Percutaneous (Endovascular) Thrombectomy Techniques

Although there are different considerations during thrombectomy procedures for AVG's and AVF's, the underlying techniques are similar. A procedural outline is presented at the end of the chapter. Since many of the thrombectomy techniques will result in some embolization of clot to the lungs, it is important to consider a patient's ability to tolerate the procedure. Considerations include:

1. The potential for the patient to have a PFO. This right to left shunt can be a gateway to catastrophic embolization to the arterial system.
2. Relative and absolute contraindications to thrombolytic therapy (listed below).
3. If the patient has severely compromised respiratory function such as severe chronic obstructive pulmonary disease.

In addition, intravenous heparin *should* be given to prevent production of more thrombus or rethrombosis of the access (unless the patient has heparin-induced thrombocytopenia). In general, unfractionated heparin 50–70 U/kg is given as a bolus. The half life of heparin is 60 min, but is prolonged in renal failure patients. Administration of antibiotics prior to intervention is more an operator preference with some interventionalists concerned about chronic bacterial colonization of the clotted access. No definite evidence of preprocedure antibiotic benefit has been demonstrated. Common doses are cefazolin 1 g IV or vancomycin 500 mg IV. A step-by-step guide to the thrombectomy techniques discussed below is presented in Appendix 1.

Complications, although rare, are potentially fatal (<1%) and include:

1. Septic embolism (if an occult-infected access is treated).
2. Pulmonary embolism.
3. Arterial embolism.
4. If thrombolytics used, clinically significant bleeding and/or intracranial hemorrhage (considered very rare, <0.1% since not delivered systemically).
5. Access or outflow vein rupture.
6. Hemolysis with hemoglobinuria and pancreatitis depending upon the mechanical device used for thrombectomy.
7. Volume overload.
8. Pseudoaneurysm formation.

Lyse and Wait

"Lyse and wait" [5]. Despite limited literature experience, this technique has become more widely used for AV grafts and AV fistulas. The original "lyse and wait" technique was described utilizing 250,000 U of UK; however, strategies with alternative lytic agents continue to evolve. Currently, for "lyse and wait," 2–6 mg tissue plasminogen activator (tPA) or 3 IU of Retavase with 3,000–5,000 U heparin given IV has been advocated. The drugs are injected into the graft 20 min to 2 h before the patient enters the procedure room. The intraaccess position of the sheath can be confirmed prior to injection by a small amount of blood return through the sheath or unrestricted passage of a 0.018 or 0.035 in. straight-tipped soft wire (more reliable). During the injection, both ends of the graft are compressed manually in an effort to prevent peripheral arterial and central venous emboli (see Fig. 15.3).

Once the patient enters the procedure room, partial or full thrombolysis may be found. Although the technique may be considered time saving, a prospective randomized trial comparing "lyse and wait" to mechanical lysis demonstrated no advantage in room or procedure time [6]. Similar techniques were described in the early eighties

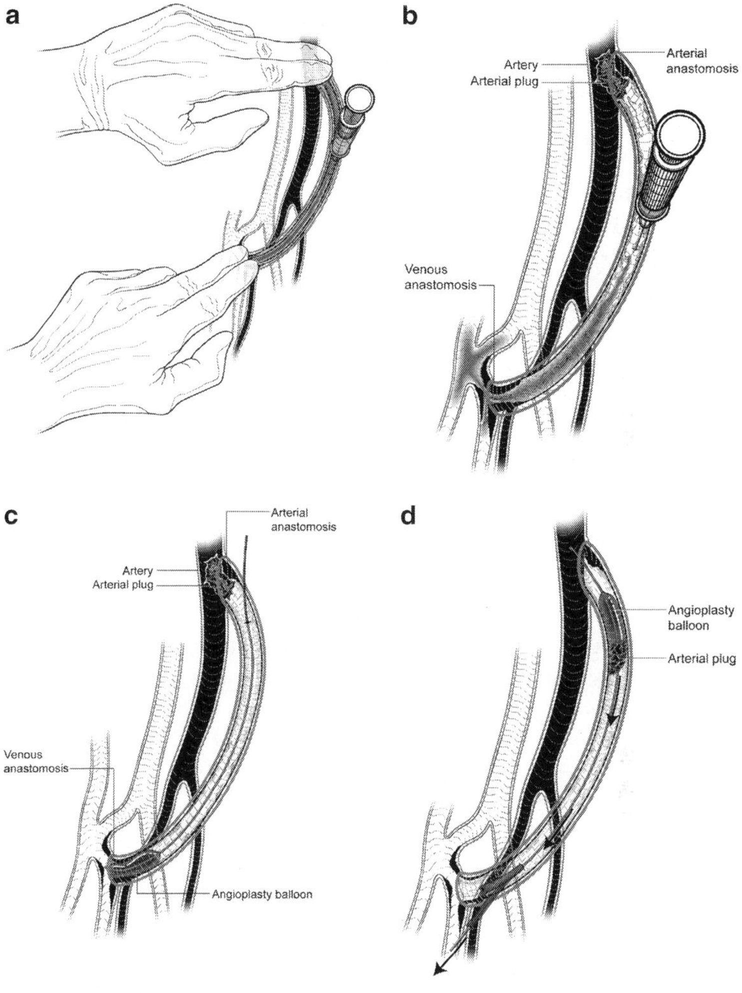

Fig. 15.3 Lyse and wait. (**a**) A small catheter is inserted into the access, and after compression of both the arterial anastomosis and venous outflow/anastomosis, thrombolytic is infused into the clot. (**b**) Clot lysis occurs over 20–60 min. (**c**) Venous anastomotic stenosis is dilated. (**d**) Arterial plug at arterial anastomosis is removed reestablishing flow within the access

mostly with streptokinase, but were abandoned due to high complication rates and poor results [7]. In addition, the status of the underlying anatomy may be unknown, i.e., the venous outflow may not be amenable to PTA prior to lytic administration. It is imperative that the patient is observed while "waiting" as significant bleeding through dialysis needle puncture sites can be encountered, especially with concurrent high-grade venous anastomotic lesions.

Infusion Thrombolysis

Infusion thrombolysis is still used by some, but abandoned by most due to high cost, long procedure time and complications associated with it. This involves infusing a thrombolytic into the access in low does over an 8–12-h period. A common dose is 1 mg of tPA or 100,000 U of urokinase per hour.

Pulse Spray

Most published literature describes the techniques and result for Urokinase. TPA is actually faster and should have the same safety profile as Urokinase if dose-equivalent amounts are used (1 mg tPA has activity of approximately 100,000 U Urokinase). The doses used now vary widely: some centers are now using 3–6 mg of tPA [8], while others are using up to 20 mg tPA. Whatever the dose, generally, heparin is not mixed with the tPA because it may cause the drug to precipitate out of solution. Heparin is, therefore, given into a central vein after the venous outflow has been assessed or through a peripheral IV. In AVF's, this technique involves passing a catheter through the entire length of thrombus and pulse spraying the entire dose over a 5-min period followed by balloon maceration of residual clot. Experience with Retavase is limited with dosing of up to 5 IU (see Fig. 15.4).

When thrombolytics are to be used, relative and absolute contraindications to their use should be reviewed for each patient [9–11].

Absolute:

1. Active clinically significant bleeding
2. Intracranial hemorrhage
3. Infected dialysis access

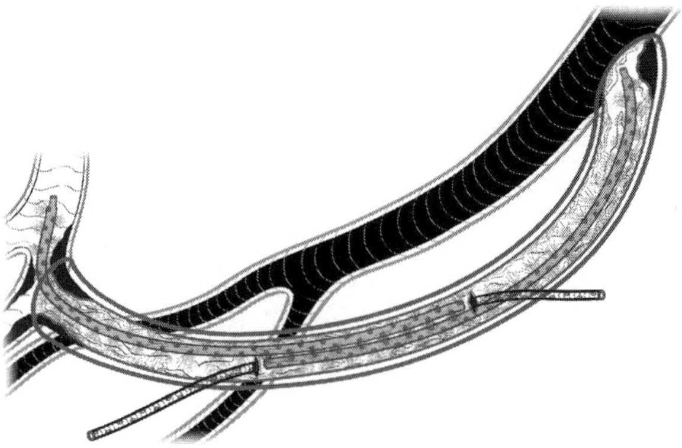

Fig. 15.4 Pulse-spray thrombolysis. Crossed infusion multisidehole catheters are placed with care taken not to have the arterial-directed catheter cross the arterial anastomosis/plug which may result in arterial embolism

Relative:

1. Cardiopulmonary resuscitation within past 10 days
2. Major nonvascular surgery or trauma within past 10 days
3. Uncontrolled hypertension: >180 mmHg systolic or >110 mmHg diastolic blood pressure
4. Intracranial tumor
5. Recent eye surgery
6. Neurosurgery (intracranial, spinal) within past 3 months Intracranial trauma within 3 months
7. Recent gastrointestinal bleeding (<10 days)
8. Established cerebrovascular event (including transient ischemic attacks within past 2 months)
9. Recent internal or noncompressible hemorrhage
10. Hepatic failure, particularly in cases with coagulopathy
11. Bacterial endocarditis
12. Diabetic hemorrhagic retinopathy

These contraindications are mostly based on consensus opinion and are also more relevant to continuous infusion therapy. For the aforementioned procedures, a relatively small dose is given over a short period of time with little systemic effect. Hence, most relative contraindications are not of concern, but should not be discounted without consideration.

Mechanical Devices

There are a number of mechanical thrombectomy devices on the market. They either macerate the clot with spinning wires or with jets of saline and particle debris is either aspirated through sheaths or the devices themselves. These include the Angiojet, Amplatzer Device, Arrow PTD device, Cleaner Rotational Thrombectomy catheter, Oasis Catheter Thrombex PMT (Edwards LifeSciences, Irvine, CA), the rotating pigtail catheter [12], and multiple other devices (Table 15.1). The Gelbfish device is based on the suction thrombectomy technique with newer devices recently introduced. Other devices can exert a direct mechanical effect to macerate clot such as the Arrow Trerotola PTD (Arrow International, Reading, PA) [13], Cleaner Rotational Thrombectomy Catheter (Rex Medical, Conshohocken, PA), and the Castaneda or the Cragg thrombolytic brush (MicroTherapeutics, San Clemente, CA) [14].

Other mechanical devices work using the Venturi effect for creating a vortex. The hydrodynamic vortex is either created by a powerful jet spray of saline or by a high-speed micropropeller. These devices include the Hydrolyser [15, 16], Clotbuster and Helix (Microvena, White Bear Lake, MN) [17–19], Angiojet [20], and the Oasis thrombectomy catheter [21]. The resulting thrombus slurry is either aspirated through the sidearm of the placed sheaths or allowed to embolize to the lungs with the exception of manual thromboaspiration. The Trellis device is a combination of multiple techniques. The device has two occlusion balloons along the shaft used to isolate the thrombosed segment to be treated. Thrombolytic may then be infused. The shaft between the two balloons acts as a coiled wire and can be spun leading to maceration of clot. The debris can then be aspirated through an aspiration port between the two balloons.

When using mechanical devices, the operator should be cognizant of the potential for significant blood loss. This can occur from aspiration of blood and mechanical fragmentation and destruction of blood cells. Use mechanical devices with caution.

Sharafuddin and Hicks [22–24] reviewed mechanical details of many of the above devices. One study also examined size distal particle embolization between four devices and found that particles >1,000 μm occurred with the Amplatz thrombectomy device [25].

Table 15.1 Characteristic of thrombectomy devices/lytic infusion catheters

Device	Indicated use	Sheath size (French)	Over-the-wire (inch)	Fragmentation	Aspiration
Mechanical thrombectomy					
Arrow-Trerotola	AVG/AVF	5–7	Available (0.025)	Yes	Yes (through sheath)
Artegraft – Dclot	AVG	6	No	Yes	Yes (through sheath)
Cordis – Hydrolyser	AVG	6	Yes (0.018)	Yes	Yes
Covidien Trellis-8 and 6	–	6–8	Yes (0.035)	Yes	Yes (also allows pharmacological thrombolysis)
Medrad Angiojet Ultra AVX	AVG/AVF	6	Yes (0.035)	Yes	Yes
Ev3 Helix/Clotbuster	AVG/AVF	7	No	Yes	No
Spectranetics ThromCat	AVF/AVG	6	Yes (0.018)	Yes	Yes
Rex Medical Cleaner	AVG	6	No	Yes	Yes (through sheath)
Aspiration only catheters					
		Over wire		Wire size	
Lumen Biomedical – Xtract Aspiration Catheter		5–6 Fr	Yes	0.014 in.	Yes
Vascular Solutions – Pronto Short Extraction Catheter		6	Yes	0.014 in.	Yes
Infusion catheters					
Angiodynamics-Speedlyser		5		0.018	
EV3-Cragg McNamara Valved Infusion Catheter		4/5		0.035/0.038 in.	
Merit Medical – Mistique Infusion Catheter		5		0.035/0.038 in.	

No studies have determined if any device is better than any other. However, there are some commonalities. Use of these devices does not require concomitant use of thrombolytics, which is considered desirable in a small subset of patients with relative contraindications to use of thrombolytics. Also, all the devices still require removal of the arterial plug, although the Arrow PTD device has been shown to be effective for this purpose as well. The arterial plug is removed by using the basket as a snare to pull out the arterial plug. Finally, all the devices are relatively more expensive than the cost of thrombolytics alone and medical cost is a consideration.

Thromboaspiration

Manual thromboaspiration involves no thrombolytic agent or device. The thromboaspiration technique uses 7–9 Fr large-lumen angled catheters, which are advanced over wires through previously inserted sheaths. Also, angled guiding sheaths can be used. Clots are then aspirated by connecting the catheter to a large-volume syringe (>30 cc) and aspirating while moving the catheter back and forth into the thrombus. The angled catheter is then removed and the clot is ejected from the catheter and then reinserted to remove more clot. The venous limb is declotted first followed by the arterial limb. The potential disadvantage of this method is loss of large volumes of blood [26, 27]. For patients that cannot tolerate thrombolytic therapy, this technique is a viable option with relatively high technical success and adequate patency outcomes (see Fig. 15.5).

Summary

Advantages of mechanical thrombectomy devices over pharmacological thrombolysis are decreased procedure times and reduced bleeding complications as thrombolytic agents are not used. Disadvantages

Fig. 15.5 Thromboaspiration technique (Modified from Turmel-Rodriques et al. [27]). Using 7 or 8 Fr angled open-ended or aspiration catheters (non-tapered), clot can be aspirated using 20–50 syringes to generate sufficient pressure. Clot can be also be aspirated around angles and pseudoaneurysms

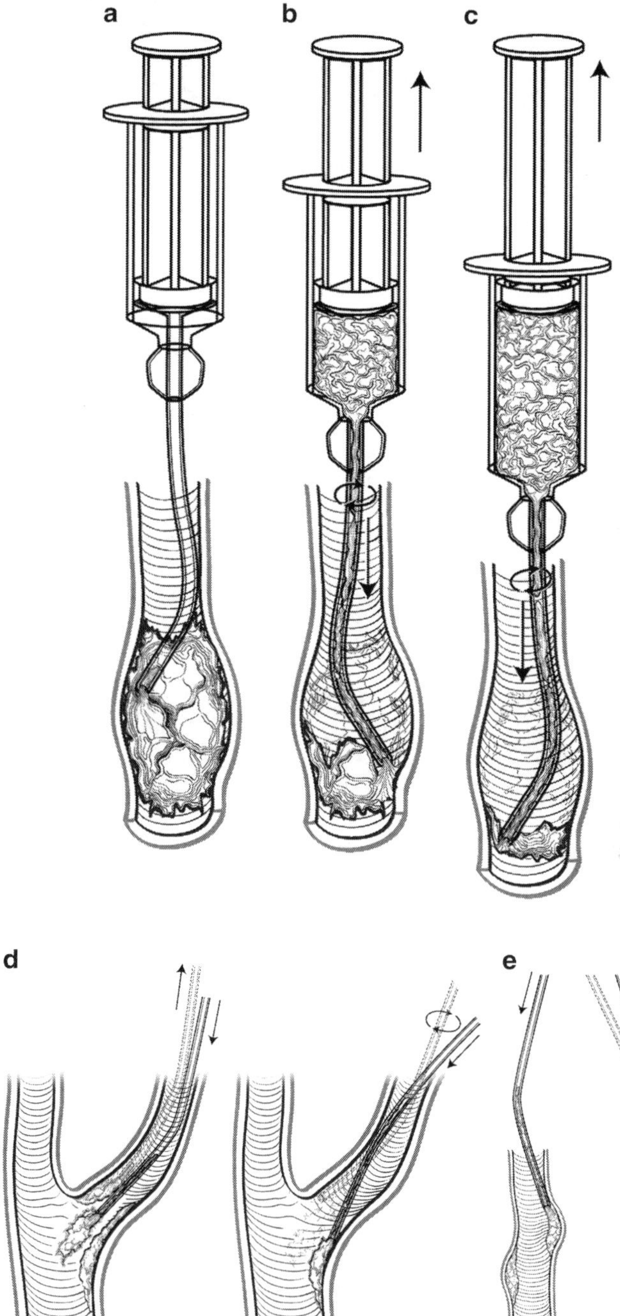
a
b
c
d
e

primarily are related to costs of the devices. Overall, these differences aside, there is no evidence that any device or method confers greater success of the procedure and improved patency of the access following thrombectomy/thrombolysis [28].

Arterial Steal

Access-related critical ischemia occurs in 3–5% of patients after construction of arteriovenous access for hemodialysis [29]. It can present as hand pain, tissue loss, and loss of neurologic function and occurs more commonly in diabetics, women, and patients with brachial artery fistulas. The difference diagnosis includes monomelic neuropathy and carpal tunnel syndrome. Diagnosis is confirmed by photoplethysmography of the digits in the involved hand. A digital pressure of less than 60 mmHg is concerning for ischemia. Digital pressures may drop even further on dialysis. Once digital ischemia is confirmed, the workup for arterial steal includes a complete assessment of that extremity's arterial tree and an evaluation of the fistula flow rate.

Duplex ultrasonography is helpful in uncovering arterial and venous stenotic lesions within the arm. It is also particularly useful in determining the direction of flow within the radial artery distal to radial cephalic fistulas. A change in flow direction from retrograde to antegrade in the distal radial artery with compression of the fistula confirms the classically described palmar arch steal by the fistula from the ulnar artery. However, there are limitations of Duplex ultrasound. It can miss critical central lesions both in the subclavian artery and central veins. Therefore, selective arteriography should be performed in all extremities prior to treatment of arterial steal.

Occasionally, minor symptoms, such as hand coolness or intermittent numbness, can be treated with covering the hand and limiting exposure to cold. These minor complaints will often improve over time with the physiologic arterial dilatation that occurs in response to the increased flows to the arm. However, more severe symptoms of rest pain or sensorimotor dysfunction must be dealt with expeditiously to avoid gangrene. Options for treatment of access-related arterial steal include ligation or coiling of the distal radial artery, fistula lengthening, banding, interposition grafting, distal revascularization with interval ligation (DRIL), revision using distal inflow (RUDI), and proximalization of the arterial inflow (PAI). The choice between these options is based on severity of the symptoms, fistula flow rate, availability of other veins both for conduit or alternative fistula sites, and the experience and capabilities of the treating physician or availability of referral services.

Percutaneous Options

All hemodynamically significant arterial stenoses from the aortic arch to the arterial anastomosis should be treated primarily, usually with balloon angioplasty by appropriately trained physicians. Orificial subclavian artery stenoses are best treated with balloon expandable stents, although self-expanding stents can be used. If arterial steal symptoms persist following correction of arterial inflow lesions, further intervention is often needed.

For arterial steal associated with radial cephalic fistulas, ligation or transcatheter coil embolization of the radial artery just distal to the arteriovenous anastomosis improves digital perfusion by eliminating retrograde flow from the palmar arch in the hand. Prior to obstructing the radial artery flow, it is critical to determine ulnar artery flow to all fingers. This can be suggested by observing flow to the hand with radial artery compression, but must be confirmed radiologically prior to embolization. This can easily be done by balloon occluding the distal radial artery, obtaining an ulnar arteriogram, and simultaneously measuring digital pressures. If adequate digital perfusion is confirmed in all fingers, the radial artery just distal to the arteriovenous anastomosis can be coil embolized [30].

During embolization, care must be taken not to allow the coil to migrate into the hand; a simple protective step is to inflate a blood pressure cuff above systolic pressure on the upper arm during deployment to limit flow through the radial artery and fistula. Short coils that are at least 1 mm larger than the distal radial artery should be employed and packed into the artery beyond the anastomosis, but not into the hand. Tornado coils (0.035 in.) are preferred. Coils are deployed by loading them into the catheter and pushing them forward with a pusher wire with a very soft tip so that, upon exit of the wire, the tip does not spasm the vessel. In addition, the catheter should be stabilized during deployment of the coil with slight forward pressure so that as the coil exits, the catheter does not push back resulting in improper coil deployment location. Embolization of large accessory or collateral veins arising off the fistula has also been performed in a small group of patients ($n=5$) with success [31].

Alternatively, the radial artery can be ligated just distal to the arteriovenous anastomosis through a small stab incision under local anesthesia, saving the cost of a coil and assuring accurate occlusion. An added benefit of ligation is that it can easily be reversed if ischemia worsens over the next several hours. Results are good in properly selected patients, with symptom resolution in 86% of patients [30]. These patients require close observation of digital perfusion following the procedure to be certain symptoms improve. A strong disadvantage of this procedure is that when symptoms persist or later recur, ligation of the fistula will no longer salvage the hand, necessitating radial artery surgical reconstruction.

There are many techniques which are utilized to optimize and standardize banding results, including plication over a catheter, banding over an angioplasty balloon (Miller procedure) [32], or overwrap of a fistula with a known size graft. Minimally invasive limited ligation endoluminally assisted revision (Miller) has been associated with excellent symptomatic relief without thrombosis by the original authors, but their results have not been replicated [32]. Through a small 1–2 cm skin incision near the arterial anastomosis (2–3 cm away), the fistula is bluntly dissected free of surrounding tissues. A 4–5 mm balloon catheter is expanded to full pressure in the juxta-anastomotic region and a 2–0 monofilament stitch is passed around the vessel containing the inflated balloon and tied. Size is determined and roughly equal or slightly smaller than the downstream artery (see Fig. 15.6). The balloon is deflated and if there are persistent symptoms of steal, the procedure is repeated with another ligature placed within 5 mm of the original ligature. The skin incision is then closed with 2–0 nylon sutures. The procedure is relatively simple, with little morbidity, and done as at outpatient under local anesthesia. Whichever technique is used, optimal banding success requires intraoperative measurement of both access flow rates and digital perfusion [33].

Surgical Options

Fistula lengthening may be useful in short fistulas with minimal ischemic symptoms, but is more commonly used as part of PAI. Banding is particularly useful for accesses with elevated flows (>1.2 L/min)

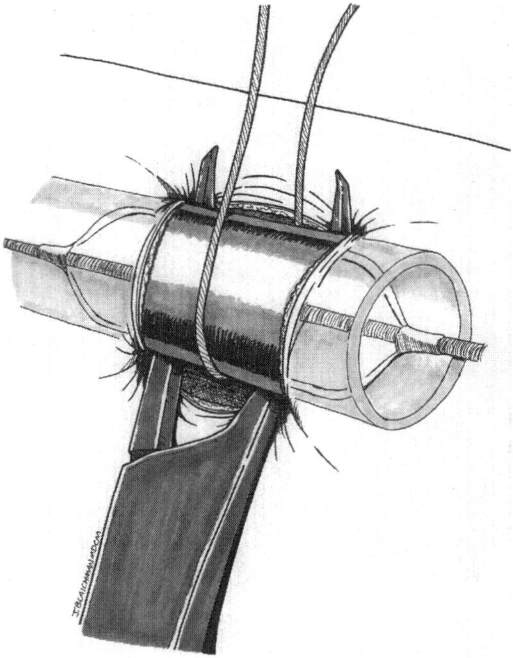

Fig. 15.6 Percutaneous banding technique for reduction of flow to reduce arterial steal

and can be used for high-output cardiac failure associated with dialysis access as well. However, in situations with modest fistula flows and digital ulceration, banding is less likely to resolve the digital ischemia adequately. Interposition grafting using a tapered 4–7 mm PTFE graft can also be used to increase outflow resistance within the access circuit to improve digital perfusion. This is particularly useful when the access is already prosthetic.

The DRIL procedure involves construction of an arterial bypass, preferably with a valved vein conduit, from above the AV anastomosis to an artery beyond the access site [34]. When native arterial continuity exists, the artery is ligated distal to the AV anastomosis, but proximal to the anastomosis of the bypass graft (see Fig. 15.7). The results of the DRIL for relief of ischemia are excellent, with 90% of patients receiving substantial or complete relief of ischemic symptoms and 75% healing ischemic lesions without amputation [35]. Additionally, the procedure is durable. The brachial artery bypass

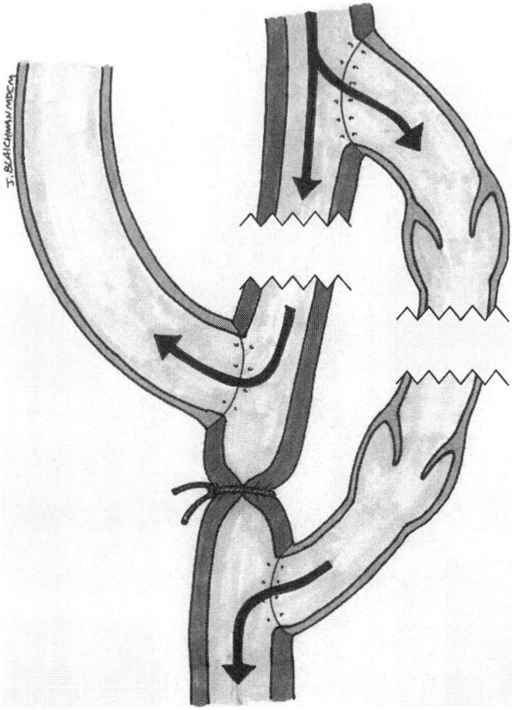

Fig. 15.7 DRIL bypass. The bypass typically originates up to 20 cm away from the access arterial origin

primary patency is 80% at 4 years, while the fistulae have primary patency rates of 83% at 1 year [35].

Alternatives to the DRIL procedure which do not require ligation of the axial artery are PAI [36] or RUDI [37]. PAI involves converting the arterial supply of the arteriovenous access to a more proximal artery using a prosthetic graft. Like the DRIL procedure, PAI is particularly useful in patients with modest fistula flow rates and significant steal symptoms. When performed in patients with severe ischemic symptoms, ulcerations, or gangrene, PAI improved symptoms in all patients, with immediate resolution in 84% [36]. Mean distal arterial pressure increased from 32±9 mmHg preoperatively to 63±8 mmHg post-PAI. Mean access flows did not change significantly. Patency of the grafts was also excellent (primary 87 and 67%, secondary 90 and 78% at 1 and 3 years, respectively). RUDI involves ligation of the distal fistula with reconstruction from a more distal arterial inflow using a vein bypass graft. It also has the advantage over the DRIL procedure in that it does not involve ligation of the axial artery. Experience with RUDI is more limited and results are variable, with high fistula failure rates in some studies [38].

In circumstances of considerable gangrene, the arteriovenous access may need to be abandoned. In this setting, arterio-arterial bypasses, for example ipsilateral axillo-axillary or fem-femoral bypasses, particularly around stenotic arterial lesions, have also been used in patients with severe peripheral artery disease with AV access created steal [39]. These bypasses have good patency rates (73% primary and 96% secondary at 1 year) with few interventions (0.47 procedures per year). Ligation of a fistula with or without further arm revascularization often improves symptoms and heals ischemic lesions, at the expense of access loss.

In summary, while banding or plication is effective in treating arterial steal in patients with relatively high flow fistulae and mild ischemic symptoms, the DRIL or PAI procedures have gained more widespread adoption in patients with moderate flow rates and rest pain or digital gangrene.

Dilation-Resistant Stenoses or the Waist that Does not Efface

It is not uncommon to encounter stenoses that are resistant to balloon angioplasty particularly in dialysis fistulas and grafts [40, 41] where higher inflation pressures often exceeding 20 atm are required. In an effort to obtain a technically successful dilation, there are a variety of methods/devices available.

Ultra-high-Pressure Balloons

For venous stenoses that are refractory to dilation with conventional angioplasty balloons, dilation with high-pressure balloons may allow successful treatment of the stenosis. These devices include the Blue Max 20 (Boston Scientific, Natick, MA) and the Powerflex Extreme (Cordis, Nutley, NJ). These devices are capable of dilation to 20 atm of rated burst pressure, although some interventionalists will routinely exceed this limit by several atmospheres. Ultra-high-pressure balloons are also available, such as the Conquest and Atlas balloons (C.R. Bard, Covington, GA). These balloons are constructed of Kevlar but maintains a low profile, and the 8 mm balloon can be inserted through a conventional 6 Fr vascular sheath. The rated burst pressure is 27 atm for the Conquest balloon and 18 atm for the larger diameter Atlas balloon, although in our practice we have routinely inflated the Conquest balloon to 35 atm without balloon disruption. A recent study supports this practice [42]. This can result in successful treatment of lesions that do not respond to conventional or other high-pressure angioplasty balloons. However, clear patency advantage in fistulas or grafts has not been demonstrated [43].

Parallel Wire Balloon Technique

A novel yet inexpensive method for dealing with a resistant stenosis in patients with synthetic grafts or fistulas is the parallel wire technique. This involves placing a guidewire between the balloon catheter and the stenosis. A new angioplasty balloon (VascuTrak, C.R. Bard, Covington, GA) is specifically designed for this purpose as well. During inflation, the wire is thought to crack or cut the intima, allowing for a controlled tear of the intima with conventional angioplasty balloons. This technique has also been used effectively in autogenous fistulas [44] for improved technical success, but no proven patency improvement (see Fig. 15.8).

Cutting Balloons

Cutting balloons have small atherotomes imbedded within the balloon material and are forced outward with inflation. The atherotome “scores” the vessel wall cutting through fibrous tissue and allows for a technically successful angioplasty for lesions resistant to normal pressure angioplasty. However, repeat POBA may be required, and with ultra-high pressure balloons now available, there is little use for them. No studies to date, including a randomized prospective multicenter study, have found a patency benefit to using these devices [45].

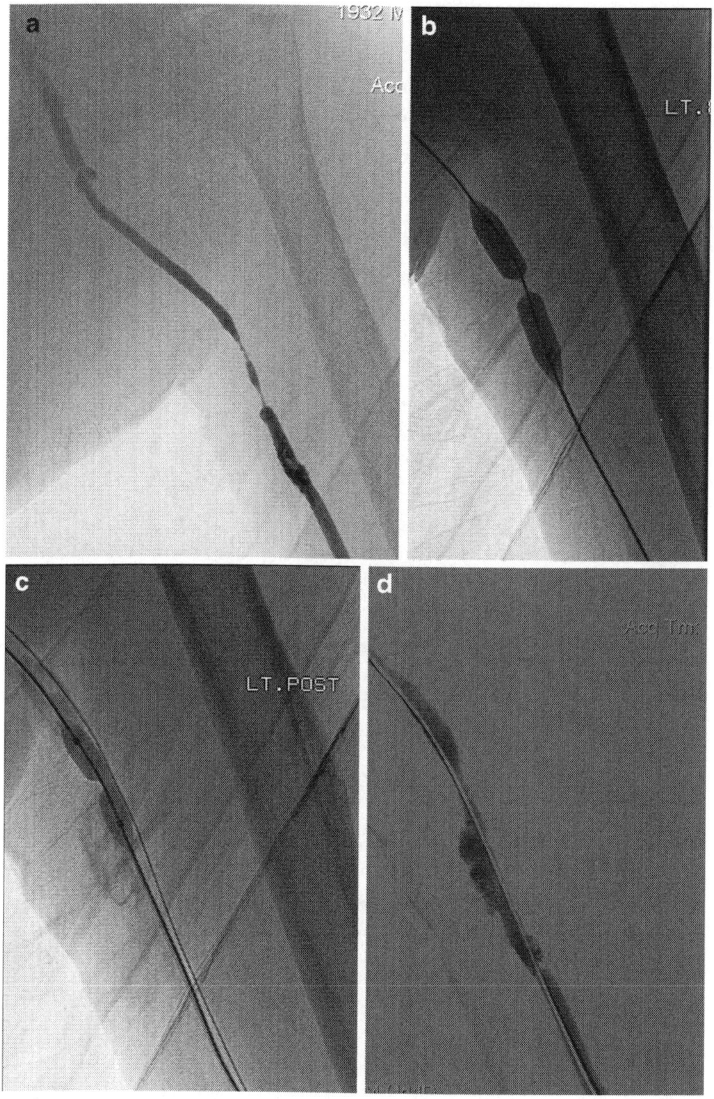

Fig. 15.8 Parallel wire balloon dilation. (**a**) Focal basilic vein stenosis. (**b**) Despite dilation with an 8 mm PTA balloon inflated to 30 atm, a tight focal stenosis persists. (**c**) A 0.018 in. mandril wire is placed across the stenosis and the balloon is reinflated. (**d**) Resultant parallel wire dilation results in dilation of stenosis

Stents

Stents are *not* indicated for resistant stenoses, as the radial force of a stent will not overcome the stenosis in the short- or long-term. The adage that "a stent is only as good as your first angioplasty" should be borne in mind when considering stent placement. At present, stent placement should be reserved for circumstances in strict accordance with the DOQI guidelines [46].

Elastic Recoil

Elastic recoil has been defined by many interventionalists as renarrowing within minutes of a successfully dilated (no residual waist along the balloon) venous stenosis. If, after successfully effacing the waist on the balloon, sufficient elastic recoil occurs to render the angioplasty unsatisfactory (i.e. ≥30%), the initial approach used by most is either prolonged inflation times (5 min or more) for one or two more inflations or progressive balloon enlargement up to 2 mm larger than the original balloon size used (in the absence of pain during inflation with the original balloon).

Although some interventionalists and most stent device companies are advocating for stent placement of elastic recoil lesions, there has been no study to indicate any improved outcomes. In fact, there has been no study that properly defines, quantifies, qualifies, and determines outcomes of elastic recoil in dialysis grafts and fistulas. Although this is an indication to stent by K/DOQI practice standards, this statement is a consensus statement in the absence of any significant data. An option is reexamining the access with Transonics at the next dialysis treatment, and if there continued decreased flows, the patient is referred for repeat intervention (see Fig. 15.9). If this is still unsuccessful, stents may be considered in selected instances.

Pseudoaneurysms

Within dialysis grafts, pseudoaneurysms are in areas of graft degeneration often from frequent needle punctures. By K/DOQI Guideline 27, they require treatment when the pseudoaneurysm:

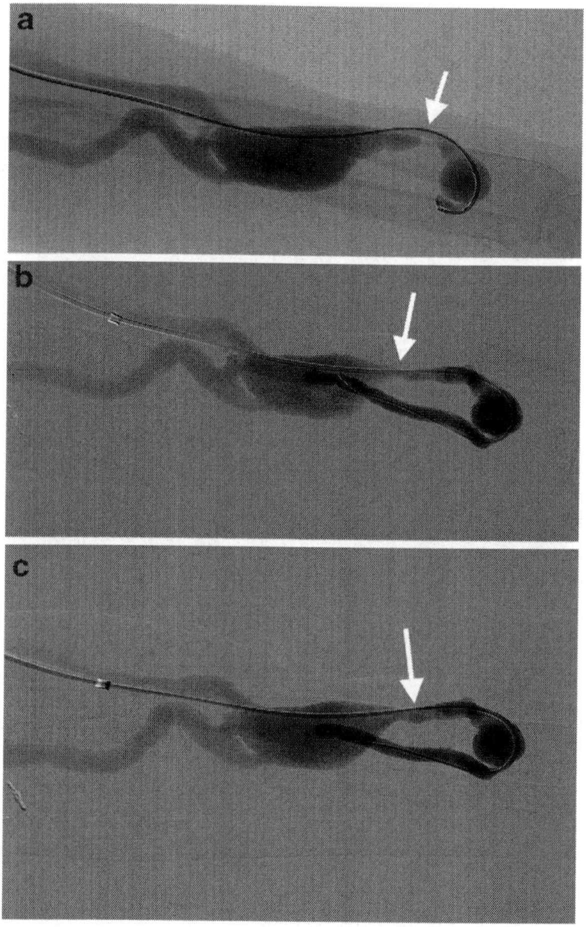

Fig. 15.9 Argument against elastic recoil. (**a**) Focal stenosis (*arrow*) in proximal radiocephalic fistula. (**b**) Five minutes after dilation with 6 mm PTA balloon, there is recurrent narrowing (*arrow*) or elastic recoil. (**c**) 15 min after PTA, elastic recoil has resolved (*arrow*)

1. Is characterized by rapid expansion in size (Evidence/Opinion)
2. Exceeds twice the diameter of the graft (Opinion)
3. Threatens viability of the overlying skin (Opinion) and
4. Is infected (Evidence)

Within fistulas, the etiology of aneurysm formation is less clear, but they are usually associated with increased fistula pressure from outflow stenoses. Within both access types, these areas represent potential rupture and therefore a potential medical emergency.

Physical examination and an appropriate history will help determine if there is a need for intervention or observation. One simple maneuver is to pinch the skin over the pseudoaneurysm. If you can pinch it, there is redundancy to the tissue and a low risk of rupture. If the skin is shiny, taut, appears stretched, and/or has a blood clot on top of it, then intervention is likely required acutely. Consultation with an access surgeon is advised.

Arterial Pathology

A little considered cause of AVF or AVG dysfunction is arterial inflow lesions. While many interventionalists interrogate the arterial anastomosis, further upstream pathology can exist. Such pathology can contribute to repeated thrombosis of the access, failure of an AVF to mature, insufficient flows for proper dialysis, and "Steal syndrome" Some of these specific problems are discussed in the relevant chapters. However, there are some general considerations.

Arterial lesions can arise not uncommonly from the subclavian artery onwards (see Fig. 15.10) [47] (and from the abdominal aorta downwards for lower body access sites). A simple way to assess for a possible arterial stenosis/occlusion is to place a catheter via the dialysis access retrograde into the feeding artery and measure the arterial pressure. This can be compared to the cuff blood pressure in the opposite arm.

If an arterial inflow lesion is suspected, further assessment can be obtained by passing a catheter retrograde up the feeding artery through the access to the level where pathology is no longer suspected. If this is done, a 4 Fr catheter is recommended and care should be taken to prevent spasm of the artery when advancing the catheter. Another option is to assess arterial flow with a proper arterial Doppler ultrasound examination or a CT arteriogram.

Although techniques for interventions on arterial stenoses are similar to those for venous stenoses within AV accesses, there are potentially more severe complications that can occur for the operator who is not properly trained and performs arterial interventions routinely. For the practicing interventionalist who is not familiar with arterial interventions, dilating the feeding artery or arterial anasto-mosis to the access should be the limit of intervention. Such interventions are beyond the scope of this book and appropriate consultation should be sought.

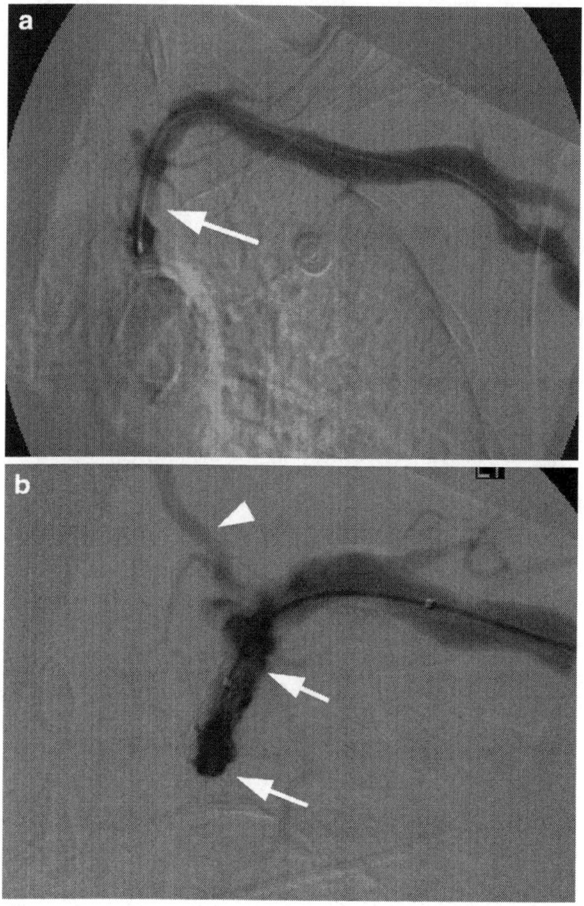

Fig. 15.10 Patient with poor flows through upper arm graft. (**a**) A catheter is advanced to the origin of the subclavian artery which demonstrated (*arrow*) atherosclerotic osteal narrowing. (**b**) The stenosis is corrected with an 8 mm balloon expandable stent (*arrows*) with careful attention paid to not covering the vertebral artery (*arrowhead*) which would have devastating consequences for the patient

For example, if the patient has a subclavian artery osteal stenosis, primary treatment would be stent placement. Complications from an improperly performed intervention include acute ischemia of the arm, stroke via the vertebral artery, possible heart ischemic insult if the patient has an internal mammary artery bypass to the heart, and loss of the stent within the aorta.

When dilating the feeding artery or arterial anastomosis, the operator should be aware that vessel spasm and dissection are much more common than within dialysis accesses and outflow veins. Oversizing of the dilation balloon is not recommended, and in heavily calcified arteries, using a smaller balloon reduces the risk of these complications. Stenting of feeding arteries is not advised as small diameter stents in peripheral arteries have poor patency and are prone to accelerated intimal hyperplasia and thrombosis. If arterial spasm occurs, beyond conservative management, one can administer nitroglycerine intra-arterially in the area of spasm in doses of 100–300 μg in 5–10 min intervals up to a total dose of 1,000 μg. The patient's blood pressure should be monitored continuously, and if there is a significant drop in pressure, nitroglycerine doses should be discontinued.

Anticoagulation and Antiplatelet Therapy

To date, there is no clear evidence that any prophylactic medication reduces intimal hyperplasia or reduces access thrombosis rates. Some clinicians place patients who have frequently thrombosing accesses in the absence of stenoses on low-dose warfarin with the hope of preserving the access. There is no conclusive evidence to support this practice.

Other Common Considerations/Tips

External manipulation/massage assists in passage of angioplasty balloons and/or passage of thrombectomy devices/catheters through tortuous portions and pseudoaneurysms in AVF's/AVG's. Some interventionalists forgo the use of access sheaths for simple interventions. If POBA is planned, then there is no need to place a sheath. However, if multiple manipulations or more complex interventions are planned, a sheath provides a less traumatic pathway to the access as well as an ability to image the fistula during interventions. If all endovascular techniques fail, then surgical revision must be considered.

When stenosis is suspected but not clearly identified, pulling back a partially inflated angioplasty balloon across the access may indicate occult points of stenosis. Under fluoroscopic visualization, the stenosis is revealed when the balloon deforms or compresses as it crosses the stenosis. Pullback pressures through a catheter may also identify an occult lesion. During POBA of stenoses, if there is concern regarding access thromboses during prolonged inflation, injection of saline or contrast via the introduction sheath (if placed) will displace blood from the access in most cases decreasing the risk of inadvertent thrombosis.

Considerations for Primary Surgical Intervention

Angioplasty

While angioplasty of stenotic venous lesions in dialysis access circuits has a high rate of technical success, long-term patency is limited. Therefore, selected lesions may be more effectively treated surgically. Recurrent stenotic lesions will certainly recur in short order with repeated angioplasty. In these situations, consideration should be given to surgical repair with vein or PTFE patch angioplasty, interposition grafting, or transposition of the graft to another outflow vein. Short segment interposition grafts have good primary patency in this situation (71% at 1 year) [48]. Swing segment stenoses in the distal cephalic vein of radial cephalic fistulas presents a persist problem with poor long-term results following angioplasty. Again, in the setting of failed or recurrent stenosis after angioplasty, surgical correction with proximalization of the arteriovenous anastomosis is well tolerated, durable, and allows continued use of the fistula after the procedure. One-year primary and secondary patencies of proximalization of radial cephalic fistulas are 80 and 95%, respectively [49]. Optimal treatment of graft venous anastomotic stenoses also often involves more than just angioplasty. Placement of a stent graft across the venous anastomosis results in better patencies than angioplasty alone [50]. However, certain locations are not amenable to stent graft placement. These stent grafts cannot be placed across joints, across anastomoses with greater than a 90° angulation, or into branching veins where the stent graft would occlude an outflow for the graft. Surgical correction with graft extensions or patches should be considered in these settings. Alternatively, an upper arm fistula can be constructed from the outflow vein. Always consider a treatment option's effect on future fistula sites.

Thrombectomy

Surgical thrombectomy offers an excellent option to percutaneous thrombectomy or thrombolysis and is preferred in select circumstances. The preferred method depends upon local expertise, equipment, and access. When surgical correction of venous aneurysms, pseudoaneurysms from degenerated grafts, infected grafts, skin erosions, poor outflow veins, or chronic thrombus is required, the thrombectomy should be performed surgically at the same setting. All of these conditions increase the risk of failure or complications from percutaneous treatment, and such thrombectomy is unnecessary if surgery is required subsequently. For fistulas, surgical thrombectomy is as technically successful as percutaneous thrombectomy, but has better long-term patencies (51–84% primary and 69–95% secondary patency at 1 year) [51]. This is likely due to the difficulty of aspirating or removing aged thrombus from an irregularly sized vessel using current percutaneous techniques. Therefore, fistulas with large aneurysmal segments or recurrent thrombosis should be considered for surgical thrombectomy.

As stated above, percutaneous access thrombectomy can carry significant risks, particularly in regard to embolization. Percutaneous thrombectomy carries a 23–59% risk of embolization when studied with perfusion scans or pulmonary angiography [52, 53]. While mostly asymptomatic, these emboli can be significant in patients with pulmonary hypertension, severe pulmonary or cardiac disease, or PFO. Since larger thrombi can be removed through a venotomy than a catheter, flow is reversed within the vein during surgical thrombectomy; and firm, attached thrombus can be more effectively removed with open thrombectomy; surgical thrombectomy carries a much lower risk of pulmonary embolism. Therefore, surgical thrombectomy is also preferred in these high-risk patients.

Key Points

- The enemy of "good" is "better."
- PTA balloon, stent, and stent graft size is usually 1 mm larger than the adjacent normal vein segment.
- When stenting, avoid overextending the stent into normal vein segments to preserve venous capital.

- A stent/stent graft is only as good as your angioplasty for stenosis. PTA has a greater outward radial force than self-expanding stents.
- If unable to profile the arterial/venous anastomosis, rather than rotating the image intensifier, have the patient or you rotate their arm.
- It is important to image the entire access circuit from the feeding artery to the right atrium.
- Thrombosis can occasionally occur in the absence of stenosis.
- For thrombectomy and thrombolysis, it is important to remove all clot, specifically remove the entire arterial plug and dilate all significant stenoses.
- Infection of the access is an absolute contraindication to thrombectomy/thrombolysis.
- "You only get one chance to place a permanently implantable device in a patient once." Take your time and be sure of what you are doing.
- Elastic recoil is a poorly characterized event.
- If you do not routinely treat arterial pathology, do not assume interventions are similar to those performed in AV accesses. Seek appropriate consultation.

Appendix 1. AV Graft/AV Fistulae Thrombectomy

Pulse Spray

- The area containing the graft/fistula is prepared and draped to create a sterile field.
- For both straight and looped grafts, two puncture sites are required to access the entire circuit to remove all clot and the arterial plug. Puncture sites should be chosen to allow for access to both the arterial and venous portions of the graft (antegrade and retrograde access), but not so close to each other where a portion of the access is not accessible.
- Using a 25G needle, the skin at expected locations of puncture is infiltrated with 1% lidocaine.

- The graft is then punctured with either an 18/19G needle that can accommodate a 0.035 in. wire or a 21G needle from a micropuncture set at a 45–60° angle.
- The first puncture is preferably made in the arterial portion of the graft-directed antegrade towards the venous outflow.
- When performing the puncture, care should be taken to avoid puncturing the back wall of the graft. Ultrasound, if available, is a convenient tool to aid puncture.
- A wire is then advanced through the needle, and with fluoroscopy and/or palpation of the graft, intraluminal location is verified.
- If a 0.035 in. wire is used, a nonhydrophilic straight soft-tipped wire is preferred to push through the clot. For the micropuncture set, the wire provided is used and later upsized to a 0.035 in. wire.
- If access is primarily obtained towards the venous outflow, after placement of an appropriately sized sheath over a wire (6 Fr for routine PTA), a catheter is advanced beyond the clot and the venous outflow is assessed. Any venous outflow stenosis is treated with PTA. Some treat stenosis before pulse spray.
- Position pulse-spray catheter (s) in the graft. Most use two "crossing" catheters.
- Reconstitute agent. For tPA, 2 mg is reconstituted in 2 mL of sterile water for injection. Doses of 2–6 mg can be used. For urokinase, where available, 250,000–1,000,000 U can be used. A variety of 4–5 Fr pulse-spray catheters are available from Merit Medical, EV3, and Angiodynamics.
- The thrombolytic agent is then pulsed in through the catheter in 0.5–1 cc forceful injections. Use a 3-cc syringe or smaller to generate high pressure to force thrombolytic into the clot every 10–30 s.
- After pulse spray, if a second sheath has not been placed, this is now done within the venous limb of the graft directed towards the arterial plug. Care should be taken to avoid pushing the arterial plug into the feeding artery when placing this sheath (4–5 Fr).
- Depending on the length of untreated clot within the arterial limb, a pulse-spray catheter can be advanced to but not beyond the arterial plug and further thrombolytic can be delivered.
- Thrombolytic dwell time should be at least 15 min.
- The arterial plug is then removed by either suction aspiration or by using a Fogarty balloon catheter (4 Fr).
- If a Fogarty catheter is used, the catheter is passed into the feeding artery and the balloon should be inflated to the point of slightly

molding along the arterial wall and in this inflated state, pulled across the arterial anastomosis.
- Gentle suction is placed on the sheath so that the arterial plug is aspirated upon withdrawal of the Fogarty catheter.
- Assess using physical examination of the graft. A thrill or pulse should be present (see endpoint determination).
- Treat residual clot in the graft with balloon maceration and/or external compression.
- After all possible clot is removed, the arterial inflow can be assessed by inflating a balloon within the outflow and refluxing contrast gently back across the arterial anastomosis to assess for stenosis and/or residual clot.
- Perform a final fistulogram from the arterial inflow to the right atrium and treat any remaining significant stenoses. Make sure to profile each anastomosis and ensure all significant stenoses have been dilated and no residual clot persists particularly at the arterial anastomosis.

Lyse and Wait

This methodology is often desirable as this technique allows for delivery of the thrombolytic agent prior to the patient arriving within the procedure room. In general, the thrombolytic is delivered 30–45 min before the procedure, and over that time interval, another procedure can be performed. By the time the patient enters the procedure room, most of the clot has dissolved thereby reducing the in-room procedure time. The methodology is very similar to the pulse spray methodology with the following exceptions:

- A small area of the access is prepared and draped in a sterile fashion within the holding or triage area.
- Access is obtained to the access with an angiocatheter or micropuncture set within the arterial limb of the graft or arterial anastomosis with the catheter directed towards the venous outflow. Intraaccess location should be verified either by attempting to aspirate clot, passing a wire into the access and withdrawing it and checking the wire for adherent clot, or visualizing the wire using ultrasound.
- The thrombolytic is then injected into the access with firm digital pressure applied at the arterial anastomosis to occlude it and prevent pushing clot into the artery. The venous outflow is also

compressed to allow the thrombolytic to be forced throughout the clot within the access.

- When the patient is taken to the procedure room, the entire access is prepared and draped sterilely and a fistulogram is performed (very gentle injection of contrast so pressure is not introduced into the graft) through the catheter within the access.
- If outflow stenoses are found, the catheter is exchanged over a wire and exchanged for an appropriately sized sheath to accommodate the devices needed for treating the stenoses/occlusion.
- A second puncture is performed towards the arterial inflow and access is obtained to remove the arterial plug at the arterial anastomosis.
- Occasionally, the arterial plug can be removed or dislodged with external massage of the arterial anastomosis towards the outflow.

Mechanical Devices (Modify According to each Individual Device After Reviewing the IFU)

With use of mechanical devices, sterile preparation of the access is required and sheaths are placed into the access to allow access to all clot.

- Apply the mechanical thrombolytic device to the venous end of graft or fistula (some prefer this step before placing an "arterial" sheath; others find it easier to place both wires and cross them before passing the sheaths). In fistulas, external compression of aneurysms onto the thrombectomy device may aid in clearing thrombus from these areas.
- Place the "arterial" sheath.
- Apply mechanical device to arterial end of the access.
- If applicable, aspirate after each pass (PTD).
- Treat the arterial plug (Fogarty, occlusion balloon, device, adherent thrombectomy catheter).
- Assess and treat any significant peripheral venous outflow stenosis with PTA.
- After the clot is removed, the arterial inflow can be assessed by inflating a balloon within the outflow and refluxing contrast gently back across the arterial anastomosis to assess for stenosis and/or residual clot.

- Assess patency using physical exam of the access. A thrill or pulse should be present (see endpoint determination).
- Treat any residual clot with the device or balloon maceration as necessary.
- Perform a final fistulogram from arterial inflow to the right atrium.

Balloon-Assisted Thromboaspiration

- Place a 6 or 7 Fr removable hub "venous" sheath if available. Remove hub and aspirate clot if possible.
- Replace hub. If a hub removing sheath is not available, a sheath should be used where the side arm allows for aspiration. I prefer to use the Performer sheath (Cook Medical, Bloomington, IN) which has a large sidearm port.
- Place a 6 Fr "arterial sheath."
- Pass a 5 Fr Fogarty catheter along arterial limb to near anastomosis. Inflate balloon and pull back toward sheath while aspirating on 6/7 Fr sheath with hub removed or aspirating via the sidearm. Another option is to place a 20-cc Luer lock syringe on the sheath sidearm and pull the plunger back to the point where it locks in the withdrawn position maintaining continuous suction.
- Repeat step 3, passing the balloon beyond arterial anastomosis.
- Assess the access for pulsatility to confirm inflow. If inflow is absent, repeat the balloon thrombectomy until pulsatility is restored.
- Pass the 5 Fr Fogarty catheter through venous sheath beyond central limit of remaining clot.
- Inflate the balloon and withdraw catheter while aspiring through the sidearm of sheath (s).
- Repeat steps as necessary.
- Assess residual clot burden; if large, use a mechanical device to complete the procedure or try external massage of the access to mobilize clot. If not, assess and treat venous outflow stenosis with PTA.
- Assess graft/fistula with physical exam. A thrill should be restored after successful PTA (see endpoint determination above).
- Treat any residual clot with Fogarty balloon, with all attempts to aspirate all clot. Perform final fistulogram from arterial inflow to right atrium and treat any significant stenoses.

Manual Catheter-Directed Thromboaspiration

- After insertion of a 7 or 8 Fr sheath into the dialysis access preferably near the arterial anastomosis directed towards the outflow, aspirate clots using a 7 or 8 Fr slightly angled (vertebral or multipurpose type) aspiration catheter. Perform as many passes as necessary until no additional clots are aspirated. Use a 20–50-cc Luer lock syringe.
- Leave a guide wire through the venous-directed sheath and place 7 or 8 Fr arterial-directed sheath into the access.
- Push, very gently, a slightly angled 5 Fr catheter over a hydrophilic guide wire into the artery and check the exact level of the arterial anastomosis.
- Aspirate clots starting from the sheath. If the catheter is clogged, flush it into gauze and reintroduce it further toward the anastomosis.
- Inject gently 2–5 mL of contrast medium through the arterial sheath during compression of the graft/fistula and look for residual clots.
- Push the angled aspiration catheter to contact any residual clots and aspirate with quick back and forth movements to detach the thrombi. Stop only when no residual clot is visible.
- When no residual clot is visible, dilate any underlying stenoses.
- To dilate before aspiration of all the thrombi increases the risk of pulmonary embolism.
- After clot is removed, the arterial inflow can be assessed by inflating a balloon within the outflow and refluxing contrast gently back across the arterial anastomosis to assess for stenosis and/or residual clot.
- Perform a final angiogram from arterial inflow to right atrium [27, 54, 55].

References

1. Trerotola SO, Ponce P, Stavropoulos SW, et al. Physical examination versus normalized pressure ratio for predicting outcomes of hemodialysis access interventions. J Vasc Interv Radiol. 2003;14(11):1387–94.
2. Sullivan KL, Besarab A, Bonn J, Shapiro MJ, Gardiner Jr GA, Moritz MJ. Hemodynamics of failing dialysis grafts. Radiology. 1993;186(3):867–72.
3. Lilly RZ, Carlton D, Barker J, et al. Predictors of arteriovenous graft patency after radiologic intervention in hemodialysis patients. Am J Kidney Dis. 2001;37(5):945–53.

4. Forauer AR, Hoffer EK, Homa K. Dialysis access venous stenoses: treatment with balloon angioplasty-1- versus 3-minute inflation times. Radiology. 2008;249(1):375–81.
5. Cynamon J, Lakritz PS, Wahl SI, Bakal CW, Sprayregen S. Hemodialysis graft declotting: description of the "lyse and wait" technique. J Vasc Interv Radiol. 1997;8(5):825–9.
6. Vogel PM, Bansal V, Marshall MW. Thrombosed hemodialysis grafts: lyse and wait with tissue plasminogen activator or urokinase compared to mechanical thrombolysis with the Arrow-Trerotola Percutaneous Thrombolytic Device. J Vasc Interv Radiol. 2001;12(10):1157–65.
7. Zeit RM. Arterial and venous embolization: declotting of dialysis shunts by direct injection of streptokinase. Radiology. 1986;159(3):639–41.
8. Rajan DK, Clark TW, Simons ME, Kachura JR, Sniderman K. Procedural success and patency after percutaneous treatment of thrombosed autogenous arteriovenous dialysis fistulas. J Vasc Interv Radiol. 2002;13(12):1211–8.
9. Rajan DK, Patel NH, Valji K, et al. Quality improvement guidelines for percutaneous management of acute limb ischemia. J Vasc Interv Radiol. 2009;20 (7 Suppl):S208–18.
10. NIH Consensus Development summary. Thrombolytic therapy in thrombosis. South Med J. 1980;73(11):1525–6.
11. Semba CP, Bakal CW, Calis KA, et al. Alteplase as an alternative to urokinase. Advisory Panel on Catheter-Directed Thrombolytic Therapy. J Vasc Interv Radiol. 2000;11(3):279–87.
12. Schmitz-Rode T, Wildberger JE, Hubner D, Wein B, Schurmann K, Gunther RW. Recanalization of thrombosed dialysis access with use of a rotating mini-pigtail catheter: follow-up study. J Vasc Interv Radiol. 2000;11(6): 721–7.
13. Trerotola SO, Vesely TM, Lund GB, Soulen MC, Ehrman KO, Cardella JF. Treatment of thrombosed hemodialysis access grafts: Arrow-Trerotola percutaneous thrombolytic device versus pulse-spray thrombolysis. Arrow-Trerotola Percutaneous Thrombolytic Device Clinical Trial. Radiology. 1998;206(2):403–14.
14. Dolmatch BL, Casteneda F, McNamara TO, Zemel G, Lieber M, Cragg AH. Synthetic dialysis shunts: thrombolysis with the Cragg thrombolytic brush catheter. Radiology. 1999;213(1):180–4.
15. Vorwerk D, Schurmann K, Muller-Leisse C, et al. Hydrodynamic thrombectomy of haemodialysis grafts and fistulae: results of 51 procedures. Nephrol Dial Transplant. 1996;11(6):1058–64.
16. Overbosch EH, Pattynama PM, Aarts HJ, Schultze Kool LJ, Hermans J, Reekers JA. Occluded hemodialysis shunts: Dutch multicenter experience with the hydrolyser catheter. Radiology. 1996;201(2):485–8.
17. Qian Z, Kvamme P, Raghed D, et al. Comparison of a new recirculation thrombectomy catheter with other devices of the same type: in vitro and in vivo evaluations. Invest Radiol. 2002;37(9):503–11.
18. Uflacker R, Rajagopalan PR, Vujic I, Stutley JE. Treatment of thrombosed dialysis access grafts: randomized trial of surgical thrombectomy versus mechanical thrombectomy with the Amplatz device. J Vasc Interv Radiol. 1996;7(2):185–92.

19. Sofocleous CT, Cooper SG, Schur I, Patel RI, Iqbal A, Walker S. Retrospective comparison of the Amplatz thrombectomy device with modified pulse-spray pharmacomechanical thrombolysis in the treatment of thrombosed hemodialysis access grafts. Radiology. 1999;213(2):561–7.
20. Vesely TM, Williams D, Weiss M, et al. Comparison of the angiojet rheolytic catheter to surgical thrombectomy for the treatment of thrombosed hemodialysis grafts. Peripheral AngioJet Clinical Trial. J Vasc Interv Radiol. 1999;10 (9):1195–205.
21. Barth KH, Gosnell MR, Palestrant AM, et al. Hydrodynamic thrombectomy system versus pulse-spray thrombolysis for thrombosed hemodialysis grafts: a multicenter prospective randomized comparison. Radiology. 2000;217(3): 678–84.
22. Sharafuddin MJ, Hicks ME. Current status of percutaneous mechanical thrombectomy. Part I. General principles. J Vasc Interv Radiol. 1997;8(6): 911–21.
23. Sharafuddin MJ, Hicks ME. Current status of percutaneous mechanical thrombectomy. Part III. Present and future applications. J Vasc Interv Radiol. 1998;9(2):209–24.
24. Sharafuddin MJ, Hicks ME. Current status of percutaneous mechanical thrombectomy. Part II. Devices and mechanisms of action. J Vasc Interv Radiol. 1998;9(1 Pt 1):15–31.
25. Muller-Hulsbeck S, Grimm J, Leidt J, Jahnke T, Heller M. Comparison of in vitro effectiveness of mechanical thrombectomy devices. J Vasc Interv Radiol. 2001;12(10):1185–91.
26. Poulain F, Raynaud A, Bourquelot P, Knight C, Rovani X, Gaux JC. Local thrombolysis and thromboaspiration in the treatment of acutely thrombosed arteriovenous hemodialysis fistulas. Cardiovasc Interv Radiol. 1991;14 (2):98–101.
27. Turmel-Rodrigues L, Sapoval M, Pengloan J, et al. Manual thromboaspiration and dilation of thrombosed dialysis access: mid-term results of a simple concept. J Vasc Interv Radiol. 1997;8(5):813–24.
28. Vashchenko N, Korzets A, Neiman C, et al. Retrospective comparison of mechanical percutaneous thrombectomy of hemodialysis arteriovenous grafts with the Arrow-Trerotola device and the lyse and wait technique. AJR Am J Roentgenol. 2010;194(6):1626–9.
29. Tordoir JH, Dammers R, van der Sande FM. Upper extremity ischemia and hemodialysis vascular access. Eur J Vasc Endovasc Surg. 2004;27(1):1–5.
30. Miller GA, Khariton K, Kardos SV, Koh E, Goel N, Khariton A. Flow interruption of the distal radial artery: treatment for finger ischemia in a matured radiocephalic AVF. J Vasc Access. 2008;9(1):58–63.
31. Kariya S, Tanigawa N, Kojima H, et al. Transcatheter coil embolization for steal syndrome in patients with hemodialysis access. Acta Radiol. 2009;50(1): 28–33.
32. Goel N, Miller GA, Jotwani MC, Licht J, Schur I, Arnold WP. Minimally invasive limited ligation endoluminal-assisted revision (MILLER) for treatment of dialysis access-associated steal syndrome. Kidney Int. 2006;70(4):765–70.
33. Scheltinga MR, Van Hoek F, Bruyninckx CM. Surgical banding for refractory hemodialysis access-induced distal ischemia (HAIDI). J Vasc Access. 2009; 10(1):43–9.

34. Schanzer H, Schwartz M, Harrington E, Haimov M. Treatment of ischemia due to "steal" by arteriovenous fistula with distal artery ligation and revascularization. J Vasc Surg. 1988;7(6):770–3.
35. Knox RC, Berman SS, Hughes JD, Gentile AT, Mills JL. Distal revascularization-interval ligation: a durable and effective treatment for ischemic steal syndrome after hemodialysis access. J Vasc Surg. 2002;36(2):250–5. discussion 256.
36. Zanow J, Kruger U, Scholz H. Proximalization of the arterial inflow: a new technique to treat access-related ischemia. J Vasc Surg. 2006;43(6):1216–21. discussion 1221.
37. Minion DJ, Moore E, Endean E. Revision using distal inflow: a novel approach to dialysis-associated steal syndrome. Ann Vasc Surg. 2005;19(5): 625–8.
38. Callaghan CJ, Mallik M, Sivaprakasam R, Iype S, Pettigrew GJ. Treatment of dialysis access-associated steal syndrome with the "revision using distal inflow" technique. J Vasc Access. 2010;12(1):52–6.
39. Zanow J, Kruger U, Petzold M, Petzold K, Miller H, Scholz H. Arterioarterial prosthetic loop: a new approach for hemodialysis access. J Vasc Surg. 2005;41(6):1007–12.
40. Trerotola SO, Kwak A, Clark TW, et al. Prospective study of balloon inflation pressures and other technical aspects of hemodialysis access angioplasty. J Vasc Interv Radiol. 2005;16(12):1613–8.
41. Vesely TM, Pilgram TK. Angioplasty balloon inflation pressures during treatment of hemodialysis graft-related stenoses. J Vasc Interv Radiol. 2006;17(4): 623–8.
42. Trerotola SO, Stavropoulos SW, Shlansky-Goldberg R, Tuite CM, Kobrin S, Rudnick MR. Hemodialysis-related venous stenosis: treatment with ultrahigh-pressure angioplasty balloons. Radiology. 2004;231(1):259–62.
43. Rajan DK, Platzker T, Lok CE, et al. Ultrahigh-pressure versus high-pressure angioplasty for treatment of venous anastomotic stenosis in hemodialysis grafts: is there a difference in patency? J Vasc Interv Radiol. 2007;18(6):709–14.
44. Fukasawa M, Matsushita K, Araki I, Tanabe N, Takeda M. Self-reversed parallel wire balloon technique for dilating unyielding strictures in native dialysis fistulas. J Vasc Interv Radiol. 2002;13(9 Pt 1):943–5.
45. Vesely TM, Siegel JB. Use of the peripheral cutting balloon to treat hemodialysis-related stenoses. J Vasc Interv Radiol. 2005;16(12):1593–603.
46. National Kidney Foundation Kidney Diseases Outcomes Quality Initiative. Clinical practice guidelines for vascular access: update 2000. Am J Kidney Dis. 2001;37(1 Suppl 1):S137–181.
47. Khan FA, Vesely TM. Arterial problems associated with dysfunctional hemodialysis grafts: evaluation of patients at high risk for arterial disease. J Vasc Interv Radiol. 2002;13(11):1109–14.
48. Georgiadis GS, Lazarides MK, Lambidis CD, et al. Use of short PTFE segments (<6 cm) compares favorably with pure autologous repair in failing or thrombosed native arteriovenous fistulas. J Vasc Surg. 2005;41(1):76–81.
49. Mickley V, Cazzonelli M, Bossinger A. The stenosed Brescia-Cimino fistula: operation or intervention? Zentralbl Chir. 2003;128(9):757–61.
50. Haskal ZJ, Trerotola S, Dolmatch B, et al. Stent graft versus balloon angioplasty for failing dialysis-access grafts. N Engl J Med. 2010;362(6):494–503.

51. Tordoir JH, Bode AS, Peppelenbosch N, van der Sande FM, de Haan MW. Surgical or endovascular repair of thrombosed dialysis vascular access: is there any evidence? J Vasc Surg. 2009;50(4):953–6.
52. Gorriz JL, Martinez-Rodrigo J, Sancho A, et al. Endoluminal percutaneous thrombectomy as a treatment for acute vascular access thrombosis: long-term results of 123 procedures. Nefrologia. 2001;21(2):182–90.
53. Swan TL, Smyth SH, Ruffenach SJ, Berman SS, Pond GD. Pulmonary embolism following hemodialysis access thrombolysis/thrombectomy. J Vasc Interv Radiol. 1995;6(5):683–6.
54. Turmel-Rodrigues L, Raynaud A, Louail B, Beyssen B, Sapoval M. Manual catheter-directed aspiration and other thrombectomy techniques for declotting native fistulas for hemodialysis. J Vasc Interv Radiol. 2001;12(12):1365–71.
55. Turmel-Rodrigues L, Pengloan J, Rodrigue H, et al. Treatment of failed native arteriovenous fistulae for hemodialysis by interventional radiology. Kidney Int. 2000;57(3):1124–40.

Chapter 16
Interventions in Dialysis Grafts

Dheeraj K. Rajan and Dirk S. Baumann

Thrombosis occurs roughly 10 times more frequently in dialysis grafts compared to autogenous fistulas. Thrombosis in AVGs is often the result of an underlying hemodynamically significant stenosis. The site of stenosis can often be determined by physical examination where inflow and outflow stenoses can be identified. Key points to evaluate by examination are the location and type of graft, presence of pseudoaneurysms, presence of dilated collateral veins particularly on the chest, and the pulsatility or thrill of flow within the graft itself. Ideally, there is a transition of pulsatility from the arterial anastomosis to a thrill towards the end of the graft. If there is pulsatility throughout the graft, one suspects an outflow stenosis. A lack of thrill by palpation commonly indicates an inflow problem. Lack of any thrill or pulsatility indicates possible thrombosis. An in-room ultrasound allows a quick examination of the dialysis access and determination of the underlying problem, thereby allowing for preplanning of interventions. Clinical examination is also the single most reliable

D.K. Rajan (✉)
Head and Associate Professor, Division of Vascular & Interventional Radiology, Department of Medical Imaging, University of Toronto, Toronto, Ontario, Canada
e-mail: Dheeraj.Rajan@uhn.on.ca

D.K. Rajan (ed.), *Essentials of Percutaneous Dialysis Interventions*, DOI 10.1007/978-1-4419-5657-6_16,
© Springer Science+Business Media, LLC 2011

indicator of procedural success following intervention, with restoration of a thrill to the distal portion of the graft associated with higher patency rates [1].

The Puncture

Access will depend to a large extent on the configuration of the graft and if the access is thrombosed. For straight or C-shaped grafts, one puncture directed towards the suspected pathology is sufficient unless thrombosis is suspected. If unsure, puncturing the arterial limb of the graft within 1–2 cm of the arterial anastomosis directed towards the venous outflow allows visualization of most of the graft. If the graft is thrombosed, two punctures in opposite directions as far apart from each other as possible are used. For loop grafts, possibilities for access include the apex technique and the "double barrel" technique. If two accesses are required to treat lesions or thrombosis, placing both accesses in the venous limb of the graft, one near the apex facing centrally and one near the venous anastomosis directed arterially, allows access to the entire graft. Alternatively, one can place a centrally directed sheath along the arterial limb and the arterially directed sheath along the venous limb ("double-barrel shotgun"). The disadvantage of this latter technique is that it does not allow straight-line access for venous angioplasty and in cases of central venous angioplasty, may not allow enough balloon catheter length to reach the stenosis (see Fig. 16.1). An advantage of the "double barrel" technique is that there is less recirculation during dialysis if sheaths are left in after the procedure.

Puncture and subsequent sheath placement should be directed towards the pathology, which is usually located at the venous anastomosis in AVG's. The simplest way to determine which side of the loop graft is the venous limb is to ask the patient. On physical exam, this can also be determined by compressing the apex of the graft with a finger and temporarily occluding flow. The side of the graft with a pulse is the arterial side, while the side without pulsatility is the venous side. If the graft is thrombosed, ultrasound may be of assistance in determining which limb is anastomosed to which vessel. Finally, one can rely on basic vascular anatomy and how a typical graft is surgically placed. For example, a forearm loop graft venous limb is typically anastomosed to the basilic vein. This is located medial to the brachial

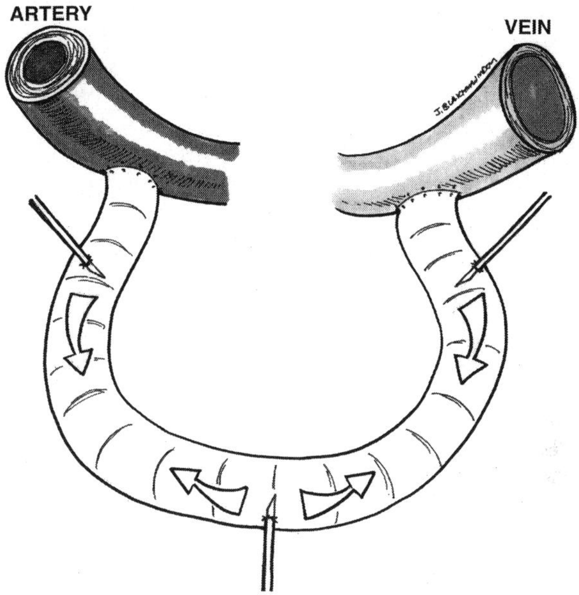

Fig. 16.1 Apex puncture and double barrel puncture directions/locations

artery. However, the venous end of the graft can also be anastomosed to the antecubital vein which lies lateral to the brachial artery (allowing outflow into both the basilic and cephalic veins). In this case, the venous limb sits lateral to the artery. Odds are the venous limb is the more medially located limb in the forearm.

Access can be achieved with a micropuncture set, single wall needle, sheath needle, or an (inexpensive) 18G Angiocath. To puncture the graft, first inject lidocaine using a 25G needle or smaller needle, and inject along a subcutaneous to subcuticular course at the planned puncture site raising a small skin wheal. Then, stabilize the graft between the thumb and first finger of one hand, palpating the walls of the graft at the planned puncture site. The needle is then inserted into the anterior wall of the graft between the two fingers until a distinct "popping" sensation is felt. The puncture should be a sufficient distance away from the lesion to be treated to allow the intervention to be performed (at least 3 cm) and at a relatively steep angle to reduce the length of subcutaneous tract (potential reduction in bleeding complications and pseudoaneurysm formation). If the patient feels pain with needle insertion after lidocaine has been given, there is a chance that you have passed through the front and back wall of the graft. The needle should be withdrawn slowly until flowing blood return occurs. In the case of a thrombosed graft, clot can be aspirated or a wire used to assess intra-graft location. For puncture into a thrombosed graft, a 0.035-in. straight soft tipped wire is preferred. A J wire may not push forward, and a stiff wire may track along the outside of the graft, giving the operator a false belief that the wire is within the graft. The 0.035-in. wire also allows for quicker transition to a sheath and/or directional catheters.

Imaging the Graft

Fistulography may be performed by puncturing the graft with a small-gauge needle or angiocatheter used for peripheral venous access and injecting contrast. Gentle hand injections of 10–15 cc of contrast over 2–3 s per "run" obtaining DSA images at two frames per second is usually sufficient in functioning grafts. Volume and rate can be modified based on the size of the vascular territory to be imaged and flow rates. Power pump injection is rarely if ever required. If one expects to be performing an intervention, using an 18G angiocath is sufficiently large enough to image the access and to accommodate subsequent passage of a 0.035 in. wire. To properly assess the central venous structures, a catheter advanced centrally may be rarely required for adequate opacification. It is also important to reflux the arterial anastomosis to exclude any hemodynamically significant inflow stenosis. This can be done by temporarily occluding the venous outflow with the aid of external compression of the venous limb (with a clamp), inflating a blood pressure cuff above the venous anastomosis to suprasystolic pressure or temporarily occluding the venous limb of the graft internally with an inflated balloon catheter. This simple technique can be performed during balloon angioplasty of a venous stenosis with injection of contrast through the access sheath, which should be done slowly to avoid injecting a large amount of contrast into the arterial system. The entire access from arterial inflow to the right atrium should be assessed. If a stenosis is suspected, an oblique view should be obtained to verify an ambiguous finding. Moving the arm to a slightly abducted position may resolve axillary vein narrowing that is actually the result of soft tissue compression rather than fixed stenosis.

The majority of stenoses in synthetic dialysis grafts occur at or near the venous anastomosis [2, 3] with nearly 75% of all stenoses located within this area (see Fig. 16.2). The incidence of central venous stenoses is dependent on prior history of catheter insertions. Arterial anastomotic stenosis, although considered uncommon should be considered and imaged. Intragraft stenoses are relatively common compared to arterial stenoses and are often the result of repeated needle punctures in the same location. A simple trick to determine if there is a more central arterial lesion is to measure arterial pressure within the feeding artery of the graft and obtain a blood pressure measurement in the opposite arm. A greater than 10 mmHg systolic gradient may indicate central arterial pathology. Any stenosis greater than 50% angiographically, particularly in the presence of venous collaterals, is considered hemodynamically significant. If both an arterial and

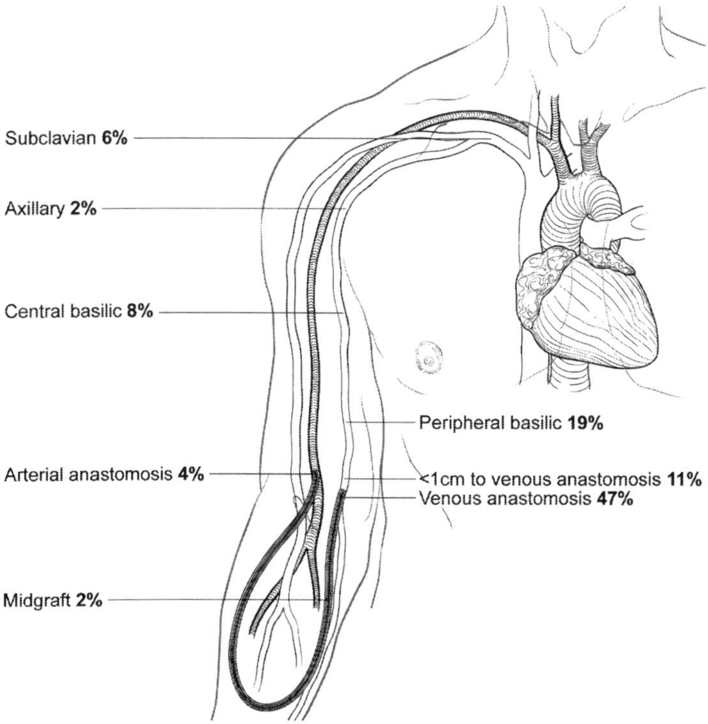

Fig. 16.2 Location and prevalence of stenoses in patients with loop forearm grafts (Modified from Kanterman et al. [2])

venous anastomotic or limb stenosis are suspected, two punctures may be required. In the case of loop grafts, a single perpendicular puncture at the apex of the graft will allow access to both limbs of the graft as well as the inflow and outflow vessels as mentioned above.

Angioplasty

For angioplasty, the proper balloon catheter diameter can be determined by the normal diameter of the vein proximal to the stenosis or distal to the stenosis excluding the area of poststenotic dilatation. As mentioned in Chap. 14, PTFE grafts are either tapered or nontapered. Tapered grafts are 4 mm at the arterial limb and 6–7 mm at the venous limb. Therefore, to oversize a stenosis by 1 mm, an 8-mm diameter balloon is used at the venous anastomosis and a 5 mm at the arterial stenosis. Intragraft stenoses are usually treated with 6- to8-mm balloons. Nontapered PTFE grafts are 6 mm throughout and therefore usually require 7-mm balloons at the venous and arterial end. For angioplasty of the feeding artery, balloon catheters with diameters of 4–6 mm are usually sufficient. Occasionally, stenoses are resistant to high-pressure balloon catheters, and ultra high-pressure balloon catheters are required to completely efface the lesion (>20 atm inflation pressures). Also "cutting" balloons may be used for lesions that do not efface with high-pressure balloons although improved patency has not been obtained with these devices. Another method is the parallel wire balloon technique where the wire is reversed back along the outer part of the balloon catheter and acts as a blade during balloon expansion [4]. A 0.014- or 0.018-in. wire works best (also see Chap. 15). Residual narrowing greater than 30% usually indicates insufficient dilation, and the region is redilated with the same balloon diameter or a larger balloon usually 1 mm greater in diameter than the previous balloon used. If stenosis persists, despite effacement of the waist, obtaining direct pressure measurements across the lesion may help clarify the effectiveness of the angioplasty. The treatment is considered hemodynamically success obtained if there is less than a 10 mm Hg systolic pressure gradient across the residual stenosis. It is not our practice to administer heparin routinely for simple angioplasty.

For other vein segments to be dilated, the corresponding normal adjacent vein segment diameter should be used as a reference in choosing balloon sizes. Wire access should be maintained across the lesion angioplastied until you are satisfied with the treatment. If wire access is lost across the lesion treated, potential complications such as vessel rupture may become impossible to address immediately to the detriment of the patient. POBA is also used to treat in-stent stenosis where intimal hyperplastic tissue grows through the interstices of the stent.

In the setting of treating a thrombosed graft, stenosis encountered at the arterial anastomosis may be due to a residual arterial plug. An arterial plug, especially if resistant and adherent to the wall, can create a flow-compromising lesion and must be removed completely to insure success of any thrombectomy procedure. Historically, true arterial stenoses were thought to account for approximately 5% of all graft-related stenoses. However, recent studies suggest a significantly higher incidence of arterial stenoses [5]. Nevertheless, most believe that management of what looks like a stenosis at the arterial anastomosis is best performed by using thrombectomy techniques such as a Fogarty balloon, mechanical thrombolytic device, or a mechanical device designed for wall-adherent clot extraction. Some institutions believe that angioplasty of the arterial plug at the arterial anastomosis is acceptable or even preferable, while others believe this may be associated with a higher restenosis rate.

Outcome following angioplasty is varied and is approximately 60% at 6 months in multiple retrospective studies. The DOQI guideline states that effective PTA, as defined by a less than 30% residual stenosis should have a 50% primary patency at 6 months. However, recent randomized studies indicate that POBA patency is much lower than originally thought, ranging from 23–40% at 6 months [6–8]. Balloon versus surgical patch angioplasty in dialysis grafts has been examined with authors finding balloon angioplasty to be more practical or no improved patency with surgery [9–11].

Stents

The routine use of intravascular stents to treat AVG stenoses has not been shown to improve access patency. The results of stent placement for venous stenoses in dialysis access have been disappointing, and no prospective randomized trials exist to support their routine use whatsoever [12–15]. In addition, it is important to remember that stenting is only as effective at opening a stenosis as angioplasty. If the balloon fails to expand, stents have less outward force and therefore will not result in an improved outcome in such a situation.

However, stents may help in salvaging AVGs following acute PTA failure, rapid restenosis, and vessel perforation. If a stent is going to be used, self-expanding nitinol stents are highly preferred. Nitinol stents open to their predetermined length and diameter. Due to the metal characteristics of nitinol (50% nickel: 50% titanium) and stent design, these stents do not shorten or elongate significantly during deployment. When heated to body temperature, nitinol stents dilate to their predetermined diameter. Although they can be dilated to a diameter bigger than their predetermined size, the stent will recoil back down to the predetermined size. This stent type also has the advantage of conforming to the vessel and when crushed or compressed, will re-expand to its predetermined diameter and/or length. Balloon-expandable stents are not recommended (with the exception of the SVC) as they distort or change anatomy and are crushable (See Chap. 20, Fig. 16.2). They do not re-expand on their own. Wallstents are still used in some parts of the world. Although they are self-expanding, the length is variable depending on vessel diameter. When delivered, the location of the back end of the stent is not consistent. Furthermore, due to the structure of the stent, point compression at one location of the stent causes a vector of force away from that point of stenosis that may result in the stent migrating forward or backward from the stenosis after deployment or the so-called watermelon seed effect.

If a stent is going to be placed, it is very important to follow strict sterile procedures and to have meticulous technique. *You have one chance to place something properly that becomes a permanent device in a patient's body*. A wire of sufficient length and rigidity should be in place to allow for smooth exchange and delivery of the stent system without losing access to the lesion. A general rule is to use a wire that is double the length of the delivery system. Ideally, the wire should be placed into the IVC to prevent arrhythmias during manipulation of the wire. Although hydrophilic wires are good for crossing lesions, they can easily pull out of the lesion due to their low friction. An overly floppy wire leads to redundancy in the wire which may translate into an improperly placed stent.

Indications

Specific situations where stents are indicated are (1) flow-limiting dissections, (2) vein rupture not controlled with conservative measures, (3) failure of angioplasty to open an occluded venous segment and

(4) limited residual access sites with a contraindication to surgery or for lesions that are surgically inaccessible and fail PTA (two PTAs within 3 months). This last indication is subjective as stents may cause more harm in the long term. For flow-limiting dissections resulting from POBA, self-expanding stents may be used to salvage the access, preserving access function. Post-PTA venous rupture is not an uncommon event with reported rupture rates of 2–5% [13, 16]. When rupture does occur, conservative treatments can include reversal of anticoagulation, observation, balloon tamponade, external compression of the rupture site, stent deployment, or intentional graft thrombosis. The latter option is considered least desirable since it results in loss of the access, necessitates the placement of temporary access, and requires construction of an alternative permanent access. Stent deployment may be safe and effective in cases of rupture by providing a smooth low-resistance channel for blood flow [17, 18] (see Fig. 16.3). Patency rates are similar to stents placed in peripheral veins for reasons other than rupture [16].

For flow-limiting dissections, conservative measures include short-term (minutes) observation or repeat angioplasty to tack down the flap (>1 min). If these fail, then stenting can be considered. For the last scenario, if an occluded segment of vein is traversed and angioplasty fails to reestablish a patent lumen, then stenting can be performed of the occluded segment. This is common for occluded central vein segments as discussed in Chap. 20. Although stenting provides initial high technical success and initial primary patency, its mode of failure is neointimal hyperplasia throughout the length of the stent. Also, use of stents can convert a focal stenosis into a stent long stenosis (see Fig. 16.4). Therefore, stenting should be limited to the confines of the previous stenosis. Lastly, stents are not indicated to trap thrombus. If the clot dissolves with autolytic pathways, here is a potential risk of the stent becoming a free-floating device within the vein and becoming a migration risk.

In-Stent Stenosis

There are no approved therapies for in-stent stenosis. The most common treatment is POBA although other treatments including use of cutting balloons, freezing balloons, stents, and atherectomy devices have been tried. None has been found to be convincingly

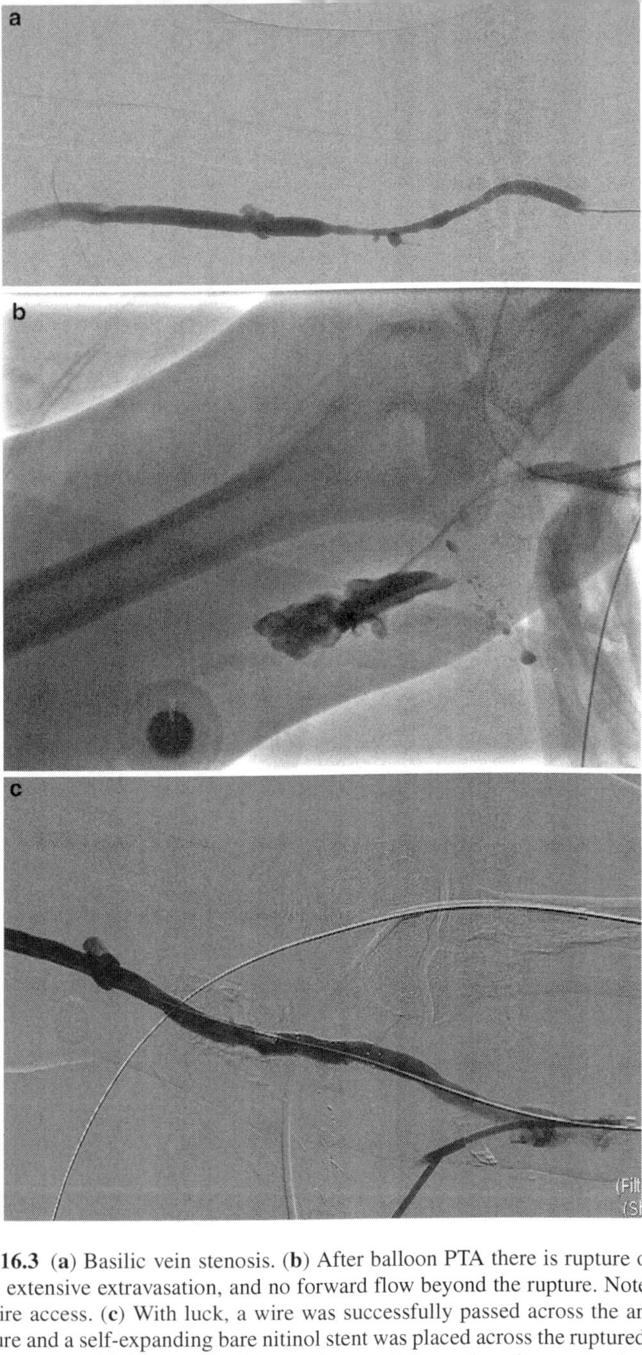

Fig. 16.3 (**a**) Basilic vein stenosis. (**b**) After balloon PTA there is rupture of the vein, extensive extravasation, and no forward flow beyond the rupture. Note loss of wire access. (**c**) With luck, a wire was successfully passed across the area of rupture and a self-expanding bare nitinol stent was placed across the ruptured vein segment, reestablishing normal flow and preventing continued extravasation

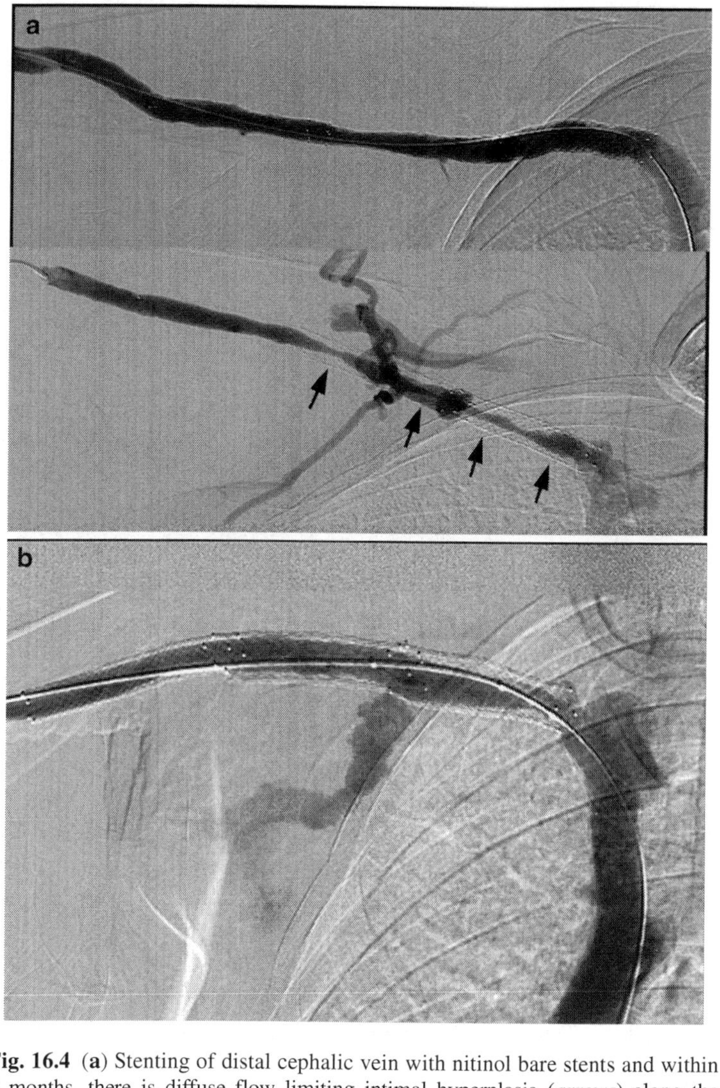

Fig. 16.4 (**a**) Stenting of distal cephalic vein with nitinol bare stents and within 3 months, there is diffuse flow limiting intimal hyperplasia (*arrows*) along the entire length of the stents. (**b**) Balloon angioplasty results in venous rupture despite presence of stents. (**c**) Ruptured vein segment salvaged with stent graft which was used because of coexistent intimal hyperplasia

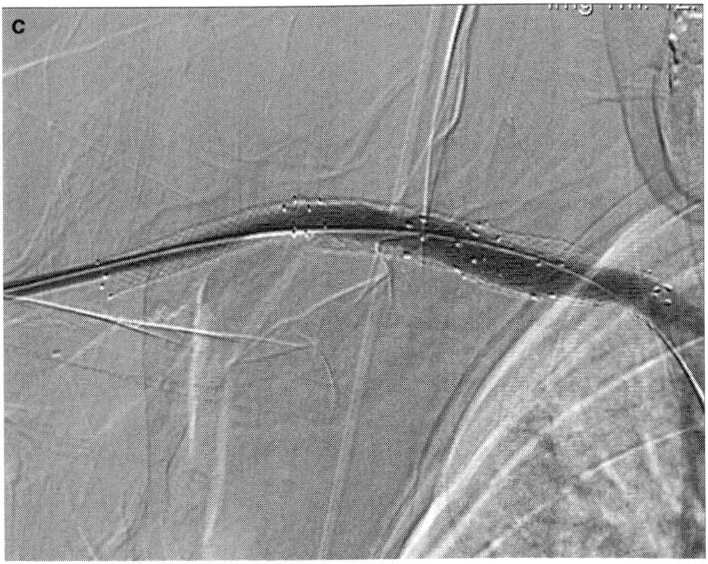

Fig. 16.4 (continued)

effective as all one is doing is pushing tissue against a metal scaffold already in place. When determining the balloon or stent size to be used, one should use the size of the stent already placed as a reference. Placing a stent larger than this or using a PTA balloon larger than this confers no added benefit as one cannot expand durably beyond the diameter of the background stent (unless balloon expandable). Stent grafts can be considered and may hold some durable promise. Again, the device diameter placed should not exceed the diameter of the underlying stent. Depending on the amount of hyperplasia present, this situation may actually require a device that is 1–2 mm smaller in diameter to prevent graft material infolding within the stent graft.

Stent Grafts

Although use of stents and most stent grafts in dialysis access is considered off-label within North America, the Bard Flair stent graft is an "on label" approved device in North America for primary use for venous anastomotic stenosis in patients with arm dialysis grafts. Relative contraindications include anastomoses with an angulation greater than 90° and placement of the device across a joint space at the elbow or shoulder. Although a randomized multicenter prospective study of this device found it to be statistically superior to POBA at the venous anastomosis of dialysis grafts [7], the results should not be extrapolated to use of these devices in other areas of the access circuit or fistulas.

Stent grafts can also be used off label within North America to exclude pseudoaneurysms within dialysis grafts (see Fig. 16.5), treat

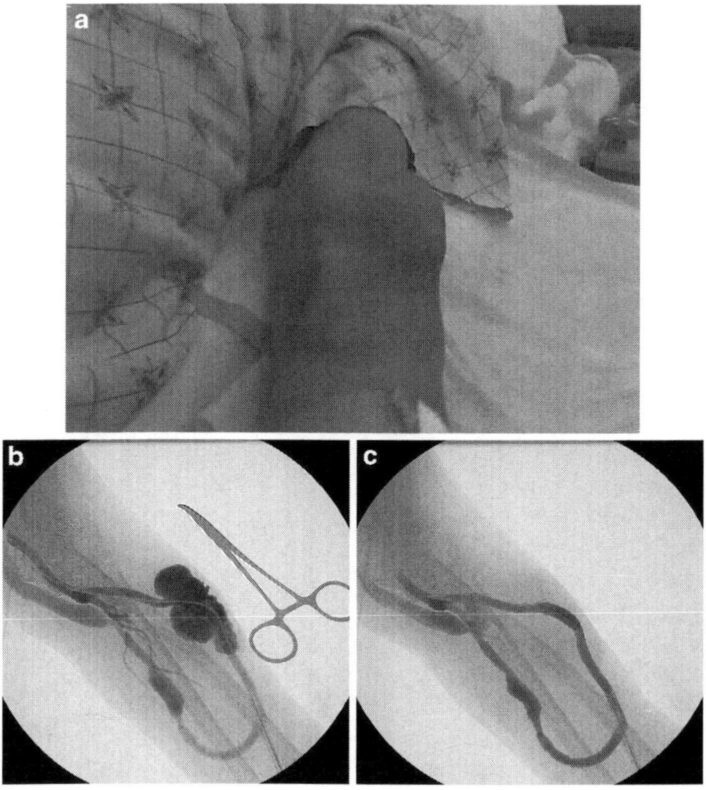

Fig. 16.5 (**a**) Rapidly expanding pseudoaneurym of dialysis graft with doubling in size within 48 h. (**b**) Fistulogram demonstrates large wide-necked pseudoaneurysm. Hemostat in image was used as a reference for sizing. (**c**) Pseudoaneurysm is excluded with two 7-mm Fluency (CR Bard) stent grafts

in-stent stenosis, keep occluded venous segments open, and cover ruptured venous segments. Although there are many uses, until further studies are conducted for these indications, stent grafts should be reserved for situations where other proven options have failed.

Since stent grafts can have either a polytetrafluoroethylene or Dacron covering, prophylactic gram positive coverage prior to insertion is recommended either with Ancef 1 g or vancomycin 1 g if the patient is allergic to penicillin. Prophylactic or postprocedure anticoagulation is not required.

Sizing is similar to that for stents where size of the next normal adjacent segment is used as the reference. Stent grafts have lower friction than uncovered stents, and therefore, care should be taken when deploying and dilating these devices as they are prone to migration. At the time of insertion, all manipulation through the device should be fluoroscopically monitored. After deployment, the stent graft should be dilated with a balloon of the same diameter to properly seat the device. Device length should be chosen so that there is at least one centimetre overextension beyond the lesion being covered. There are many different manufacturers of stent grafts with some devices more rigid than others. In general, the devices are more rigid than uncovered stents and are therefore prone to kinking when approaching or exceeding 90° angles which should be avoided.

If traversing degenerating grafts with pseudoaneurysms, there is the possibility of the device kinking within the pseudoaneurysm and therefore pulling into it. In addition, oversizing of the stent graft should be avoided with maximum oversizing by 1 mm. Oversizing of the stent graft leads to infolding of the graft material with proliferative fibrosis filling in the folds which actually results in a narrower lumen (see Fig. 16.6). Following deployment, the pseudoaneurysm should be aspirated to reduce the size and future deformity of the pseudoaneurysm. Although this has been successful in published reports, patency is somewhat limited for this indication (20% at 6 months) [19]. Although off label, there are anecdotal reports of dialysis needles being passed through stent grafts.

Before any stent or stent graft is placed, it is important to consider future accesses in the patient. Often, due to high flow from the current access, outflow veins thicken or mature, which is also termed "arterialization" and can be used to form new accesses particularly arteriovenous fistulas. Also, since "arterialization" has occurred, clinical success of fistula placement is much higher, and these fistulas

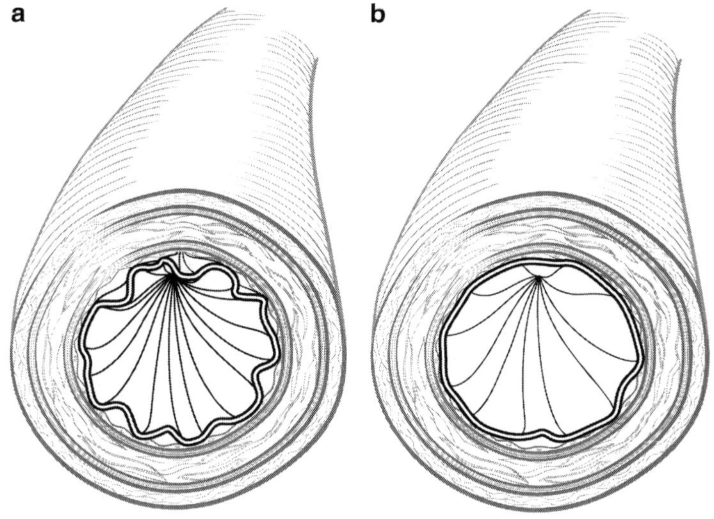

Fig. 16.6 Stent graft sizing. (**a**) Device placed is 2 mm larger than target vessel diameter. As a result, the stent graft infolds with resultant intimal hyperplasia within the folds and actual decrease of luminal diameter. (**b**) Device placed is oversized by 1 mm with no resultant infolding and maintained luminal diameter

can often be accessed much earlier (within a couple of weeks) than primarily created AVF's. An important question to ask is if the device might compromise or damage arterialized outflow vein segments. If so, stent or stent graft placement should be avoided, so that the outflow vein can be used for a new access rather than maintaining a poorly functioning one. Also, as mentioned in the previous chapter, the interventionalist should consider the benefits versus risks of using these devices in patients with acute ongoing infections as there is a slight risk that they may become infected, particularly when associated with pseudoaneurysms.

Thrombolysis/Thrombectomy for Dialysis Grafts (Also See Chap. 15)

Acute thrombosis of AVGs is a clinically avoidable situation. With the aid of routine monitoring and clinical examination, hemodynamically significant stenoses can be detected and treated with prophylactic

PTA prior to access thrombosis. In general, a graft with flow rates of less than 600 mL per minute is at greater risk of thrombosis. It is prudent to treat dysfunctional grafts prior to thrombosis as the outcome of grafts is significantly better after dilation or revision of stenoses than following surgical or radiological declotting [20–22]. Other considerations include the cost, time, and associated morbidity of treating clotted access versus POBA. However, graft thrombosis is not always avoidable. When it happens, one can attempt to declot a graft up to three weeks after thrombosis. For thrombosis of a newly created graft (less than 30 days old), one should attempt percutaneous declotting with caution. Patency following percutaneous thrombectomy of these newly constructed grafts is very poor when compared with mature graft thrombectomy, likely reflecting an underlying technical problem with placement of the graft.

A number of methods, other than surgical thrombectomy, for declotting AVGs have been described. These can be categorized as pharmacological, mechanical, and thromboaspiration. A variety of mechanical devices now exist that can be used to declot AVGs and have also been used with varying success in autogenous fistulas. Patient/thrombus characteristics somewhat influence what technique or device is to be used. Considerations include: (1) graft configuration, (2) age of the thrombus, (3) the presence of intragraft stenoses and/or pseudoaneurysms, and (4) the extent of thrombus extension up into the native vein. For example, if clot extends into the native veins, a mechanical device may be more practical to deal with the clot burden than thrombolysis. With thrombosed grafts, there are three basic problems that have to be dealt with. Almost all thromboses are related to significant outflow stenosis that requires dilation. Secondly, one has to deal with the clot that has formed within the graft and lastly, an arterial plug that forms at the arterial anastomosis of the graft (see Fig. 16.7).

The basic principals of graft thrombolysis regardless of method are (see Fig. 16.8):

1. Crossed catheter access
2. Fragmentation/maceration or pulverization of all clot within the graft
3. Aspiration of the particulate clot debris to minimize embolization to the pulmonary circulation
4. Treatment of any significant underlying stenosis and
5. Removal of the arterial plug (which is resistant to thrombolysis)

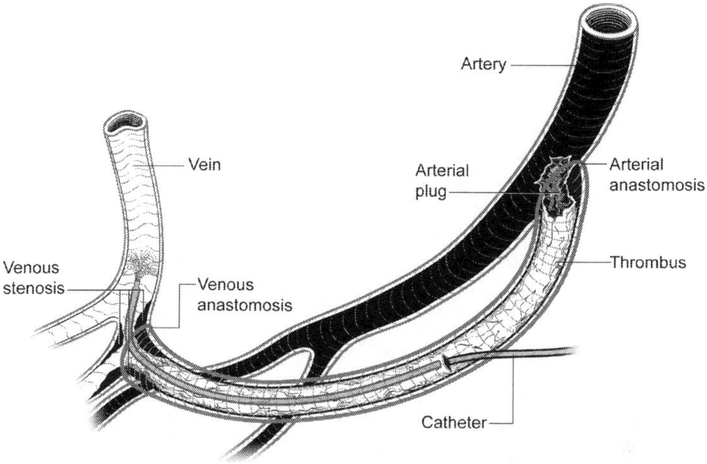

Fig. 16.7 Anatomy of thrombosis within a dialysis graft. Thrombosis related to outflow stenosis at the venous anastomosis with acute clot back to the arterial anastomosis where an arterial plug (distinct from thrombus) has formed. Catheter has been advanced into the venous outflow beyond the clot to assess status of outflow veins prior to initiating thrombus removal

Prior to embarking on the thrombolysis procedure, an outflow venogram is performed to exclude a central venous occlusion or other lesion, which would preclude successful thrombectomy (see Fig. 16.7). In addition, this step verifies that interventions are being performed on the venous side of the access and not mistakenly the arterial side.

Once thrombus is removed from the graft (average volume of clot within an upper arm dialysis graft is 3.2 mL [23]), an arterial plug is often found at the arterial anastomosis of thrombosed grafts. The arterial plug is a firm, rubbery plug composed of fibrin and red blood cells and is located at the arterial anastomosis in all thrombosed hemodia-lysis grafts [23]. The plug is often <0.5 mL and there is minimal risk of allowing it to embolize to the lungs. This plug must be removed during the thrombectomy procedure as it is nonresponsive to enzymatic thrombolysis. The arterial plug can be removed with a 4 Fr Fogarty balloon or an over-the-wire 5 Fr Fogarty catheter (Edwards LifeSciences, Irvine, CA), an angioplasty balloon, or a thromboaspiration device/catheter. When using the Arrow Trerotola PTD, the basket can be uncovered beyond the plug and gently withdrawn into the plug (evidenced by narrowing of the basket) before

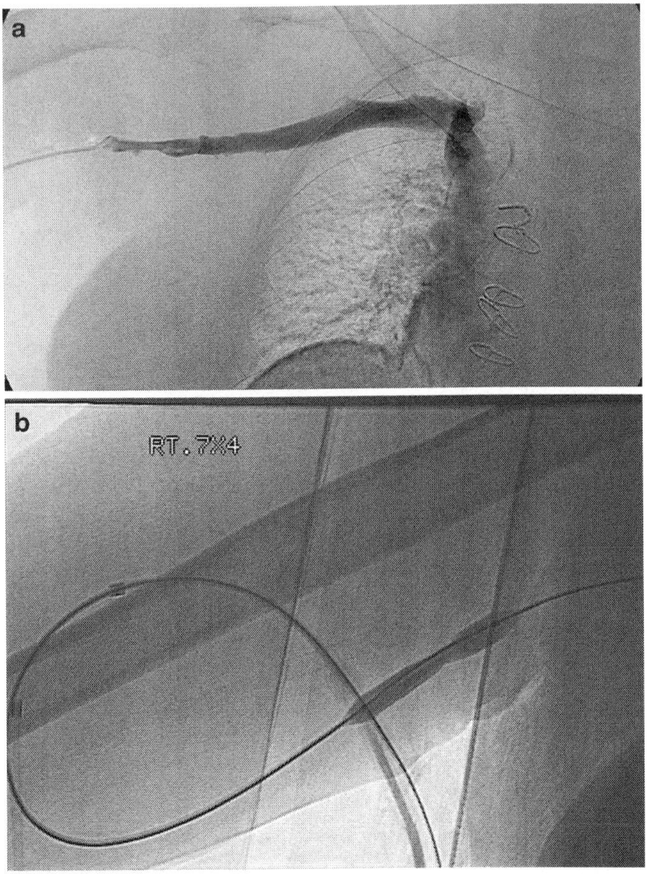

Fig. 16.8 Lyse and Wait declotting of dialysis graft. After delivery of the thrombolytic, (**a**) a catheter is advanced beyond the venous anastomosis and contrast is injected to verify patency of the outflow veins. (**b**) A new puncture towards the arterial anastomosis is then performed, and using a Fogarty catheter, the arterial plug is removed, reestablishing flow within the graft. The venous anastomosis is then dilated. (**c**) With the balloon inflated at the venous anastomosis (*arrowhead*), the graft is gently refluxed to assess the arterial limb of the graft and to assess the arterial anastomosis. A portion of the arterial plug (*arrow*) remains and requires removal. (**d**) Completion fistulogram demonstrates no residual significant stenosis or clot

activating the motor to remove the plug. In cases of difficult plugs where residual adherent clot is present, the Fogarty adherent clot catheter can be a valuable tool. Multiple passes are often required to fully dislodge the plug.

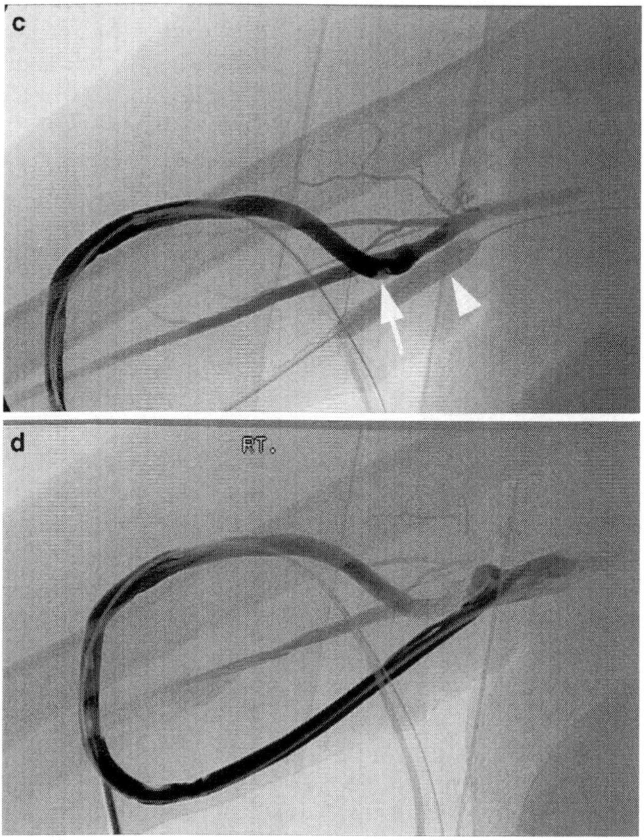

Fig. 16.8 (continued)

Careful attention is required to prevent the plug from dislodging and passing into the feeding artery. Although emboli into the feeding artery are usually asymptomatic [24] and conservative therapy is typically sufficient, occasionally infusion of thrombolytics or suction thrombectomy may be required to remove the embolus. A method of "backbleeding" to clear the feeding artery of a dialysis graft has also been described [25]; the artery proximal to the anastomosis is occluded with a balloon or manual compression, reversing the direction of arterial flow beyond the balloon to dislodge the embolus retrograde into the graft.

If any inflow, intragraft, and/or outflow stenoses are detected that are considered hemodynamically significant, these are subsequently angioplastied. Residual thrombus can be removed with additional passes of the thrombectomy device, pulled over to the venous outflow, or macerated with balloon catheters. K\DOQI guidelines have also indicated that regardless of the method of declotting, a minimum of 40% primary patency should be observed at 3 months [20].

Pharmacological Thrombolysis

In the early 1980s, streptokinase was used with some success but common use was limited by local bleeding complications and allergic reactions [26–28]. Since these early reports, many modifications in the techniques and pharmacological agents used to pharmacologically thrombolyse grafts have occurred.

The "lyse and wait" technique involves inserting an angiocatheter (under sterile conditions) near the arterial anastomosis directed towards the venous outflow [29]. The graft is then compressed at the venous and arterial anastomoses during injection of the thrombolytic agent (over 30 s) to confine the agent to the thrombosed graft. After "waiting" for 20–40 min, the patient is brought to the angiography suite and the procedure is continued to identify and treat any underlying hemodynamically significant stenoses (see Fig. 16.8).

The "pulse-spray" technique uses two crossed tapered catheters with multiple side holes with forceful injection of thrombolytic agent into the clot [30]. One catheter is placed from the venous limb of the graft towards the arterial limb without crossing the arterial anastomosis. The second catheter is placed from the arterial limb directed towards the venous limb of the graft.

The initial agent used for pharmacological thrombolysis was urokinase with an original dose of 250,000 IU (Abbokinase; Abbott Laboratories, Chicago, IL). Since urokinase was withdrawn by the U.S. Food and Drug Administration from 1999 until 2002, other thrombolytic agents came into use including reteplase (Retavase; EKR Therapeutics, Bedminister, NJ) and alteplase (t-PA, Activase; Genentech Inc., San Francisco, CA). Reteplase has been approved by the FDA for use in patients with acute myocardial infarction. The dose for declotting grafts is 2–5 U with "lyse and wait" or pulse spray techniques. Heparin is administered separately because heparin causes precipitation of reteplase. The most commonly used lytic agent today is recombinant tissue-type plasminogen activator (t-PA).

Doses of t-PA range from 1 to 6 mg. As with reteplase, heparin cannot be combined with t-PA in the same syringe as both will precipitate out. The role of GP IIb/IIIa inhibitors used in combination with lytic drugs for declotting hemodialysis grafts has not yet been formally evaluated.

Mechanical Thrombectomy

Typically mechanical declotting that utilizes mechanical devices is more expensive than pharmacological declotting due to device costs (minimum of US$ 600/procedure). Mechanical devices are discussed in Chap. 15. Dual access is required for thrombolysis/thrombectomy with mechanical devices. The arterial plug must be removed with pharmacomechanical and pharmacological methods as described above. Finally, the underlying stenosis also needs to be treated.

Outcomes of Thrombolysis

Outcomes vary between different pharmacological methods and lytic agents used to thrombolyse grafts. Multiple large studies have shown that surgical thrombectomy and revision have 1-year secondary patency rates of 75–98% [31–35]. However, many of these studies create a new or surgically revise the venous anastomosis, which makes direct comparison to percutaneous methods difficult. The disadvantage of prior surgical intervention was that each graft revision, extension, or new graft occurs at the expense of normal vein whereas percutaneous thrombectomy preserves normal vein. Newer surgical techniques patch over the area of intimal hyperplasia with little use of normal adjacent vein.

There is no clear advantage or disadvantage of any of the above methods for declotting dialysis grafts. Pharmacological thrombolysis is associated with higher bleeding complications [22, 36] whereas mechanical thrombolysis devices are more costly. The use of some mechanical devices may result in a significant amount of blood loss and/or embolization of clot. Technical success and outcomes are summarized in Table 16.1.

Table 16.1 Technical success rates and primary patency after percutaneous graft declotting (series mixing grafts and autogenous fistulas are excluded)

Method	Technical success (%)	Primary patency
Pulse spray	90–92	41%/3 months [38]
UK [37, 38]	88	50%/3 months
rt-PA [39]		
"Lyse and Wait" [29]	94	–
Amplatz Thrombectomy Device [40, 41]	89–93	47–65%/1 month 50%/3 months [41]
Angiojet [42]	73	32/15% 1/3 months
Arrow-Trerotola PTD [43]	95	39%/3 months
Hydrolyser [44]	84	57/48% 1/3 months
Cragg/Castaneda Brush [45]	93	37%/3 months
Oasis thrombectomy device [38]	95	69/40% 1/3 months
Manual Thromboaspiration [22]	98	84/63% 1/3 months
Comparison "lyse and wait" to Arrow PTD [46]	98–99	Mean patency 5.4 months for both
Angiojet [47]	91	57/43% at 3/6 months
Angiojet [48]	99	70/40% at 1/6 months

Access Abandonment

If the access is to be abandoned and requires occlusion, prior to embarking on such an absolute measure, one should assess what access sites the patients have and their overall access plan over their expected life span. If the patient is limited in options, surgical revision or stent grafts may be considered. One can terminate an access many ways nonsurgically. Methods to do so percutaneously are discussed in Chap. 17.

Surgical Interventions

Whenever performing a dialysis access intervention, preprocedural planning is paramount for directing therapy and preserving critical venous real estate. Initially, the patient's access history must be determined. If possible, the exact site of the venous anastomosis and any recent interventions should be established. While examination of a graft is not always as revealing as examining a fistula, important information must be gained prior to the intervention to guide the study, particularly cannulation site and direction of cannulation. Evaluation should also note potential future venous sites for fistula construction. Finally, prior to intervention, a discussion with the dialysis center, the nephrologist and the patient may elucidate other concerns about the access which need to be addressed.

During the procedure, consideration must be given to not only the most expeditious treatment of the offending lesion, but also the expected treatment outcome and its impact on future dialysis options. For the most common stenosis, a venous anastomotic stenosis, extension of the graft with a Bard FLAIR stent graft into the normal caliber outflow vein has been shown in a prospective, randomized trial to be superior to balloon angioplasty [7]. However, these stent grafts cannot be placed across joints and into anastomoses with greater than 90° of angulation. Additionally, these grafts should not be placed if they would obstruct an outflow vein which could be used for a future fistula. For example, forearm loop brachial artery grafts are usually constructed to the antecubital (median cubital) vein. This vein has outflow into both the upper arm basilic and cephalic veins. Stent grafting across one of these outflow veins from the antecubital vein may cause thrombosis of that vein, eliminating the use of this vein in the future for an upper arm fistula. Similar venous anatomy can occur in the outflow of upper arm grafts as well. In these situations where angioplasty has failed or stent grafting is contraindicated, surgical correction is preferred. Surgical options include vein or PTFE patch angioplasty, graft extension into the vein more proximally, or transposition of the graft to another adjacent vein. Finally, a forearm graft can be converted to an upper arm fistula using the now matured upper arm outflow vein. Unless it requires transposition, this outflow vein can often be cannulated immediately, obviating the need for catheter placement. While balloon angioplasty is simple and safe, it is often not the best option for treatment of failing arteriovenous grafts.

With the increased technical success of modern combined pharmacomechanical thrombectomy, using tissue plasminogen activator and newer thrombectomy devices, the outcomes over the last decade of endovascular treatment of thrombosed arteriovenous grafts have approached that of surgical management [49]. However, the preferred method depends upon the local expertise, availability of trained and interested specialists, and ease of access to the appropriate surgical or interventional suite. Cost comparisons between these newer techniques and surgery have also not been performed. In settings where the newer treatment options and devices are not available, endovascular graft thrombectomy results are inferior to surgery [50], and surgical thrombectomy is recommended. Additionally, when surgical correction of lesions is expected, surgical thrombectomy will be more expeditious. Examples would include degenerated grafts with associated pseudoaneurysms needing interposition grafting or replacement, recurrent thrombosis with poor venous outflow requiring graft transposition to another vein, or grafts with known chronic thrombus, particularly seen around needle cannulation sites. In this latter situation, open thrombectomy with the use of adherent clot extraction catheters or even uterine curettes is more effective than percutaneous techniques at removing this strongly adherent, fibrous graft intimal lining. In patients with severe pulmonary and cardiac disease, surgical thrombectomy lowers the risk of pulmonary embolism, reported to be as high as 23–59% in patients studied after percutaneous thrombectomy [51, 52]. While most of these are asymptomatic, death rates of 5% were reported in a small group of patients with underlying pulmonary and cardiac disease [52]. Surgical thrombectomy lowers this risk, because larger thrombi are removed through the venotomy than possible through a sheath and flow reversal during the procedure prevents embolization. Thus, surgical thrombectomy offers advantages over endovascular management in certain situations.

Key Points

- When dilating a stenosis at the venous anastomosis or within the graft, contrast injection through the access sheath will allow easy visualization of the arterial anastomosis.
- If prolonged balloon inflation is required, and there is a concern for graft thrombosis, injection of saline through the sheath will remove blood from the graft and reduce chances of thrombosis.
- Always keep your wire across the lesion being treated until satisfied with the outcome.
- PTA of the entire graft during declotting will ensure removal or compression of all clots if residual clot is present. This should be done only if necessary and after flow is reestablished within the graft.

- No evidence supports routine use of stents in dialysis access, but their use in selected situations may permit graft salvage.
- Stents in time convert a focal stenosis to a stent-length stenosis, and there is no approved therapy for in-stent stenosis.
- It is always easier, cheaper, and more time efficient to angioplasty a failing graft than declotting/thrombectomizing one.
- The FLAIR stent graft primarily placed at the venous anastomosis for stenosis has been found to be significantly superior to POBA for primary patency.

References

1. Trerotola SO, Ponce P, Stavropoulos SW, et al. Physical examination versus normalized pressure ratio for predicting outcomes of hemodialysis access interventions. J Vasc Interv Radiol. 2003;14(11):1387–94.
2. Kanterman RY, Vesely TM, Pilgram TK, Guy BW, Windus DW, Picus D. Dialysis access grafts: anatomic location of venous stenosis and results of angioplasty. Radiology. 1995;195(1):135–9 [Erratum appears in Radiology. 1995;196(2):582].
3. Turmel-Rodrigues L, Pengloan J, Blanchier D, et al. Insufficient dialysis shunts: improved long-term patency rates with close hemodynamic monitoring, repeated percutaneous balloon angioplasty, and stent placement. Radiology. 1993;187(1):273–8.
4. Fukasawa M, Matsushita K, Araki I, Tanabe N, Takeda M. Self-reversed parallel wire balloon technique for dilating unyielding strictures in native dialysis fistulas. J Vasc Interv Radiol. 2002;13(9 Pt 1):943–5.
5. Khan FA, Vesely TM. Arterial problems associated with dysfunctional hemodialysis grafts: evaluation of patients at high risk for arterial disease. J Vasc Interv Radiol. 2002;13(11):1109–14.
6. NKF-K/DOQI. III. Clinical practice guidelines for vascular access: update 2000. Am J Kidney Dis. 2001;37(1 Suppl 1):S137–181.
7. Haskal ZJ, Trerotola S, Dolmatch B, et al. Stent graft versus balloon angioplasty for failing dialysis-access grafts. N Engl J Med. 2010;362(6):494–503.
8. Vesely TM, Siegel JB. Use of the peripheral cutting balloon to treat hemodialysis-related stenoses. J Vasc Interv Radiol. 2005;16(12):1593–603.
9. Bitar G, Yang S, Badosa F. Balloon versus patch angioplasty as an adjuvant treatment to surgical thrombectomy of hemodialysis grafts. Am J Surg. 1997;174(2):140–2.
10. McCutcheon B, Weatherford D, Maxwell G, Hamann MS, Stiles A. A preliminary investigation of balloon angioplasty versus surgical treatment of thrombosed dialysis access grafts. Am Surg. 2003;69(8):663–7. discussion 668.

11. Lemson MS, Tordoir JH, van Det RJ, et al. Effects of a venous cuff at the venous anastomosis of polytetrafluoroethylene grafts for hemodialysis vascular access. J Vasc Surg. 2000;32(6):1155–63.
12. Gray RJ, Horton KM, Dolmatch BL, et al. Use of Wallstents for hemodialysis access-related venous stenoses and occlusions untreatable with balloon angioplasty. Radiology. 1995;195(2):479–84.
13. Patel RI, Peck SH, Cooper SG, et al. Patency of Wallstents placed across the venous anastomosis of hemodialysis grafts after percutaneous recanalization [see comments]. Radiology. 1998;209(2):365–70.
14. Vogel PM, Parise C. SMART stent for salvage of hemodialysis access grafts. J Vasc Interv Radiol. 2004;15(10):1051–60.
15. Kariya S, Tanigawa N, Kojima H, et al. Peripheral stent placement in hemodialysis grafts. Cardiovasc Intervent Radiol. 2009;32(5):960–6.
16. Rajan DK, Clark TW. Patency of Wallstents placed at the venous anastomosis of dialysis grafts for salvage of angioplasty-induced rupture. Cardiovasc Intervent Radiol. 2003;26(3):242–5.
17. Rundback JH, Leonardo RF, Poplausky MR, Rozenblit G. Venous rupture complicating hemodialysis access angioplasty: percutaneous treatment and outcomes in seven patients. AJR Am J Roentgenol. 1998;171(4):1081–4.
18. Funaki B, Szymski GX, Leef JA, Rosenblum JD, Burke R, Hackworth CA. Wallstent deployment to salvage dialysis graft thrombolysis complicated by venous rupture: early and intermediate results. AJR American Journal of Roentgenology. 1997;169(5):1435–7.
19. Vesely TM. Use of stent grafts to repair hemodialysis graft-related pseudoaneurysms. J Vasc Interv Radiol. 2005;16(10):1301–7.
20. NKF-DOQI. Clinical practice guidelines for vascular access. National Kidney Foundation-Dialysis Outcomes Quality Initiative. Am J Kidney Dis. 1997;30(4 Suppl 3):S150–91.
21. Hodges TC, Fillinger MF, Zwolak RM, Walsh DB, Bech F, Cronenwett JL. Longitudinal comparison of dialysis access methods: risk factors for failure. J Vasc Surg. 1997;26(6):1009–19.
22. Turmel-Rodrigues L, Pengloan J, Baudin S, et al. Treatment of stenosis and thrombosis in haemodialysis fistulas and grafts by interventional radiology. Nephrol Dial Transplant. 2000;15(12):2029–36.
23. Winkler TA, Trerotola SO, Davidson DD, Milgrom ML. Study of thrombus from thrombosed hemodialysis access grafts. Radiology. 1995;197(2):461–5.
24. Trerotola SO, Johnson MS, Shah H, Namyslowski J, Filo RS. Incidence and management of arterial emboli from hemodialysis graft surgical thrombectomy. J Vasc Interv Radiol. 1997;8(4):557–62.
25. Trerotola SO, Johnson MS, Shah H, Namyslowski J. Backbleeding technique for treatment of arterial emboli resulting from dialysis graft thrombolysis. J Vasc Interv Radiol. 1998;9(1 Pt 1):141–3.
26. Goldberg JP, Contiguglia SR, Mishell JL, Klein MH. Intravenous streptokinase for thrombolysis of occluded arteriovenous access. Its use in patients undergoing hemodialysis. Arch Intern Med. 1985;145(8):1405–8.
27. Klimas VA, Denny KM, Paganini EP, et al. Low dose streptokinase therapy for thrombosed arteriovenous fistulas. Trans Am Soc Artif Intern Organs. 1984;30:511–3.

28. Rodkin RS, Bookstein JJ, Heeney DJ, Davis GB. Streptokinase and transluminal angioplasty in the treatment of acutely thrombosed hemodialysis access fistulas. Radiology. 1983;149(2):425–8.
29. Cynamon J, Lakritz PS, Wahl SI, Bakal CW, Sprayregen S. Hemodialysis graft declotting: description of the "lyse and wait" technique. J Vasc Interv Radiol. 1997;8(5):825–9.
30. Bookstein JJ, Fellmeth B, Roberts A, Valji K, Davis G, Machado T. Pulsed-spray pharmacomechanical thrombolysis: preliminary clinical results. AJR Am J Roentgenol. 1989;152(5):1097–100.
31. Miller PE, Carlton D, Deierhoi MH, Redden DT, Allon M. Natural history of arteriovenous grafts in hemodialysis patients. Am J Kidney Dis. 2000;36(1):68–74.
32. Anderson CB, Sicard GA, Etheredge EE. Bovine carotid artery and expanded polytetrafluroethylene grafts for hemodialysis vascular access. J Surg Res. 1980;29(2):184–8.
33. Sabanayagam P, Schwartz AB, Soricelli RR, Lyons P, Chinitz J. A comparative study of 402 bovine heterografts and 225 reinforced expanded PTFE grafts as AVF in the ESRD patient. Trans Am Soc Artif Intern Organs. 1980;26:88–92.
34. Raju S. PTFE grafts for hemodialysis access. Techniques for insertion and management of complications. Ann Surg. 1987;206(5):666–73.
35. Sabanayagam P. 15-year experience with tapered (4-7mm) and straight (6mm) PTFE angio-access in ESRD patients. Chicago: W.L. Gore & Associates and Precept Press; 1995.
36. Vogel PM, Bansal V, Marshall MW. Thrombosed hemodialysis grafts: lyse and wait with tissue plasminogen activator or urokinase compared to mechanical thrombolysis with the Arrow-Trerotola Percutaneous Thrombolytic Device. J Vasc Interv Radiol. 2001;12(10):1157–65.
37. Valji K, Bookstein JJ, Roberts AC, Oglevie SB, Pittman C, O'Neill MP. Pulse-spray pharmacomechanical thrombolysis of thrombosed hemodialysis access grafts: long-term experience and comparison of original and current techniques. AJR Am J Roentgenol. 1995;164(6):1495–500. discussion 1501–1493.
38. Barth KH, Gosnell MR, Palestrant AM, et al. Hydrodynamic thrombectomy system versus pulse-spray thrombolysis for thrombosed hemodialysis grafts: a multicenter prospective randomized comparison. Radiology. 2000;217(3): 678–84.
39. Falk A, Mitty H, Guller J, Teodorescu V, Uribarri J, Vassalotti J. Thrombolysis of clotted hemodialysis grafts with tissue-type plasminogen activator. J Vasc Interv Radiol. 2001;12(3):305–11.
40. Uflacker R, Rajagopalan PR, Vujic I, Stutley JE. Treatment of thrombosed dialysis access grafts: randomized trial of surgical thrombectomy versus mechanical thrombectomy with the Amplatz device. J Vasc Interv Radiol. 1996;7(2):185–92.
41. Sofocleous CT, Cooper SG, Schur I, Patel RI, Iqbal A, Walker S. Retrospective comparison of the Amplatz thrombectomy device with modified pulse-spray pharmacomechanical thrombolysis in the treatment of thrombosed hemodialysis access grafts. Radiology. 1999;213(2):561–7.

42. Vesely TM, Williams D, Weiss M, et al. Comparison of the angiojet rheolytic catheter to surgical thrombectomy for the treatment of thrombosed hemodialysis grafts. Peripheral AngioJet Clinical Trial. J Vasc Interv Radiol. 1999;10(9):1195–205.
43. Trerotola SO, Vesely TM, Lund GB, Soulen MC, Ehrman KO, Cardella JF. Treatment of thrombosed hemodialysis access grafts: Arrow-Trerotola percutaneous thrombolytic device versus pulse-spray thrombolysis. Arrow-Trerotola Percutaneous Thrombolytic Device Clinical Trial. Radiology. 1998;206(2):403–14.
44. Vorwerk D, Schurmann K, Muller-Leisse C, et al. Hydrodynamic thrombectomy of haemodialysis grafts and fistulae: results of 51 procedures. Nephrol Dial Transplant. 1996;11(6):1058–64.
45. Dolmatch BL, Casteneda F, McNamara TO, Zemel G, Lieber M, Cragg AH. Synthetic dialysis shunts: thrombolysis with the Cragg thrombolytic brush catheter. Radiology. 1999;213(1):180–4.
46. Vashchenko N, Korzets A, Neiman C, et al. Retrospective comparison of mechanical percutaneous thrombectomy of hemodialysis arteriovenous grafts with the Arrow-Trerotola device and the lyse and wait technique. AJR Am J Roentgenol. 2010;194(6):1626–9.
47. Littler P, Cullen N, Gould D, Bakran A, Powell S. AngioJet thrombectomy for occluded dialysis fistulae: outcome data. Cardiovasc Intervent Radiol. 2009;32(2):265–70.
48. Kakkos SK, Haddad GK, Haddad J, Scully MM. Percutaneous rheolytic thrombectomy for thrombosed autogenous fistulae and prosthetic arteriovenous grafts: outcome after aggressive surveillance and endovascular management. J Endovasc Ther. 2008;15(1):91–102.
49. Tordoir JH, Bode AS, Peppelenbosch N, van der Sande FM, de Haan MW. Surgical or endovascular repair of thrombosed dialysis vascular access: is there any evidence? J Vasc Surg. 2009;50(4):953–6.
50. Green LD, Lee DS, Kucey DS. A metaanalysis comparing surgical thrombectomy, mechanical thrombectomy, and pharmacomechanical thrombolysis for thrombosed dialysis grafts. J Vasc Surg. 2002;36(5):939–45.
51. Gorriz JL, Martinez-Rodrigo J, Sancho A, et al. Endoluminal percutaneous thrombectomy as a treatment for acute vascular access thrombosis: long-term results of 123 procedures. Nefrologia. 2001;21(2):182–90.
52. Swan TL, Smyth SH, Ruffenach SJ, Berman SS, Pond GD. Pulmonary embolism following hemodialysis access thrombolysis/thrombectomy. J Vasc Interv Radiol. 1995;6(5):683–6.

Chapter 17
Interventions in Dialysis Fistulas

Dheeraj K. Rajan and Dirk S. Baumann

As in dialysis grafts, the underlying cause of failures or thromboses in functional dialysis fistulas is most often venous stenosis. Primary percutaneous treatment remains POBA. Management of dysfunctional autogenous fistulas presents a number of challenges not encountered with arteriovenous grafts. Attempts at percutaneous intervention require substantially more effort and time, which is often rewarded with durable patency that exceeds dialysis grafts. There is often a steep learning curve associated with management of dysfunctional fistulas, particularly when declotting them. It is a disservice to a patient with an AV fistula not to consider a trial of endovascular therapy for both failed mature and immature fistulas prior to abandoning them.

D.K. Rajan (✉)
Head and Associate Professor, Division of Vascular & Interventional Radiology, Department of Medical Imaging, University of Toronto, Toronto, Ontario, Canada
e-mail: Dheeraj.Rajan@uhn.on.ca

D.K. Rajan (ed.), *Essentials of Percutaneous Dialysis Interventions*, DOI 10.1007/978-1-4419-5657-6_17,
© Springer Science+Business Media, LLC 2011

Autogenous Fistulas That Fail to Mature

Compared to AVGs, there is higher initial technical failure rate for autogenous hemodialysis fistulas to mature to the point of durable use. Preoperative venous mapping with venography, ultrasound, and in the future magnetic resonance venography (MRV) assist in identifying suitable veins and identifying potential problems such as central venous stenosis.

Fistulas can fail to mature for a number of reasons. These reasons include the following: (1) failure for the vein to "arterialize," (2) large and/or multiple venous collaterals reducing flow through the cephalic vein, (3) insufficient size of the cephalic vein, and (4) technical factors at the time of surgery. Further percutaneous management is discussed in Chap. 18.

Dysfunctional Mature Autogenous Fistulas

A mature or functioning autogenous fistula is defined by K/DOQI by a "Rule of 6's": (1) the fistula has a flow of approximately 600 mL/min, (2) is less than 0.6 cm below the surface of the skin, and (3) has a minimal diameter of 0.6 cm.

Percutaneous interventions within a functioning fistula are technically more challenging for a number of reasons, some of which are as follows:

1. A thin and mobile venous wall
2. Irregular anatomy, often resulting in difficulty clinically and angiographically identifying the anastomosis
3. An underlying stenosis can occur anywhere from the feeding artery to the superior vena cava
4. An underlying stenosis that is often tight and difficult to cross
5. Venous collaterals which may make it difficult to define the anatomy of the fistula
6. Acute angulation at the anastomosis between the artery and vein which may be difficult to cross
7. Venous aneurysms

Interventions that are commonly performed are angioplasty and percutaneous declotting of dysfunctional autogenous fistulas. Stenting or stent-grafting is reserved for failure of angioplasty in the setting of a threatened loss of access.

Stenoses of the arterial inflow are responsible for an overall flat fistula, which is difficult to cannulate without the help of a tourniquet and/or ultrasound guidance. Stenoses of the venous outflow are typically responsible for a "too convenient" fistula, which is much too visible and easy to puncture, but with subsequent increased compression times after dialysis and formation of aneurysms. These aneurysms, which are common in cannulation sites after some months of dialysis, are ideal examination points because the skin is even thinner at their level: an aneurysm under tension indicates an outflow stenosis, and an abnormally flat and depressible aneurysm indicates an inflow problem. In cases of stenosis developing between the two cannulation sites, the "arterial" aneurysm is tough or full whereas the "venous" aneurysm is soft. In addition, stenoses in cannulation areas can make routine needling impossible. Collateral vessels indicate resistance to flow in AVFs and may represent areas of stenosis. Unlike AVGs, multiple and tandem stenoses are common in AVFs.

The Puncture

Unlike grafts, there is often no reassuring thickened tubular wall that is palpable. Depending on the location and number of stenoses, the fistula can be flat, segmentally dilated or dilated along its entire length. If the fistula is flat, externally compressing the distal outflow will cause the fistula to dilate up allowing one to palpate an area to puncture. This can be done with digital compression or a tourniquet applied to the upper arm. Another trick is to simply identify the course of the fistula based on previous needle punctures and to identify a location based on this course. Another method is to use ultrasound guidance to identify the fistula and aid in puncture. As with grafts, lidocaine should be injected at the site of expected puncture subcutaneously and subdermally. Also, the puncture should be a sufficient distance away from the lesion to be treated to allow the intervention to be performed (at least 3 cm) and at a relatively steep angle to reduce the length of subcutaneous tract (potential reduction in bleeding complications and aneurysm formation).

Imaging

It is important to image fistulas properly and the whole outflow circuit as well as the inflow artery. This can be done by inserting a small catheter into the fistula or a small angiocatheter, preferably 18 gauge if intervention is probable as this size allows passage of a 0.035 in. wire. Imaging can also be performed by primarily placing a sheath if the type and location of intervention is known prior to puncture. Overlying collateral veins can obscure stenoses in the access circuit, and occasionally orthogonal views are needed to identify an area of stenosis. Imaging in a two dimensional plane does not always reveal pathology in a three dimensional space (see Fig. 19.7, Chap. 19). For imaging of radiocephalic fistulas, it is important to profile the inflow artery anastomosis and juxta-anastomotic region of the fistula (first 3–5 cm of the fistula beyond the anastomosis). The preferred way is to enter the fistula retrograde (opposite to direction of flow) near the elbow and advance a catheter into the radial artery passing the catheter retrograde within the artery. A 4 Fr Kumpe catheter works well but given the acute angulation of the anastomosis, this may be difficult. Another option is to inflate a blood pressure cuff along the upper arm. This will allow for reflux of contrast across the anastomosis. A disadvantage with this method is collaterals may fill preferentially without adequately opacifying the anastomosis.

Lastly, arterial punctures are an option. A small catheter such as a 25 gauge angiocatheter or a 3 Fr catheter can be inserted into the brachial artery at the elbow level antegrade for radiocephalic fistulas (see Fig. 17.1) and retrograde for upper arm fistulas which allows for opacification of the entire circuit from an arterial injection of contrast. Another approach is via the radial artery at the wrist. Again, routine interventions from this approach are not recommended as there is a small risk of loss of the radial artery. From this point, a small catheter can be advanced retrograde to the arteriovenous anastomosis (see Fig. 17.2). Routine intervention via the brachial approach was associated with a higher complication rate (12%) [1] although a recent study where transradial interventions were performed on radiocephalic AVFs was not associated with any radial artery complications [2]. Arterial spasm is occasionally encountered and can be treated with 0.1–0.2 mg aliquots of nitroglycerine (1 mg mixed with 9 mL of normal saline) administered directly into the spasmed artery at 1–5 min intervals with no more than a total of 1 mg delivered. Overdosage can lead to cardiovascular collapse. A femoral venous

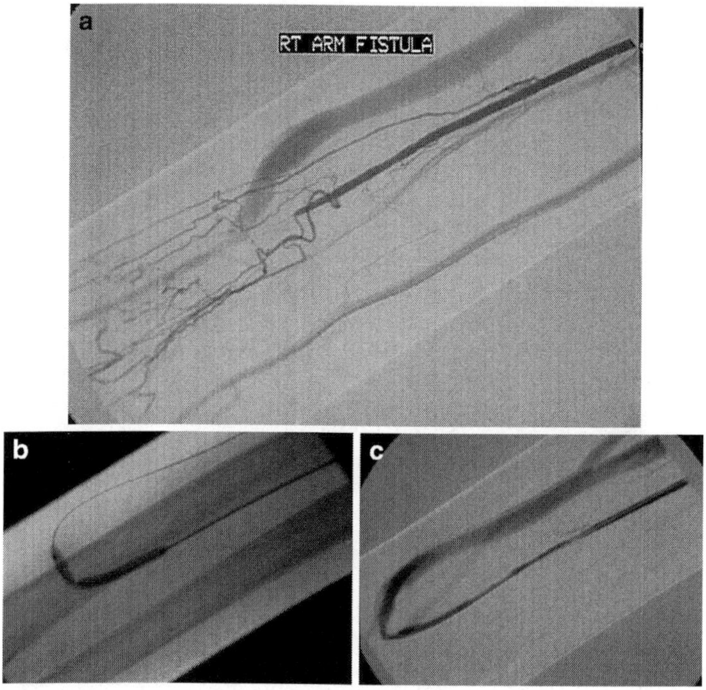

Fig. 17.1 (**a**) Inflow radial artery is occluded with collateral supply via the ulnar artery filling the fistula. (**b**) Via the brachial approach, with a 0.18 in. OTW 4 mm PTA balloon, the radial artery is reopened (**c**) for direct flow to the fistula

cannulation offers a good approach for upper arm fistulas, especially if central venous lesions cannot be crossed from the arm. This approach allows advancement of the catheter through the fistula and into the arterial inflow for correction of both arterial inflow and venous outflow stenoses with one cannulation. Additionally, it permits more remote catheter manipulation, lowering radiation exposure to the operator. A final approach is accessing arm fistulas via a jugular vein puncture and passing retrograde into the fistula. This is an unnecessarily complicated approach but can be considered in unique situations. Collateral vessels indicate resistance to flow in AVFs and may represent areas of stenosis; Unlike AVGs, multiple and tandem stenoses are common in AVFs.

For brachiocephalic fistulas, collateral vessels are less prominent. The direction of puncture for imaging the circuit is dependent on

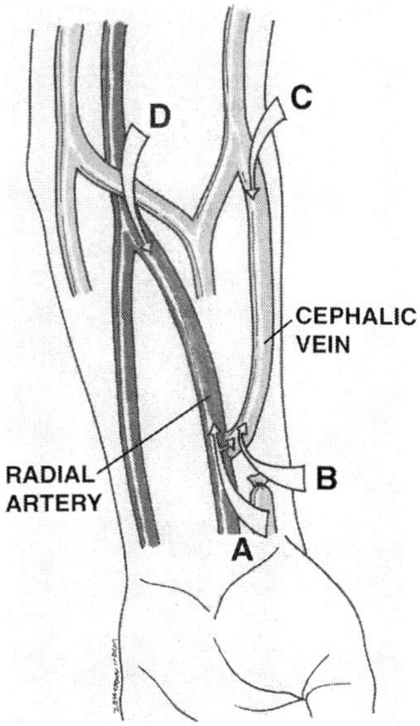

Fig. 17.2 Puncture sites for imaging and possible intervention in radiocephalic fistulas. A – Radial artery, B – Juxta-anastomotic region of the fistula, C – Retrograde into the fistula near the elbow. D – Brachial artery over epicondyle

suspected location of pathology. If an outflow stenosis is suspected, during angioplasty, the arterial anastomosis can be refluxed when the balloon is occluding the outflow through the access sheath. If a retrograde puncture is performed, a small catheter can be advanced into the brachial artery retrograde from the fistula. An angled hydrophilic wire such as the Terumo Glidewire greatly facilitates advancement of a catheter retrograde into either the brachial or radial arteries.

As with grafts, gentle hand injections of 10–15 cc of contrast over 2–3 s per "run" obtaining DSA images at 2 frames/s are usually sufficient in patent fistulas. Volume and rate of contrast injection are modified based on size of vascular territory to be imaged and flow rates. Power pump injection is rarely if ever required.

Angioplasty

Unlike dialysis grafts, the most common location of stenosis is dependent on the type of fistula present. Clinical exam is a significant aid in determining the site of initial puncture. If the fistula is pulsatile, an outflow stenosis is present. If the fistula is flat or has no thrill, an inflow lesion is suspected. Palpating along the length of the fistula may reveal points of stenosis as hardened areas to touch. Elevating the arm is also effective in demonstrating inflow problems. If the fistula flattens with elevation, the patient has an inflow lesion. If the fistula is tender to the touch and erythematous with no thrill and has a rope like feel to it, thrombosis should be suspected. An in-room ultrasound examination of the fistula adds significant information such as location of stenoses, location of collateral veins, course of the fistula, and possible length of thromboses. One should be cognizant of the possibility of multiple stenoses in fistulas that will impact access puncture location for interventions.

For radiocephalic AVFs, a retrograde puncture close to the elbow will allow access to most stenoses whereas an antegrade approach near the AV anastomosis in brachiocephalic AVFs allows access to most stenoses (see Fig. 17.3). For radiocephalic fistulas, the most common location of stenosis is within 5 cm of the arteriovenous anastomosis or also known as the juxta-anastomotic region with over 60% in this location (see Fig. 17.4) with 75% of stenoses occurring distal or peripheral to the elbow [3]. Two studies have noted that cephalic arch stenosis (the perpendicular portion of the cephalic vein in the region of the delto-pectoral groove, prior to its junction with the axillary vein) was common among patients with upper arm fistulas (see Fig. 17.5). Specifically, a patient with a dysfunctional brachiocephalic fistula was 37 times more likely to harbor this lesion than a patient with a dysfunctional radiocephalic fistula with a prevalence of 39–55% was noted within upper arm fistulas vs. 2–7% in forearm autogenous fistulas [4, 5]. For transposed brachiobasilic fistulas, the most common location is at the swing point of the basilic vein [6] (see Fig. 17.3). For ulnar-basilic and transposed radiobasilic fistulas, the most common location of stenosis is the juxta-anastomotic region (52 and 44% respectively) [7].

Balloon catheter size is determined by location of the stenosis. For stenoses involving the arteriovenous anastomosis and/or the first 5 cm of the cephalic vein, typical balloon sizes used are 4–7 mm diameter balloons. I use a nonhydrophilic stiff wire for angioplasty as this is less likely to fall out of the patient or slip away from the lesion and a stiffer wire straightens out the acute angulation of some anastomoses allowing for easier tracking of the balloon and angioplasty. When dilating near the arterial anastomosis with a balloon with a diameter >2 mm larger than the artery, care should be taken to avoid a portion of the balloon inflating within the artery. A balloon with short shoulders is advantageous in this area, allowing

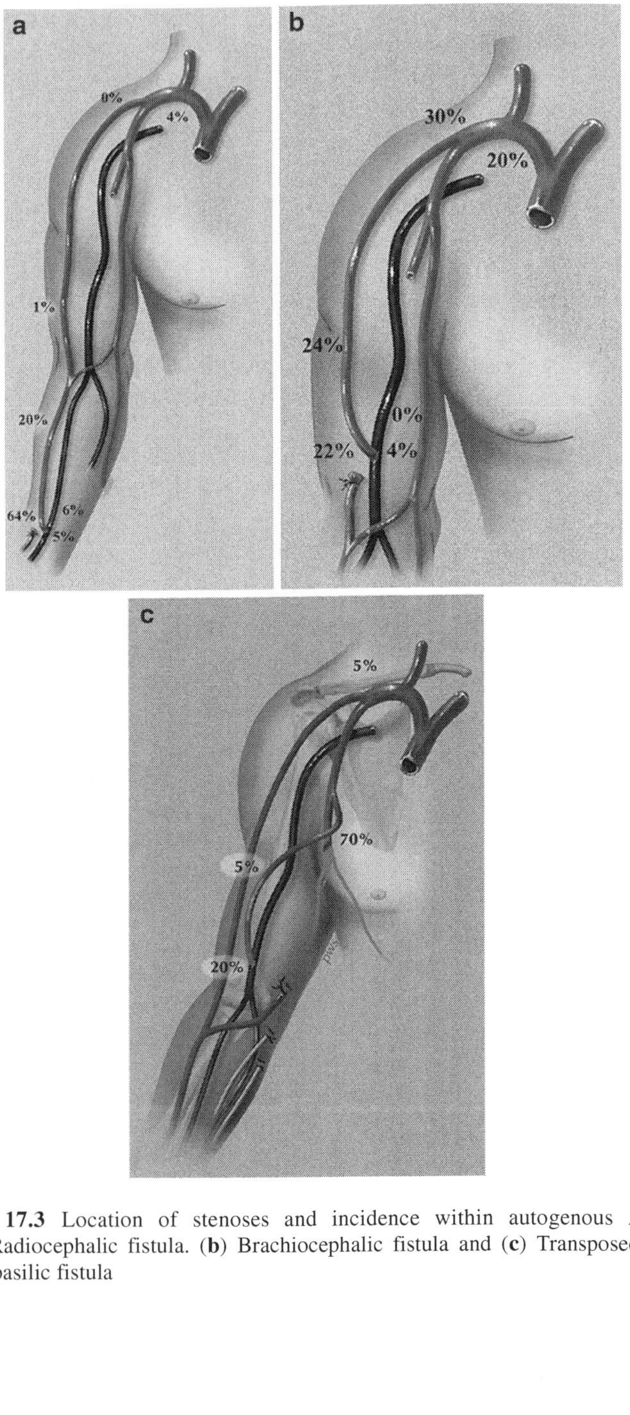

Fig. 17.3 Location of stenoses and incidence within autogenous AVFs. (**a**) Radiocephalic fistula. (**b**) Brachiocephalic fistula and (**c**) Transposed brachiobasilic fistula

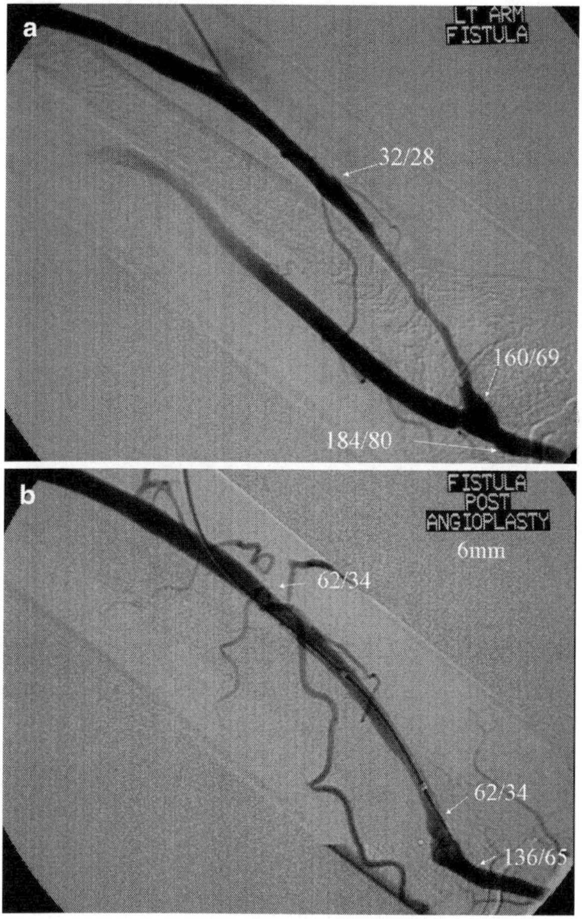

Fig. 17.4 Most common location of stenosis in the radiocephalic fistula is the juxta-anastomotic region. (**a**) Significant pressure gradient is measured. (**b**) Following 6 mm PTA, pressure gradient is eradicated and thrill is reestablished within the fistula. In another patient, (**c**) radiocephalic fistula with JAS resistant to high pressure POBA. (**d**) Initial dilation with cutting balloon (predates larger sizes). (**e**) Postcutting balloon POBA to 7 mm with no resistance. (**f**) No residual stenosis after POBA touchup

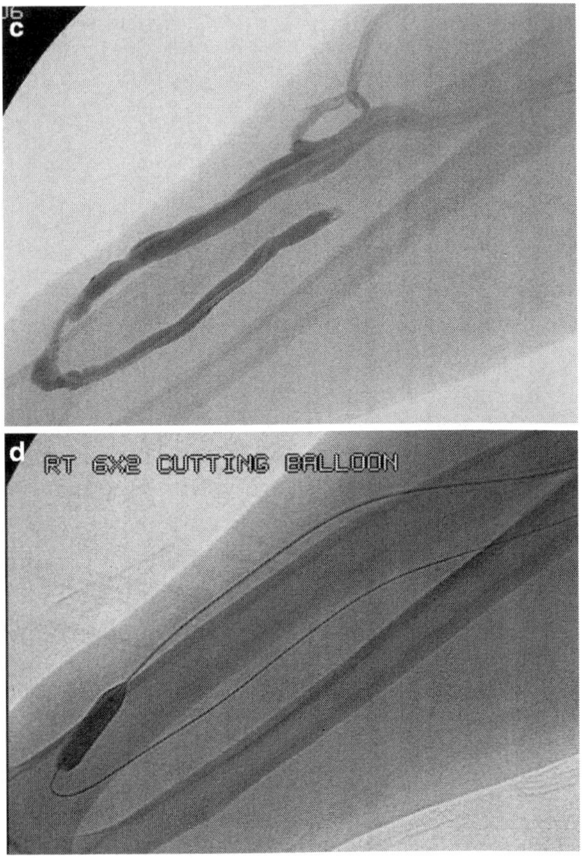

Fig. 17.4 (continued)

for dilatation right up to the AV anastomosis. Inadvertent overdilation of the artery can lead to spasm, thrombosis, rupture, and/or dissection leading to loss of the fistula.

In selected cases where crossing of tight stenoses from the venous side is not possible, a directional hydrophilic guidewire may be passed from a brachial arterial approach and used to cross the lesion in an antegrade direction. The guidewire tip can then be snared from the venous side enabling passage of balloons and other devices from this access rather than the arterial access. External manipulation of the fistula may aid in the passage of balloon catheters. Another alternative is to use a lower profile 0.018-in. wire and angioplasty system.

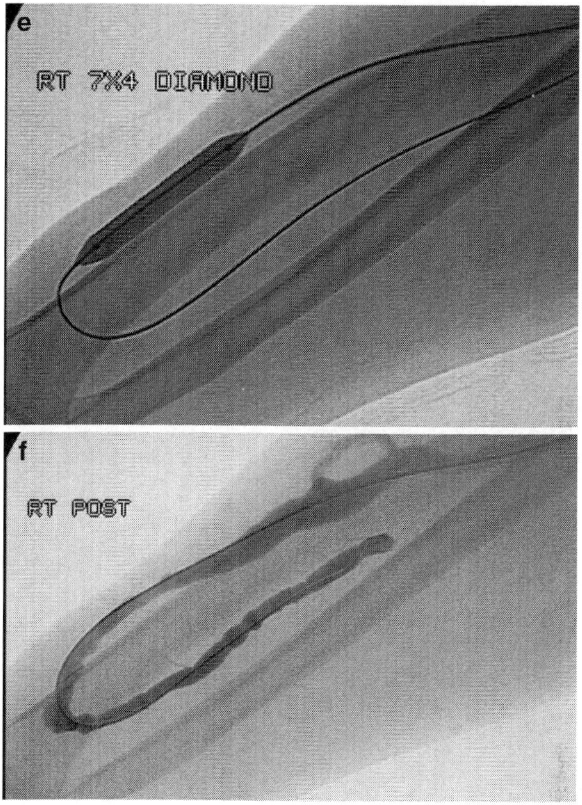

Fig. 17.4 (continued)

Given that many of these systems are 4 Fr in size, interventions can be performed from the brachial artery and radial artery approach for arm fistulas, albeit with a higher complication rate associated with the brachial puncture site. Stenoses along the outflow cephalic vein typically can be dilated from 7 to 10 mm.

Cephalic arch stenosis is very resistant to balloon angioplasty and frequently requires the use of high-pressure balloons. This lesion is also prone to rupture with a reported rupture rate of 6% (see Fig. 19.2, Chap. 19) [4]. The most common balloon catheter used to dilate this lesion is 8 mm diameter. Further discussion is presented in Chap. 19. Central venous stenosis and occlusion management are discussed in Chap. 20.

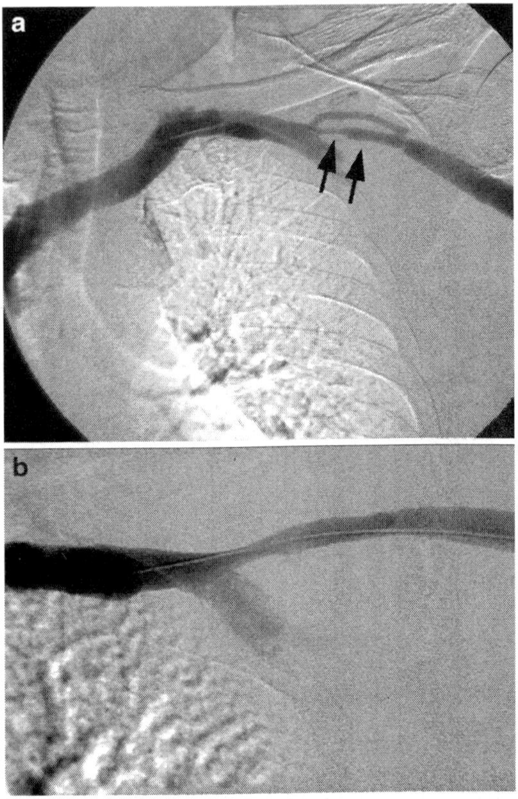

Fig. 17.5 (**a**) Uncomplicated cephalic arch stenosis (*arrows*) more commonly found in brachiocephalic fistulas. (**b**) Following 8 mm POBA, stenosis is corrected

Outcomes of POBA

Multiple studies examining outcomes for autogenous hemodialysis fistulas reported success rates ranging from 91 to 95% and 1-year primary patency rates from 39 to 62% depending on the type of fistula [1, 3, 5, 8] (Table 17.1). Secondary patency rates range from 82 to 86% were achieved at 1 year but with more frequent reintervention in the upper arm (11 months vs. 18 months) [3, 5]. The article by Turmel-Rodrigues et al. also reported the influence of the age of the vascular access on the outcome: the older the fistula at the time of the first dilation, the better the results. Manninen et al. [1] reported a 58 and 44%

Table 17.1 Patency rates following percutaneous angioplasty for nonthrombosed autogenous hemodialysis fistulas

				Primary patency			Secondary patency	
References	Fistula type	No.	Success (%)	6 Month (%)	12 Month (%)	24 Month (%)	6 Month (%)	12 Month (%)
Manninen et al. [1][a]	Forearm	53	91	58	44	40	90	85
Clark et al. [8]	Forearm/upper arm	53	94	55	26		82	82
Lay et al. [39]	Forearm	31	90	77	64		85	81
Turmel-Rodrigues et al. [5]	Forearm	155	95	67	51	37	–	85
	Upper arm	65	97	57	35	24	–	82
Rajan et al. [3]	Radiocephalic	94	98 overall	75	62		88	86
	Brachiocephalic	57		51	39		89	85

[a]Includes 12 thrombosed fistulas

primary patency rate at 6 months and 1 year. Secondary patency was 85 and 79% at 1 and 2 years. Procedures were performed on radiocephalic fistulas only, and 12 thrombosed fistulas were included in the outcome analysis. This study also reported significantly poorer outcomes when stenoses were located near the anastomosis and when the feeding artery was "small" [1]. Clark et al. [8] examined 53 dysfunctional nonthrombosed fistulas and observed primary and secondary patency rates of 55 and 82% at 6 months and 26 and 82% at 12 months with radiocephalic, brachiocephalic, and brachiobasilic fistulas combined as a single group. In our study, we found that there was no significant difference in secondary outcome following angioplasty for dysfunctional autogenous fistulas regardless of type of fistula, location and number of stenoses, and age of the patient. We have observed that dysfunctional brachiocephalic fistulas require more frequent interventions than radiocephalic fistulas, an observation that is consistent with studies by Turmel-Rodrigues and Clark et al. [3, 5, 8].

The current anatomic success standard of postangioplasty residual stenosis of less than 30% applies to dialysis grafts. In dysfunctional autogenous fistulas, the vein is subject to spasm, elastic recoil, or other factors, which may result in persistent residual stenosis greater that 30%. Clark et al. [8] found no difference in long-term patency among fistulas with >30% residual stenosis compared to anatomically successfully treated stenosis. This suggests that the current standard of anatomic success for angioplasty may not be applicable to autogenous fistulas.

Vascular Stenting

Current practice guidelines published by the Society of Interventional Radiology (SIR) and K/DOQI recommend placement of stents for failed angioplasty, recurrent central vein stenosis within less than 3 months, and rupture of the outflow vein [9]. Also, less than 30% residual stenosis following angioplasty is recommended [10] although this standard for venous angioplasty is uncertain. While stenting was previously recommended for failed angioplasties with a residual stenosis greater than 30%, there is no data to show increased long-term patency with stents in this setting. Further evaluation of this standard is warranted to avoid potential overuse of stents with questionable long-term patency in hemodialysis patients [11–13].

Given the known poor patency of stents in veins, we reserve stenting in dialysis fistulas only when it is absolutely necessary to maintain immediate patency of the dialysis fistula. These indications are flow-limiting dissection, acute occlusion not corrected with repeat angioplasty and venous rupture that is not controlled with conservative measures. Consider avoiding stenting or stent grafting areas that may compromise or damage arterialized vein segments that can be used for a new access rather than maintaining a poorly functioning one.

Placing stents or stent grafts within patients who are septic or have an active significant ongoing infection possibly predisposes these devices to becoming infected. As they are permanently implanted, the interventionalist should consider the benefits vs. risks of using these devices in this clinical scenario. Lastly, as mentioned in the Chap. 16, stents are not indicated to trap thrombus as there is potential migration risk.

Clotted Autogenous Hemodialysis Fistulas

Anatomy of Thrombosis: Thrombosis of an AV fistula is very different from that of its synthetic graft (AVG) counterpart. Whereas thrombosis is typically limited to the graft, thrombosis within a fistula typically occurs from the anastomosis to the next point of collateral vein circulation. Occasionally, the thrombosed segment may lie in the cephalic vein between two points of collateral venous circulation. The thromboses can be short segment or long segment depending on location and number of stenoses. Compared to declotting of AVGs, thrombosed fistulas are more difficult to access and declot. Many situations may exist which significantly impact on the difficulty of this procedure. These considerations include the following:

1. A thin venous wall which is occasionally difficult to palpate
2. Anatomy is highly variable making localization of anastomosis difficult
3. Stenosis can occur anywhere from the feeding artery to the SVC
4. Multiple collaterals can be deceptive
5. Aneurysms are more common in fistulas with clot of varying ages present within them and may be colonized with bacteria
6. The anastomosis may be sharply angulated making it impossible to traverse from the fistula
7. Larger clot burden compared to dialysis grafts
8. The feeding artery may be thrombosed

Depending on the size of the cephalic vein, the amount of clot may be substantial compared to AVGs. Attempts to puncture the true fistula may be difficult due to the decompressed nature of the fistula. Also, in an attempt to puncture the fistula, the wrong vein may be entered and the thrombosed segment may not be crossed. The native fistula has no rigid artificial wall to guide direction of a wire or thrombectomy device. Given that AVFs utilize native veins, concern regarding perforation exists.

Management

Thrombosed fistulas can be reopened successfully typically within 48 h with recent reports of success within 14 days [14, 15]. However, preference is for treatment within 0–72 h. Beyond 14 days, inflammatory and sclerotic changes become more prominent and the fistula is more prone to rupture sometimes extensively during intervention. A percutaneous attempt should be made prior to surgical attempts as surgical thrombectomy was usually limited by lack of appropriate equipment to treat all underlying lesions. However, with the introduction of C-arm fluoroscopy capabilities in some OR suites within the United States, these limitations have been overcome in selected practices. Prior to embarking on thrombolysis, it is important to ascertain whether the fistula is mature or not and has been used for effective hemodialysis treatment. Infection of the fistula is also an absolute contraindication.

Declotting of AVFs is typically performed as an outpatient procedure, with IV sedation and pain medication provided as required. Patients often have significant local tenderness due to reactive phlebitis in the region of thrombosis. This should not be confused with infection. If infection is present, the patient often has constitutional symptoms of infection and will likely have an elevated white blood cell count. Also, clinical signs of redness, tenderness, and heat often precede thrombosis by multiple days when the fistula is infected. Preprocedure antibiotics remain at the discretion of the treating physician as there is no evidence for or against this practice. Patients should be heparinized to prevent propagation of clot and rethrombosis during the procedure. With successful declotting, no form of chronic anticoagulation is necessary. Establishing adequate flow can be difficult. If flow within the fistula appears sluggish, it may be beneficial to discuss possible further surgical thrombectomy with a surgeon. Re-angioplasty any remaining underlying stenosis within a few days may also be considered.

Methods of Declotting and Outcomes

Prior to embarking on declotting of a fistula, it is important to recognize that although a fistula may appear clotted, some may contain a short segment occlusion rather than thrombus. In such cases traversal of the occlusion using a directional catheter (e.g., 4 Fr Kumpe) and glidewire with subsequent POBA in most cases is sufficient to restore patency with no need for thrombolytics or mechanical thrombectomy devices. This simple maneuver is also sufficient for short segmental thrombus where POBA macerates the thrombus (see Fig. 17.6).

Unlike percutaneous therapy of thrombosed AV grafts, there have been relatively few studies that have described methods for declotting autogenous fistulae. Reported methods have included systemic or local administration of streptokinase, urokinase, tPA, and surgical thrombectomy (see Fig. 17.7). Technical success rates with local or systemic infusion of thrombolytics alone ranged from 33 to 90%. Surgical declotting of autogenous fistulas has met with varied success, often at the expense of native venous segments in prior studies. Bone and Pomajzi [16] described 22% cumulative patency at 6 months with surgical thrombectomy alone. However, a recent review suggests similar outcomes between surgical techniques and endovascular techniques in fistulas [17].

Mechanical devices and other pharmacomechanical and aspiration techniques are discussed in Chap. 15. An on-label approved device for AVFs that is preferred is the Arrow PTD device. The Arrow-Trerotola device is a spinning nitinol basket that breaks up or macerates the clot and then one aspirates the broken up clot through the access sheaths (see Fig. 17.8). It is available as an over the wire or non-over-the-wire device. The over-the-wire device is useful for tight angulations and the wall contact nature of the device helps strip clot from aneurysms occasionally with the aid of external massage/compression.

Declotting is only part of the revascularization process. In most cases, balloon angioplasty was also required to dilate underlying shunt stenosis. Location of stenoses has been discussed above. Our experience suggests that large aneurysms may produce poorer outcome

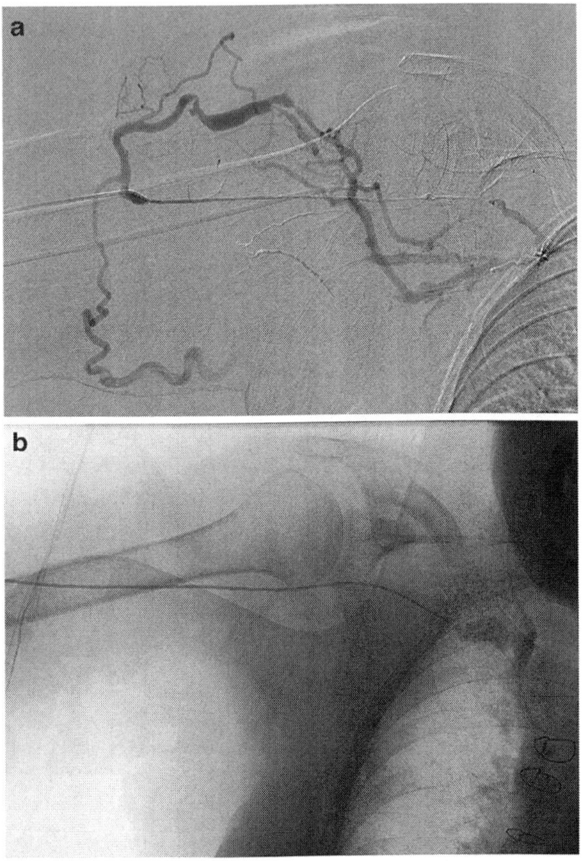

Fig. 17.6 Patient presents for dialysis catheter insertion after another center determines the brachiocephalic fistula is thrombosed and unsalvageable. (**a**) Fistulogram from patent proximal one third of fistula demonstrates chronic occlusion of the distal two third of the cephalic vein. (**b**) Using a 4 Fr Kumpe catheter and glidewire, the occlusion is traversed. (**c**, **d**) After 8 mm PTA of the occluded cephalic vein and 12 mm PTA of the innominate vein stenosis, rapid flow is reestablished with no required catheter insertion or thrombectomy/thrombolysis

and lead to acute failure, possibly from propagation of residual clot within the aneurysm [18] leading to eventual rethrombosis. There are potential ways to deal with retained clot within aneurysms. One may externally massage the area to dislodge clot or roll a syringe along the aneurysm or fistula, as one would use a rolling pin to roll out dough.

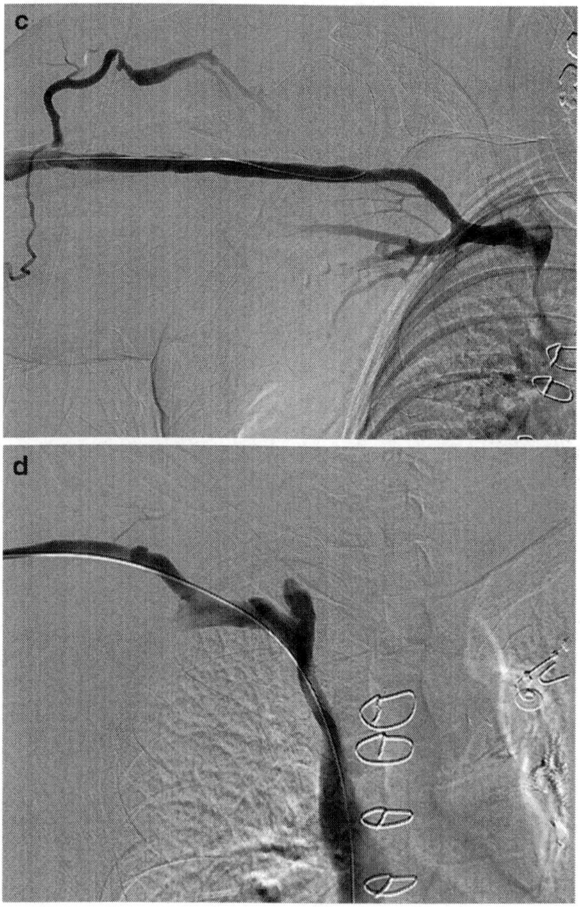

Fig. 17.6 (continued)

Wetting the overlying skin reduces friction. This method has been described as the "Rajan Rolling Pin Technique" (see Fig. 17.9). Aneurysms can be excluded with stent grafts. This is an off-label indication within the United States, and there is minimal but positive evidence to consider this in bailout situations. One should be aware however that aneurysms often contain old clot that can be colonized by bacteria. Therefore, there is some concern for potential infection of the stent graft. Another method involves making a small <5 mm incision into the aneurysm and using small forceps, extracting the old

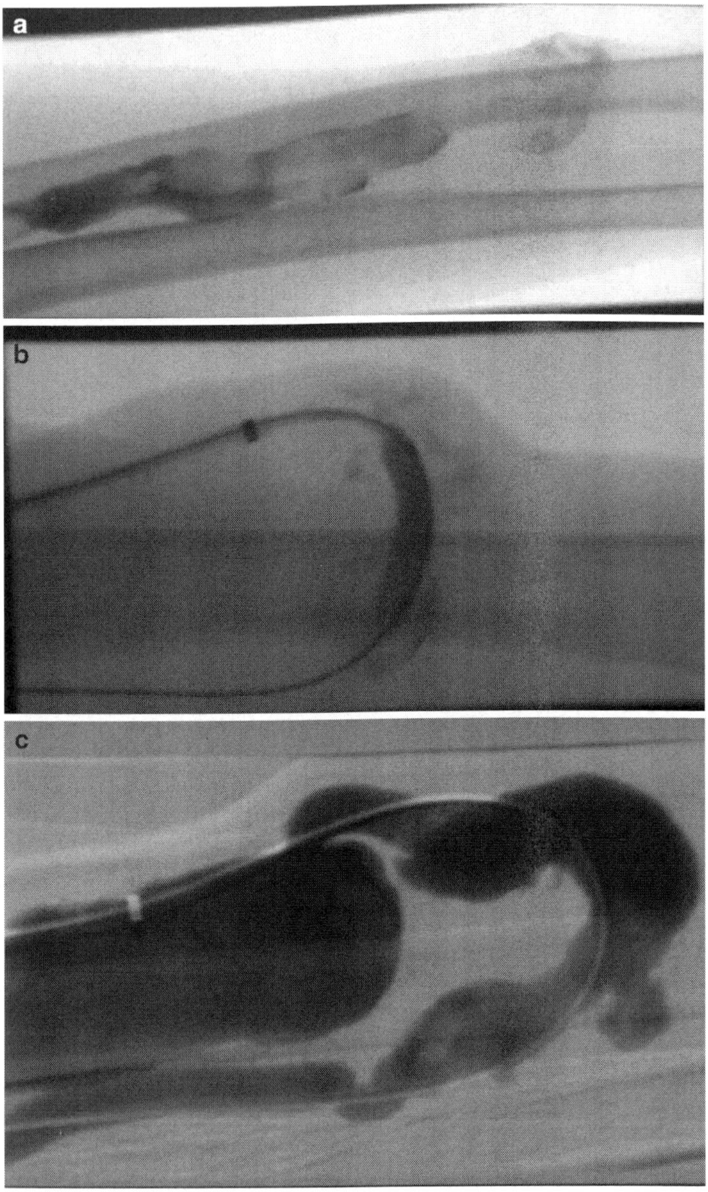

Fig. 17.7 Radiocephalic end to end fistula functioning for 19 years presents with first episode of thrombosis. (**a**) Fistula is punctured where not thrombosed in a retrograde direction. Injection of contrast demonstrates a significant amount of

clot by grabbing it and taking out small chunks or squeezing it out. After extraction, the incision is closed with a monofilament single purse string or interrupted stitch.

Improved clinical success later in our experience has come from modifications in our approach to clotted fistulae. Perhaps most important is perseverance. Declotting of AV fistulae compared to grafts requires more time, effort, and patience. We also now routinely use ultrasound to aid in access to the fistula and to identify the thrombosed segment of the fistula and length of thrombosis. External manipulation of the fistula also facilitates passage of a wire and/or catheter through aneurysms, stenosis, and acute angulations of vessels common to AV fistulae. We routinely perform an outflow venogram prior to declotting to assess for any outflow lesions. If these lesions are not correctable percutaneously, further intervention is abandoned.

Advantages of percutaneous therapy over surgical thrombectomy are many. Percutaneous declotting can be performed as an outpatient procedure without use of operating room facilities and thereby may reduce direct costs. In addition, underlying lesions that may result in fistula thrombosis can occur anywhere from the subclavian artery to the superior vena cava. All of these lesions can be detected and treated precisely and systematically using facilities available in the modern angiography suite. The contour of the declotted fistula may be irregular in spite of maximal clot removal, these wall irregularities generally correct and become smooth on repeat studies at approximately 2 weeks.

Tips

1. Declotting fistulas is often difficult and requires significantly more time than declotting dialysis grafts. When first starting to do these, allot 2–3 h. Frustration from lack of time can translate into failure. Give yourself enough time.

Fig. 17.7 (continued) clot in the proximal portion of the fistula. Note extensive calcifications in the region of the arteriovenous anastomosis. (**b**) After pulse-spray infusion of 4 mg of tPA, external massage and angioplasty of an underlying stenosis with a 6 mm noncompliant balloon, and balloon thrombectomy of residual clot with a Fogarty catheter, (**c**) the fistula has brisk flow. Note the multiple aneurysms and tortuosity of the peripheral fistula that highlights difficulties in declotting fistulae. The fistula continues to function maintained with PTA and no further clotting episodes 9 years later

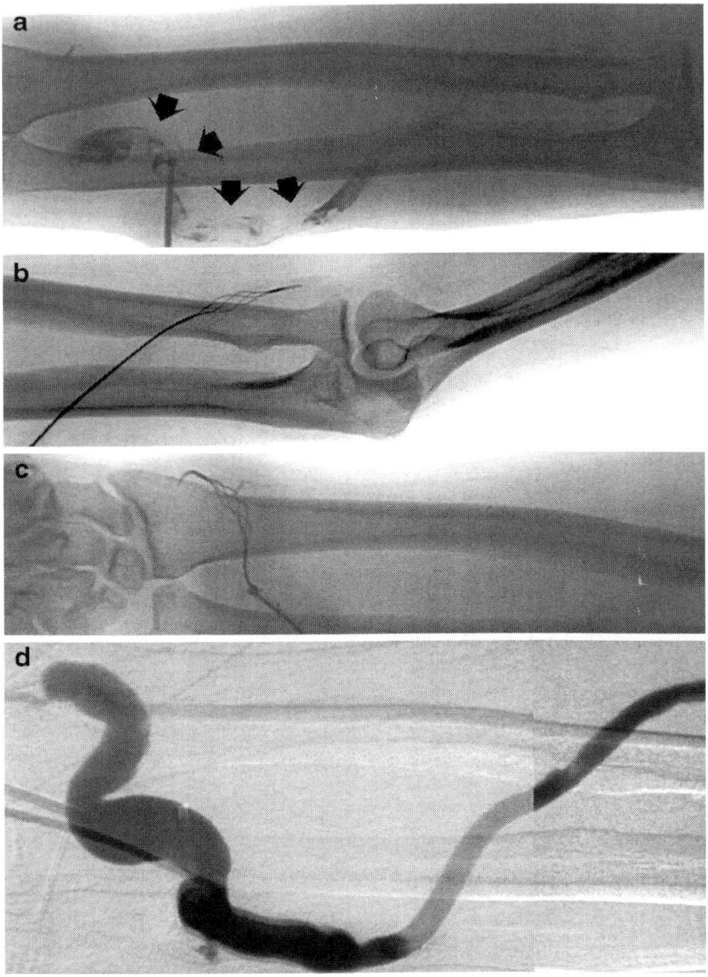

Fig. 17.8 Thrombectomy AV fistula with Arrow-Trerotola Percutaneous Thrombectomy Device (PTD) (Case provided courtesy of Dr. Timothy I. Clark). Mature radiocephalic fistula which thrombosed 72 h earlier. (**a**) The fistula has been accessed in a retrograde direction near the anastomosis. Contrast outlines extensive clot burden within tortuous segment of fistula (*arrows*). (**b**) Through a 6-Fr sheath, the PTD was positioned to the level of the anastomosis. The rubber tip of the device is in the radial artery. The device basket was opened across the arterial plug and pulled back into the fistula prior to initiating thrombectomy. To overcome the tortuous anatomy, the sheath had been advanced to this position over a guidewire and then withdrawn to move the PTD into position. An over-the-wire

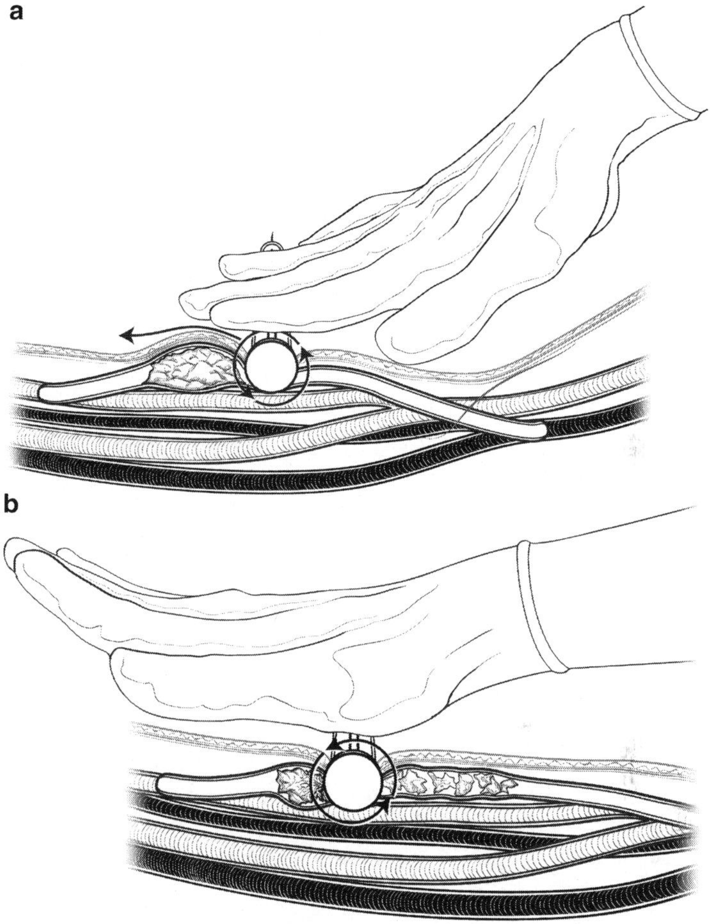

Fig. 17.9 The "Rajan rolling pin technique." Clot is fragmented and mobilized within the access and areas of aneurysmal dilation. The skin is wetted to reduce friction and an empty syringe is rolled back and forth across the area of thrombosis. Care should be taken to prevent rolling or pushing clot across the arterial anastomosis

Fig. 17.8 (continued) device can also be used. Aspiration is maintained through the side arm of the sheath during activation of the PTD. (**c**) After several passes of the PTD in the initial portion of the access, an antegrade puncture is made with passage of the PTD in this direction. (**d**) Completion fistulograms showing complete patency of the access. Underlying areas of stenosis revealed after PTD thrombectomy have been treated with 6 and 8 mm angioplasty

2. Placing a tourniquet or blood pressure cuff on the upper arm may allow dilation of the outflow vein facilitating entry into the fistula. Occasionally, ultrasound-guided puncture may be required. A preliminary ultrasound, with or without Doppler evaluation, in the angiographic suite can assist in determining the course of the main draining vein and determine the extent of the thrombosis and the location of collaterals. This can help in planning the puncture site. During attempted crossing of the thrombosed segment, external manipulation may assist in passage of the wire. Also, previous puncture sites of the fistula can be used as a guide to determine if the correct course of the fistula is being traversed.
3. When transvenous access is not possible, imaging of the fistula can be performed by inserting a 22-gauge angiocatheter or 3 Fr inner cannula of a micropuncture set into the brachial artery for antegrade imaging. This approach is associated with a relatively high complication rate of 12% in one study [1, 19] and should be reserved for special cases. This method of access also limits therapeutic options as placement of large sheaths is likely difficult and increases puncture site complications substantially. The combination of an angled (4 or 5 Fr) catheter and a hydrophilic guide wire frequently makes it possible to pass the stenosis. Using the hydrophilic guide wire, the next step is then to enter the introducer-sheath, which has previously been placed in the fistula in a retrograde fashion. The guide wire is then pushed selectively into the introducer-sheath to contact the hemostatic valve while the introducer-sheath is slowly removed [1]. Some sheaths (Cordis) allow removal of the hemostatic valve and allow retrograde passage of wire without sheath removal. The guide wire inserted via the brachial artery re-emerges therefore from the fistula, through the skin and above the stenosis. The introducer-sheath is reintroduced over the guide wire to facilitate dilation of the stenosis with a balloon pushed from the fistula instead of the brachial artery, thus limiting the size of the hole in the artery.
4. External manipulation can be used to dislodge clot from the fistula and/or aneurysms if the aforementioned procedures fail to do so. This method can also be used to guide catheters or thrombectomy devices through the fistula.
5. Use of a "safety guide wire" [20]: when the fistula is tortuous, with stenoses, sharp angulations, and/or aneurysms, or when blind predilation is necessary to allow the passage of a thrombectomy device (such as a thromboaspiration catheter), repeat passes with

catheters or devices are likely to be difficult. Similarly, thrombectomy or dilation maneuvers in the anastomotic area can damage the feeding artery. In such cases, a guide wire is passed through the introducer-sheath into the feeding artery or into the superior vena cava depending on the location of the area of concern. After placement of this "safety guide wire," which should not be a hydrophilic guide wire prone to spontaneous inadvertent removal, a second guide wire is passed through the same sheath. The sheath is then removed and repositioned only over the second "working" guide wire, leaving the safety guide wire exiting directly through the skin beside the introducer-sheath. While thrombectomy and dilation maneuvers can be performed through the sheath, the safety guide wire is a fluoroscopic landmark of the anatomy of the fistula and potentiates rapid reopening of the fistula by passing a dilation balloon or a stent over it if complications occur.

In Summary

Declotting of AVFs requires more time and patience compared to AVGs. Therapy is more challenging owing to difficulty in palpation, variation in anatomy, clot burden, aneurysm formation, and multiplicity of lesions. Although many methods for declotting have been described, how one re-establishes function is less important. What remains most important for durable success is to (1) *remove all possible clot* and (2) *treat all underlying lesions* to the point of angiographic (<30% residual stenosis) or pressure success. Management of fistulae has a large learning curve and requires significant patience.

Outcomes

Manual thromboaspiration with angioplasty has been described by Turmel-Rodrigues with technical success rates of 93 and 76% for lower and upper arm fistulae respectively. Primary patencies of 89, 70, and 49% at 3, 6, and 12 months respectively for lower arm fistulae were observed. For upper arm fistulae, primary patency at 3, 6, and 12 months was 36, 18, and 9%. Secondary patency rates in the forearm and upper arm were 89 and 76% respectively at 3 months, 84 and 68% at 6 months, and 81 and 50% at 1 year [21].

Results of studies using mechanical thrombectomy devices used in conjunction with angioplasty have yielded technical success rates of 76–100% with 36–70% and 18–60% primary patency rates at 3 and 6 months respectively and 60–80% assisted primary patency at 6 months [22–26] (Table 17.2).

Liang et al. [15] using a combination of balloon angioplasty and infusion of urokinase achieved primary and secondary patency values of 81 and 84% at 6 months. Our personal experience has generated modest outcomes due to a high initial failure rate [27] (Table 17.3).

Unique Situations

Aneurysms

Although many refer to the areas of aneurysmal dilation within fistulas as pseudoaneurysms, this terminology is incorrect as all vessel wall layers are present and therefore these areas of dilation or bulging are true venous aneurysms. Some patients eventually develop aneurysms or more appropriately venous varices of their AVFs. The pathophysiology behind aneurysms is unknown although the two main theories are that they are the result of multiple punctures in the same location and/or venous outflow stenosis. Regardless of the underlying cause, they can become very large and beyond cosmetic concerns, they can become focal points of thrombosis or catastrophic rupture. Otherwise, there is no indication to treat them specifically. Aneurysms can become points of flow stenosis and retain varying ages of clot within them. They can become the underlying cause of access thrombosis. If this is the case of thrombosis, techniques discussed above and below may deal with this problem. For impending rupture, the clinical signs are a very thin shiny skin overlying the aneurysm occasionally with a small clot or eschar on the skin. This represents a potential emergency and should be recognized as such. Prior to repair, the patient should be immediately instructed in how to control exsanguination if this site were to begin bleeding. There is no single method to treat aneurysms. Beyond surgical alternatives mentioned below, unproven options include (1) abandoning the access, (2) reducing the flow through the access, and (3) converting part of the fistula into a graft by placing stent grafts across the aneurysms.

Table 17.2 Outcomes following mechanical device use for thrombosed AVFs

	Device used	Patients/fistula declotted	Average intervention time	Technical success (%)	Primary patency 3 months (%)	Primary patency 6 months (%)	Primary patency 1 year (%)	Others
Turmel-Rodrigues et al. [21]	Thrombo-aspiration	73 Fistulas, 56 forearm (fa), 17 upper arm (ua)	134 min – fa, 119 min – ua	93 fa, 76 ua	89 fa, 36 ua	70 fa, 18 ua	49/9 fa/ua	Secondary 1 year patency 81%/50%, 3% complications
Haage et al. [24]	Hydrolyzer, Amplatz thrombectomy devices or balloon maceration	54 Fistulas	–	89	63	52	27	51% Secondary patency at 1 year
Overbosch et al. [23]	Amplatz thrombectomy catheter	22 Fistulas, 37 AVGs	60–90 min	89 for fistulas	Median primary patency of 14 weeks			15% Complications
Vorwerk et al. [40]	Hydrolyser (Cordis)	19 Fistulas, 15 AVGs	–	84	Cumul patency for both 37% 6 months, 32% 1 year			20% Complications
Schmitz-Rode et al. [25]	Rotating Pigtail	15 Fistulas, 11 AVGs	118 min	100	65	47		
Rocek et al. [22]	Arrow-Trerotola	10 Fistulas	126.1 min	100	70	60		Assisted primary patency at 6 months 80%
Littler et al. [41]	Angiojet (Possis)	44 Fistulas, 20 AVGs		91	AVF-61, AVG-57	AVF-34, AVG-43		10% Complications, two cases of arterial embolization

Table 17.3 Outcomes following pharmacomechanical therapy for thrombosed AVFs

Pharmacomechanical	Method used	Patients/fistula declotted	Average intervention time	Technical success (%)	Primary patency 3 months (%)	Primary patency 6 months (%)	Primary patency 1 year (%)	Others
Liang et al. [15]	Thrombolytics and PTA	42	–	90	–	81	70	84 and 80% Secondary patency at 6/12 months, 10% complications
Rajan et al. [27]	Thrombolytics and PTA	25	104 min	73	36	28	24	44% Secondary patency after 3 months, 7% complications
Zaleski et al. [42]	Thrombolytics with PTA	17	1.7 h	82		71	64	93% Secondary patency at 6/12 months
Poulain et al. [43]	Thrombolytics, PTA, and thrombo-aspiration	16 Fistulas, 23 AVGs, 18 bovine carotid grafts		59			Overall 59% functioning at 1 year	
Schon and Mishler [14]	Thrombolytics with PTA	15	101 min	94				81% Long-term patency – defined as greater than 30 days
Clark et al. [8]	Thrombolytics with PTA	12	–	66	60			67/44% Secondary patency at 6/12 months, 8% complication

Ways to Occlude the Access

If the access is to be abandoned, prior to embarking on such an absolute measure, one should assess what access sites the patient has and their overall access plan over their expected lifespan. If the patient is limited in options, surgical revision or stent grafts may be considered. One can terminate an access in many ways nonsurgically. One is to simply pass a monofilament stitch around the access near the arterial anastomosis through the skin and tie the stitch down to close the access (see Fig. 17.10). Another method is to occlude the fistula with coils or an Amplatzer Plug (AGA Medical). Both of these methods have higher risk as the access is high flow and the embolic devices may embolize to the lungs. To avoid this, flow can be temporarily

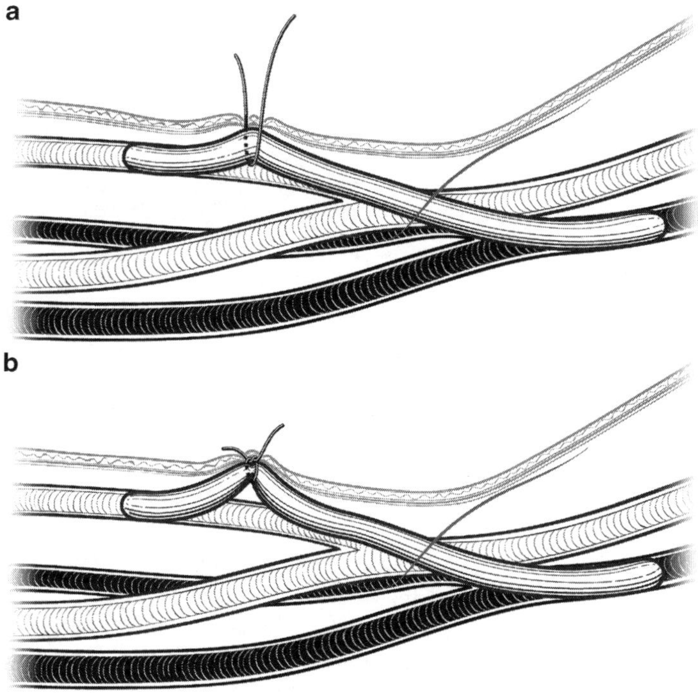

Fig. 17.10 (**a**) Monofilament stitch on tapered needle is passed through the skin, under the access and back though the skin. (**b**) The stitch is then tied, thereby occluding the access. This method can also be used to occlude venous collaterals close to the skin surface rather than using coils (more costly and irritating to patients)

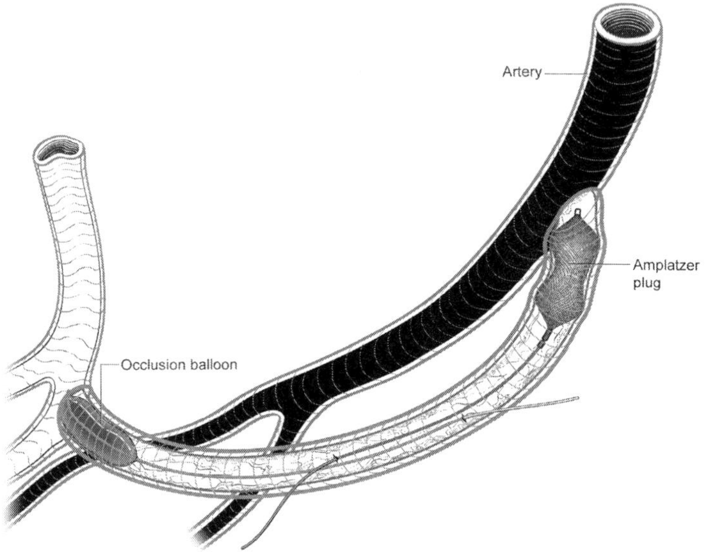

Fig. 17.11 Occlusion of the access. An occlusion balloon is placed toward the venous outflow of the access and inflated to arrest flow and prevent embolization. Via a second puncture directed toward the arterial inflow, the Amplatzer plug is delivered and deployed near the anastomosis within the access. The size of the plug used should be at least 2 mm larger than the target area of the access. After deployment, the occlusion balloon is deflated slowly with intermittent injection of contrast to document flow termination within the access prior to complete removal

stopped with an occlusion balloon within the fistula while coils or the plug are deposited close to the arterial anastomosis (see Fig. 17.11) and then slowly deflated to make sure distal embolization does not occur. If an Amplatzer plug is to be used, the device diameter should be at least 2 mm larger than the graft or fistula segment diameter is to be placed in. For coils, a similar size for initial coils to be placed is used followed by smaller coils to fill in the center of the coil mass as bigger coils tend to fill along or lie along the vein or graft wall. When deploying either device, one must be vigilant to ensure the devices do not move into or embolize into the feeling artery. Lastly, embolization should absolutely not be used if the access is infected. These are permanent foreign devices that will act as ongoing sources of infection. Clearly surgical ligation is cheapest when available, but another simple and relatively cheap alternative is thrombin injection into the fistula. While employing compression of the inflow portion of the

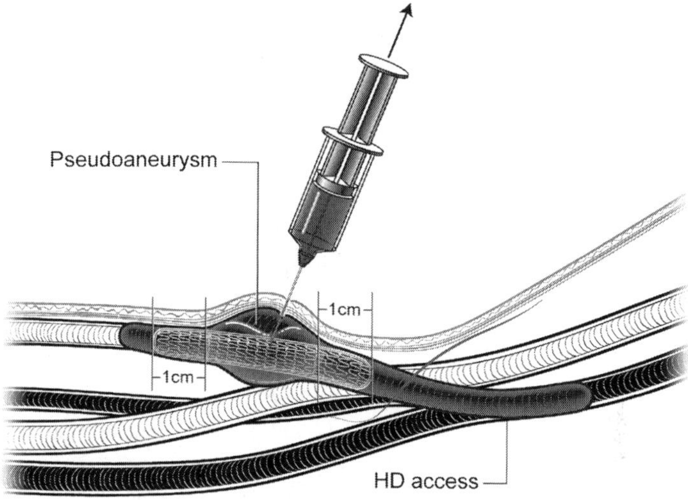

Fig. 17.12 After insertion of an appropriately sized stent graft with sufficient (>1 cm) overlap with the normal caliber vessel on either side, liquid contents of the now excluded aneurysm are aspirated

fistula, the fistula can be cannulated and injected with 1,000–5,000 U of thrombin. This results in immediate thrombosis of the fistula, much like when used in femoral pseudoaneurysm thrombosis.

Stent Grafts and Aneurysms of AVFs

There is limited literature on the use of stent grafts to exclude aneurysms although there are initial promising selected cases. If one is going to exclude the aneurysm with a stent graft, there are some considerations when doing so. Prophylactic antibiotics should be given prior to insertion as the aneurysm often has thrombus within it that is chronically colonized with bacteria. The stent graft should extend or be long enough to extend to normal vein segments on either side with a minimum of 1 cm coverage within the normal segments on either side. After deployment, a small needle should be inserted into the aneurysm to remove blood within it and decompress it (see Fig. 17.12). Following deployment, some time (at least a week) should be given to allow the area stented to heal or fibrose prior to puncturing the stent graft for dialysis. There has been no formal study on if or how long stent grafts grafts can be punctured for dialysis although anecdotally, this is done frequently. If traversing aneurysms, there is the possibility of the device kinking within the aneurysm and therefore pulling into it. In addition, oversizing of the stent graft should be avoided with maximum oversizing by 1 mm as mentioned in Chap. 16. A potential future but rare complication to consider from placing stent grafts is the risk of fractured strut extrusion through the skin related to dialysis needles placed though the device.

Stent Grafts to Salvage Fistulas

There is no properly conducted randomized study that demonstrates benefits of stent grafts in fistulas. However, there is a single randomized although somewhat poorly constructed study that demonstrated superiority over stenting within the cephalic arch (Chap. 19). In addition there are two limited retrospective studies that suggest that stent grafts in fistulas have superior patency to angioplasty alone when used to salvage the fistula [28, 29]. Stent grafts can be used at sites of balloon-induced vein rupture as a method of salvage, to cover aneurysms and to exclude thrombus (see Fig. 17.13). In situations where acute loss of fistula patency is expected, particularly in failed thrombectomy of dialysis fistulas, stent grafts may salvage the access with patency exceeding 80% at 6 months. Multiple overlapping devices effectively convert a fistula into a combination of graft and fistula or as some have coined the term "graftula." Again, one should consider the permanent nature of the devices, antibiotic prophylaxis, possible exclusion of future accesses, and appropriate sizing.

Occluded Outflow

Some portions of fistulas occasionally continue to function if collaterals are present. Often pressures are high and inadequate dialysis is possible. Unstudied techniques for salvage offer an alternative when there are limited or no options for other accesses in the patient. One option is sharp needle puncture into an adjacent vein and then bridging the tract with a stent or stent graft (see Case 1, Chap. 29). Another alternative that has been tried with unpublished success is to dilate

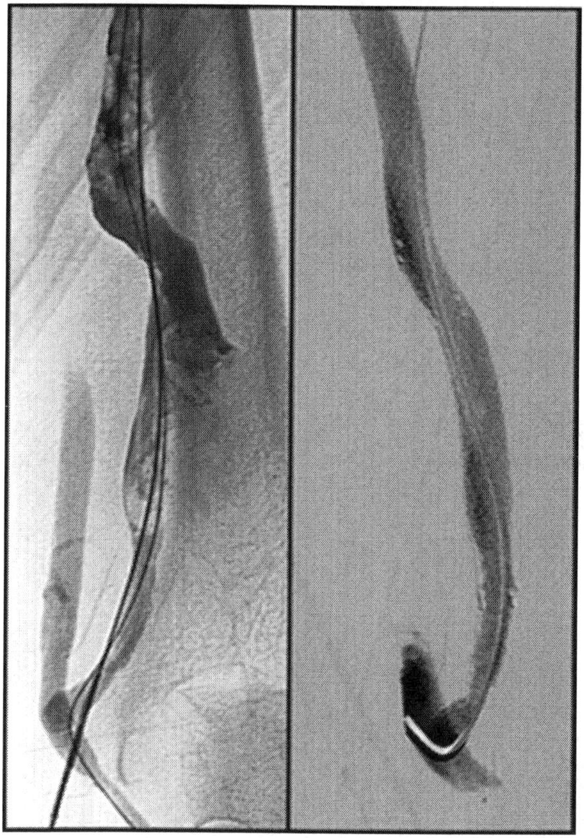

Fig. 17.13 Thrombosed brachiocephalic fistula. Retained clot within aneurysms inhibiting flow. After placement of two stent grafts, rapid flow is reestablished by excluding the clot filled pseudoaneurysms

outflow collaterals with the hope that dilation will lead to better outflow and reduced pressures. The technique is similar to sequential balloon maturation of outflow veins discussed in Chap. 18.

The Megafistula

This is often the result of very high flow through the fistula with possible outflow stenosis. Short of abandoning the fistula, surgical banding to reduce flow can be attempted by a surgeon or percutaneously [30].

Another method is attempting percutaneous banding discussed in Chap. 15. Finally, surgical alternatives exist including placing an interposition graft within the fistula. It is unclear if these patients have an underlying elastase abnormality or if there is any other underlying molecular causes.

If thrombosis is to occur, the clot burden can exceed 50 cc. Care when thrombectomizing the fistula has to be taken to avoid embolization to the lungs as the volume is sufficient to cause a potentially fatal pulmonary embolism. An option rarely discussed is considering overnight infusion of thrombolytic agent within the thrombus with a multi-sidehole infusion catheter. For tPA, 0.5–1.0 mg/h (concentration of 1 mg/10 cc) is infused and for urokinase, a concentration of 3,000 U/mL is used with a rate of 60,000–120,000 U/h. A subtherapeutic continuous infusion of heparin concurrent with tPA and therapeutic heparin infusion with urokinase is recommended to prevent pericatheter thrombus formation and rethrombosis. Also, if continuous infusion is undertaken, blood work should be obtained every 4–6 h including a CBC, coagulation profile, and fibrinogen level to monitor risk for bleeding and anticoagulation. Subtherapeutic levels of heparinization are determined with PTT which should be below 70 s and therapeutic range is 70–90 s. For fibrinogen levels, if fibrinogen drops below 100 mg/dL or there is a greater than 50% drop in levels between current and the previous value, this indicates higher risk of spontaneous bleeding for the patient. This is a resource-intensive method requiring an actively monitored overnight bed stay to monitor for hemorrhagic complications. The risk of intracranial hemorrhage is <1%. However, within a clotted megafistula, this may be the best way to salvage the access without surgical thrombectomy and/or significant pulmonary embolism. The Trellis device (Covidien) is very effective at single setting thrombolysis of large diameter thrombosed fistulas, while lowering the risk of pulmonary embolism due to its balloon-controlled segment of thrombolysis.

Surgical Treatment Alternatives to Fistula Angioplasty

During the procedure, consideration must be given to not only the quickest treatment of the offending lesion but also the expected treatment outcome and its impact on future dialysis options. While balloon angioplasty of a stenotic lesion is effective in the short term, safe, and relatively inexpensive, it is not always the only or best option. Recurrent stenotic lesions will certainly recur with repeated balloon angioplasty. Surgical revision with short segment interposition grafts (either autologous or PTFE) yields good primary patency (71% at 1 year in a prospective cohort of stenotic and thrombosed fistulas) [31]. Swing segment lesions in the distal transposed segments of radial cephalic fistulas frequently recur within months of angioplasty [32]. These lesions can be easily treated with proximalization of the radial cephalic anastomosis, while still allowing proximal cannulation and use of the fistula for hemodialysis. Technical success of up to 100% has been reported with 1 year primary and secondary patencies of 80 and 95%, respectively [33]. Finally, when considering treatment of immature fistulas, remember that there are several possible reasons for inadequacy of a dialysis fistula. While most commonly the vein has failed to enlarge adequately for use, the vein may also be too deep or tortuous for cannulation. Enlarging such a vein with angioplasty will not address the underlying problem and likely not improve cannulation of the fistula. Instead, superficialization or transposition of the vein, with dilatation if needed, is the more appropriate therapy. Most importantly, avoid unnecessary treatment and possible damage to potential future venous access sites. Always consider a treatment option's effect on future fistula sites.

Surgical Thrombectomy for Thrombosed Fistulae

The results of surgical thrombectomy compare favorably to that of percutaneous methods for the treatment of thrombosed fistulae. In a recent review of 36 large studies treating thrombosed arteriovenous fistulae, Tordoir et al. [17] found similar, good technical success rates for various methods of thrombectomy, including surgical (80–100%). With both surgical and percutaneous methods, lower arm fistulae were more effectively treated than upper arm fistulae (roughly 95% vs. 75%). However, both primary and secondary patency rates for surgery were better than with percutaneous treatments with pharmacomechanical thrombectomy and angioplasty (51–84% primary and 69–95% secondary surgical patency at 1 year). Surgery is particularly beneficial over endovascular treatment in forearm fistula thrombosis (70–80% primary and 85–95% secondary at 1 year patency). These procedures are performed as outpatient procedures under local anesthesia, often in less than 1 h. Due to the high cost of the mechanical thrombectomy devices and thrombolytics, surgical treatment, if available, may also be cheaper. Finally, a combined surgical thrombectomy with endovascular treatment of remote lesions is often most expeditious and successful.

Percutaneous thrombectomy techniques risk pulmonary embolism and should be avoided in patients with significant pulmonary or cardiac disease. The risk likely varies with the technique used and may be limited with certain devices such as the Arrow-Trerotola thrombectomy device [34] or the Trellis device (Covidien), which allows proximal balloon control of the venous outflow during the thrombectomy/thrombolysis. Larger diameter fistulae, especially those with aneurysmal segments, are at particular risk for embolization. The clot burden is significant; sometimes over 250 mL. Layered thrombus of older age in these larger segments is also not as effectively removed percutaneously, permitting later embolization once flow is re-established. The exact incidence is unknown, but several studies demonstrate a 23–59% risk of pulmonary embolism using perfusion scans and/or pulmonary angiography [35, 36]. While most of these pulmonary emboli are initially asymptomatic, deaths have been reported in patients with underlying pulmonary and cardiac disease [36]. Repeated procedures should also be avoided, to prevent consequences, such as pulmonary hypertension, from the cumulative effects of these emboli. Surgical thrombectomy can also result in pulmonary emboli, but to a lesser degree due to reversal of flow in the vein during thrombectomy, the ability to retrieve larger thrombi through the open incision, and the improved capability to remove thrombus, especially firm, attached, aged thrombus, using adherent clot catheters.

The ideal method of treating thrombosed fistulae depends upon available resources and talent. When surgery is expected to be required after thrombectomy, in large diameter fistulae or fistulae with large aneurysms, in patients with significant pulmonary disease, and in the setting of failed percutaneous thrombectomy, surgical thrombectomy should be the primary approach. In fistulae with older thrombus, surgical therapy with more aggressive adherent clot extractors is more effective. Often, however, a combined surgical thrombectomy with remote endovascular treatment is necessary. Although prospective, randomized trials are needed to resolve the issue in other situations, data now indicates surgical treatment of thrombosed fistulae has similar technical success to; may be safer, quicker, and cheaper than; and has better long-term results than percutaneous methods.

Surgical Treatment of Venous Aneurysms

Native fistulae can develop venous aneurysms, usually as a result of upstream venous obstruction or needle cannulation, which require surgical treatment to prevent rupture and exsanguination. Whenever aneurysmal segments of a fistula develop, the fistula should be evaluated and any obstructions treated to slow progression of the aneurysmal degeneration. Other segments of the fistula should be used for cannulation sites to prevent further skin damage and rupture. Attempts should be made to salvage aneurysmal fistulae, especially in patients who are young or with limited options for fistula construction. While short aneurysmal segments with normal caliber adjacent vein can be converted to grafts with intraluminal stent grafts, many of the aneurysmal fistulae are quite large (>3 cm) and do not have an adequate landing zone for the stent graft ends. Placement of stent grafts also limits cannulation zones, carries a significant chance of stent graft infection, and often does not improve the cosmetic appearance of the aneurysm. Alternatives for surgical correction of dialysis fistula aneurysms include aneurysmorrhaphy with suture or stapled closure and an optional prosthetic wrap, plication, and replacement of an aneurysmal section with an interposition vein or PTFE graft. Recently, surgical correction with reduction and reconstruction with foreshortening of the aneurysmal fistula has been described with excellent results [37]. This method is particularly useful for the megafistula with elevated flows related to diffuse aneurysmal enlargement. Along with the repair of the aneurysm, the vein is often transposed and the damaged overlying skin excised. Despite long operative times (mean 188 min), these procedures had little associated morbidity, maintained autogenous fistulae, gave durable results (primary patency 14 months, secondary patency 16.5 months), and improved the appearance of the fistula, something that bothers the patient more than any other symptom [37, 38].

If aneurysm growth continues, a new access site should be constructed, if possible, prior to the need to abandon this aneurysmal fistula to limit the need for a catheter. For example, if an upper arm transposed basilic fistula is becoming severely aneurysmal, a contralateral fistula should be created and allowed to mature prior to abandonment of the original basilic fistula. For extremely enlarged aneurysms, those with overlying skin breakdown, or infected fistulas, ligation is necessary. All associated branches into the aneurysm should be ligated to prevent refilling of the aneurysm with subsequent persistent thrombus. Alternatively, the entire aneurysm and redundant, necrotic skin can be excised. Although more invasive than endovascular repair, surgical correction of fistula aneurysms is more durable and cosmetic than endovascular repair, while maintaining an all autogenous fistula with its associated benefits.

Summary

Whenever performing a dialysis access intervention, preprocedural planning, intraprocedural re-evaluation, and postprocedural follow-up are all critical to providing the highest potential for long-term patency and function. Initially, the patient's access history must be determined. If possible, the review of the history should include the original surgical operative report, reports of any previous noninvasive (Duplex ultrasound or transonic flow measurements) or invasive (fistulogram) procedures and details of the current dysfunction of the fistula. Examination of a fistula by an experienced and careful clinician will nearly always reveal the site of the problem leading to fistula dysfunction. This is critical for planning the type of procedure (surgical or endovascular), the site of access (either surgical or percutaneous), and the direction of access. A thorough consideration of information from the dialysis center, nephrologist, and patient will allow for a safe, expeditious, and effective procedure, whether surgical or endovascular.

Key Points

- Abandonment of a thrombosed or immature fistula without a trial of endovascular treatment is a disservice to the patient.
- Fistula declotting can be time consuming and frustrating. Give yourself extra time to do them and take your time.
- Ultrasound of a clotted fistula helps determine the extent of thrombus and how one is going to manage the thrombectomy procedure.

- Extrinsic compression of the fistula can aid passage of devices and mobilize clot in declotting procedures.
- A semirigid wire passed retrograde through the fistula and retrograde up into the feeding artery straightens out the anastomosis aiding passage of an angioplasty balloon.
- Interventions via the brachial or radial artery, if necessary, can be performed with 0.018 in. platforms to reduce arterial puncture size and therefore potential complications.
- Maintain wire position across the lesion(s) being treated until satisfied with the outcome.
- Routine use of stents is not associated with improved long-term outcomes.
- It is always easier, cheaper, and more time efficient to angioplasty a failing fistula than declotting one.
- Stent grafts should be reserved for salvage situations until further evidence validates use in fistulas.

References

1. Manninen HI, Kaukanen ET, Ikaheimo R, et al. Brachial arterial access: endovascular treatment of failing Brescia-Cimino hemodialysis fistulas – initial success and long-term results [see comments]. Radiology. 2001;218(3):711–8.
2. Wu CC, Wen SC, Chen MK, et al. Radial artery approach for endovascular salvage of occluded autogenous radial-cephalic fistulae. Nephrol Dial Transplant. 2009;24(8):2497–502.
3. Rajan DK, Bunston S, Misra S, Pinto R, Lok CE. Dysfunctional autogenous hemodialysis fistulas: outcomes after angioplasty – are there clinical predictors of patency? Radiology. 2004;232(2):508–15.
4. Rajan DK, Clark TW, Patel NK, Stavropoulos SW, Simons ME. Prevalence and treatment of cephalic arch stenosis in dysfunctional autogenous hemodialysis fistulas. J Vasc Interv Radiol. 2003;14(5):567–73.
5. Turmel-Rodrigues L, Pengloan J, Baudin S, et al. Treatment of stenosis and thrombosis in haemodialysis fistulas and grafts by interventional radiology. Nephrol Dial Transplant. 2000;15(12):2029–36.
6. Oliver MJ, McCann RL, Indridason OS, Butterly DW, Schwab SJ. Comparison of transposed brachiobasilic fistulas to upper arm grafts and brachiocephalic fistulas. Kidney Int. 2001;60(4):1532–9.
7. Natario A, Turmel-Rodrigues L, Fodil-Cherif M, et al. Endovascular treatment of immature, dysfunctional and thrombosed forearm autogenous ulnar-basilic and radial-basilic fistulas for haemodialysis. Nephrol Dial Transplant. 2010;25(2):532–8.

8. Clark TW, Hirsch DA, Jindal KJ, Veugelers PJ, LeBlanc J. Outcome and prognostic factors of restenosis after percutaneous treatment of native hemodialysis fistulas. J Vasc Interv Radiol. 2002;13(1):51–9.
9. Aruny JE, Lewis CA, Cardella JF, et al. Quality improvement guidelines for percutaneous management of the thrombosed or dysfunctional dialysis access. Standards of Practice Committee of the Society of Cardiovascular & Interventional Radiology. J Vasc Interv Radiol. 1999;10(4):491–8.
10. Gray RJ, Sacks D, Martin LG, Trerotola SO. Reporting standards for percutaneous interventions in dialysis access. Technology Assessment Committee [see comments]. J Vasc Interv Radiol. 1999;10(10):1405–15.
11. Gray RJ, Horton KM, Dolmatch BL, et al. Use of Wallstents for hemodialysis access-related venous stenoses and occlusions untreatable with balloon angioplasty. Radiology. 1995;195(2):479–84.
12. Vorwerk D, Guenther RW, Mann H, et al. Venous stenosis and occlusion in hemodialysis shunts: follow-up results of stent placement in 65 patients. Radiology. 1995;195(1):140–6.
13. Vesely TM, Hovsepian DM, Pilgram TK, Coyne DW, Shenoy S. Upper extremity central venous obstruction in hemodialysis patients: treatment with Wallstents. Radiology. 1997;204(2):343–8.
14. Schon D, Mishler R. Salvage of occluded autologous arteriovenous fistulae. Am J Kidney Dis. 2000;36(4):804–10.
15. Liang HL, Pan HB, Chung HM, et al. Restoration of thrombosed Brescia-Cimino dialysis fistulas by using percutaneous transluminal angioplasty. Radiology. 2002;223(2):339–44.
16. Bone GE, Pomajzi MJ. Management of dialysis fistula thrombosis. Am J Surg. 1979;138(6):901–6.
17. Tordoir JH, Bode AS, Peppelenbosch N, van der Sande FM, de Haan MW. Surgical or endovascular repair of thrombosed dialysis vascular access: is there any evidence? J Vasc Surg. 2009;50(4):953–6.
18. Glanz S, Bashist B, Gordon DH, Butt K, Adamsons R. Angiography of upper extremity access fistulas for dialysis. Radiology. 1982;143(1):45–52.
19. Trerotola SO, Turmel-Rodrigues LA. Off the beaten path: transbrachial approach for native fistula interventions. Radiology. 2001;218(3):617–9.
20. Turmel-Rodrigues L, Raynaud A, Louail B, Beyssen B, Sapoval M. Manual catheter-directed aspiration and other thrombectomy techniques for declotting native fistulas for hemodialysis. J Vasc Interv Radiol. 2001;12(12):1365–71.
21. Turmel-Rodrigues L, Pengloan J, Rodrigue H, et al. Treatment of failed native arteriovenous fistulae for hemodialysis by interventional radiology. Kidney Int. 2000;57(3):1124–40.
22. Rocek M, Peregrin JH, Lasovickova J, Krajickova D, Slaviokova M. Mechanical thrombolysis of thrombosed hemodialysis native fistulas with use of the Arrow-Trerotola percutaneous thrombolytic device: our preliminary experience. J Vasc Interv Radiol. 2000;11(9):1153–8.
23. Overbosch EH, Pattynama PM, Aarts HJ, Schultze Kool LJ, Hermans J, Reekers JA. Occluded hemodialysis shunts: Dutch multicenter experience with the hydrolyser catheter. Radiology. 1996;201(2):485–8.
24. Haage P, Vorwerk D, Wildberger JE, Piroth W, Schurmann K, Gunther RW. Percutaneous treatment of thrombosed primary arteriovenous hemodialysis access fistulae. Kidney Int. 2000;57(3):1169–75.

25. Schmitz-Rode T, Wildberger JE, Hubner D, Wein B, Schurmann K, Gunther RW. Recanalization of thrombosed dialysis access with use of a rotating mini-pigtail catheter: follow-up study. J Vasc Interv Radiol. 2000;11(6):721–7.
26. Turmel-Rodrigues LA. Hemodialysis access declotting: a native fistula is not a prosthetic graft. J Vasc Interv Radiol. 2000;11(1):135–7.
27. Rajan DK, Clark TW, Simons ME, Kachura JR, Sniderman K. Procedural success and patency after percutaneous treatment of thrombosed autogenous arteriovenous dialysis fistulas. J Vasc Interv Radiol. 2002;13(12):1211–8.
28. Bent CL, Rajan DK, Tan K, et al. Effectiveness of stent-graft placement for salvage of dysfunctional arteriovenous hemodialysis fistulas. J Vasc Interv Radiol. 2010;21(4):496–502.
29. Gupta M, Rajan DK, Tan KT, Sniderman KW, Simons ME. Use of expanded polytetrafluoroethylene-covered nitinol stents for the salvage of dysfunctional autogenous hemodialysis fistulas. J Vasc Interv Radiol. 2008;19(6): 950–4.
30. Miller GA, Goel N, Friedman A, et al. The MILLER banding procedure is an effective method for treating dialysis-associated steal syndrome. Kidney Int. 2010;77(4):359–66.
31. Georgiadis GS, Lazarides MK, Lambidis CD, et al. Use of short PTFE segments (<6 cm) compares favorably with pure autologous repair in failing or thrombosed native arteriovenous fistulas. J Vasc Surg. 2005;41(1):76–81.
32. Falk A. Maintenance and salvage of arteriovenous fistulas. J Vasc Interv Radiol. 2006;17(5):807–13.
33. Mickley V, Cazzonelli M, Bossinger A. The stenosed Brescia-Cimino fistula: operation or intervention? Zentralbl Chir. 2003;128(9):757–61.
34. Trerotola SO, Johnson MS, Schauwecker DS, et al. Pulmonary emboli from pulse-spray and mechanical thrombolysis: evaluation with an animal dialysis-graft model. Radiology. 1996;200(1):169–76.
35. Gorriz JL, Martinez-Rodrigo J, Sancho A, et al. Endoluminal percutaneous thrombectomy as a treatment for acute vascular access thrombosis: long-term results of 123 procedures. Nefrologia. 2001;21(2):182–90.
36. Swan TL, Smyth SH, Ruffenach SJ, Berman SS, Pond GD. Pulmonary embolism following hemodialysis access thrombolysis/thrombectomy. J Vasc Interv Radiol. 1995;6(5):683–6.
37. Woo K, Cook PR, Garg J, Hye RJ, Canty TG. Midterm results of a novel technique to salvage autogenous dialysis access in aneurysmal arteriovenous fistulas. J Vasc Surg. 2010;51(4):921–5.
38. Quinn RR, Lamping DL, Lok CE, et al. The Vascular Access Questionnaire: assessing patient-reported views of vascular access. J Vasc Access. 2008;9(2): 122–8.
39. Lay JP, Ashleigh RJ, Tranconi L, Ackrill P, Al-Khaffaf H. Result of angioplasty of Brescia-Cimino haemodialysis fistulae: medium-term follow-up. Clin Radiol. 1998;53(8):608–11.
40. Vorwerk D, Schurmann K, Muller-Leisse C, et al. Hydrodynamic thrombectomy of haemodialysis grafts and fistulae: results of 51 procedures. Nephrol Dial Transplant. 1996;11(6):1058–64.
41. Littler P, Cullen N, Gould D, Bakran A, Powell S. AngioJet thrombectomy for occluded dialysis fistulae: outcome data. Cardiovasc Interv Radiol. 2009;32(2):265–70.

42. Zaleski GX, Funaki B, Kenney S, Lorenz JM, Garofalo R. Angioplasty and bolus urokinase infusion for the restoration of function in thrombosed Brescia-Cimino dialysis fistulas. J Vasc Interv Radiol. 1999;10(2 Pt 1):129–36.
43. Poulain F, Raynaud A, Bourquelot P, Knight C, Rovani X, Gaux JC. Local thrombolysis and thromboaspiration in the treatment of acutely thrombosed arteriovenous hemodialysis fistulas. Cardiovasc Interv Radiol. 1991;14(2): 98–101.

Chapter 18
The Immature or Failure to Mature Fistula

Abigail Falk and Dheeraj K. Rajan

Introduction

One of the inherent problems with hemodialysis fistula creation and hence bias towards creating them is a relatively high failure rate of maturation of 25–33% within North America [1]. This happens despite preoperative screening for selection of the best artery and vein [2, 3]. With the introduction of the Fistula First Initiative, there has been increased emphasis on primary placement of an autogenous hemodialysis fistula within the United States with a correspondent increase in number of nonmaturing fistulas and interest in techniques to salvage them.

Fistulas can fail to mature for a number of reasons. These reasons include: (1) failure for the vein to "arterialize," (2) large and/or multiple venous collaterals reducing flow through the fistula vein, (3) insufficient size of the fistula vein, and (4) technical factors at the time of surgery. The most common underlying cause is anatomic lesions that may exist anywhere in the access circuit. The ideal situation for fistula development would be inflow pressure high enough

A. Falk (✉)
American Access Care, Brooklyn, New York, USA
e-mail: Abigailfalk123@pol.net

D.K. Rajan (ed.), *Essentials of Percutaneous Dialysis Interventions*,
DOI 10.1007/978-1-4419-5657-6_18,

© Springer Science+Business Media, LLC 2011

to overcome low venous resistance. K/DOQI indicates that a fistula considered sufficient for dialysis should have the so-called rule of 6s: (1) blood flow >600 mL/min, (2) access vein diameter >6 mm and (3) the access vein depth should be <6 mm from the skin surface. K/DOQI guidelines also recommend that if the fistula fails to mature within 6 weeks, fistulography or another imaging study is necessary to determine the cause [4].

Imaging

As discussed in Chap. 17, autogenous fistulas can have multiple areas of stenosis, and it is important to assess the entire access circuit including the feeding artery. An initial examination with ultrasound can reveal areas of stenosis, venous diameter, thrombosis, accessory/collateral vessels, and assess flow rates. Ultrasound thereby aids in determining interventions required and site of puncture and also in a majority of cases is required to provide guidance for access to the fistula. In select cases or if ultrasound is not available, a small arterial catheter (3 Fr inner dilator, 21G IV catheter, 4 Fr sheath) assists greatly in assessing the fistula. This approach has several advantages: (1) when refluxing contrast across the arterial anastomosis from the venous approach is not possible in the presence of a JAS and/or accessory veins, (2) arterial inflow is better assessed, (3) provides the best view of the entire access including flow characteristics. When performing fistulography, beyond imaging the entire access circuit including the feeding artery, it is very important to obtain orthogonal views to exclude occult stenoses that may not be evident in a single plane.

Salvage Techniques

To reach the objective of converting an immature fistula to a functioning fistula, beyond conservative measures such as hand/arm exercises (which can increase blood flow and vessel size), percutaneous management is primarily based on balloon angioplasty of arteries and veins with occasional need for sequential dilation, embolization or ligation of accessory veins, and occasional thrombectomy. These procedures can be performed on an outpatient basis and heparinization is rarely required (transarterial interventions if large sheaths are used and for declotting procedures). Procedures can be performed safely as early as 4 weeks after surgical creation.

Angioplasty

Stenoses within the arteries can be the result of atherosclerotic or diabetic disease or acquired lesions such as clamp injury. Also, the feeding artery may simply be anatomically small (see Fig. 18.1). Venous stenoses commonly occur at sites of vessel mobilization or swing points and prior sites of venipuncture. Within radiocephalic fistulas, the most common lesion is within the juxta-anastomotic region as in functioning RC fistulas (see Fig. 18.2). Also, the venous outflow may simply be anatomically small as well. Fistulas that fail to mature may have at least one stenotic lesion within their access circuit, and often have multiple lesions (see Fig. 18.1). Venous stenoses and accessory veins are the most common lesions found in these fistulas. Table 18.1 describes stenosis locations associated with fistulas that fail to mature.

Inflow lesions, if identified, may be amenable to PTA via a retrograde fistula approach. Diffuse/extensive inflow disease may necessitate abandoning the site. Arterial stenotic lesions may be the result of calcified vessels unable to dilate. For such cases, it is important to not

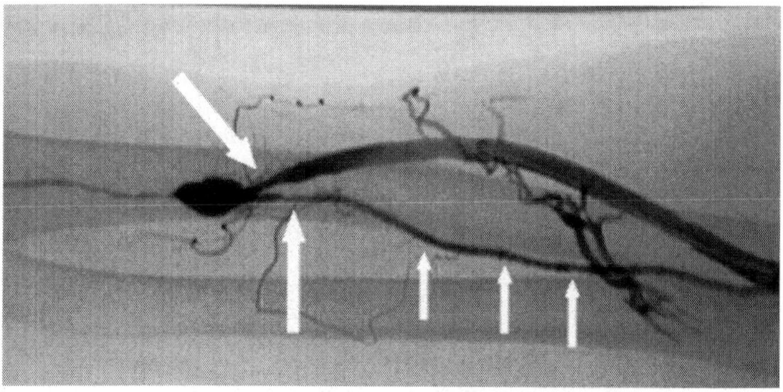

Fig. 18.1 Multiple problems within an RC fistula that failed to mature. *Small arrows* outline a diseased and diffusely small radial artery in this diabetic patient. *Large arrows* point to focal arterial stenosis and a juxta-anastomotic venous stenosis

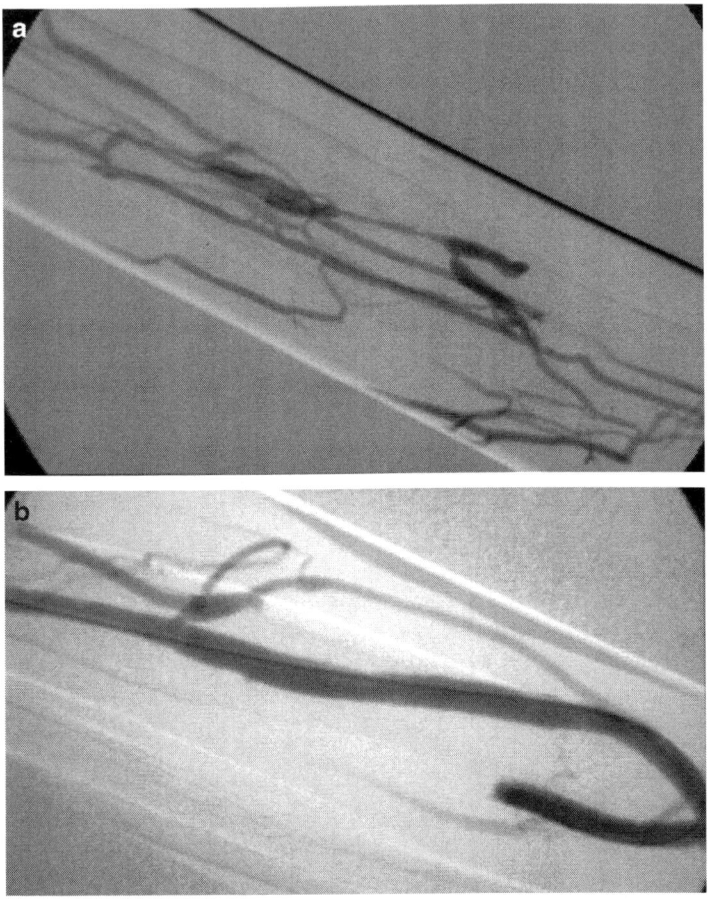

Fig. 18.2 (**a**) RC fistula that had failed to mature after 3 months. Multiple collaterals are present with no clear dominant channel. Via a retrograde transvenous approach, the AV anastomosis was crossed and a suspected JAS was angioplastied with a 5 mm PTA balloon. (**b**) Following PTA, collateral pathways collapsed, and a clear outflow cephalic vein is now seen. The fistula became functional 2 weeks later

oversize the PTA balloon 1 mm greater than the vessel diameter as complications of arterial PTA has significantly higher morbidity than venous lesions.

For venous stenotic lesions, standard PTA techniques are used for focal lesions.

Table 18.1 Location of lesions in nonmaturing fistulas

References	Number of fistulas	Arterial inflow (%)	Arterial anastomosis (%)	Swing point (%)	Outflow vein (%)	Central vein (%)	Accessory vein (%)	Multiple (%)
Turmel-Rodrigues et al. [8]	69		6	55	39		0	25
Beathard et al. [1]	100	4	38	43	36	9	46	40
Falk [12]	65	8	6	25	33	2	19	29
Nassar et al. [13]	118	5	47	64	59	8	29	71
Clark et al. [14]	101	6	4	38	49	3	4	42

Sequential Dilation

For long segments of stenosis or simply an anatomically small outflow fistula vein sequential dilation may be attempted [5, 6]. Sequential dilation, or what is sometimes called balloon-assisted maturation (BAM), is a technique of serial dilations of the vein over short intervals of time. A common algorithm is to initially dilate the sclerotic or small vein to 5 mm and then at 2-week intervals increase the balloon diameter by 1–2 mm until a satisfactory vein diameter and functionality is achieved. Using 8–10 cm length balloons improves technical success and reduces procedure time (see Fig. 18.3). Dilation time is typically <20 s/dilation to reduce the chance of

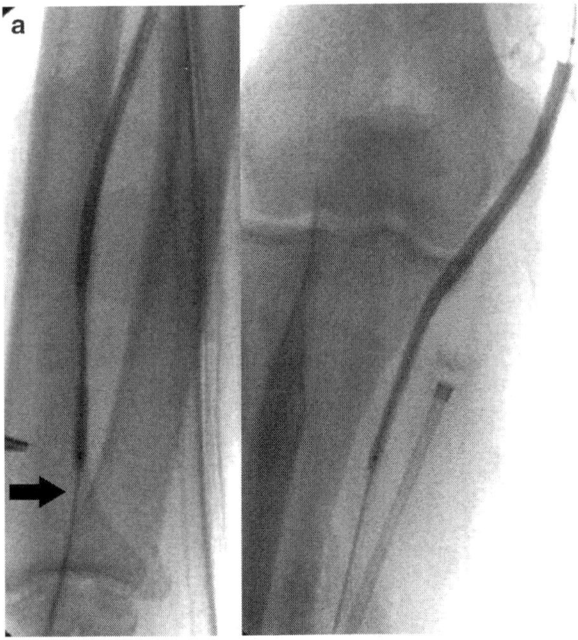

Fig. 18.3 One-year-old nonmaturing right radiocephalic fistula. The fistula thrombosed 6 weeks prior to intervention. Ultrasound showed minimal thrombus. The mid forearm cephalic vein was patent with 3 mm diameter. Four thousand units of heparin given with no tPA (**a**) 3 mm × 10 cm angioplasty initially from distal radial artery approach (*arrow*) to cross occluded swing point segment. (**b**) Retrograde cephalic vein approach 2 weeks later. A 4 mm PTA was performed to dilate arterial anastomosis followed by 6 and 7 mm PTA to dilate body of cephalic vein. (**c**) Completion fistulogram shows widely patent RC fistula

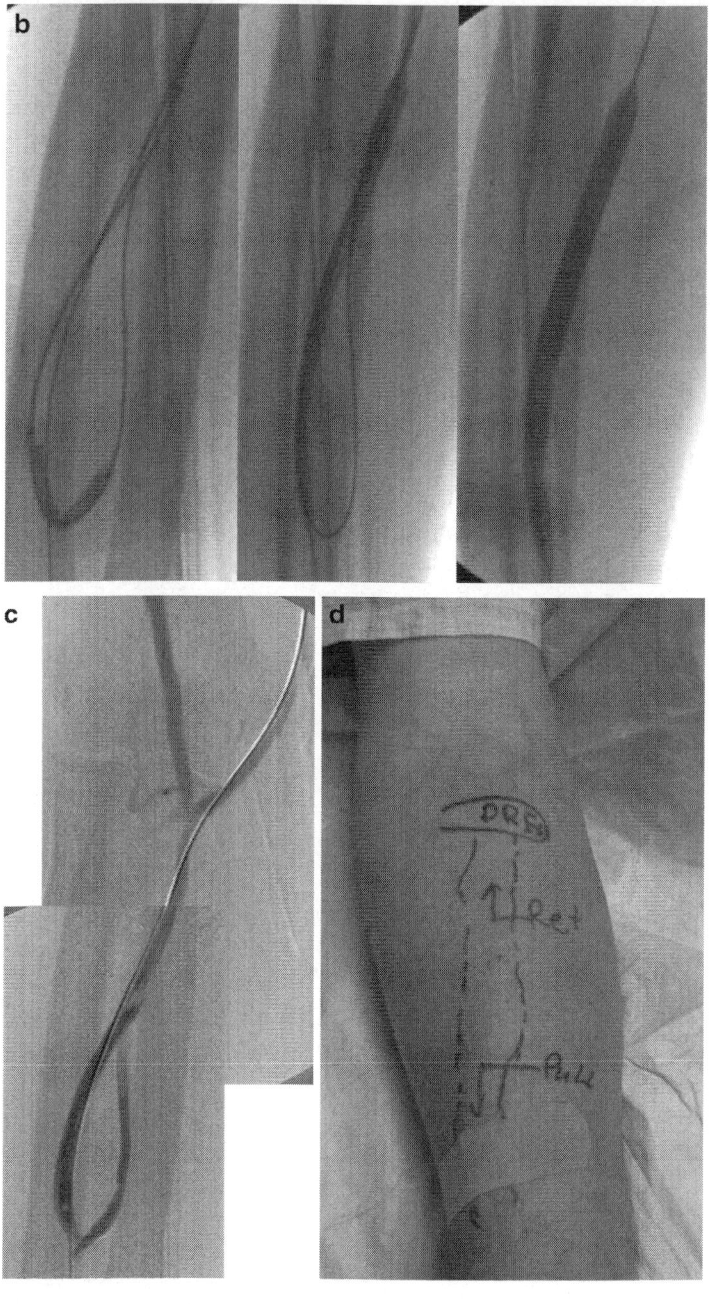

Fig. 18.3 (continued) with a good thrill within it. (**d**) With indelible marker, the fistula was marked as well as points of puncture, i.e., instructions to use fistula. Images courtesy of American Access Care, New York

thrombosis. In addition, shutting down or occluding flow to the AVF by compressing the anastomosis during vein dilations is recommended so that incoming blood does not leak out of venous tears and cause large areas of ecchymosis during the procedure. Also balloon dilation is performed central to peripheral to reduce the likelihood of blood extravasation as it is easier to pull back a balloon than push it forward. Lastly, with radiocephalic fistulas, if there is an option to place the wire within the deep veins of the upper arm, do so to promote flow into the deep (larger, healthier) veins rather than the upper arm cephalic vein to avoid long-term problems.

Approach

Depending on the location of lesions and interventions to be performed, a transarterial approach via the brachial or radial arteries (as mentioned in Chap. 17) using 0.018 in. PTA balloons may be advantageous (see Fig. 18.3a). This approach allows for visualization of the entire circuit and facilitates crossing of the anastomosis, and all lesions, with the exception of central venous lesions, can be treated via this one puncture. Central venous interventions require 6–10 Fr devices which are associated with a much higher risk of arterial injury. Complications from the arterial approach include hematomas, pseudoaneurysm formation, arterial spasm, and dissection and can occur in up to 12% of brachial punctures although recent studies have found this to be much lower particularly with a retrograde radial approach compared to an antegrade brachial approach [7]. Spasm can often be overcome with intra-arterial injection of nitroglycerin. However, central venous lesions are rarly if ever a cause of fistula non-maturation.

Accessory/Branching Veins

Accessory/branching veins may result in poor fistula maturation due to numerous outflow pathways. If necessary, embolization/ligation of these veins may be performed at the same time as venous dilation although some interventionalists believe that treating accessory/collateral veins is not necessary [8]. Hence, we first attempt balloon dilation of stenoses; then, if the fistula fails to mature, ligation/embolization may be considered.

Management of competing veins consists of venous "ligation." This can be performed surgically or percutaneously with suture ligation and/or embolization. Suture ligation is best suited for superficially located veins given minimal distance for subcutaneous dissection. Coils within superficial veins can be irritating to patients (see Fig. 18.4) and possibly erode through the skin. Coil embolization is best suited for deep collateral/accessory veins as cutdown suture ligation is more difficult with potential risks of nerve/muscle and tendon injury.

The technique for ligation is as follows: roadmap the accessory vein and mark the overlying skin. The patient may then be referred to have the vein surgically ligated (small skin incision and permanent suture ligature), or this can be performed within the procedure room. Rather than marking the skin, a wire or balloon can be advanced into vein of concern. The point of ligation should be at least 5 mm from its origin off the fistula to prevent peri-inflammatory changes from the ligation from causing stenosis of the fistula at a later time. This point can be determined with fluoroscopy and angiographic runs. A cutdown onto the wire/balloon is then performed and nonabsorbable

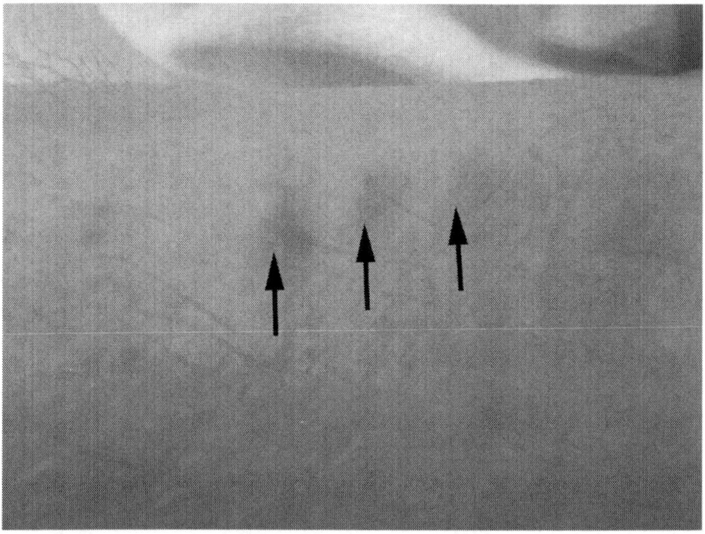

Fig. 18.4 Superficial accessory vein was coil embolized to promote maturation of the fistula. The patient complained of ongoing irritation after embolization. *Arrows* point to coil clearly deforming the skin

2-0 or 3-0 silk or polypropylene skin sutures (×2) are tied around the vein after withdrawal of the balloon/wire to permanently occlude it [9] (see Fig. 18.5). The skin can then be closed with interrupted 3-0 or 4-0 monofilament stitches. A variation of this method is to simply pass a monofilament stitch transcutaneously around the wire/balloon and tie the knot onto the skin after removal of the wire/balloon. The stitch can then be removed >14 days later and no cutdown is required (see Fig. 18.6).

For deeper accessory vein(s), they can be selected and occluded with embolization coils. Appropriate-sized coils should be used to ensure that they occlude the collateral/accessory vein; they do not embolize to the lungs due to undersizing and are not too long where

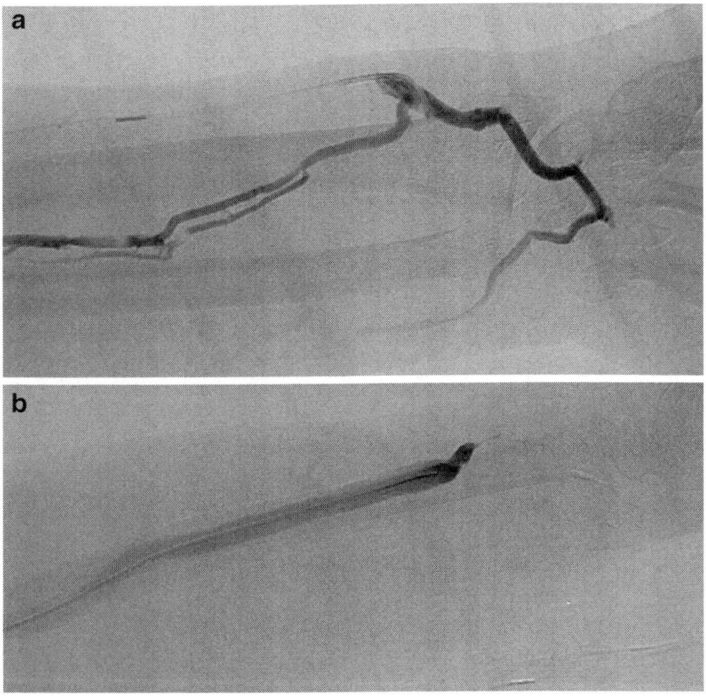

Fig. 18.5 Patient with RC fistula created 3 months earlier. Despite JAS PTA 1 month earlier, the fistula does not have sufficient flows. (**a**) A large accessory vein was siphoning flow from the cephalic vein outflow. (**b**) The accessory vein was isolated with a 4 Fr catheter and a cutdown was performed where the catheter was palpated with subsequent suture ligation of the vein

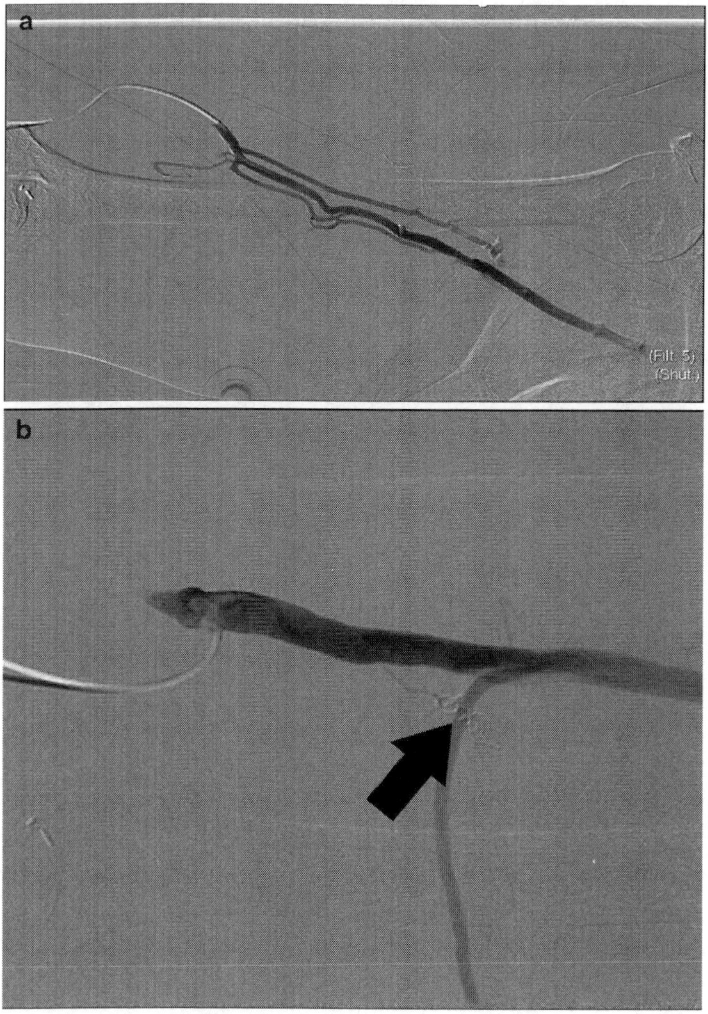

Fig. 18.6 Nonmaturing BC fistula with multiple superficial and deep collateral veins. (**a**) Large deep accessory vein with multiple branches arising off proximal fistula. (**b**) This was embolized with a single 6 mm Nestor coil (*arrow*) in the main truck away from the fistula outflow with no continued flow in the accessory vein. (**c**) Superficial collateral vein is selected with a catheter. (**d**) Catheter is externally palpated and using the catheter as a guide, (**e**) an external monofilament suture was placed around the accessory/collateral vein through the skin and tied, thereby occluding the vein, and flow is now via the cephalic vein. *Arrow* points to embolization of deep venous collateral

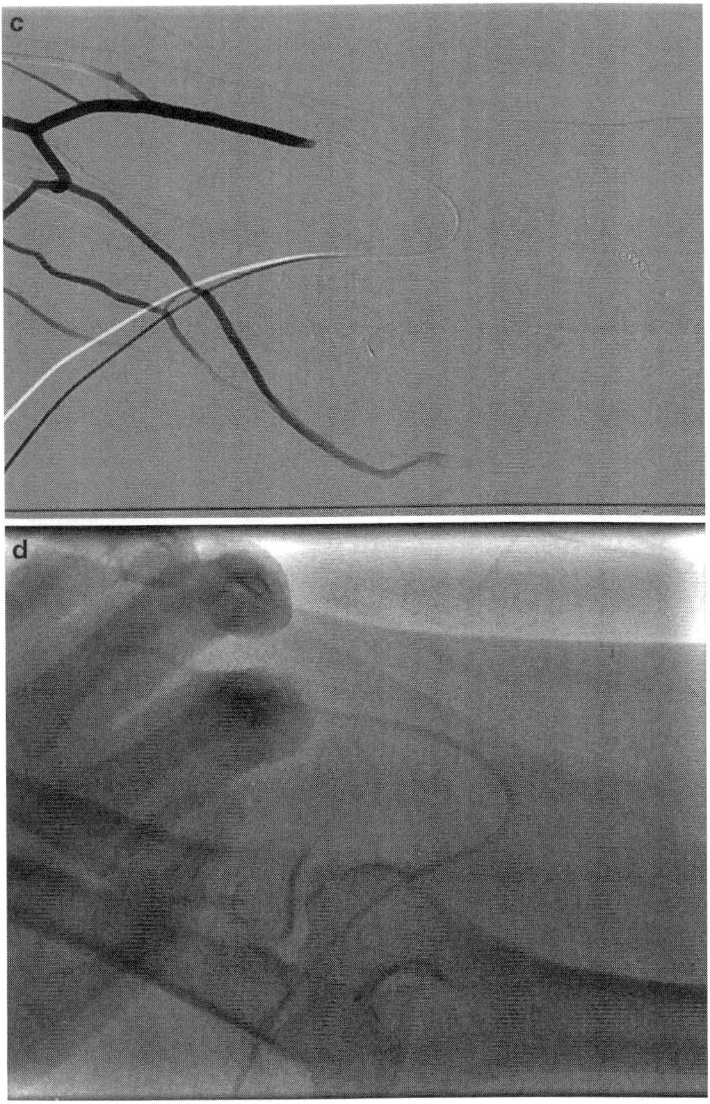

Fig. 18.6 (continued)

the coil extends back into the fistula causing stenosis or occlusion. Fibered coils should be used, should be at least 2 mm larger in diameter than the vein being embolized, should be packed into the vein to sufficiently occlude flow, and should be placed a sufficient

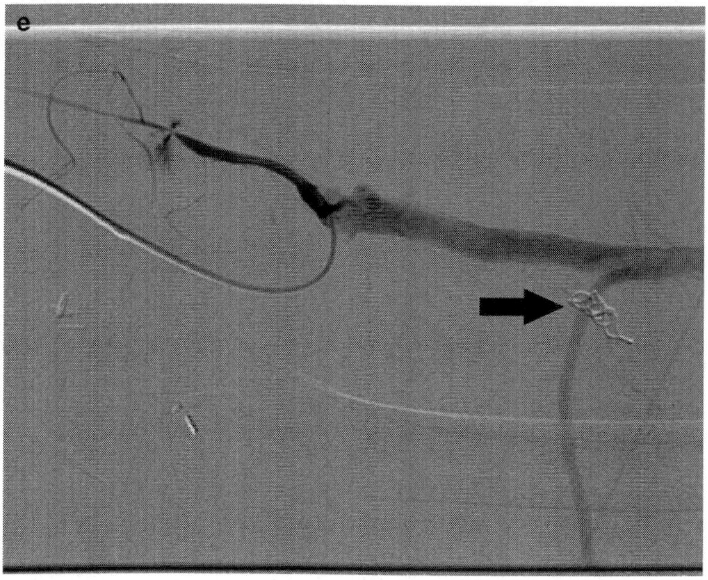

Fig. 18.6 (continued)

distance from the fistula (>5 mm) to prevent inflammation from the embolization causing stenosis formation in the fistula (see Fig. 18.6). Nestor coils are recommended.

Median Cubital Vein Ligation

If development of fistula remains poor after accessory vein ligation, then median cubital vein ligation can be performed to increase venous resistance. The median cubital vein is mapped with fistulography and skin marked. Via a small surgical incision, the vein is identified and ligated with a 4-0 silk suture [10].

Mainstream Banding

Mainstream banding or temporary banding of the main venous channel is reserved for cases where all other salvage techniques fail and is rarely necessary. The banding technique involves placement of a 4 mm balloon in the venous outflow above the elbow. The balloon-inflated vein is isolated via a cutdown, and a 3-0 Vicryl suture is wrapped around the vein/balloon. The balloon is deflated and removed, yielding venous stenoses. This is a "temporary" band, as the suture absorbs in 3 weeks [10] Dissolvable stiches are known to cause an inflammatory reaction which may translate permanent stenosis.

Thrombectomy

If the immature AVF is thrombosed, then one can perform a thrombectomy with simple PTA maceration of the clot in most cases. There is typically a minimal amount of thrombus usually located at the juxta-anastomotic region. Use heparin in this case.

Follow-Up

As treated immature AVFs often require multiple interventions to convert them into functional fistulas, they are more prone to becoming dysfunctional in shorter periods of time. It is recommended to have the fistula reexamined every 3 months after maturity to maintain patency.

Surgical Options

Surgical interventions include patch angioplasty, hybrid creation of a combination of fistula and graft, reanastomosis, or creation of a new fistula.

Outcomes

Overall, the percutaneous salvage rate of immature fistulas is reported as 75–95% with primary patency of 30–60% and secondary patency of 75–90% at 1 year. Outcomes of multiple studies are summarized in Table 18.2. Overall complications via the transvenous

Table 18.2 Salvage of nonmaturing fistulas

References	Number of fistulas	Fistula age (months)	Interventions	Salvage rate (%)	1 Year patency
Beathard [10]	63	4.2	Venous PTA, ligation and banding, 8 arterial inflow excluded, 1.5 procedures/fistula	82.5	75% Secondary
Turmel-Rodrigues et al. [8]	69	2.5	Venous PTA, 17 aspiration thrombectomies, no embolization/ligation of collaterals	97	39% Primary, 79% secondary
Faiyaz et al. [9]	17	4.0	Venous ligation only 1.7 procedures/fistula	88	
Tordoir et al. [2]	17	4.0	6 Venous PTA short segment stenosis, 6 surgery (hybrid, reanastomosis), no thrombectomy	47	
Beathard et al. [1]	100	4.7	Arterial venous ligation or coil embolization, 1.6 lesions/fistula	92	68% Secondary
Shin et al. [15]	19	1.8	Venous PTA, 3 venous ligations	74	61% Primary, 82% secondary
Falk [12]	65	2.7	Arterial and venous PTA, venous ligation, banding, thrombectomy, 1.7 procedures/fistula	74	
Nassar et al. [13]	118	4	PTA, embolization	83	62% Primary, 93% secondary
Song et al. [16]	22	2.7	PTA, central venous stents	96	28% Primary, 85% secondary
Clark et al. [14]	101	2.5	PTA, venous ligation	88	34% Primary, 75% secondary
Asif et al. [17]	41		Arterial/venous PTA, 1.7 procedures/fistula	95	46% Primary, 94% secondary

approach are 9.3% of which 5.5% are hematomas and 2.2% are venous ruptures [11].

In summary, nonmaturing fistulas require multiple interventions to elevate them to the level of maintained functionality. The frequent number of interventions has led some to equate these fistulas as equivalent to poorly functioning grafts vs. others who consider the frequent interventions as fiscally sound practice. Fistulas that have failed to mature that present thrombosed have particularly poor primary patency rates.

Key Points

- Frequent reinterventions are required. Schedule follow-up appointments.
- Improper imaging leads to missed lesions. Image the whole circuit in multiple projections.
- An average of two to three interventional sessions are required before a fistula matures sufficiently for use.
- The salvage techniques should be performed sequentially until the desired end point of fistula functionality is encountered. These steps may require up to 6 weeks before the fistula becomes functional. After the fistula has been in use for 2 weeks, the catheter, if the patient has one, should be removed.
- Consider not fully treating more central lesions and/or minor cephalic arch lesions and minor distal swing segment lesions (in brachial-transposed basilic AVF) so that the AVF will mature and be easier to cannulate (under a little outflow resistance).
- Marking puncture points along the fistula with indelible marker improves success of access at the time of dialysis.

References

1. Beathard GA, Arnold P, Jackson J, Litchfield T. Aggressive treatment of early fistula failure. Kidney Int. 2003;64(4):1487–94.
2. Tordoir JH, Rooyens P, Dammers R, van der Sande FM, de Haan M, Yo TI. Prospective evaluation of failure modes in autogenous radiocephalic wrist access for haemodialysis. Nephrol Dial Transplant. 2003;18(2):378–83.

3. Patel ST, Hughes J, Mills JL, Sr. Failure of arteriovenous fistula maturation: an unintended consequence of exceeding dialysis outcome quality Initiative guidelines for hemodialysis access. J Vasc Surg. 2003;38(3):439–45; discussion 445.
4. Vascular Access Work Group. Clinical practice guidelines for vascular access. Am J Kidney Dis. 2006;48 Suppl 1:S176–247.
5. De Marco Garcia LP, Davila-Santini LR, Feng Q, Calderin J, Krishnasastry KV, Panetta TF. Primary balloon angioplasty plus balloon angioplasty maturation to upgrade small-caliber veins (<3 mm) for arteriovenous fistulas. J Vasc Surg. 2010;52(1):139–44.
6. Miller GA, Goel N, Khariton A, et al. Aggressive approach to salvage non-maturing arteriovenous fistulae: a retrospective study with follow-up. J Vasc Access. 2009;10(3):183–91.
7. Wu CC, Wen SC, Chen MK, et al. Radial artery approach for endovascular salvage of occluded autogenous radial-cephalic fistulae. Nephrol Dial Transplant. 2009;24(8):2497–502.
8. Turmel-Rodrigues L, Mouton A, Birmele B, et al. Salvage of immature forearm fistulas for haemodialysis by interventional radiology. Nephrol Dial Transplant. 2001;16(12):2365–71.
9. Faiyaz R, Abreo K, Zaman F, Pervez A, Zibari G, Work J. Salvage of poorly developed arteriovenous fistulae with percutaneous ligation of accessory veins. Am J Kidney Dis. 2002;39(4):824–7.
10. Beathard GA, Settle SM, Shields MW. Salvage of the nonfunctioning arteriovenous fistula. Am J Kidney Dis. 1999;33(5):910–6.
11. Voormolen EH, Jahrome AK, Bartels LW, Moll FL, Mali WP, Blankestijn PJ. Nonmaturation of arm arteriovenous fistulas for hemodialysis access: a systematic review of risk factors and results of early treatment. J Vasc Surg. 2009;49(5):1325–36.
12. Falk A. Maintenance and salvage of arteriovenous fistulas. J Vasc Interv Radiol. 2006;17(5):807–13.
13. Nassar GM, Nguyen B, Rhee E, Achkar K. Endovascular treatment of the "failing to mature" arteriovenous fistula. Clin J Am Soc Nephrol. 2006; 1(2):275–80.
14. Clark TW, Cohen RA, Kwak A, et al. Salvage of nonmaturing native fistulas by using angioplasty. Radiology. 2007;242(1):286–92.
15. Shin SW, Do YS, Choo SW, Lieu WC, Choo IW. Salvage of immature arteriovenous fistulas with percutaneous transluminal angioplasty. Cardiovasc Interv Radiol. 2005;28(4):434–8.
16. Song HH, Won YD, Kim YO, Yoon SA. Salvaging and maintaining non-maturing Brescia-Cimino haemodialysis fistulae by percutaneous intervention. Clin Radiol. 2006;61(5):404–9.
17. Asif A, Roy-Chaudhury P, Beathard GA. Early arteriovenous fistula failure: a logical proposal for when and how to intervene. Clin J Am Soc Nephrol. 2006;1(2):332–9.

Chapter 19
Cephalic Arch Stenosis

Dheeraj K. Rajan, Timothy I. Clark, and Dirk S. Baumann

The cephalic arch represents the portion of the cephalic vein in the shoulder as it traverses the deltopectoral groove, through the clavipectoral fascia, and passes below the clavicle and joins the axillary vein. Occasionally, an accessory cephalic arch is present. Rarely, the cephalic arch empties into the internal or external jugular vein. This area has a particular propensity for stenosis: the causes are likely multifactorial. Hypotheses regarding pathophysiology include unfavorable shear stress mechanisms related to high flow and angulation of the vein segment leading to intimal injury and subsequent stenosis. Another theory focuses on the relative immobility of the cephalic arch within the deltopectoral groove related to fascial planes (see Fig. 19.1). The theory is that these fascial planes constrain the vein and prevent remodeling to accommodate the high flows of the dialysis access.

Regardless of the pathophysiology, cephalic arch stenosis represents one of the more problematic lesions seen in percutaneous interventions for dialysis fistulas and occasionally dialysis grafts. This lesion is

---

D.K. Rajan (✉)
Head and Associate Professor, Division of Vascular & Interventional Radiology, Department of Medical Imaging, University of Toronto, Toronto, Ontario, Canada
e-mail: Dheeraj.Rajan@uhn.on.ca

D.K. Rajan (ed.), *Essentials of Percutaneous Dialysis Interventions*, DOI 10.1007/978-1-4419-5657-6_19,
© Springer Science+Business Media, LLC 2011

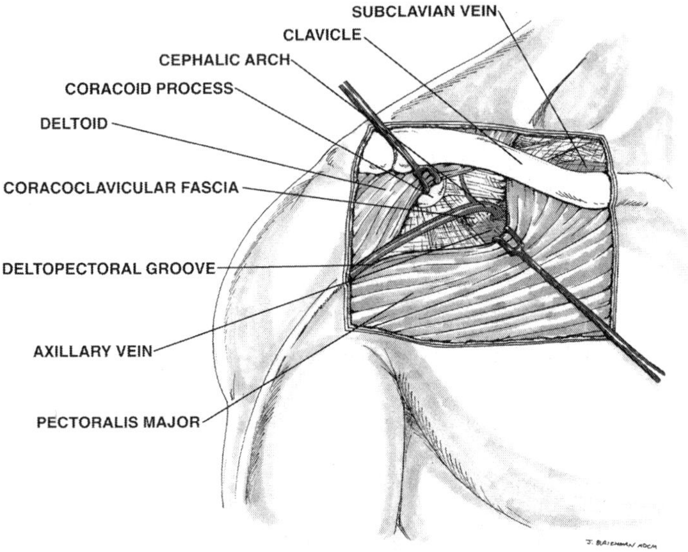

Fig. 19.1 Anatomy of the shoulder adjacent to the cephalic arch

primary seen in patients with brachiocephalic fistulas. This area is prone to spasm, rupture, and frequent restenosis with poor primary intervention patency. In addition, stenosis at this location typically requires higher inflation pressures (greater than 15 atm) to achieve technical success with POBA [1].

Primary treatment or standard of care remains POBA (see Fig. 19.2). Uncovered stenting in this area is not recommended, and there is no evidence to suggest improved patency with stenting compared to POBA for this lesion. Also, as mentioned previously, uncovered stents convert a focal lesion into a stent-length lesion as intimal hyperplasia develops along the length of the stent (see Fig. 19.3). Uncovered stents in this area are also prone to fracture. In addition, no effective therapies have been proven to be effective against in-stent stenosis. Initial studies do suggest that stent grafts may have a role in this specific lesion. This role has not been adequately determined. Other devices have also not been effectively evaluated in this location.

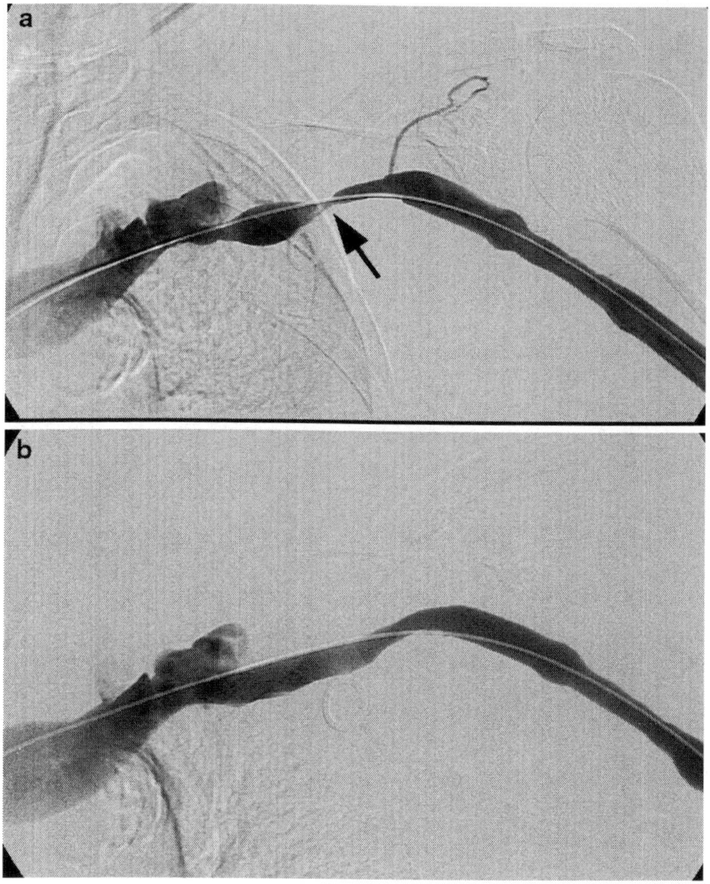

Fig. 19.2 (**a**) Cephalic arch stenosis (*arrow*). (**b**) After 8 mm PTA, no significant stenosis persists

Interventions

When cephalic arch stenosis is present, prior to intervening, a wire should traverse the stenosis and be of sufficiently long length to allow exchange of devices as necessary. A nonhydrophilic wire length of at least 145 cm should be used and be of sufficient rigidity to allow for easy tracking of balloon catheters. If stenting/stent grafting is possibly required, a wire length of at least 180 cm is recommended to

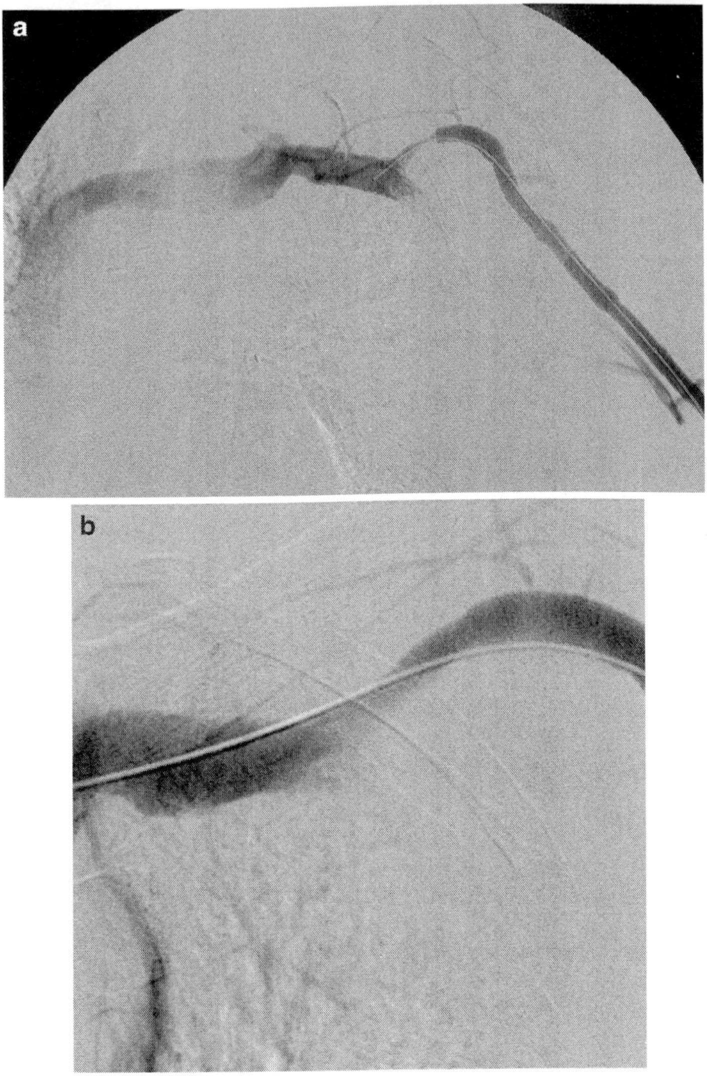

Fig. 19.3 (**a**) Cephalic arch stenosis successfully dilated (**b**) with 8 mm PTA balloon. (**c**) One month later, patient returns and after 6 mm PTA there is massive rupture of the cephalic arch with a rapidly expanding hematoma and increasing patient pain. (**d**) Ruptured segment is salvaged with an 8-mm nitinol stent. The stent does not extend into the axillary vein. (**e**) Three months later, the patient returns with aggressive intimal hyperplasia along the entire length of the stent (*arrows*). (**f**) The hyperplasia is dilated with an 8-mm balloon. (**g**) Post PTA, although intraluminal diameter is improved, intimal hyperplasia persists (*arrows*)

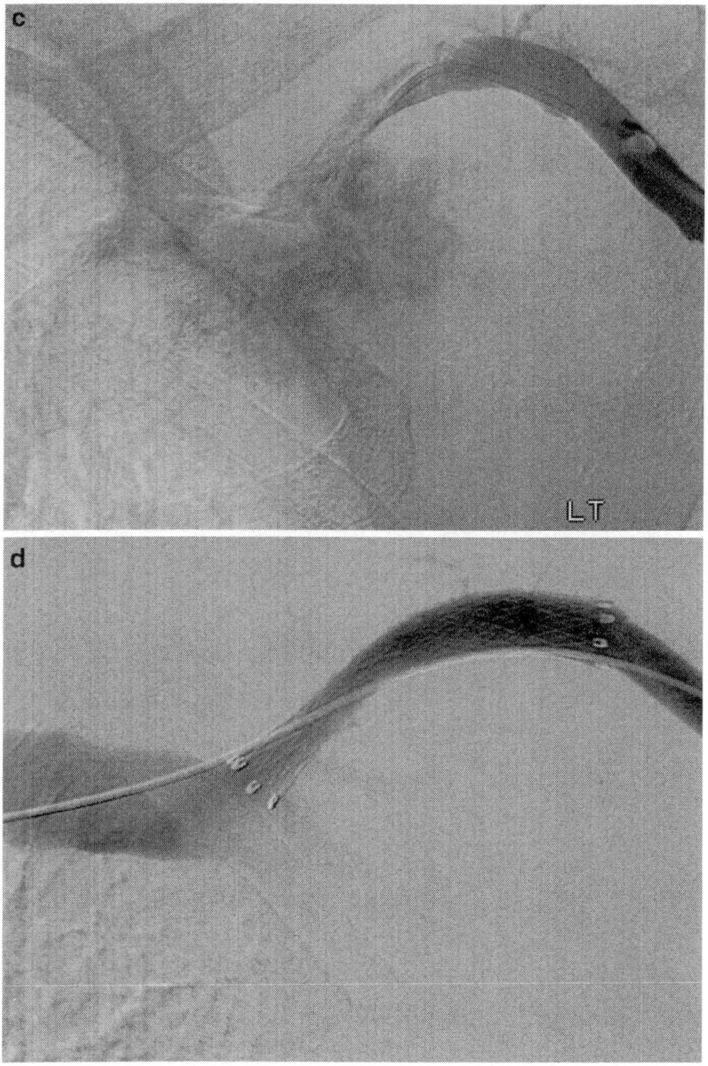

Fig. 19.3 (continued)

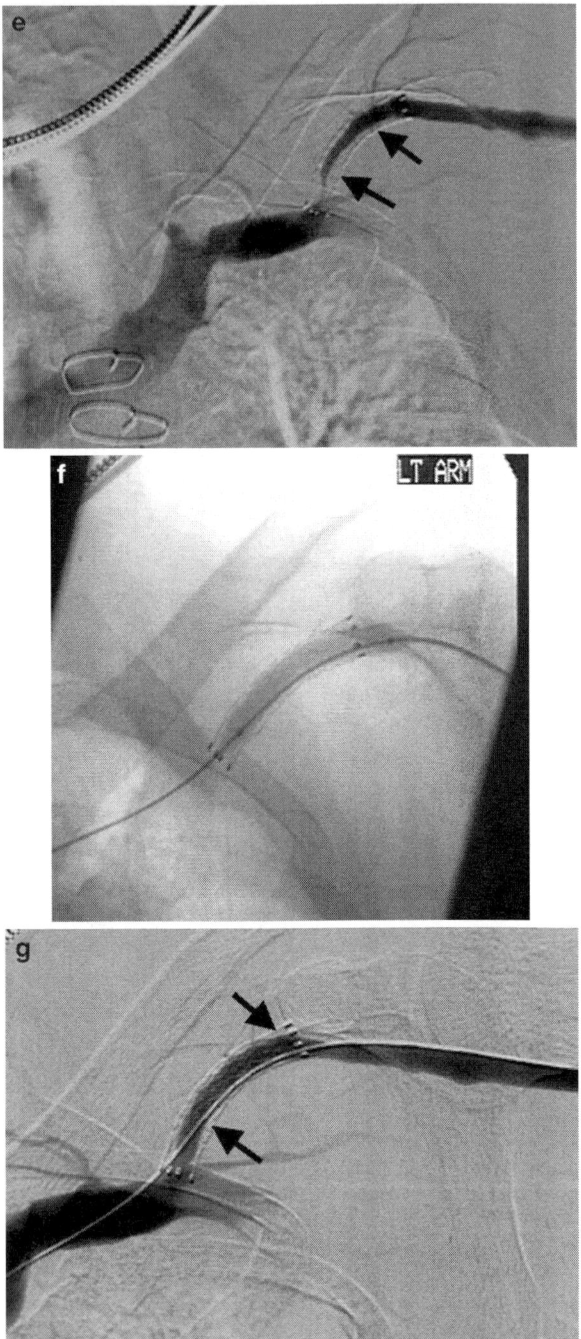

Fig. 19.3 (continued)

accommodate the length of delivery systems. Hydrophilic wires are not recommended as they tend to fall out easily or pull back away from the lesion. As cephalic arch stenosis is prone to rupture, all efforts should be made to maintain the wire across the stenosis. If rupture occurs, reattempting to cross the site of rupture may not be possible and loss of the fistula is likely.

Balloon diameters range from 6 to 12 mm diameters in this location. The balloon size is determined by the size of the adjacent diameter of normal vein. The standard angioplasty balloon size is 8 mm in diameter and 40 mm in length. When 20-mm length balloons are used, they tend to slip off or away from the lesion. Longer lengths should be avoided so as to limit damage to surrounding normal intima. Inflation pressures greater than 15 atm is often required. Care should be taken to not undersize the balloon leading to insufficient dilation of the stenosis, and oversizing will result in rupture of the vein and potential loss of the dialysis access. Some interventionists have deliberately ruptured the cephalic arch by oversizing the angioplasty balloon and subsequently stented the cephalic arch. There is no evidence to suggest this practice results in improved patency. Furthermore, there is some early evidence to suggest that stents are prone to fracturing at this location (see Figs. 19.4 and 19.5) beyond the common problem of in-stent intimal hyperplasia. Also, extension of the stent into the axillary vein can impair venous return from the ipsilateral arm.

If technical success is not obtained with POBA, other techniques may be considered. These include using a parallel wire technique where the 0.018 in. wire is placed parallel to the angioplasty balloon and acts as a cutting atherotome. A cutting balloon may also be considered in this area (see Fig. 19.6). Other devices that may be considered are ultra–high-pressure balloons or the use of a stent or stent graft in this area. If a stent or a stent graft is to be placed, multiple views should be taken of the cephalic arch as it enters the axillary vein. The junction should be properly profiled to prevent inadvertent extension of the device in the axillary vein (see Fig. 19.7). This complication may lead to thrombosis or stenosis of the axillary vein, preventing future access creation in that arm.

If elastic recoil is seen following angioplasty, generally no further intervention is performed unless recoil leads to flow limitation. In severe cases where loss of the access is considered highly likely, stenting/stent grafting are options. For flow-limiting dissections, where flow within the fistula is sluggish, stenting/stent grafting is

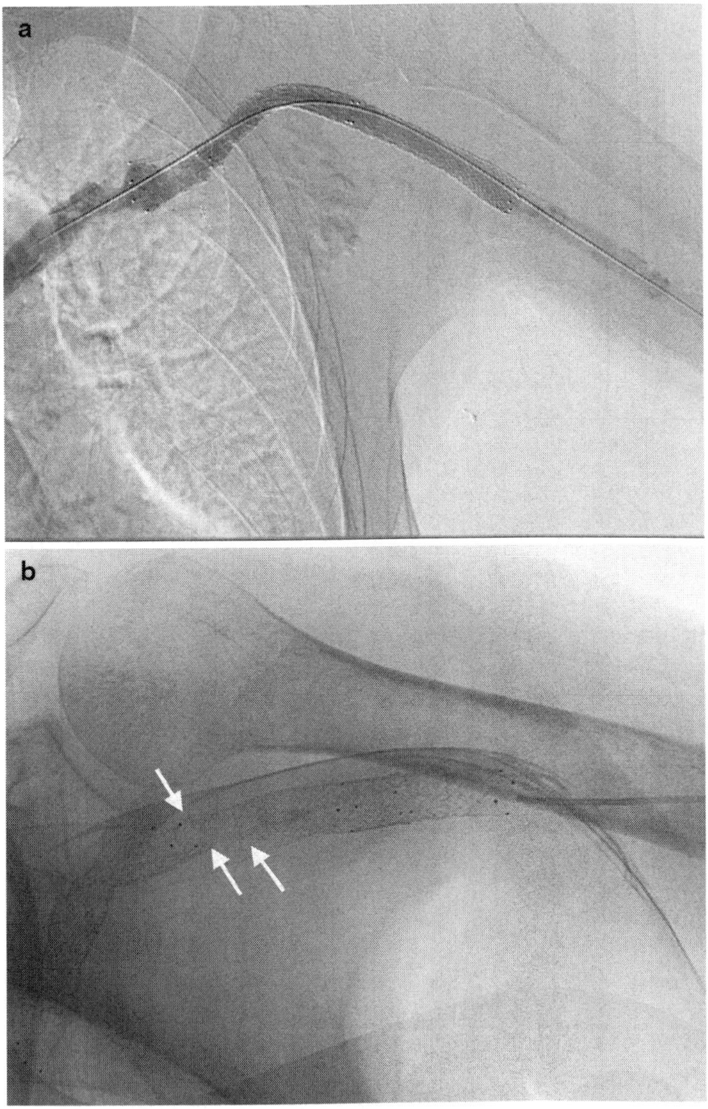

Fig. 19.4 (**a**) Cephalic arch stenosis stented with 10×60 mm nitinol stent and 14×60 mm nitinol stent into the innominate vein. (**b**) Patient returns 14 weeks later, and cephalic arch stent has torn apart (*arrows*). (**c**) Flow reestablished after placement of 10×60 mm stent graft (Fluency-CRBard) across stent fracture

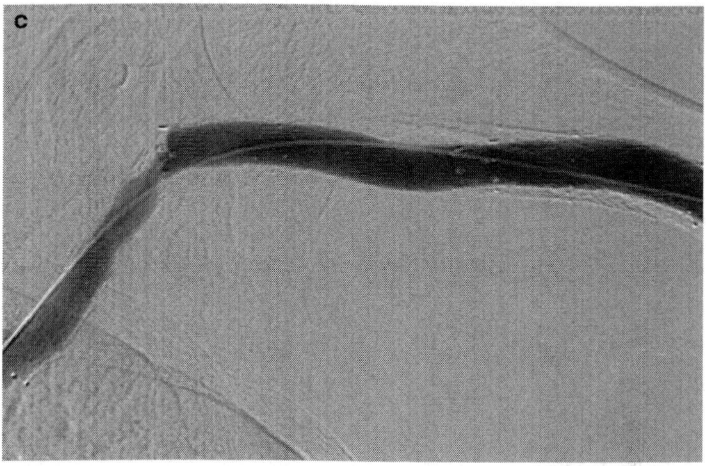

Fig. 19.4 (continued)

also an option. When rupture occurs (up to 10% of cases), options depend on severity of the rupture. If the rupture is very small with limited extravasation, two trials of balloon tamponade (5 min each) will allow most small venous tears to seal. Alternatively, heparin if given can be reversed, and the site of rupture can be observed over the next 5 min to see if the rupture resolves and there is no expanding hematoma. Also, external pressure may be applied to limit extravasation. If the rupture is large, there is an expanding hematoma, the surrounding hematoma is threatening loss of the access due to outflow vein compression, or the patient has worsening pain/neuralgia, salvage with stenting or stent/grafting should be considered.

If a stent or stent graft is used, the device should match the size of inflation balloon used or the size of the adjacent normal vein segment and cover the length of the lesion. The most common size used is an 8×40 mm device. Only self-expanding stents/stent grafts should be used and be of sufficient flexibility to conform to the anatomical arch, not distort it. Prior to considering placing the device, one should consider the potential risk for the device to migrate forward into the axillary vein with shoulder movement. Such migration may jeopardize future accesses within that arm. Balloon-expandable stents should not be used in this location, and they are prone to crushing with resultant loss of the access.

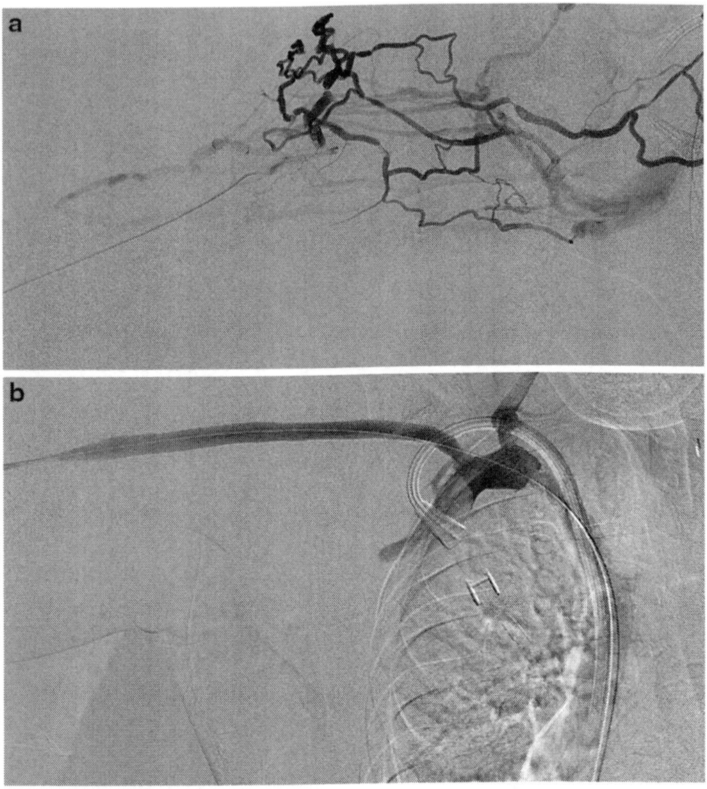

Fig. 19.5 (**a**) Occluded distal cephalic vein and arch in a patient with a BC AVF. (**b**) After crossing the occlusion, balloon PTA failed to open the occlusion and the area was stented with self-expanding nitinol stents to reestablish laminar flow. (**c**) Two months later, the patient presents with arm swelling, high pump pressures, and high recirculation. Initial film demonstrates fracture of the stent (*arrow*) at the arch. (**d**) Multiple attempts to cross the area of fracture failed with resultant loss of the fistula

Outcomes of Interventions

Primary patency after angioplasty is at 6 months is 42% [1] which compares to 51–75% at 6 months for other locations within dialysis fistulas [2, 3]. Assisted primary and secondary patencies with repeat angioplasty are acceptable with up to 75% secondary patency at 12

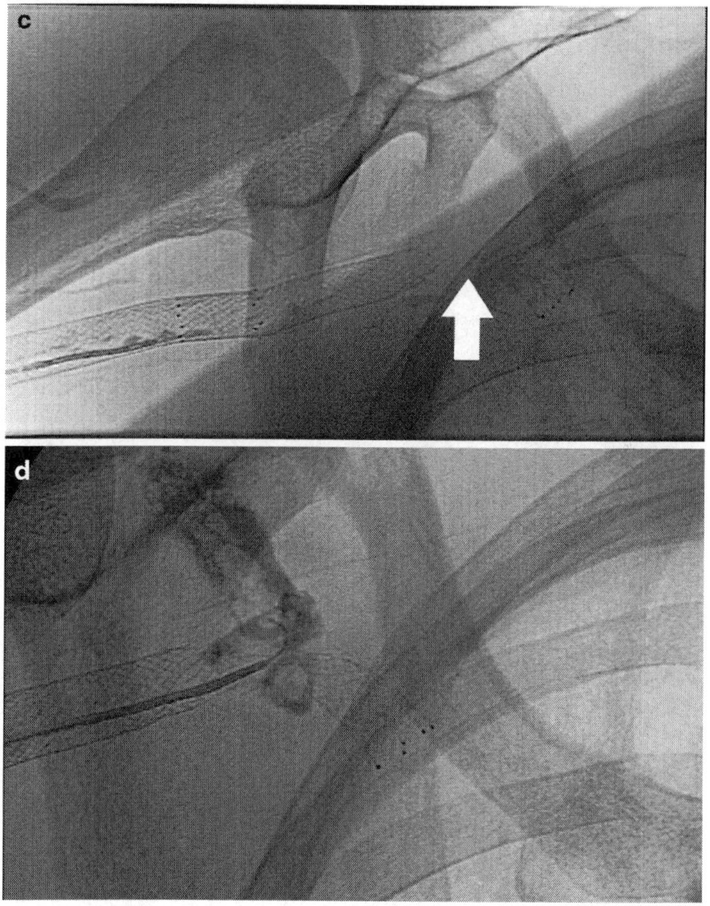

Fig. 19.5 (continued)

months [1]. In addition, other technologies have been introduced including stents and stent grafts. In a single randomized prospective study, 6-month primary patency between stents and stent grafts was 39% vs. 82%. Stent patency was equivalent to historical PTA outcomes [4]. However, this study has many limitations and should not be considered a defining outcome.

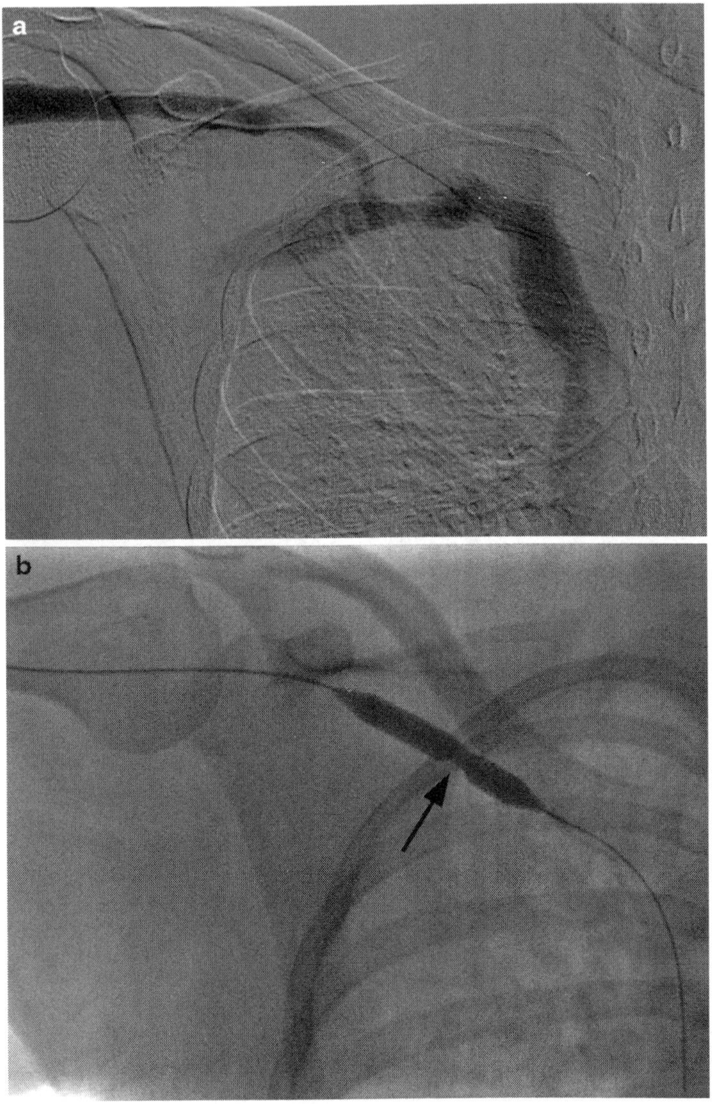

Fig. 19.6 (**a**) Standard cephalic arch stenosis. (**b**) Despite use of a Conquest (CR Bard) 8 mm angioplasty balloon inflated to 40 atm, a waist (*arrow*) is still present, indicating suboptimal angioplasty. (**c**) A 0.018 in. stainless steel mandril wire is advanced across the lesion and repeat inflation eradicates the previous waist at 22 atm. (**d**) Postangioplasty imaging reveals successful dilation of prior stenosis

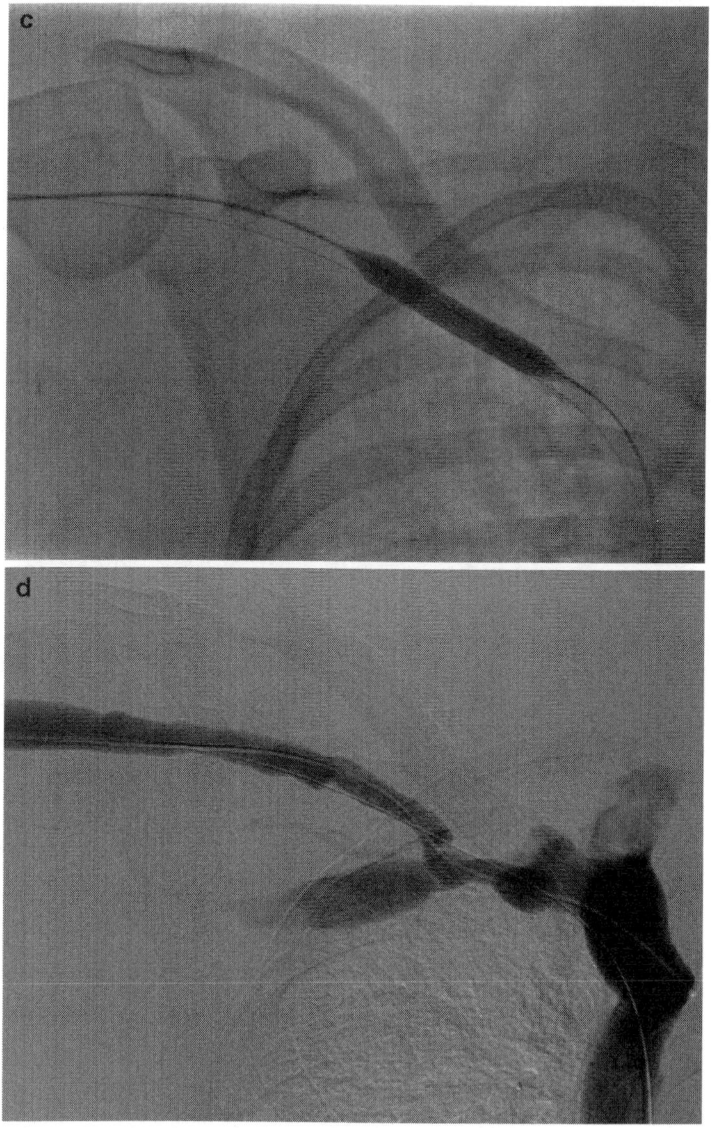

Fig. 19.6 (continued)

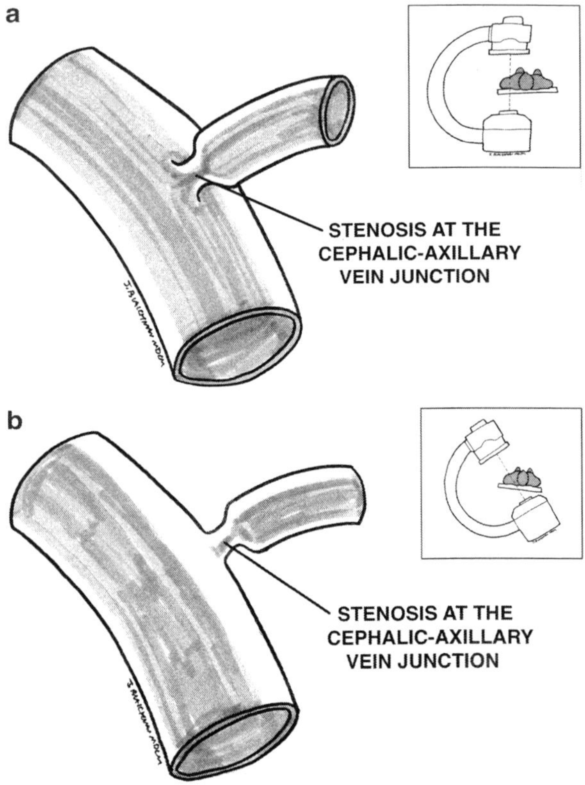

Fig. 19.7 (**a**) If the vein junction (or even anastomoses) is not properly profiled, in one projection no stenosis may be apparent. (**b**) With proper angulation and imaging, the actual stenosis and junction between the axillary and cephalic veins is properly visualized also preventing extension of a stent/stent graft into the axillary vein if required

Surgical Interventions

Since results of endovascular treatment of cephalic arch stenoses are poor even when compared to other dialysis access treatment, surgical correction of cephalic arch stenoses should at least be considered prior to endovascular intervention. When a lesion cannot be effaced safely with balloon angioplasty, surgical correction offers a means of fistula salvage with an acceptable medium-term patency. Surgical treatment limits potential rupture and adjacent vein injury as well. Surgical correction of cephalic arch rupture permits repair of the rupture site and improvement of the stenosis without the need for prosthetic implantation. Depending upon the site of rupture, surgery also avoids extension of a stent graft into the axillary vein which can obstruct future basilic and axillary vein fistula outflow. Finally, surgical treatment of cephalic arch stenosis should be performed in the setting of recurrent in situ or in-stent restenosis. The probability of recurrent stenosis is very high in patients with cephalic arch stenoses. This recurrent restenosis can lead to fistula thrombosis, making fistula salvage less likely. Indeed, surgical revision yields better primary (69% 6 month) and secondary patency rates (92% 1 year) than balloon angioplasty in the same accesses [5]. The higher risk of complications along with the poorer outcomes associated with endovascular treatment of cephalic arch stenosis make surgical treatment a viable option.

Surgical options for treatment of cephalic arch stenosis are varied, depending upon the extent of the disease, the availability of other veins, and the need for preservation of the current fistula. Extrinsic compression of the cephalic vein as it passes through the coracoclavicular fascia can be eliminated by incising the fascial bands. Often, however, this alone is not enough to allow for unimpeded flow through the vein, and surgical correction is still necessary for the remaining stenosis. Vein patch angioplasty of the stenosis can be performed. Although these are viable options, short-, medium-, and long-term patency of these procedures has not been studied. The cephalic vein can also be transposed onto the axillary or basilic veins. If transposition to the basilic or axillary vein would limit useable length of the fistula, an interposition graft can be constructed to the axillary or jugular veins. These surgical options should be considered when treating cephalic arch stenoses, especially for recurrent lesions.

Key Points

- Cephalic arch stenosis is more prevalent in upper arm fistulas and often requires higher inflation pressures to dilate it. It is more prone to rupture than other locations of stenosis.
- If stenting/stent grafting is required, one should avoid extending the device into the axillary vein, thereby eliminating future access options within the ipsilateral arm.
- Surgical options exist and should be considered in select cases.

References

1. Rajan DK, Clark TW, Patel NK, Stavropoulos SW, Simons ME. Prevalence and treatment of cephalic arch stenosis in dysfunctional autogenous hemodialysis fistulas. J Vasc Interv Radiol. 2003;14(5):567–73.
2. Turmel-Rodrigues L, Pengloan J, Baudin S, et al. Treatment of stenosis and thrombosis in haemodialysis fistulas and grafts by interventional radiology. Nephrol Dial Transplant. 2000;15(12):2029–36.
3. Rajan DK, Bunston S, Misra S, Pinto R, Lok CE. Dysfunctional autogenous hemodialysis fistulas: outcomes after angioplasty – are there clinical predictors of patency? Radiology. 2004;232(2):508–15.
4. Shemesh D, Goldin I, Zaghal I, Berlowitz D, Raveh D, Olsha O. Angioplasty with stent graft versus bare stent for recurrent cephalic arch stenosis in autogenous arteriovenous access for hemodialysis: a prospective randomized clinical trial. J Vasc Surg. 2008;48(6):1524–31.
5. Kian K, Unger SW, Mishler R, Schon D, Lenz O, Asif A. Role of surgical intervention for cephalic arch stenosis in the "fistula first" era. Semin Dial. 2008;21(1):93–6.

Chapter 20
Central Venous Interventions

Dheeraj K. Rajan, Timothy I. Clark, and Dirk S. Baumann

Central venous stenosis (CVS) and occlusions in the hemodialysis patient are unique clinical problems that arise mainly from previous central venous catheter insertions, particularly from the subclavian vein approach and left-sided approaches [1–4]. As a result of this observation, K/DOQI recommends placement of more permanent venous access and avoiding catheter-based dialysis when possible [5]. Insertion of pacemaker wires, central venous ports, and peripherally inserted central catheters (PICC) also contribute to an increased incidence of central venous lesions. This is perhaps one of the most significant problems to be addressed in the near future for dialysis patients as they live longer from advances in medical therapy and interventions. Despite consensus guidelines such as K/DOQI and widespread use of venous mapping, most patients present or declare themselves as having a significant central venous stenosis after an access is placed on the side of the lesion.

D.K. Rajan (✉)
Head and Associate Professor, Division of Vascular & Interventional Radiology, Department of Medical Imaging, University of Toronto, Toronto, Ontario, Canada
e-mail: Dheeraj.Rajan@uhn.on.ca

D.K. Rajan (ed.), *Essentials of Percutaneous Dialysis Interventions*, DOI 10.1007/978-1-4419-5657-6_20,
© Springer Science+Business Media, LLC 2011

Treatment is appropriate when a patient presents with hemodynamic and/or clinical indications for intervention. Angiographic evidence of stenosis alone is NOT an indication for intervention. Clinical indications include signs of cerebral venous hypertension, arm swelling (see Fig. 20.1), arm pain, neck swelling, breast swelling, and facial swelling/edema. Pleural effusions are also possible. Hemodynamic problems include high venous pressures, increased recirculation and increased hemostasis times with removal of the dialysis needles, and rarely thromboses of the access. Eventually, patients may develop aneurysmal dilation and/or tortuosity of their access.

When symptomatic central venous stenoses are encountered, they should initially be treated with balloon angioplasty. Asymptomatic lesions are best left untreated. One group found that treatment of asymptomatic CVS greater than 50% was associated with a more rapid stenosis and escalation of lesions compared to no angioplasty [6]. There is a growing consensus among interventionalists that angioplasty within the central veins accelerates the rate of restenosis. Although most published literature discusses treatment efficacy of central venous occlusion, a majority of lesions are not complete occlusions. The best means for dealing with central venous stenosis

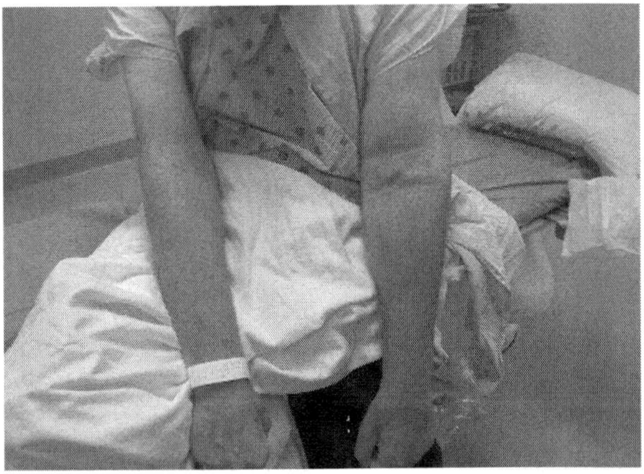

Fig. 20.1 Unilateral arm swelling in a patient with a brachiocephalic fistula and subclavian vein occlusion

is to avoid it altogether by using the internal jugular vein (preferably the right) as the exclusive access for dialysis catheters.

Diagnosis

A combination of clinical findings and imaging finding contribute to diagnosis. Including the clinical signs mentioned above, digital subtraction venography with contrast remains the standard for imaging diagnosis. It has improved sensitivity and specificity compared to duplex ultrasound. Moreover, translesional pressure gradients may be recorded at the time of catheterization. CO_2 angiography is poor for visualizing central venous structures, and other imaging modalities have not been assessed completely for assessing this problem.

A little-considered entity that may appear as stenosis of the left innominate vein is extrinsic compression by the innominate artery or an ectatic aortic arch. Extrinsic compression occurs due to the arterial lumen being more pressurized than the venous lumen thereby compressing the lumen. This external compression that appears as a stenosis is not necessarily functionally significant. Other parameters on dysfunction beyond venography findings should exist before considering treatment [7].

Intervention Options

Percutaneous options for central venous stenosis/occlusion include angioplasty, stenting, recanalization techniques for complete occlusion, and to do nothing. For stenosis alone, POBA remains the mainstay of treatment as no other devices have conclusively shown any improved overall patency. For occlusions, prior to intervening, one should be assured that the occlusion is not acute occlusive thrombus. If so, the guidewire will traverse the area of occlusion very easily, and minimal collaterals will be present. In such cases, thrombectomy (via previously described techniques in Chap. 15) should be performed first. For chronic occlusions, multiple techniques can be utilized to reopen the vein segment. However, this is a relatively high-risk procedure with potentially fatal complications and should be undertaken with due diligence and precaution where appropriate support services are available, particularly cardiothoracic surgery. However, given that these patients often have platelet dysfunction and multiple mediastinal venous collaterals with high blood flow, any surgical intervention acutely often is futile and results in the untimely death of the patient.

One should also consider the impact of the intervention prior to performing it. Percutaneous interventions have a very poor primary patency and therefore should be avoided if not indicated. For central lesions, if the patient presents acutely with arm or neck swelling, this will likely improve over weeks as collaterals develop. This will also improve function of the access. The question to ask oneself is: will the intervention durably improve the patient's clinical situation or should you wait to see if they improve by themselves? Also, if the patient has developed a number of collaterals, opening up the occluded segment may not be of any value as the collaterals have compensated for the occlusion. Central lesions are rarely the cause for access thrombosis. There is nothing wrong with the patient having mildly elevated pressures during dialysis compared to performing an intervention of them that places them on the path of multiple repeated interventions and eventual failure of the access.

Techniques

Stenosis

It is important to visualize the central lesion as best as possible to determine locations of significant collaterals and other adjacent vein segments. A venogram performed from the dialysis access is often not sufficient and better imaging and anatomy definition can be obtained by advancing a catheter close to the lesion and performing the venogram through the catheter (see Fig. 20.2).

For stenotic areas, a glidewire and directional catheter combination is used to cross the stenosis (see Fig. 20.3). Once crossed, advancing a wire into the IVC provides an additional level of secure access across the lesion. Leaving a wire within the heart can predispose to arrhythmias, possible tricuspid valve damage, and theoretically, cardiac perforation. When leaving a wire in the IVC, a stiff nonhydrophilic

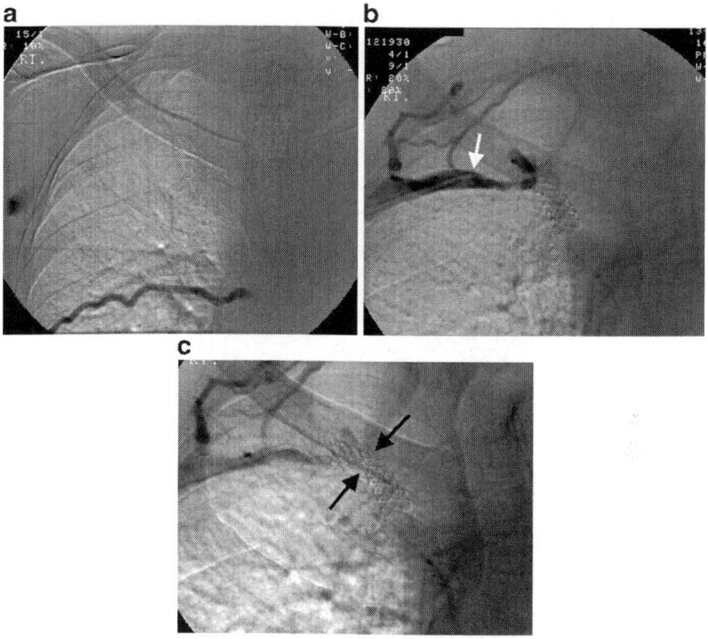

Fig. 20.2 (**a**) Venogram performed peripherally fails to demonstrate location of pathology centrally. (**b**) After advancing a catheter centrally (*arrow*), location of pathology is now clearly identified. (**c**) Crushed balloon expandable stent causing occlusion of the vein. *Arrows* indicate point of compression

wire is recommended. This type of wire is less prone to migration and allows for better tracking of balloons and stent platforms.

For subclavian stenoses, standard balloon diameters are 10–14 mm; for innominate vein stenoses, the range is 10–16 mm, and the superior vena cava required sizes ranging from 12 to 20 mm. Stenting or stent grafting is reserved for flow-limiting dissections, flow-limiting elastic recoil (as evident by persistent collaterals), and ruptures. Self-expanding nitinol stents should be used as balloon-expandable stents are prone to crushing and Wallstents are prone to migration during deployment, eccentric loading (stenosis) that can lead to concentric narrowing, and decreased radial strength and resultant poor patency.

If there is elastic recoil or early restenosis, a decision should be made with respect to managing the recurrent stenosis with a stent

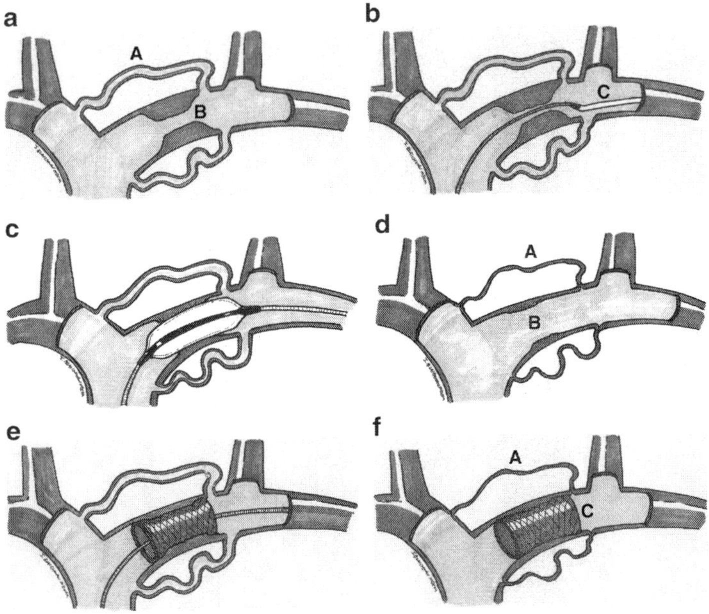

Fig. 20.3 (**a–d**) Standard dilation of central venous stenosis. A – Venous collaterals. B – Central stenosis. C – Directional catheter. (**e**, **f**) Stent deployment for rupture or elastic recoil. Venous collaterals (A) deflate once stenosis is sufficiently treated

vs. repeated balloon dilation (see Fig. 20.3e, f). A stent is usually necessary for complete occlusions. This practice is supported by the K/DOQI. When deploying a stent, it is critical to avoid compromising branch veins that may be needed for a future dialysis catheter, i.e., contralateral innominate, ipsilateral internal or external jugular, etc. Stent oversizing is mandatory to avoid delayed migration or dislodgment. Generally, the stent should be oversized by approximately 10% for optimal wall apposition. The use of stents shorter than 40 mm in length is problematic due to the risk of migration due to insufficient vessel wall contact. Furthermore, another concern regarding stents placed within the subclavian veins more centrally is that they are prone to repeated episodes of compression between the costoclavicular ligament and first rib, the so called "pinch-off" syndrome. Fractures of bare stents have been observed in this location (see Fig. 20.4).

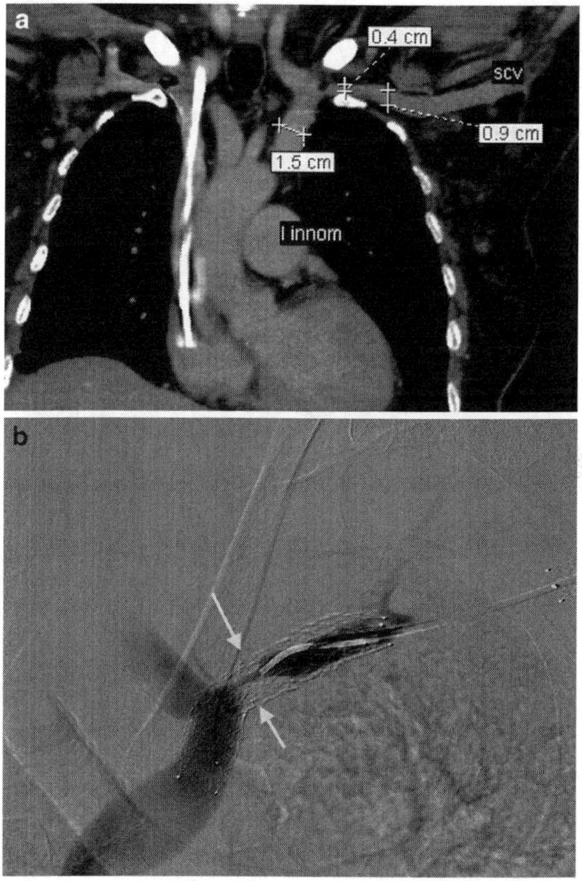

Fig. 20.4 (**a**) Contrast-enhanced CT of the chest. Coronal imaging demonstrates degree of normal anatomical (>50%) compression of the SCV as it crosses the first rib and costoclavicular ligament with arms above the head. This is not a fixed stenosis but represents a focal point of intermittent mechanical compression. (**b**) A patient with BC AVF underwent dilation of SCV stenosis with failure of POBA and subsequently stented with 12×60 mm nitinol self-expanding stent. The patient returns 3 months later with swollen arm. The nitinol stent is fractured (*arrows*) at pinch-off point between costoclavicular ligament and first rib. (**c**, **d**) Fluency stent graft is placed across the tear, and patency of internal jugular vein is maintained. The patient remains asymptomatic 12 months later

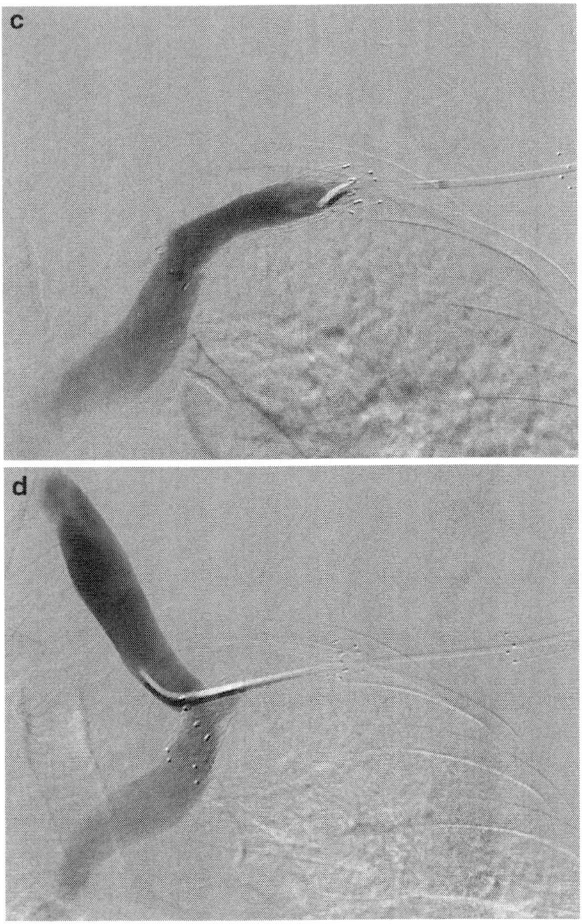

Fig. 20.4 (continued)

Occlusions

The typical method for crossing an area of occlusion is to identify a focal beak-like area of narrowing prior to the occlusion and attempt to pass a hydrophilic guidewire across the occlusion with the aid of a directional catheter (see Fig. 20.5). It is preferred to access the lesion from the access or supra-atrial veins as manipulation is easier with limited room and a shorter distance as opposed to working from the

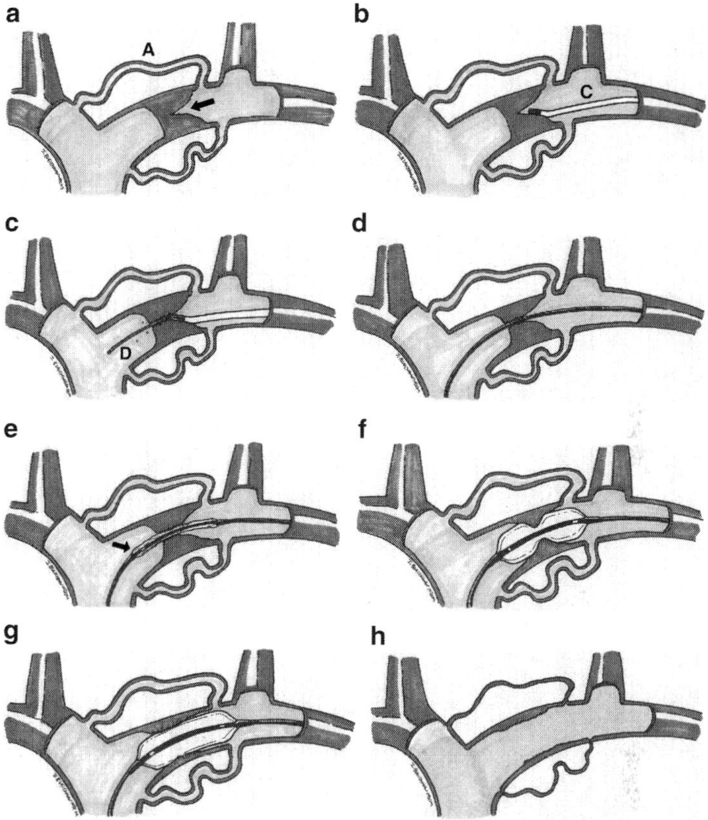

Fig. 20.5 Standard approach for treatment of central venous occlusions. A – Venous collateral, C – directional catheter, D – guidewire. *Arrow* in (a) represents beaklike narrowing at the origin of the occlusion. *Arrow* in (e) represents centering of balloon catheter across area of occlusion. Following adequate dilation, collaterals deflate

femoral approach through the atrium. Once the occlusion is crossed, an exchange for a stiffer wire is required to facilitate passage of a balloon catheter across the occlusion. Balloon size is typically 10–14 mm. In a majority of cases, a web-like constriction is visualized and prolonged inflation and/or high-pressure balloon catheters are required to overcome the occlusion. Serial dilation starting with a small balloon diameter, usually a 4 mm diameter balloon and increasing balloon diameter is recommended to exclude perforation between dilation steps. Recently, the availability of ultra–high-inflation

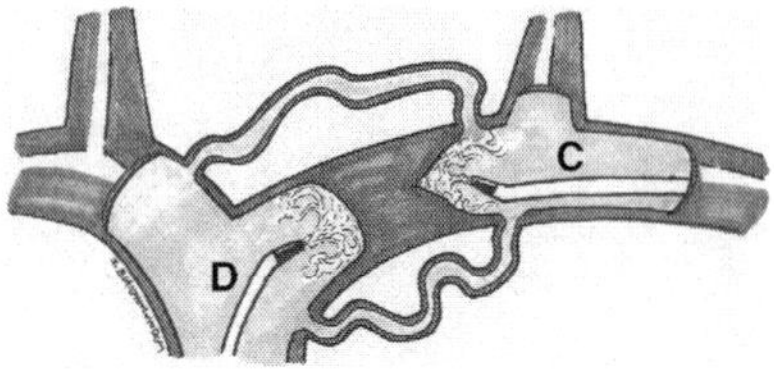

Fig. 20.6 Exact length and location of occlusion determined via approaches from the arm and the leg prior to intervention, C – Directional catheter from the access, D – directional catheter from femoral access

pressure balloons (Atlas, Bard, Covington, GA) has enabled complete effacement of the waist of the lesion at rated burst pressures in the 18-atm range.

For occlusions that cannot be crossed with traditional methods, an alternative percutaneous approach is sharp recanalization. This method can be performed from a single upper arm approach for short lesions. More difficult occlusions often require an upper extremity and femoral approach and imaging in multiple planes (obliquities) to ensure that the needle used is crossing the area of occlusion [8–10]. Contrast is injected at the site of occlusion from either side of the occlusion to determine the location and length and to guide the direction of puncture (see Fig. 20.6). Before embarking on sharp recanalization, one should understand that there is the potential to puncture into the mediastinal or pleural or pericardial spaces and the aorta. With flows from arm accesses reaching up to 2 L/min, bleeding into these areas is potentially fatal.

The initial sharp device that can be used for puncture is the back end of a glidewire. Other devices that can be used include the directional sheath needle combinations from transjugular intrahepatic portosystemic shunt (TIPS) kits. Examples include the Haskal set (Cook Medical, Bloomington, IN), the Rosch Uchida Set (Cook) and the Colapinto needle. One can also use a transseptal cardiac puncture needle. A new device that holds promise is the Powerwire (Baylis Medical, Mississauga, ON). This is a directional wire which delivers radiofrequency energy to the tip of the wire, allowing it to burn its way though tissues. Advantages include directionality and less trauma, thereby potentially less complications.

Tricks that can be utilized include placing an open loop snare (Ensnare or loop snare; 5–15 mm) on the other side of the occlusion and using it as a target to aim for with the needle or wire (see Fig. 20.7a). Another assisting method is to inflate an angioplasty balloon adjacent to the site of occlusion. This allows for improved

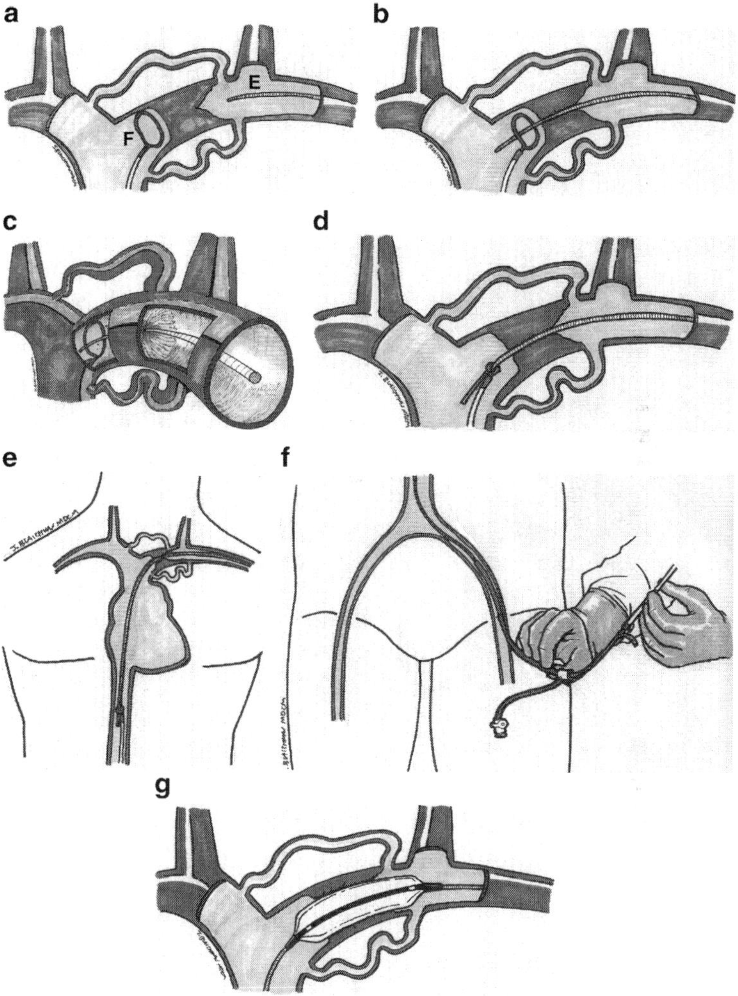

Fig. 20.7 (**a**) Via femoral venous access, a loop snare is advanced up to the central side of the occlusion and used as a target for sharp needle puncture across the occlusion (F – loop snare, E – glidwire or needle). (**b–d**) Wire or wire through needle is captured with the loop snare while ensuring that puncture is across the central part of the occlusion. (**e**, **f**) If required, wire can be pulled out though the femoral puncture, thereby having wire access established from the arm to the groin with external control of both ends of the wire ("Body floss"). (**g**) "Body Floss" access allows maximum control of interventions including POBA and stenting

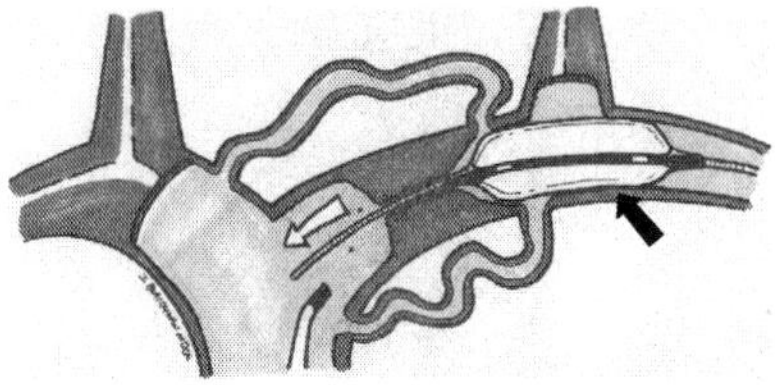

Fig. 20.8 Angioplasty balloon (*black arrow*) is inflated to provide stability to advance glidewire and to assist in centering the wire to cross the occlusion (*white arrow*)

stability, pushability, and centering of the guidewire lumen to the long axis of the occluded vein segment and the back end of the glidewire can then be passed through the balloon wire lumen centered through the lesion (see Fig. 20.8).

If a wire was used to transverse the area of occlusion, intraluminal location can be verified by snaring the wire from the other side if dual access was obtained. If not, a 4 Fr hydrophilic catheter can be advanced over the wire across the occlusion and contrast can be used to verify intraluminal location. Once intraluminal location is verified and a catheter traverses the occlusion, a stiffer wire should be advanced through the catheter into the IVC. Through and through access from the arm access through to the femoral sheath (called a "body floss") provides the most stability but is often not required. This technique requires snaring the wire and pulling it though the femoral sheath (see Figs. 20.7 and 20.9). A sufficiently long wire should be utilized to allow maintained location within the IVC. This method is significantly helpful in creating a stable track to advance devices across the lesion that might not otherwise pass through.

Following establishment of secure access across the occlusion, sequential dilation starting with small balloons to large balloons should be undertaken with intervening venograms to exclude extraluminal passage.

Only in cases of rupture, occlusion, and technical failures to improve flow do we place a self-expanding stent. Self-expanding stents have the advantage of being crush resistant and return to their normal size if they are compressed. Use of balloon-expandable stents has been associated with compression (see Fig. 20.2) and spontaneous migration, and they should not be used [11, 12]. If a large rupture has occurred or there is obvious bleeding into the pericardial/mediastinal or pleural spaces and an expanding hematoma, then placement of a stent graft is performed for clinical salvage of the complication. The size of the stent or stent graft is determined by the size of the adjacent normal vein segment but is approximately

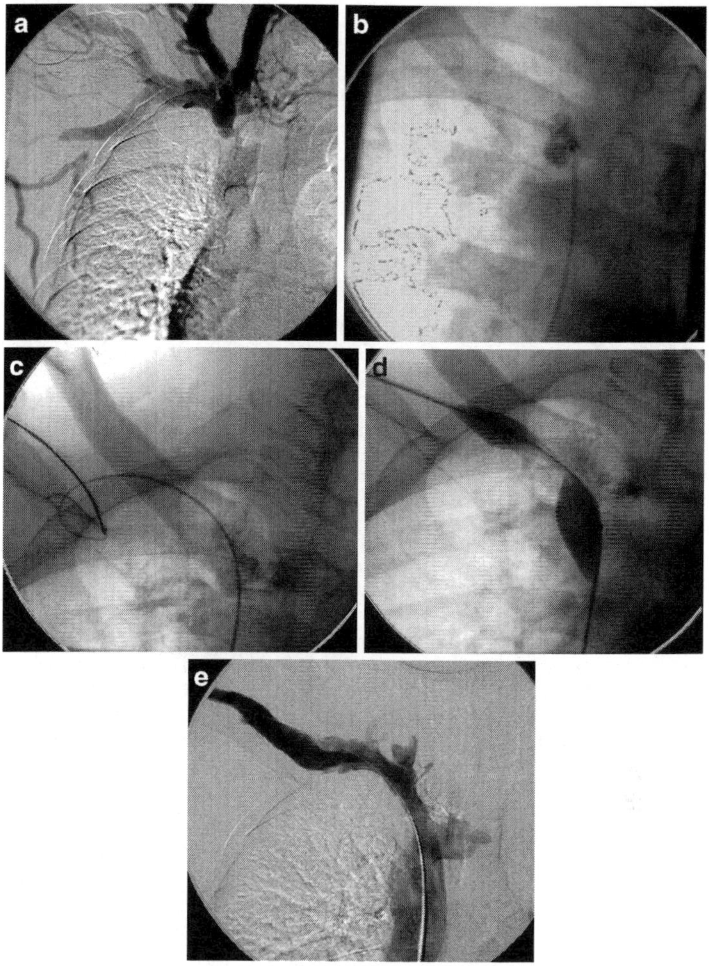

Fig. 20.9 Patient with upper arm access presents with face, neck, and arm swelling. (a) Complete occlusion of the right innominate vein. (**b**) Multiple attempts were made to traverse the occlusion with the soft end and back end of the glidewire from the access without success. A femoral vein puncture was performed and using a directional catheter, the back end of the glidewire (sharp needle equivalent) was used to puncture across the occlusion. After a catheter was advanced over the wire through the occlusion, the wire from the femoral approach was snared and pulled out through the dialysis access, thereby establishing a "Body floss" with the wire extending from the access out through the femoral vein. (**c**) Angioplasty was then performed serially with venograms performed from the access between each size increase to assure no venous rupture. (**d**) Final dilation was performed with a 14×40 mm Atlas balloon (CR Bard). (**e**) Completion venogram demonstrates rapid flow and no residual stenosis. No stenting was required

the sizes mentioned above for corresponding vein segments. When placing either of these devices, it is absolutely imperative to avoid covering uninvolved vein segments such as the internal jugular vein or the innominate/SVC junction (see Fig. 20.10).

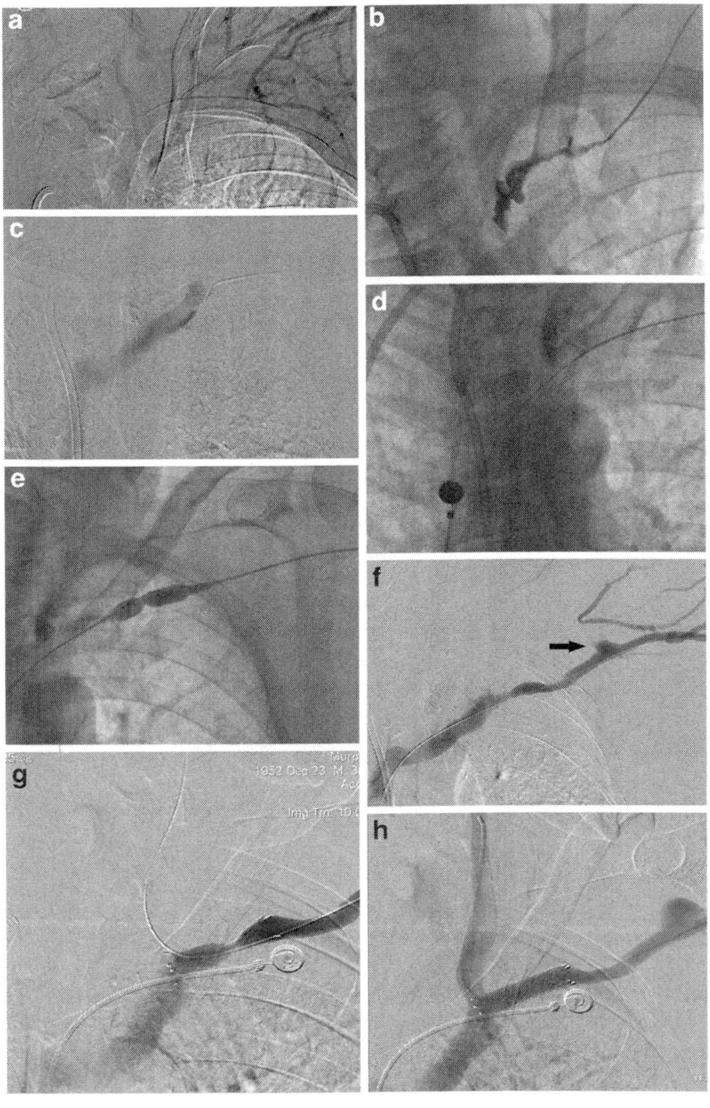

Another not yet proven alternative is to dilate central vein collaterals to improve flow and improve the patient's hemodynamic or clinical problems (see Fig. 24.5, Chap. 24).

SVC Syndrome

This represents a spectrum of clinical severity leading up to a medical emergency from minimal return of blood from the upper extremities and brain leading to elevated venous pressures, dyspnea, and elevated venous pressure within the brain, eventually leading to death from cerebral edema. Within the dialysis patient, the most common cause is occlusion of the SVC and/or both brachiocephalic veins. The underlying cause is venous injury from prior catheter insertions starting a cascade of stenosis followed by occlusion. Percutaneous treatment is as above. If the patient has an SVC occlusion and this is successfully traversed, balloon dilation should be attempted first as the patient may have a simple fibrous web occlusion. If there is acute thrombus in addition to the lesion, a short course of mechanical or pharmacological thrombolysis should be attempted to reduce the area that requires stenting and to prevent pulmonary embolism.

In most cases, POBA is not sufficient, and stenting will be required. Prior to POBA or stenting, one should carefully map or determine the length of pathology and proximity to the right atrium

Fig. 20.10 Patient had BC AVF placed 2 months earlier and 2 days after placement felt popping in shoulder and arm swelled up. The fistula has never been used. (**a**) Initial fistulogram shows extensive venous collaterals and occlusion of the cephalic arch SCV. (**b**) Initial attempts with glidewire result in entry into mediastinum. (**c**) Eventually, area of occlusion was traversed and entry into the innominate vein was verified with contrast hand injection. (**d**) Stiff 180 cm non-hydrophilic wire is advanced through the catheter across the pathology in case stenting would be required. (**e**) PTA with 10×40 mm balloon. (**f**) Reestablished flow with decompression of collaterals. Focal rupture (arrow) was managed conservatively and did not require further intervention. (**g**) Patient returns 2 months later with swollen arm. Focal stenosis at SCV stented with 10×40 mm Fluency stent graft (concern for fracture of bare stent at this location) with resumption of normal flow (**h**) after dilation of stent graft. Note preservation of internal jugular vein and healed site of previous venous rupture in (**f**)

and left brachiocephalic vein. If a stent is to be placed, it should not extend into the right atrium, and efforts should be made to avoid jailing out or covering the left innominate vein if it is open. Occasionally, stenting the SVC and left innominate vein into the SVC may be required (kissing stents) to maintain patency of the innominate vein.

Stenting the SVC is the one instance where a balloon-expandable stent can be used. However, the SVC can have a diameter that exceeds 22 mm. Balloon-expandable stents have the advantage of having a much larger hoop or outward strength than self-expanding stents. If one is going to be used, the preferred stent is the Palmaz stent. It is important to understand the sizing of this stent prior to deployment as it shortens with greater diameter. If a self-expanding stent is used, a sufficient diameter should be used. A stent diameter of >12 mm and <20 mm is recommended. For occluded innominate veins, reopening a single innominate vein is sufficient for decompressing the venous hypertension. Both sides reopened are rarely needed.

Pacemaker-Induced Stenosis/Occlusion

In rare instances, patients can present with central stenosis/occlusion of the subclavian and/or innominate veins from inserted pacemaker leads (see Fig. 20.11). It remains unclear if it is safe to angioplasty/stent these areas as there is concern for pacer lead dysfunction/infection. Although there is no defining literature regarding the safety of doing so, limited anecdotal reports and two retrospective studies suggest that it is safe to do so with limited primary patency of <20% (PTA)-45% (stenting) at 6 months [13, 14].

Literature

Outcome following balloon angioplasty for central venous stenosis has a good initial success rate with minimal complications. However, initial success and patency is lower than for peripheral venous stenoses. Technical success rates range from 70 to 100% with mean patency at 6 months ranging from 29 to 42% [15, 16] or average

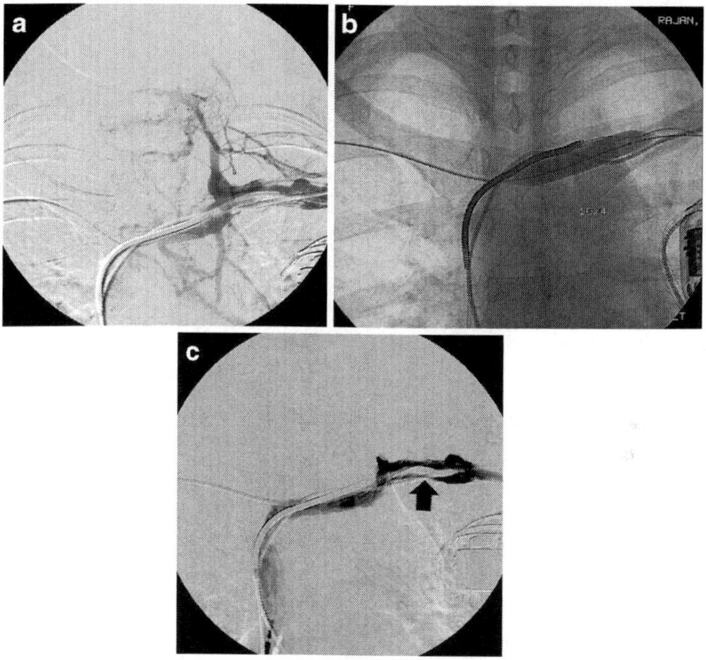

Fig. 20.11 Patient with left upper arm AVF and dual lead pacemaker presents with arm swelling and inability to access fistula due to swelling. (**a**) Initial venogram demonstrates occlusion of the left innominate vein, narrowing of the LSCV, and multiple venous collaterals. (**b**) The innominate and subclavian veins are dilated with a 10-mm PTA balloon. (**c**) Post PTA, rapid flow is reestablished with decompression of collaterals. Note fibrous tissue around leads in SCV (*arrow*)

restenosis in 7.6 months [17], which is relatively poor compared to a range of 38–63% 6-month cumulative primary patency following angioplasty for peripheral stenoses [15, 18–20].

Outcome following angioplasty/stenting of central venous stenosis in hemodialysis patients is somewhat limited and difficult to compare with no established reporting standards prior to 1999 [21]. With Wallstents, five studies have been reported for central venous stenosis/occlusion [4, 22–25] with three studies mixing results with peripheral stenoses [4, 22, 23]. Technical success was between 96 and 100%. Primary patency ranged from 42 to 84% at 6 months but was less than 31% at 12 months in all five studies [4, 22–25]. Multiple repeat interventions are required to maintain patency. Although stenting has good technical outcomes, multiple interventions are required to achieve satisfactory secondary patency outcomes.

Overall primary patency for endovascular interventions including angioplasty and/or stenting range from 14 to 67% at 12 months [3, 10, 26]. Stent grafts primarily with the Fluency and Viabahn devices are another unexplored option, and patency has not yet been properly studied although anecdotal reports suggest patencies that exceed POBA and bare metal stenting.

Surgical Interventions for Central Venous Occlusion

Surgical options for bypass of central venous occlusions are limited, but viable in clinically symptomatic patients with limited remaining venous access. As stated previously, the best treatment for central venous stenoses related to dialysis access is prevention. Placement of central venous catheters, PICC lines, and pacemaker wires into the subclavian veins must be avoided in all patients with chronic kidney disease. If required, central venous catheters should be placed via the right internal jugular vein if at all possible.

Symptomatic subclavian venous stenosis or occlusion can be treated with bypass or jugular vein transposition. Bypasses can be performed from the axillary vein to the ipsilateral jugular vein, ipsilateral innominate vein or contralateral axillary vein. Potential bypass conduit includes an 8 mm PTFE graft, saphenous vein, or deep or superficial femoral vein. These bypasses are quite effective at eliminating arm swelling and have relatively good patency results in comparison to angioplasty [27, 28]. If patent, transposition of the ipsilateral jugular vein to the axillary vein can also be performed with little morbidity and excellent symptom relief [29]. Lastly, a HeRO device can be used to maintain an upper arm fistula/graft if the central venous lesion can be crossed but develops rapid recurrent stenosis.

Innominate vein stenoses are more difficult to treat surgically. Axillary vein or artery to contralateral axillary vein bypasses with PTFE graft or saphenous vein can be performed when endovascular treatment is not possible or has already failed. Primary and secondary patency rates of axillary-to-axillary PTFE bypasses are quite good (72 and 89% at 1 year, respectively) given the large size of the axillary vein [30]. Alternatively, arterioarterial bypasses, for example axilloaxillary or femorofemoral bypasses, with ligation of the artery between the anastomoses of the loop bypass have also been used in patients with central vein stenosis or severe peripheral artery disease with arterial steal [31]. These bypasses have good patency rates (73% primary and 96% secondary at 1 year) with few interventions (0.47 procedures/year). In patients who have exhausted all other venous access, bypass to the right atrial appendage results in good AVF functional results (mean patency 15.4 months) with acceptable morbidity and mortality [32]. Finally, if other options are exhausted, ligation of an arteriovenous fistula may be necessary. Ligation nearly always eliminates symptoms of arm swelling and venous hypertension. Since results of endovascular treatment are limited, surgical options are well recognized and efficacious alternatives for the treatment of central venous stenosis.

Summary

Central interventions are becoming more prominent as dialysis patients live longer. With the Fistula First initiative, there has actually been an increased use of dialysis catheters while fistulas mature (or fail). Given that the number one cause of central vein problems are prior catheter insertions, it is reasonable to assume central interventions will increase. Beyond POBA, most interventions are relatively advanced and should not be discounted as simple. Complex interventions should be performed in a tertiary referral center for the benefit of the patient. Although stent grafts are not approved in North America for use in such interventions, stocking a few of these devices is highly recommended as they provide added confidence for a bail-out or salvage of a potentially catastrophic situation.

Key Points

- The best treatment for CVO/CVS remains prevention of insertion of central venous devices.
- Angiographic stenosis alone is not an indication to intervene. There should be at least one additional clear hemodynamic or clinical indication to intervene.

- Obtaining a CT venogram of chest may allow better characterization of central venous lesions and assist in treatment plan.
- Use an exchange length wire or wire sufficiently long enough to prevent loss of access across the lesion when exchanging for devices after you have successfully traversed the lesion.
- For central venous interventions, particularly CVO, placing a long sheath up to the lesion improves technical success of the intervention.
- POBA is standard of care.
- Complex central venous occlusions should be treated at centers with appropriate backup surgical services.
- Stent grafts may salvage a potentially fatal complication. Keeping a few immediately available is prudent when attempting advanced central interventions.
- When performing complex central venous interventions, one should always be aware of the potential complication of pericardial tamponade.
- If you are unsuccessful, someone else may be successful.
- Central venous occlusion is rarely a cause for fistula thrombosis.
- A patent radiocephalic fistula may function well even in the presence of CVS/CVO. Mild symptoms in such patients may not warrant intervention.

References

1. Surratt RS, Picus D, Hicks ME, Darcy MD, Kleinhoffer M, Jendrisak M. The importance of preoperative evaluation of the subclavian vein in dialysis access planning. AJR Am J Roentgenol. 1991;156(3):623–5.
2. Criado E, Marston WA, Jaques PF, Mauro MA, Keagy BA. Proximal venous outflow obstruction in patients with upper extremity arteriovenous dialysis access. Ann Vasc Surg. 1994;8(6):530–5.
3. Maskova J, Komarkova J, Kivanek J, Danes J, Slavikova M. Endovascular treatment of central vein stenoses and/or occlusions in hemodialysis patients. Cardiovasc Interv Radiol. 2003;26(1):27–30.
4. Oderich GS, Treiman GS, Schneider P, Bhirangi K. Stent placement for treatment of central and peripheral venous obstruction: a long-term multi-institutional experience. J Vasc Surg. 2000;32(4):760–9.

5. Eknoyan G, Levin NW, Eschbach JW, et al. Continuous quality improvement: DOQI becomes K/DOQI and is updated. National Kidney Foundation's Dialysis Outcomes Quality Initiative. Am J Kidney Dis. 2001;37(1):179–94.
6. Levit RD, Cohen RM, Kwak A, et al. Asymptomatic central venous stenosis in hemodialysis patients. Radiology. 2006;238(3):1051–6.
7. Itkin M, Kraus MJ, Trerotola SO. Extrinsic compression of the left innominate vein in hemodialysis patients. J Vasc Interv Radiol. 2004;15(1 Pt 1):51–6.
8. Farrell T, Lang EV, Barnhart W. Sharp recanalization of central venous occlusions. J Vasc Interv Radiol. 1999;10(2 Pt 1):149–54.
9. Athreya S, Scott P, Annamalai G, Edwards R, Moss J, Robertson I. Sharp recanalization of central venous occlusions: a useful technique for haemodialysis line insertion. Br J Radiol. 2009;82(974):105–8.
10. Rajan DK, Saluja JS. Use of nitinol stents following recanalization of central venous occlusions in hemodialysis patients. Cardiovasc Interv Radiol. 2007;30(4):662–7.
11. Bjarnason H, Hunter DW, Crain MR, Ferral H, Miltz-Miller SE, Wegryn SA. Collapse of a Palmaz stent in the subclavian vein. AJR Am J Roentgenol. 1993;160(5):1123–4.
12. Gray RJ, Dolmatch BL, Horton KM, Romolo JL, Zarate AR. Migration of Palmaz stents following deployment for venous stenoses related to hemodialysis access. J Vasc Interv Radiol. 1994;5(1):117–20.
13. Asif A, Salman L, Carrillo RG, et al. Patency rates for angioplasty in the treatment of pacemaker-induced central venous stenosis in hemodialysis patients: results of a multi-center study. Semin Dial. 2009;22(6):671–6.
14. Saad TF, Myers GR, Cicone J. Central vein stenosis or occlusion associated with cardiac rhythm management device leads in hemodialysis patients with ipsilateral arteriovenous access: a retrospective study of treatment using stents or stent-grafts. J Vasc Access. 2010;11(4):293–302.
15. Beathard GA. Percutaneous transvenous angioplasty in the treatment of vascular access stenosis. Kidney Int. 1992;42(6):1390–7.
16. Lumsden AB, MacDonald MJ, Isiklar H, et al. Central venous stenosis in the hemodialysis patient: incidence and efficacy of endovascular treatment. Cardiovasc Surg. 1997;5(5):504–9.
17. Kovalik EC, Newman GE, Suhocki P, Knelson M, Schwab SJ. Correction of central venous stenoses: use of angioplasty and vascular Wallstents. Kidney Int. 1994;45(4):1177–81.
18. Kanterman RY, Vesely TM, Pilgram TK, Guy BW, Windus DW, Picus D. Dialysis access grafts: anatomic location of venous stenosis and results of angioplasty [erratum appears in Radiology. 1995;196(2):582]. Radiology. 1995;195(1):135–9.
19. Safa AA, Valji K, Roberts AC, Ziegler TW, Hye RJ, Oglevie SB. Detection and treatment of dysfunctional hemodialysis access grafts: effect of a surveillance program on graft patency and the incidence of thrombosis. Radiology. 1996;199(3):653–7.
20. Turmel-Rodrigues L, Pengloan J, Blanchier D, et al. Insufficient dialysis shunts: improved long-term patency rates with close hemodynamic monitoring, repeated percutaneous balloon angioplasty, and stent placement. Radiology. 1993;187(1):273–8.

21. Gray RJ, Sacks D, Martin LG, Trerotola SO. Reporting standards for percutaneous interventions in dialysis access. Technology Assessment Committee [see comments]. J Vasc Interv Radiol. 1999;10(10):1405–15.
22. Gray RJ, Horton KM, Dolmatch BL, et al. Use of Wallstents for hemodialysis access-related venous stenoses and occlusions untreatable with balloon angioplasty. Radiology. 1995;195(2):479–84.
23. Vorwerk D, Guenther RW, Mann H, et al. Venous stenosis and occlusion in hemodialysis shunts: follow-up results of stent placement in 65 patients. Radiology. 1995;195(1):140–6.
24. Vesely TM, Hovsepian DM, Pilgram TK, Coyne DW, Shenoy S. Upper extremity central venous obstruction in hemodialysis patients: treatment with Wallstents. Radiology. 1997;204(2):343–8.
25. Haage P, Vorwerk D, Piroth W, Schuermann K, Guenther RW. Treatment of hemodialysis-related central venous stenosis or occlusion: results of primary Wallstent placement and follow-up in 50 patients. Radiology. 1999; 212(1):175–80.
26. Kim YC, Won JY, Choi SY, et al. Percutaneous treatment of central venous stenosis in hemodialysis patients: long-term outcomes. Cardiovasc Interv Radiol. 2009;32(2):271–8.
27. Bhatia DS, Money SR, Ochsner JL, et al. Comparison of surgical bypass and percutaneous balloon dilatation with primary stent placement in the treatment of central venous obstruction in the dialysis patient: one-year follow-up. Ann Vasc Surg. 1996;10(5):452–5.
28. Suliman A, Greenberg JI, Angle N. Surgical bypass of symptomatic central venous obstruction for arteriovenous fistula salvage in hemodialysis patients. Ann Vasc Surg. 2008;22(2):203–9.
29. Puskas JD, Gertler JP. Internal jugular to axillary vein bypass for subclavian vein thrombosis in the setting of brachial arteriovenous fistula. J Vasc Surg. 1994;19(5):939–42.
30. Morsy MA, Khan A, Chemla ES. Prosthetic axillary-axillary arteriovenous straight access (necklace graft) for difficult hemodialysis patients: a prospective single-center experience. J Vasc Surg. 2008;48(5):1251–4.
31. Zanow J, Kruger U, Petzold M, Petzold K, Miller H, Scholz H. Arterioarterial prosthetic loop: a new approach for hemodialysis access. J Vasc Surg. 2005;41(6):1007–12.
32. El-Sabrout RA, Duncan JM. Right atrial bypass grafting for central venous obstruction associated with dialysis access: another treatment option. J Vasc Surg. 1999;29(3):472–8.

Chapter 21
Hemodialysis Access Interventions: An Asian Perspective

Farah G. Irani, Bien-Soo Tan, Manish Taneja, Richard Lo, and Kiang Hiong Tay

Introduction

The prevalence of end stage renal disease (ESRD) in Singapore is high, and is on an upward trend due to the high incidence of diabetes and an aging population. The crude rates (CR) for ESRD incidence increased from 213.2 per million population (pomp) in 1999 to 295.3 pomp in 2006 [1].

The renal transplant program is limited by the availability of organs with most being cadaveric transplants. In 2006, there were 124 new renal transplant recipients (CR 22.6 pomp) with 1,154 prevalent transplant patients (CR 306.7 pomp) [1]. Hence the main stay of renal replacement therapy in Singapore is dialysis. There were 728 (CR 193.5 pomp) new patients initiated on dialysis in 2006, with 77.9% (567 patients, CR 150.7 pomp) being on hemodialysis, and the rest on peritoneal dialysis (22.1%). The total number of patients on dialysis for the same period was 3,774

F.G. Irani (✉)
Consultant, Interventional Radiology Center, Department of Diagnostic Radiology, Singapore General Hospital, Singapore
e-mail: farah.gillan.irani@sgh.com.sg

D.K. Rajan (ed.), *Essentials of Percutaneous Dialysis Interventions*,
DOI 10.1007/978-1-4419-5657-6_21,
© Springer Science+Business Media, LLC 2011

(CR 1,003.0 pomp) with hemodialysis accounting for 81.2% (3,063 patients, CR 670 pomp) [1]. Renal replacement therapy therefore has a significant financial impact on the economy, with an estimated cost of S$241 million/year [2].

In Singapore, the main causes of ESRD are diabetic nephropathy (59.6%) and primary glomerulonephritis (17.3%). Patients have associated co-morbid conditions like ischemic heart disease (38.2%), cerebrovascular disease (15%), peripheral vascular disease (10.7%), and hepatitis B (3.8%) [1]. These factors make for a fragile high risk patient, making any intervention very challenging.

As hemodialysis is the main stay of renal replacement therapy in Singapore, vascular access creation and maintenance are high volume procedures for both the vascular surgeons and the interventional radiologists. The presence of concomitant vasculopathies as a result of diabetes makes intervention in these patients complicated and challenging.

Hemodialysis

In Singapore, hemodialysis is predominantly via the native arteriovenous fistula (AVF), with creation of an arteriovenous graft (AVG), only considered if a patent has exhausted his/her native veins or has poor native veins. Native AVFs require at least 6 weeks to mature before they can be used [3]. As most patients present late in the Asian population (due to cultural sensibilities), preemptive AVF creation is not common. Hence initiation of hemodialysis is via a tunneled dialysis catheter, inserted into an internal jugular vein in a majority of cases.

As most of our patients are of small body habitus, we generally tend to use a 19 cm tip to cuff catheter for the right side, and a 23 cm tip to cuff catheter for the left side. In an ideal situation, all patients with CKD should have preemptive AVF creation, so as to avoid the need for tunneled catheter insertion, and hence possible central vein stenosis. We try and mitigate the incidence of central vein stenosis due to tunneled dialysis catheters, by inserting them on the side opposite to the side of AVF creation, unless there are no available neck veins.

Prior to creation of an AVF, most patients have a Doppler ultrasound (US) of the upper arm veins to judge for size and patency.

The commonest type of AVF created is the radial-cephalic (RC) AVF at the wrist. The left upper limb is the commonest site of placement, as the right is the dominant hand in most patients. Should the wrist RC AVF fail, the patient would then go onto creation of a brachial–cephalic (BC) AVF at the elbow if a mid forearm RC AVF is not possible. Failure of the BC AVF would lead to the creation of a brachial-basilic transposition (BBT) AVF, either as a single procedure or a two stage procedure.

Interventional Radiology

As most of our patients are quite young when they start hemodialysis (mean age 58.2 years) and require arteriovenous (AV) access for a long time, we are quite aggressive in AVF salvage, be it percutaneous or surgical. In our public healthcare setting, all patients co-pay, and therefore treatment costs are a consideration in deciding the type of equipment and devices used.

For a start, the failure to mature rate for an AVF can be quite high with rates ranging from 11 to 60% [4–6]. The KDOQI guideline [3] of the rule of 6s (i.e., 6 mm vein, 6 weeks for maturation, <6 mm under the skin and 600 mL flow) for an AVF to provide adequate and good dialysis does not hold true in the Asian population. As our vessels are smaller, AVFs may take longer to mature, necessitating longer duration of catheter directed dialysis.

We perform sequential balloon dilatation and coiling of large draining tributaries to help accelerate maturation [7]. Failure to mature is mainly seen in RC AVFs. If at the end of 6 weeks an AVF is non palpable or cannot support insertion of a needle, it is then deemed as failure to mature. Following a fistulogram, we generally access the vein with ultrasound guidance and a 21G micropuncture needle. A 4 or 5 Fr sheath is inserted and after the culprit vein is traversed, angioplasty is initially performed with a 4 mm balloon, and if required, further upsized by 1 mm. The AVF is reassessed at 1 month. If the initial intervention is not adequate, then we redilate the AVF with a larger balloon if possible. If the retrograde transvenous approach should fail, then the antegrade transarterial approach can be attempted [8].

Due to the chronicity of the disease and the long term recurring costs, most patients tend to dialyze within the community in voluntary welfare centers which are manned by nurses [2]. Hence, access of AVFs is at their most prominent points recurrently leading to formation of aneurysms. Presence of these aneurysms associated with varying shear stress on the venous walls, uremia, and repeated low grade inflammation from repeated needling results in the development of venous stenoses which can result in AVF failure. There are ongoing educational initiatives to address this issue. We do not place stent grafts to exclude the aneurysms. However, as discussed in Chap. 17, in cases where impending rupture is of concern, our access surgeons will plicate the fistula, or place a short jump graft to exclude the aneurysm.

We generally intervene when blood flow rates are below 300 mL/min in the RC AVFs and 600 mL/min in the BC AVFs. However, if sudden precipitous fall in flow rates is noted on serial trending, intervention is performed earlier. While access monitoring techniques during dialysis are now well established, these are not universally available at the dialysis centers. As a result, patients with dysfunctional AVFs can present with advanced lesions.

Technique

In our institution, the primary imaging modality for a clinically failing access is a fistulogram. It is performed in the radiological suites by directly accessing the AVF with a 21G butterfly needle or 22G venflon and injecting contrast, and sequentially imaging the veins of the upper extremity using digital subtraction angiography. The AV anastomosis and feeding artery are imaged by refluxing contrast by inflation of a BP cuff above the access point to above systolic pressure. This method, although not physiological, gives clinically relevant information on the number, nature, and site of the stenoses.

If we proceed to intervention, then the mature AVFs are accessed with an 18G puncture needle directed either centrally or peripherally depending upon the site of stenosis/stenoses. Often enough we would require accessing the AVF via two puncture sites, both antegrade and retrograde so as to cover all the lesions. We generally insert a 6 Fr sheath as it allows for more flexibility while choosing the angioplasty balloon. We generally do not go beyond a size 7 Fr sheath in the arm veins.

We cross the stenosis using a short 4 Fr diagnostic catheter (Berenstein or Cobra 2) and a 0.035 in. hydrophilic glide wire. Intravenous heparin is administered once the lesion is crossed to prevent thrombosis. We use low doses of heparin (2,000 IU) as our patients have smaller volumes of distribution. Once the stenosis is crossed, the hydrophilic wire is exchanged for a 0.035 in. Teflon wire and angioplasty is performed using an appropriate size balloon. In the RC AVFs we generally use 4 and 5 mm balloons. In the BC AVFs we use 6 and 7 mm balloons in the juxta anastomotic segment (JAS), and larger sized balloons depending upon the diameter of the nearest normal vein.

We tend to keep the balloons inflated for longer durations (90–180 s), as this helps to better mould the stenosis and reduces elastic recoil [9]. The initial balloon of choice is a complaint balloon ,which we may inflate to beyond burst pressure in some resistant cases. However, if on completion of angiogram the residual stenosis is more than 30%, we prefer using a high pressure balloon, rather than a cutting balloon to completely efface the stenosis [10, 11]. We follow this strategy due to cost constraints within our practice model.

If the vein should rupture we use balloon tamponade technique to help seal the leak. In only exceptional cases do we deploy a stent to salvage the vein [12]. In our population, we have found that stents do not do as well in the long run, and the repeat intervention rate as a result of in-stent restenosis is quite high.

In some RC AVFs where the AV anastomosis is at a very acute angle, crossing the stenosis from the venous approach is near impossible. In these cases, we access the brachial artery at the elbow antegradely using US guidance with a 21G micropuncture needle, and insert only the inner 3 Fr dilator of the exchange sheath. Through the dilator we use a 0.018 in. hydrophilic wire to cross the AV anastomosis and stenosis. This wire is then brought out through the venous access sheath, and once through and through body floss access is obtained, all intervention is performed from the venous approach. Thus the arterial access is kept to smallest French size, thereby reducing the risk of damage to the brachial artery and its distal circulation. We however do not perform the transradial approach for treatment of dysfunctional fistulas [13, 14]. Following the intervention, the access sheaths are removed and hemostasis achieved by placement of purse string sutures which are removed on discharge.

Complex Interventions

In our experience, when patients present with dysfunctional AVFs, several lesions are usually uncovered, many of which can be of high grade stenosis. It is not uncommon that to deal with all the lesions, at least two access sites are required, using both the retrograde and antegrade approaches.

Long segment cephalic vein occlusions are seen in patients with RC and BC AVFs. These may occur early after formation of the AVF resulting in non maturation. However, they may also be seen in mature AVFs, and are identified by the presence of multiple draining veins in the forearm and over the dorsum of the wrist. As most of our patients are young when dialysis is initiated and cadaveric transplant lists are long, we are very aggressive in recanalizing these long segment occlusions and salvaging the AVFs (see Fig. 21.1).

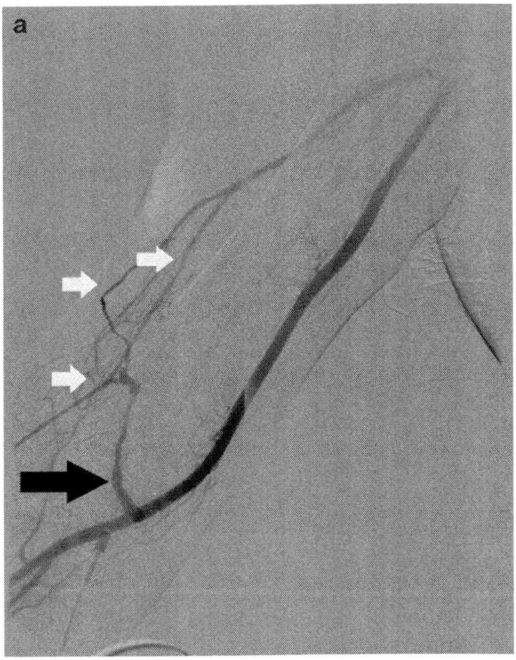

Fig. 21.1 (**a**, **b**) Fistulogram in a non-functioning right BC arteriovenous fistula (AVF) shows patent juxta-anastomotic segment (JAS) cephalic vein (*black arrow*) beyond which the cephalic vein is occluded in its entire length.

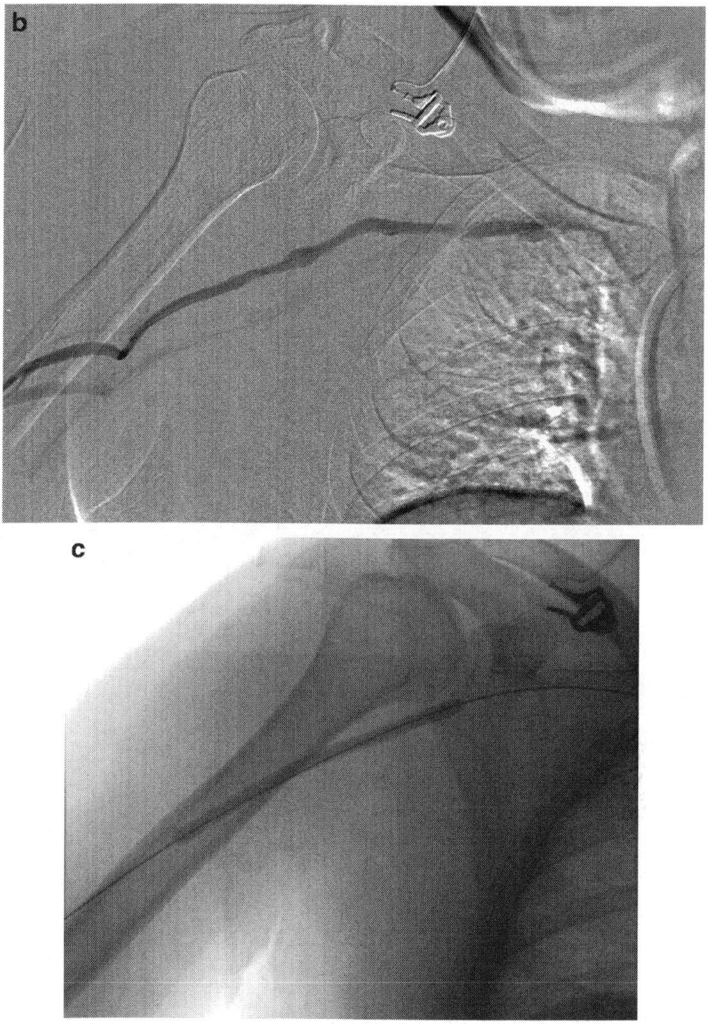

Fig. 21.1 (continued) There are multiple collaterals (*white arrows*) seen in the arm and there is reflux of contrast into the brachial artery. (**c**) Following antegrade puncture of the patent JAS, the occluded vein was recanalized and angioplastied with a 6×100 mm balloon. (**d**, **e**) Post intervention angiogram shows a widely patent cephalic vein with disappearance of the collateral veins

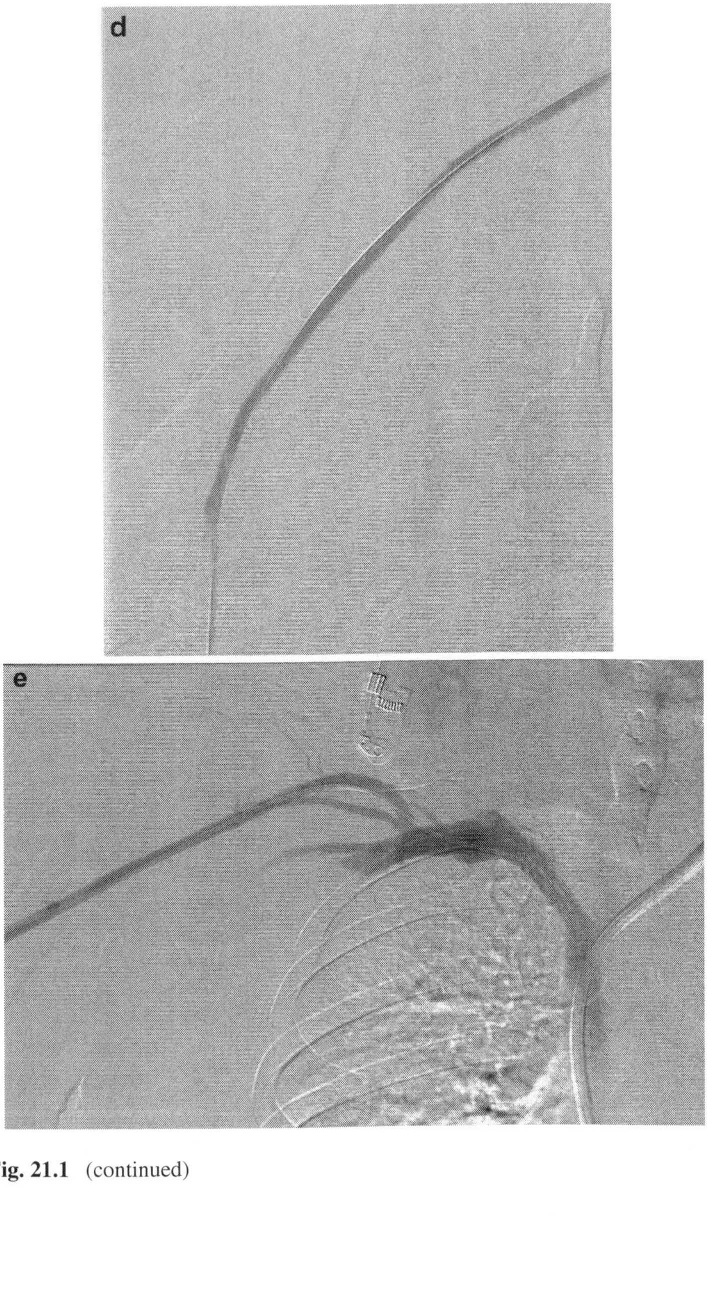

Fig. 21.1 (continued)

Following a fistulogram, the AVF is usually accessed antegradely, but retrograde access in the patent arm vein can also be utilized. After insertion of a sheath, using a 4 Fr Berenstein or C2 catheter and a 0.035 or 0.018 in. hydrophilic wire, the site of the occlusion is probed, and the catheter and wire manipulated along the expected path of the cephalic vein. In attempted recanalizations, venous perforations can occur, especially when a tiny branch vein is catheterized. If necessary, both antegrade and retrograde approaches are utilized simultaneously. With perseverance, it is possible to find the intraluminal path and recanalize the vein in the majority of cases. Once we have crossed the occlusion and the catheter is within the patent central veins (subclavian or brachiocephalic), then the entire segment is dilated. We use a 4 or 5 mm diameter, 10 cm length balloon at the initial angioplasty to minimize venous rupture. Once flow is re-established, a patent AVF will further aid in maturation of the vein. All patients are followed up in the clinic after a month to assess the AVF. If required, another intervention is organized, and at this session further upsizing of the balloon is performed similar to sequential balloon dilatation.

Thrombosed AVFs

As compared with AVGs, AVFs have a lower rate of thrombosis. Native veins due to their capacitance nature are able to withstand much slower rates of blood flow in response to a high grade stenosis before thrombosing. As per the KDOQI guidelines, it is easier to treat patent AVFs than thrombosed ones with outcomes for patent AVFs being much better. Strategies in managing occluded AVFs have been developed by other Asian centers [15, 16]. More recently, we have also been aggressively treating thrombosed AVFs, and only abandon the access following an adequate attempt at thrombolysis and angioplasty.

We use a combination of pharmacological thrombolysis (catheter directed pulse spray thrombolysis using urokinase) in conjunction with mechanical balloon maceration of the thrombus, with treatment of the underlying stenosis with angioplasty [17]. Pure mechanical thrombectomy using thrombectomy devices [18] also provides good results but as these devices are expensive, we generally use the pharmacological means. In patients in whom access is precious, surgical thrombectomy in combination with angioplasty is performed in the interventional suites. Thrombolysis in AVFs is challenging, as the presence of large thrombosed aneurysms makes complete clearing of thrombus almost near impossible. If adequate flow is reestablished through the AVF, with residual thrombus in the aneurysms, we accept the result and send the patient for dialysis and keep them anticoagulated (see Fig. 21.2). The amelioration of the stenosis and presence of flow through the AVF prevents further formation of thrombus and allows the body's natural mechanisms to resolve the thrombus.

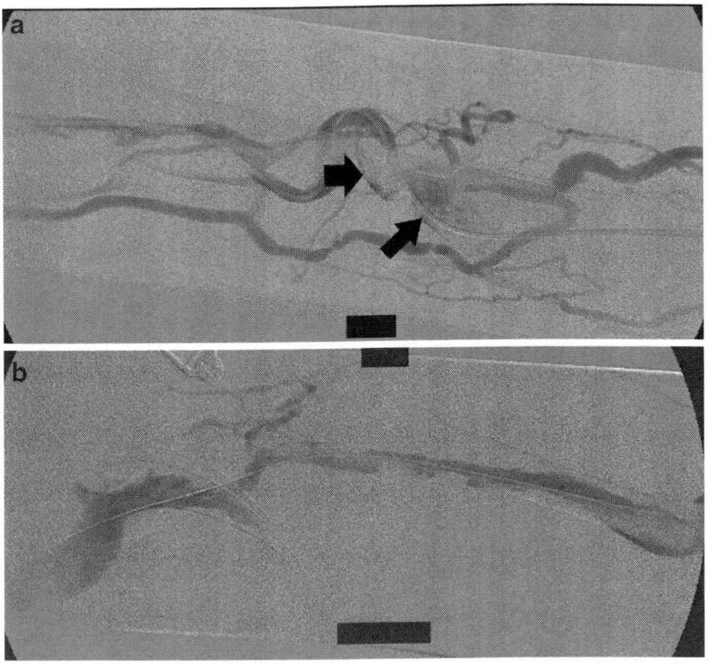

Fig. 21.2 (**a**) Fistulogram of a thrombosed left BC AVF shows no flow and multiple thrombi (*black arrows*) within the tortuous draining cephalic vein. (**b**) Following pulse spray thrombolysis and mechanical clot maceration using balloon angioplasty, final angiogram shows restoration of flow across the fistula but with residual clot within the vein. This was macerated with balloon angioplasty. (**c**) One year post intervention, the fistula is widely patent

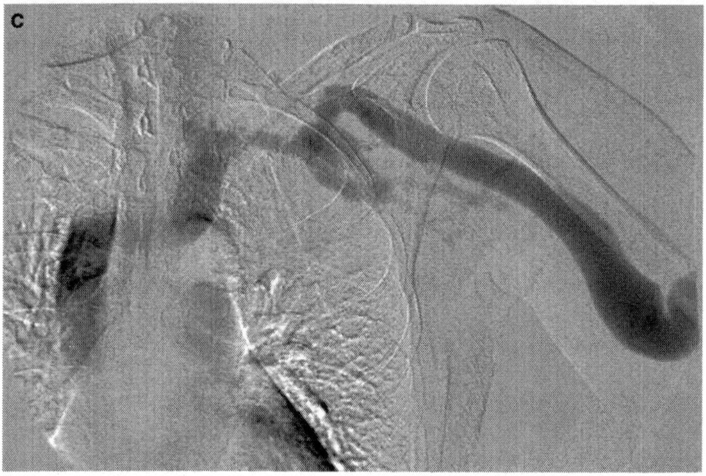

Fig. 21.2 (continued)

Central Vein Lesions

Central vein stenosis or occlusion presents with arm swelling, high venous pressures during dialysis, or increased bleeding following removal of dialysis needles. Recanalization of central vein occlusions can be very challenging and we use both the groin and arm approach. Crossing the occlusion is usually easier from the arm approach. We use a 4 Fr catheter (Berenstein or Cobra 2) with a 0.035 in. straight Teflon or a 0.035 in. stiff hydrophilic wire to cross the occlusion. We generally use 12–14 mm balloons to dilate the occlusion/stenosis and maintain balloon inflation for 3 min. Elastic recoil in the central veins can result in suboptimal angioplasty results, and repeated balloon inflation is utilized. We accept up to 50% residual stenosis in the central veins following angioplasty.

In our practice, we perform surveillance venography every 3 months in these patients. If there is significant restenosis, angioplasty is performed. This strategy helps maintain patency and allows for reintervention before the central veins completely occlude (see Fig. 21.3). We reserve stenting of central veins for patients in whom recurrence of symptoms is within 3 months, with repeat occlusion of the veins or in whom there is severe elastic recoil following angioplasty.

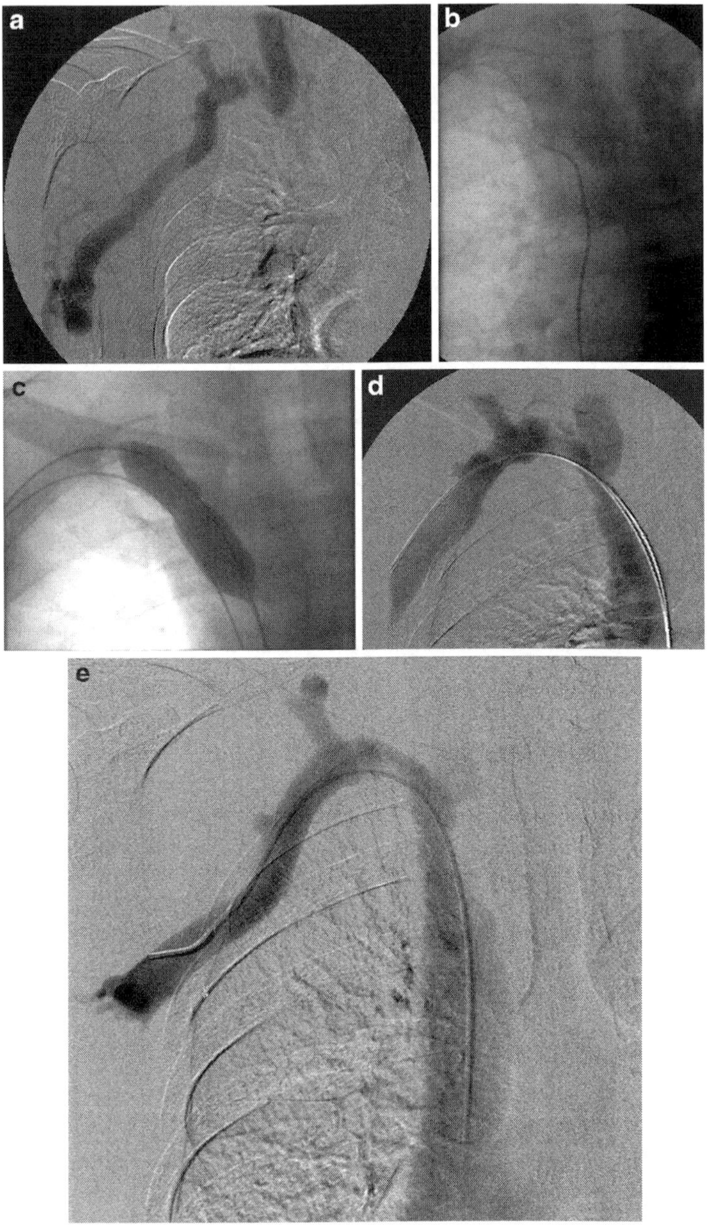
a
b
c
d
e

Particular Features of Our Patient Population

We performed an analysis of 217 consecutive patients who presented with dysfunctional AVFs from January 2009 to May 2009. The majority of the patients had RC AVFs (55%), while 33% had BC AVFs and 11% had BBT AVFs, with 81% being on the left upper limb. Multiple stenotic lesions were seen in 40% of this cohort, with multiplicity being more common in the upper arm BC and BBT AVFs.

RC AVFs tended to have a single lesion centered at the JAS. In our cohort, lesion distribution was similar to that described in a Western population by Rajan et al. [19]. In RC AVFs, 68% of the lesions were in the JAS including the AV anastomosis with 17% noted in the outflow mid forearm cephalic vein and only 8% in the central veins. In the BC AVFs, 34% were noted in the JAS, 28% in the outflow cephalic vein, 27% in the cephalic arch and 18% in the central veins. In BBT AVFs the JAS and the mid arm swing point were found to be sites of stenosis (38 and 41% respectively). Central vein stenosis was also noted in 26% of these patients.

In this cohort, a total of 447 interventions were performed in the same dialysis year to help maintain patency. We mainly used 4 and 5 mm compliant balloons in the RC AVFs, while 6 to 8 mm compliant balloons were used in the BC and BBT AVFs. In the central veins we used 12 to 15 mm compliant balloons. We reserved the use of high pressure and cutting balloons in patients who had poor outcome following balloon angioplasty with compliant balloons (16%).

It is not surprising to find that the lesion distribution for AVFs in our cohort of patients is no different from that of a Western population. However, it should be noted that there was a higher incidence of multiple lesions in our patient population (40% vs. 26%) when compared with the study by Rajan et al. Our analysis also showed

Fig. 21.3 Patient with right BBT AVF presenting with arm swelling. (**a**) Fistulogram demonstrates complete occlusion of the right brachiocephalic vein (BCV), with multiple collaterals and reflux into the right internal jugular vein. (**b**) The right BCV occlusion being crossed via the groin and arm approach. (**c**) The lesion is dilated via the groin approach with a 15×40 mm balloon. (**d**) Final angiogram shows a patent right BCV. (**e**) With surveillance venography and PTA every 3 months, the right BCV is still patent after 4 years without the need for insertion of a stent

clearly that we were dealing with a smaller caliber of vessels, which naturally is more challenging when it comes to intervention. This is not only due to the smaller Asian body habitus, but also contributed significantly by the high prevalence of diabetes.

Conclusion

In conclusion, hemodialysis interventions in the Asian population can be challenging due to the relatively small size of the vessels, multiplicity of lesions, multiple co-morbid conditions, and poor patient compliance. The distribution of lesions in the various AVFs is the same as described by other authors. As the age of onset of dialysis is younger than in the West and with a relative paucity of transplant organs, we tend to be more aggressive and perform more interventions to maintain AVF patency. Balloon angioplasty remains the mainstay of our interventional strategy as cost considerations temper the use of new expensive devices.

Key Points

- Vessel sizes are smaller in the Asian population
- Pathology is similar to the North American population

References

1. Sixth report of the Singapore Renal Registry 2005/2006. Choong Hui Lin (2008). Singapore: Ministry of Health.
2. Tan CC, Chan CM, Ho CK, et al. Health economics of renal replacement therapy: perspectives from Singapore. Kidney Int. 2005;67(S94):S19–22.
3. National Kidney Foundation. KDOQI clinical practice guidelines and clinical practice recommendations for 2006 updates: hemodialysis adequacy, peritoneal dialysis adequacy and vascular access. Am J Kidney Dis. 2006;48 Suppl 1:S1–322.
4. Yap HY, Robless PA, Lee JC, et al. Managing venous stenosis in vascular access for hemodialysis. Singapore Med J. 2007;48(1):6–10.
5. Dember LM, Beck GJ, Allon M, et al. Effect of clopidogrel on early failure of arteriovenous fistulas for hemodialysis: a randomized control trial. JAMA. 2008;299:2164–71.

6. Allon M, Lockhart MP, Lilly RZ, et al. Effect of preoperative sonographic monitoring on vascular access outcomes in hemodialysis patients. Kidney Int. 2001;60:2013–20.
7. Miller GA, Goel N, Khariton A, et al. Aggressive approach to salvage non-maturing arterivenous fistulas: a retrospective study and follow up. J Vasc Access. 2009;10(3):183–91.
8. Hong HP, Kim SK. Usefulness of percutaneous intervention with transarterial approach in the salvage of non maturing native fistulas, status post trans-venous approach failure: transarterial approach in the salvage of non maturing native fistulas. Cardiovasc Interv Radiol. 2009;32(6):1252–6.
9. Forauer A, Hoffer EK, Homa K. Dialysis access venous stenosis: treatment with balloon angioplasty – 1 versus 3 minute inflation time. Radiology. 2008;249(1):375–81.
10. Trerotola SO, Kwak A, Clark TW, et al. Prospective study of balloon inflation pressures and other technical aspects of hemodialysis access angioplasty. J Vasc Interv Radiol. 2005;16(12):1613.
11. Wu CC, Lin MC, Pu SY, et al. Comparison of cutting balloon versus high pressure balloon angioplasty for resistant venous stenoses of native hemodialysis fistulas. J Vasc Interv Radiol. 2008;19(6):877–83.
12. Rajan DK, Clark TW, Patel NK, et al. Prevalance and treatment of cephalic arch stenosis in dysfunctional autogenous hemodialysis fistulas. J Vasc Interv Radiol. 2003;14(5):567–73.
13. Wang HJ, Yang YF. Percutaneous treatment of dysfunctional Brescia-Cimino fostulae through a radial arterial approach. Am J Kidney Dis. 2006;18(4):652–8.
14. Lin YS, Li PC, Hsu JT. Feasibility of trans-radial approach in percutaneous interventions for upper arm dialysis access. Semin Dial. 2008;21(6):567–74.
15. Miyayama S, Matsui O, Taki K, et al. Occluded Brescia-Cimino hemodialysis fistulas: endovascular treatment with both brachial arterial and venous access using the pull-through technique. Cardiovasc Interv Radiol. 2005;28:806–12.
16. Liang HL, Pan HB, Chung HM, et al. Restoration of thrombosed Brescia-Cimino dialysis fistulas by using percutaneous transluminal angioplasty. Radiology. 2002;223:339–44.
17. Rajan DK, Clark TW, Simons ME, et al. Procedural success and patency after percutaneous treatment of thrombosed autogenous arteriovenous dialysis fistulas. J Vasc Interv Radiol. 2002;13(12):1211–8.
18. Shatsky JB, Berns JS, Clark TW, et al. Single centre experience with Arrow-Trerotola Percutaneous Thrombectomy Device in the management of thrombosed native dialysis fistulas. J Vasc Interv Radiol. 2005;16(12):1605.
19. Rajan DK, Bunston S, Misra S, et al. Dysfunctional autogenous hemodialysis fistulas: outcomes after angioplasty – are there clinical predictors of patency. Radiology. 2004;232(2):508–15.

Chapter 22
Pediatric Hemodialysis Interventions

Bairbre Connolly

Introduction

Background

Renal failure in children is uncommon. However, both the incidence and prevalence of end stage renal disease (ESRD) in pediatric patients is increasing worldwide. A previously quoted incident figure of 8.6/million population in 1980 has risen to 14.1/million in 2004. The prevalence has also risen from 28.3 to 81.1/million population [1]. Additional data from the UK suggests a prevalence of 69 children, aged 1–4 years/million age related population [2].

The etiologies of renal failure in children are very different to those in adults. In our institution, of children with ESRD coming to transplant, the most common diagnoses include glomerular disease (26%), obstruc-

B. Connolly (✉)
Pediatric Interventional Radiologist,
Department of Diagnostic Imaging, The Hospital for Sick Children;

Associate Professor,
Earl Glenwood Coulson Chair, Medical Imaging Department,
University of Toronto, Toronto, Ontario, Canada
e-mail: bairbre.connolly@sickkids.ca

D.K. Rajan (ed.), *Essentials of Percutaneous Dialysis Interventions*,
DOI 10.1007/978-1-4419-5657-6_22,

© Springer Science+Business Media, LLC 2011

tive uropathies (16%), hypoplastic/dysplastic diseases (16%), hereditary disease (15%) systemic diseases (9%), vascular diseases (3%) and miscellaneous causes (14%) (personal communication). The spectrum of disease entities differs amongst the younger child as compared to the older child, e.g., more boys with obstructive uropathies in the early years, and more girls with acquired diseases in the later years.

General Pediatric Considerations

As the survival of children with ESRD improves, it is important to pay attention to the sequelae (short and long term) of both the disease and its treatment. The old adage that "children are not just small adults" is particularly true in terms of management of the child with ESRD, and differs significantly in several aspects compared to adults [3–5]. Growth and nutrition are important aspects of children with ESRD, with short stature common, and protein malnutrition problematic. Supplemental nutrition through a G tube is commonly required, in order for a child to gain sufficient weight to be considered for transplant, and/or to counteract the nutritional demands of dialysis [4, 6–8]. Optimizing the timing of immunizations and use/avoidance of specific vaccinations is important [3]. Adolescence is difficult for many healthy children, but in children with ESRD compliance in terms of drugs, dialysis, and psychosocial problems are well recognized issues. School days lost are significant in terms of long term education and subsequent job opportunities [3]. The presence of catheters (peritoneal dialysis, central venous lines) creates both physical and psychological problems for children and adolescents. Graduation/transitioning to an adult facility from a pediatric nephrology program also requires attention to ensure continuity of care and ease of patient and family adjustment. Given the longer life expectancy of children, use of veins for all types of venous access carries with it potential for occlusion, stenoses, and collaterals. Such occlusions may have significant negative impact further along in the course of their disease for those who are being considered for, or require, an AV fistula. This is especially true for peripherally inserted central catheters (PICCs). Use of PICCs have become a mainstay of intravenous therapies in pediatrics in general, but their use is associated with acquired venous stenoses and thromboses. In a child with renal problems, this may negatively affect the possibility of creating and maintaining AV fistulae later in life [5].

Renal Replacement Therapy in Children

Management approach to the child with renal failure depends on several factors: the child's age, as well as the acuteness or chronicity of the renal failure. Transplant is the ideal management for children with ESRD. However, given the shortage of organs and the challenges of size in the young child, bridging or long term peritoneal dialysis (PD) or hemodialysis (HD) is frequently required [5, 9]. Choice of method of dialysis is also partly dependant on local expertise (surgical, interventional radiology), patient's age and weight, and expected duration to transplant.

Age

In the child <2 years of age, all forms of dialysis are challenging. Maintenance of dialysis catheters (PD or HD) in the child under 2 years old is difficult, and is associated with a higher incidence of catheter related problems and cumulative morbidity [10]. In the under two's, PD is considered the ideal [5, 11]. Even still, PD is associated with peritonitis, catheter displacement, and leakage. Hemodialysis is considered if/when the PD fails, if PD is contraindicated, and if awaiting transplant in the short term. Difficulties with HD in the young child pertain to the small vessel size, line blockage, low blood flows, clotting of the dialysis circuit, as well as the need to prime the circuit with blood products because of the relative proportions of the child's circulation volume to the extracorporeal circuit. There is a high incidence of catheter revisions and infections [4]. In addition, the cumulative morbidity of dialysis in children under 2 years of age, involves not just the problems arising from their dialysis catheters, but also other systemic comorbidities such as anemia, malnutrition, immunity, and effects of other congenital anomalies.

In the older child, whereas PD will preserve central veins, the efficacy of HD may be considered better than PD in terms of urea clearance. Multiple factors (e.g., long distances from the hospital) may influence the decision to opt for PD instead of HD [5, 11].

Hemodialysis

Hemodialysis can be achieved through central venous catheters, or more ideally by creation of an AV fistulae or AV graft. Unfortunately as in adults, the majority of children (over 80%) undergo HD through central venous catheters, despite the Pediatric Fistula First initiative [12]. There are compelling arguments supporting the use of fistulae, so as to preserve central vessels, avoid catheter related blood stream infections and thromboses, and an enhanced quality of life [13]. Despite some isolated individual institutional successes with the creation of AV fistulae in children, even as small as 15 kg, there remains a very low percentage of children who undergo hemodialysis through an AV fistula, in the order of 7% [14]. Given the recognized increase in morbidity, mortality, and financial costs associated with catheter related infections, thromboses and other adverse sequelae, there is a strong argument in favor of hemodialysis through an AV fistula [13]. On the other hand, there are major concerns regarding maintaining patency of fistulae in small vessels, pain of needle insertion for each dialysis, and especially the lack of surgical expertise amongst pediatric surgeons for microscope-assisted vascular anastamosis [14, 15]. The latter is a major limitation worldwide. As a consequence of all these issues, the majority of children who require dialysis are maintained on hemodialysis through central venous catheters (80–90%). The bulk of this chapter therefore will deal with the placement and management of CVCs in children, and highlight the points of difference from adult HD [16–18].

Once the decision is made to perform hemodialysis, the choice of catheter depends on the expected duration of dialysis as well as the patient's age/size. Hemodialysis is achieved through a variety of catheters placed usually in the jugular veins, and occasionally in the femoral veins (acute temporary HD). Table 22.1 outlines some possible options for choice of catheters used in our institution, and from personal communication from other institutions. The choice is determined by the flow rate required during hemodialysis. This in turn is calculated based on such parameters as the child's weight and is based on the urea clearance of 2/3/4/5 ml/min/kg body weight as well as net and maximum ultrafiltration. In the smaller child, the challenge therefore is for the vessel to be of adequate size to accommodate a relatively large hemodialysis catheter, to maintain patency of the vessel around the line, and to achieve adequate flows during dialysis.

Table 22.1 Examples of Hemodialysis catheters used in children for HD (SickKids and other institutions)

Uncuffed, non tunneled, temporary HD		Cuffed tunneled long term HD	
Patient weight (kg)	Line	Patient weight (kg)	Line
<5	Gam-Cath 6.5 Fr	<5	8 Fr Medcomp 2×5 Fr Single lumen catheters
5–15	Gam-Cath 8 Fr, 15 cm	5–20	10 Fr Medcomp Split Cath
15–35	10 Fr Quinton Mahurkar	20–35	Pediatric Quinton Permcath
>35	11.5 Fr Quinton Mahurkar	>35	Adult Quinton Permcath

These challenges pose problems from a technical point of view, a manufacturing perspective of suitable catheters, as well as for the dialysis team and machines.

IR Procedures in Children

Pediatric IR Suite

In our institution, all hemodialysis lines are placed by pediatric interventional radiologists in an interventional radiology (IR) suite. For the safe performance of IR procedures in children, the suite must be appropriately equipped to handle children [19]. For the purpose of placing HD lines, the rooms should be capable of meeting the standards for a strict sterile procedure (e.g., operating room standards). The equipment should include a tilting table, ultrasound with high frequency probe (e.g., hockey stick 15 MHz probe), fluoroscopic equipment capable of pulsed fluoroscopy (e.g., 3 or 7.5 pulses/s), with preset pediatric programs, and depending on the type/generation of equipment with a removable grid for children <20 kg. Radiation protection for the child and the operator is very important: low pulse fluoroscopy, last image hold, good shielding as the operator is closer to the source than in an adult, and hands may inadvertently be in the primary beam [20–24].

Option for sedation or anesthesia varies from institution to institution and largely depends on available anesthesiologists, local expertise for sedation, and regulatory requirements [19, 25–27]. If sedation is used, it should be provided by someone with the knowledge, skill and judgment to provide safe pediatric sedation and airway rescue. Many jurisdictions require PALS certification (see Table 22.3). The rooms must be equipped with anesthetic capabilities as the younger child will not be able to cooperate, and in many centers, including our own, the large dialysis lines are inserted with the child under some form of anesthesia. The choice of anesthesia is at the discretion of the attending anesthesiologist (e.g., full intubation, laryngeal mask, intravenous propofol) and depending on the type of line required (e.g., tunneled cuffed CVL, temporary femoral line, prior history of lines and occlusions etc.). The suites must therefore be equipped with all the different devices which the anesthesiologist may require (e.g., full range of sizes of endotracheal tubes, laryngoscopes, BP cuffs, ECG leads (neonatal and child), and capnography monitoring capabilities etc.). In addition, the suite should be equipped with a pediatric crash cart [19]. Warming equipment for smaller children is very important as the infant easily becomes hypothermic in IR procedure suites (e.g., Bair Hugger, Arizant Inc.) [19, 28]. The suites also need to carry a variety of sized wires, dilators, and peel-away sheaths to support placement of lines of all sizes for children of all weights (from 2 kg up to full adult size).

In addition to the IR suite itself, it is important to have nurses and technologists who are experienced in dealing with children. A pediatric suitable ambience is important for the provision of family centered care [19].

Technique of Catheter Placement in Children

Consent

Prior to any catheter placement, informed consent is obtained from the parents, and/or the child if of sufficient age to understand the procedure. In many jurisdictions there is no lower limit of age for legal consent. In practice, it is usually the parents who sign the consent form, but it is extremely important that the child is involved, at some level appropriate to their age and maturity and gives a verbal assent to proceed. The consent process in pediatrics is frequently lengthy and requires a detailed and thorough conversation with the parents.

In general, it can be more time consuming than with an adult, largely due to parental anxiety in their role as substitute decision makers for their child. The risks outlined include bleeding, infection, clotting, perforation, arterial puncture, pneumothorax, air embolism, clotting, poor flows despite adequate line position, arrhythmias, and pain/discomfort. We find the use of preprinted consent forms and information pamphlets very helpful for the stressed parent.

Preprocedure Blood Work

Pre-procedural blood work obtained includes a full blood count, coagulation screen, and electrolytes. It is important to be aware that in the neonate that the normal coagulation parameters vary with gestational age (see Table 22.2). The parameters we choose as acceptable limits include platelets ≤75, INR and PTT according to age [29]. The use of DDAVP prior to an invasive procedure in children with chronic renal failure, remains controversial and the evidence weak, but it is our practice to give DDAVP 30–60 min prior to an invasive procedure (e.g., renal biopsy, CVL placement) to promote platelet adhesiveness (Table 22.3) [30–32].

Technique

The procedure is performed in a strictly sterile manner. The patient is placed supine on the IR table with head down tilt, −3° to −4° of Trendelenburg. The jugular veins are examined with ultrasound (15 MHz) to ensure patency of the internal jugular veins. If both veins are patent, our first choice is the right internal jugular vein.

Table 22.2 Normal hematology parameters

Age	Hemoglobin (g/L)	Platelets ($\times 10^9$/L)	APTT (s)	INR
<6 Days	150–220	150–400	25–53	0.9–1.6
7–30 Days	140–200	150–400	25–53	0.9–1.6
<3 Months	90–135	150–400	25–53	0.9–1.6
>3 Months	100–140	150–400	23–35	0.9–1.1
5–13 Years	120–160	150–400	23–35	0.9–1.1
>13 Years	Adult values	Adult values	Adult values	Adult values

Table 22.3 Commonly used drug dosages in children (SickKids practice in IR)

Agent	Dosage
Lidocaine 1%	0.5 cc/kg
Marcaine 0.25%	1 cc/kg (max 10 cc)
Heparin 100 units/mL	<15 kg = 10 units/kg, diluted with normal saline to 1.5 mL/each lumen
	>15 kg = 1.5 mL/each lumen
Contrast (e.g., Omnipaque 300)	3 mL/kg in one bolus
	6 mL/kg over longer period time
DDAVP	0.3 μg/kg IV, 30–60 min prior
Fentanyl	1 μg/kg IV, max three doses for IR team administration
Midazolam	0.05 mg/kg IV, max three doses for IR team administration
Ketamine	0.25 mg/kg IV slowly, max three doses for IR team administration
Morphine	0.05 mg/kg IV, max q 4 hourly
Acetaminophen	15 mg/kg PO, max q 6 hourly

Other choices include left internal jugular, right or left external jugular. This area is prepped with 2% Chlorhexidine solution. In a neonate requiring hemodialysis, a weaker (0.5% Chlorhexidine) solution is used given the sensitivity of the newborn skin. The prepared area should be wide, extending from the level of the chin and down to below the level of the nipple, as the length of the external tunnel (which is dictated by the fixed length of the HD catheter) may need to be relatively quite long. It is not our practice to give routine prophylactic antibiotics. The area is then draped in the usual fashion. Adhesive drapes are useful in children because of the small surface area available for non-adhesive drapes to stay in position. They are not recommended in premature neonates, as the adhesive may remove fragile skin when the drapes are lifted.

Local anesthetic is used, either short or long acting (see Table 22.3). Using a 15 MHz hockey stick probe, the jugular vein is punctured at a level just above the clavicle. Punctures in the small child are usually performed with a micro-puncture technique and an 0.018 in. wire, subsequently upsized to an 0.035 in. wire. In the bigger child, the puncture can be made with a 19G needle, followed by an 0.035 in. wire. The puncture may be from an anterior or a lateral approach to the jugular vein. The wire is then advanced down into the SVC and right atrium. In the small child because of the short distances of the chest, it is helpful to advance the wire further into the IVC to provide better purchase, stability and support, for when it comes to dilatation.

Given the varying sizes of children it is important then to measure the tunnel accurately. As the catheters come in a variety of fixed lengths, the entry site on the chest wall will be determined by the position of the central tip. This can be measured using the floppy 0.018 in. wire centrally and subtracting the inner wire length from the total length of the catheter (tip to cuff). Alternatively, it can be estimated using fluoroscopy as a guide, by laying the catheter over the chest wall and planning the entry point of the tunnel according to the position of the cuff on the skin. The exit site is created ensuring that the nipple and rudimentary breast bud is avoided. This is especially important in young girls. In some instances the length of the external portion of the catheter may be relatively long for a small child and require the exit site to be lateral and inferior to the breast/nipple.

The tunnel is created using the provided tunneling device that comes with the kit, or an individually packaged tunneling device. To avoid damage to the tip of the larger catheters ,we sometimes will use an Argyle chest tube to tunnel with the staggered end lodged within the chest tube. To avoid an acute angle at the neck, it is our practice is to create an exaggerated square tunnel advancing from the chest entry site, cranially to the middle or lateral third of clavicle, and only then turning medially at the level of the neck incision. The catheter is then externalized through the neck incision. Once the catheter is pulled into the tunnel, the ultimate shape creates a broad, wide, smooth arc.

The appropriately sized dilator and/or peel away sheath is placed over the wire. On removal of the wire and inner introducer of the peel away sheath, it is our practice to use a hemostat on the sheath to prevent blood loss and air embolism [33, 34]. Newer valved sheaths may be provided with some lines. General anesthesia with positive pressure ventilation and Trendelenburg are helpful measures to avoid air embolism. The catheter is advanced into the sheath, and once it reaches the clamp, the clamp is removed and the sheath opened by uncrimping the sheath in the opposite direction, and the catheter is advanced down into the SVC. It is important to be gentle and careful with peeling the sheath. The jugular vein in a child is quite superficial and the soft tissues fragile (sternocleidomastoid muscle very thin), so one must be careful when splitting the peel away to tear the sheath external to the vein/skin, and not actually tear the sheath within the vein. Tearing the vein itself leads to prolonged bleeding at the neck site. Once the catheter is successfully inserted fully into the vein the sheath is removed and pressure is applied.

The position is confirmed with fluoroscopy; it is our practice also to confirm with a small injection of contrast. The catheter tip should be at the cavoatrial junction, with the distal tip in the upper right atrium [35, 36]. The location of the SVC-RA junction can be difficult to determine in children with a wide mediastinum from a large thymus. The lower level of the right main bronchus, two vertebrae below the carina, or the T6–7 vertebral levels are useful landmarks (see Fig. 22.1). Any adjustments can be made to the length by pulling gently back the catheter, approximating the cuff closer to the entry site. In neonates or small children even minimal external traction (few millimeters) can make a big difference centrally [28].

The line is then heparinized. The dosage of heparin may vary from institution to institution. Our practice is to use 10 units/kg of 100 units/mL, up to 15 kg, and diluted to the required volume of the

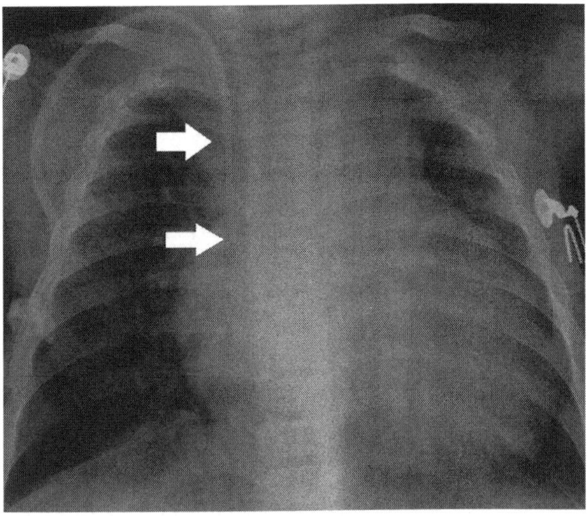

Fig. 22.1 Chest radiograph (PA) of an infant with a dual lumen dialysis line in situ through the right internal jugular vein. Note the large thymic shadow that can make it difficult to determine the position of the cavoatrial junction. Note also, the distance between the staggered ends of the line. The proximal tip (upper *arrow*) is high in the upper SVC. The distal tip (lower *arrow*) is at the upper border of the right main stem bronchus, in the distal SVC instead of the cavoatrial junction

lumen. Each lumen is individually heparinized (see Table 22.3). Over 15 kg, we use 1.5 mL of 100 units/mL (usually suffices for the volume specified on the catheter). Some centers use tPA to maintain the patency of their lines, others use an alcohol lock [37]. Usually one external dissolvable suture is placed in the neck. A second dissolvable suture is placed at the skin site making the entry site snug around the catheter and cuff. A sterile transparent dressing is then applied. An important part of the procedure in children is securing the catheter on completion of the procedure. Securement is problematic in children who will pull and tug on their lines unintentionally. Two nonabsorbable monofilament sutures applied to the wings of the catheter are helpful additional supports. The use of various securing devices (StatLock or Duoderm) may be helpful. Newer StatLock devices with a bridging component designed for dual lumen catheters have proven very useful in securing dual lumen catheters in our patient population.

Discharge

Post procedure, the children are observed for 3–4 h, until ready for discharge (awake, stable, drinking/able to maintain hydration). Observation includes monitoring of vitals and observation of the site for bleeding and swelling. Pain relief is given as required (Table 22.3). Inpatients are seen once by the IR team later in the day post procedure. Outpatients are seen by IR prior to discharge home. They are given a discharge pamphlet with discharge instructions. A follow up phone call is made by the IR clinic nurse the following day.

Challenges: Tricks of the Trade

Skin Turgor

The soft chubby skin of the neck in an infant or toddler can be difficult to puncture without loosing all visibility on ultrasound or without using excessive force. A simple tip is to look with ultrasound, decide on your spot for puncture, leave down the ultrasound, lift up the skin with your non dominant hand and pierce it with the needle, then resume sonographic guidance with the tip already below the skin. In addition, their skin has a significant stretch/elastic quality to it. After placing a line, this elasticity can cause a marked shift of the line in the tunnel, advancing inwards (becomes too long) or advancing outwards (becomes too short) as the line moves within the fatty subcutaneous tunnel.

Stagger

In small children the distance between the proximal and distal ends of a staggered catheter can be too long. It may be impossible to have both ends optimally placed, i.e., proximal one may be at the cavoatrial junction but the distal end then too low in the right atrium/IVC; alternatively the distal end may be appropriately in the upper right atrium, but the proximal one in the upper SVC/innominate vein preventing good flows (see Fig. 22.1). In some situations the operator may be forced/obliged to trim the distal staggered end to make it more appropriate especially in the neonate. NOTE: This is not a manufacturer recommendation, and may influence the recirculation rate. The issue of line length is further compounded by the child's growth - as the child grows the thorax elongates and the line becomes too short as is seen in Figure. 22.1.

Blood Loss in Children

The neonate/infant's entire blood volume is approximately 80–100 mL/kg, so bleeding or oozing when placing catheters must be kept to a minimum (Table 22.4). It behoves the interventionalist or assistant to apply digital pressure as much as possible at the neck and chest site throughout the procedure, and to use a clamp technique on the sheath or equivalent (e.g., use of newer valved sheaths) to minimize blood loss.

Choice of Line

It is important to know what volumes of flows are required for HD and what type of line is used in your institution. Our current practice is shown in the table provided, along with some choices from other

Table 22.4 Estimated blood volumes of children

Age	Total blood volume
Neonate <1 month	100 mL/kg
Infant and children	80 mL/kg
Adolescent	71–75/kg

Total blood volume (TBV) – The amount of blood in the whole body, both cells and fluid. The volume of the patient's blood is based on the patient's non edematous weight. The normal blood volume varies with age of the child.

institutions, as the choice of line varies from center to center. There is a dearth of suitable devices for the smaller child, as the pediatric market has limited financial appeal for the manufacturer. Necessity sometimes prompts one to think outside the box and use devices in an Off Label manner sometimes e.g., Dual lumen Vortex ports for certain pheresis, use of Power PICCs (e.g., 6 Fr) for dialysis in a brittle neonate. Any Off Label use must be explained to the parents. Clearance within the institution with Risk Management or submission under an submission under an Innovative Policy may be required.

Patency of Veins

Use of central veins for placement of relatively large catheters in the young child frequently results in subsequent occlusions of those veins. This becomes a major challenge in the child in whom peritoneal dialysis fails and who needs ongoing renal replacement therapy. Alternative sites such as hepatic veins, translumbar, femoral, and IVC lines have similar challenges in children as in adults.

Securement

Securing any line/device in a child is quite a challenge, as they have a tendency to pull out lines, or for them to become inadvertently dislodged, with normal childhood activity. Tape, sutures, and securing devices are all useful. Parental and nursing vigilance is however paramount.

Wires

In small babies, the length of the floppy component of the micro-puncture wire is frequently so long such that the floppy part extends from the bottom of the right atrium to the jugular vein. There is then insufficient support for dilatation, unless the wire is advanced in to the IVC. So it is helpful to negotiate into the IVC, if possible in the smaller child.

Line too Long

Not infrequently, the line may be too long in the right atrium, but if there is no further length to pull back the catheter into the subcutaneous tunnel, we will occasionally make a linear slit at the exit site in line with the tunnel, and extend the tunnel by burying the cuff in the created space/slit.

Trouble Shooting

Central venous lines in children are fraught with many problems similar to their adult counterparts e.g., fibrin sheath, infection, thrombus formation, and poor flows [38]. Assessment of poorly functioning line (low flows, poor withdrawal, multiple alarms) requires a linogram to look for fibrin sheaths, ultrasound of veins to look for clots impeding inflow and sometimes a cardiac echo of the heart to look for atrial thrombus, and confirm tip position. Our experience with the use of fibrin stripping, balloon angioplasty of fibrin sheaths, and luminal brushing in children in attempts to save access and improve dialysis flows has been mixed [39]. Occasionally, a poorly functioning line must be exchanged or removed and replaced with another line, despite no abnormality detectable on imaging. It is our practice to empirically give tPA to those lines that have difficulty with aspiration, and to perform a linogram in those with persistent problems (to identify fibrin sheaths etc.). Much of this has been dealt with in other chapters.

When concern for thrombosis is raised, initial vascular assessment is performed in children with Doppler ultrasound of the upper central venous system. A digital subtraction venogram may be required in those children with further concerns for venous thromboses not detected by ultrasound. However, the radiation dose is not insignificant and we try to avoid it if possible [40]. Now with newer equipment and the capabilities of storing fluoroscopic runs, we may be able to avoid digital subtraction venography all together. Care with contrast volume is imperative in the smaller child (see Table 22.3) [41]. Central venous occlusions in children pose similar problems for dialysis access as they do in adults, with the additional caveat that the pediatric patient has an expected longer life span requiring renal replacement therapies [42].

AV Fistulae

AV fistulae are developed for children with ESRD and also for children with hemophilia requiring frequent critical but difficult venous access. Worldwide, the creation and use of AV fistulae in children with ESRD has not been widely adopted. This reflects a variety of factors: the paucity of pediatric surgeons with an interest/focus in microvascular surgical techniques; concern about primary and secondary patency rates in young children with small vessels; in many centers the lack of pediatric IRs to provide various salvage procedures for maintaining patency of an AV fistula; and the perceived difficulties of pain and anxiety with needle access of fistulae in children [14, 15, 43]. Despite these problems there are several pediatric centers which experience good success with AV fistulae [14, 44]. In 1998 Bagolan reported a 90% success with AV fistulae in children, including children <15 kg. With increasing use of microsurgical techniques results have improved, reducing the failure-to-mature rate from 30% to approximately 10%. Distal forearm fistulae in children >20 kg (radial-cephalic), elbow or upper arm (brachial-cephalic, or brachial-basilic) or lower limb (femoral-saphenous) in smaller children are all possibilities. Bourquelot in 2003 reported a 96% immediate patency of AV fistulae in 380 children (1–16 years; 4–48 kg) and a 24 month patency of 85% for radial-cephalic, 72% for brachial-basilic and 47% brachial-cephalic fistulae. In general, vessels of 3 mm in diameter are required and an oblique end-to-side anastomosis of 7–10 mm is created.

As pediatric radiologists we play a role pre and post fistula creation. Assessment of the vessels prior to the creation of the fistula may include detailed diagnostic ultrasound to assess patency, distensibility or elasticity, as well as arm or leg venography to exclude central stenoses or venous obstruction [45–48]. Once the fistula is created and mature (approximately 4 months), our role as interventionalists involves salvage procedures of thrombectomy, thrombolysis and/or angioplasty to optimize secondary patency rates. These salvage procedures are dealt with in detail in Chap. 17. In addition to the problems recognized to occur with fistulae in adults, limb growth disturbances may also occur in children.

Worldwide, there is a growing number of pediatric centers with microvascular surgical and interventional radiology expertise, so the prevalence of AV fistulae for dialysis may increase in the future, in line with the aim of the DOQI and Canadian guidelines for prevalence of AVF to reach 40–60% [48–50]. Experience in adults has shown that the creation of a multidisciplinary vascular access team optimizes the incidence, creation, maintenance, and salvage of AVFs. As pediatric interventional radiologists we can play a major role as members of such a multidisciplinary team [14, 49].

Key Points

- Hemodialysis is provided primarily by catheters for a number of patient and technical factors.
- Blood volumes in children are much smaller than in adults. Small blood loss volumes can be associated with significant morbidity.

Acknowledgment I wish to thank Mukesh Gajaria, Chief Technologist in the Dialysis / Apharesis Unit at SickKids, for his assistance.

References

1. US Renal Data System. USRDS 2006 Annual Report; Pediatric ESRD. Am J Kidney Dis. 2007;49 Suppl 1:S159–72.
2. Lewis MA, Shaw J, Sinha MD, et al. UK Renal Registry 12th Annual Report (December 2009): chapter 14: demography of the UK paediatric renal replacement therapy population in 2008. Nephron Clin Pract. 2010;115 Suppl 1:c279–88.

3. White CT, Trnka P, Matsell DG. Selected primary care issues and comorbidities in children who are on maintenance dialysis: a review for the pediatric nephrologist. Clin J Am Soc Nephrol. 2007;2(4):847–57. Review.
4. Shroff R, Wright E, Ledermann S, et al. Chronic hemodialysis in infants and children under 2 years of age. Pediatr Nephrol. 2003;18(4):378–83.
5. Schroder C, Geary D. Dialysis modality choice and initiation in children (Chapter 53). In: Geary DF, Schaefer F, editors. Comprehensive pediatric nephrology. Philadelphia: Mosby/Elsevier; 2008. p. 817–22.
6. Sienna JL, Saqan R, Teh JC, et al. Body size in children with chronic kidney disease after gastrostomy tube feeding. Pediatr Nephrol. 2010;25(10):2115–21.
7. Rees L, Shaw V. Nutrition in children with CRF and on dialysis. Pediatr Nephrol. 2007;22(10):1689–702. Review.
8. Ramage IJ, Geary DF, Harvey E, et al. Efficacy of gastrostomy feeding in infants and older children receiving chronic peritoneal dialysis. Perit Dial Int. 1999;19(3):231–6.
9. Sheth RD, Brandt ML, Brewer ED, et al. Permanent hemodialysis vascular access survival in children and adolescents with end-stage renal disease. Kidney Int. 2002;62(5):1864–9.
10. Paul A, Fraser N, Manoharan S, et al. The challenge of maintaining dialysis lines in the under twos. J Pediatr Urol. 2011;7(1):48–51.
11. Warady B, Andrews W. Peritoneal Dialysis Access (Chapter 54). In: Geary DF, Schaefer F, editors. Comprehensive pediatric nephrology. Philadelphia: Mosby/Elsevier; 2008. p. 823–34.
12. Chand DH, Valentini RP. International pediatric fistula first initiative: a call to action. Am J Kidney Dis. 2008;51(6):1016–24.
13. Rehman R, Schmidt RJ, Moss AH. Ethical and legal obligation to avoid long-term tunneled catheter access. Clin J Am Soc Nephrol. 2009;4(2):456–60. Review.
14. Chand DH, Bednarz D, Eagleton M. A vascular access team can increase AV fistula creation in pediatric ESRD patients: a single center experience. Semin Dial. 2009;22(6):679–83.
15. Chand DH, Valentini RP, Kamil ES. Hemodialysis vascular access options in pediatrics: considerations for patients and practitioners. Pediatr Nephrol. 2009;24(6):1121–8. Review.
16. Valentini RP, Geary DF, Chand DH. Central venous lines for chronic hemodialysis: survey of the Midwest Pediatric Nephrology Consortium. Pediatr Nephrol. 2008;23(2):291–5.
17. Peynircioglu B, Ozkan F, Canyigit M, et al. Radiologically placed tunneled internal jugular catheters in the management of chronic hemodialysis and long-term infusion therapies in the pediatric population. J Vasc Interv Radiol. 2007;18(7):875–81.
18. Vo JN, Hoffer FA, Shaw DW. Techniques in vascular and interventional radiology: pediatric central venous access. Tech Vasc Interv Radiol. 2010;13(4):250–7.
19. Baskin K, Hogan M, Sidhu M, et al. Developing a Clinical Pediatric Interventional Practice: A Joint Clinical Practice Guideline from the Society of Interventional Radiology and the Society of Pediatric Radiology SIR. Standards of Practice Committee. In press.

20. Connolly B, Racadio J, Towbin R. Practice of ALARA in the pediatric interventional suite. Pediatr Radiol. 2006;36 Suppl 2:163–7.
21. Sidhu M, Goske MJ, Connolly B, et al. Image gently, step lightly: promoting radiation safety in pediatric interventional radiology. AJR Am J Roentgenol. 2010;195(4):W299–301.
22. Sidhu M, Strauss KJ, Connolly B. Radiation safety in pediatric interventional radiology. Tech Vasc Interv Radiol. 2010;13(3):158–66.
23. Sidhu MK, Goske MJ, Coley BJ, et al. Image gently, step lightly: increasing radiation dose awareness in pediatric interventions through an international social marketing campaign. J Vasc Interv Radiol. 2009;20(9):1115–9.
24. Sidhu M, Coley BD, Goske MJ, et al. Image gently, step lightly: increasing radiation dose awareness in pediatric interventional radiology. Pediatr Radiol. 2009;39(10):1135–8.
25. Sidhu MK et al. Pediatric interventional radiology workforce survey summary. Pediatr Radiol. 2007;37(1):113–5.
26. Phan H, Nahata MC. Clinical uses of dexmedetomidine in pediatric patients. Paediatr Drugs. 2008;10(1):49–69.
27. Gozal D, Mason KP. Pediatric sedation: a global challenge. Int J Pediatr. 2010;2010:701257.
28. Laffan EE, McNamara PJ, Amaral J, et al. Review of interventional procedures in the very low birth-weight infant (<1.5 kg): complications, lessons learned and current practice. Pediatr Radiol. 2009;39(8):781–90.
29. Dipchand A, Friedman J. The Hospital for Sick Children. Handbook of pediatrics. 11th ed. Toronto: Saunders; 2009. p. 848–52.
30. Kobrinsky NL, Israels ED, Gerrard JM, et al. Shortening of bleeding time by 1-deamino-8-D-arginine vasopressin in various bleeding disorders. Lancet. 1984;1(8387):1145–8.
31. Franchini M. The use of desmopressin as a hemostatic agent: a concise review. Am J Hematol. 2007;82(8):731–5. Review.
32. Hedges SJ, Dehoney SB, Hooper JS, et al. Evidence-based treatment recommendations for uremic bleeding. Nat Clin Pract Nephrol. 2007;3(3):138–53. Review.
33. Haskal ZJ. Air embolism during tunneled central catheter placement performed without general anesthesia in children: a potentially lethal complication. J Vasc Interv Radiol. 1999;10(10):1416.
34. Morello FP, Donaldson JS, Saker MC, et al. Air embolism during tunneled central catheter placement performed without general anesthesia in children: a potentially serious complication. J Vasc Interv Radiol. 1999;10(6):781–4.
35. Connolly B, Mawson JB, MacDonald CE, et al. Fluoroscopic landmark for SVC-RA junction for central venous catheter placement in children. Pediatr Radiol. 2000;30(10):692–5.
36. Baskin KM, Jimenez RM, Cahill AM, et al. Cavoatrial junction and central venous anatomy: implications for central venous access tip position. J Vasc Interv Radiol. 2008;19(3):359–65.
37. Gittins NS, Hunter-Blair YL, Matthews JN, et al. Comparison of alteplase and heparin in maintaining the patency of paediatric central venous haemodialysis lines: a randomised controlled trial. Arch Dis Child. 2007;92(6): 499–501.

38. Chand D, Ramage I. Hemodialysis vascular access: complications and outcomes (Chapter 56). In: Geary DF, Schaefer F, editors. Comprehensive pediatric nephrology. Philadelphia: Mosby/Elsevier; 2008. p. 855–65.
39. Faintuch S, Salazar GM. Malfunction of dialysis catheters: management of fibrin sheath and related problems. Tech Vasc Interv Radiol. 2008;11(3): 195–200. Review.
40. Miksys N, Gordon CL, Thomas K, et al. Estimating effective dose to pediatric patients undergoing interventional radiology procedures using anthropomorphic phantoms and MOSFET dosimeters. AJR Am J Roentgenol. 2010;194(5): 1315–22.
41. Heran MK, Marshalleck F, Temple M, et al. Joint quality improvement guidelines for pediatric arterial access and arteriography: from the Societies of Interventional Radiology and Pediatric Radiology. Society of Interventional Radiology Standards of Practice Committee; Society of Pediatric Radiology Interventional Radiology Committee. Pediatr Radiol. 2010;40(2):237–50.
42. Powell S, Chan TY, Bhat R, et al. A retrospective comparative study of tunneled haemodialysis catheters inserted through occluded or collateral veins versus conventional methods. Cardiovasc Interv Radiol. 2010;33(4): 744–50.
43. Bourquelot P, Raynaud F, Pirozzi N. Microsurgery in children for creation of arteriovenous fistulas in renal and non-renal diseases. Ther Apher Dial. 2003;7(6):498–503.
44. Tannuri U, Tannuri AC, Watanabe A. Arteriovenous fistula for chronic hemodialysis in pediatric candidates for renal transplantation: technical details and refinements. Pediatr Transplant. 2009;13(3):360–4.
45. Brittinger WD, Walker G, Twittenhoff WD, et al. Vascular access for hemodialysis in children. Pediatr Nephrol. 1997;11:87–95.
46. Bagolan P, Spagnoli A, Ciprandi G, et al. A ten-year experience of Brescia-Cimino arteriovenous fistula in children: technical evolution and refinements. J Vasc Surg. 1998;27:640–4.
47. Malovrh M. The role of sonography in the planning of arteriovenous fistulas for hemodialysis. Semin Dial. 2003;16(4):299–303.
48. Lok C, Oliver M. Overcoming barriers to arteriovenous fistula creation and use. Semin Dial. 2003;16(3):189–96.
49. National Kidney Foundation. NFK–DOQI clinical practice guidelines for vascular access. Am J Kidney Dis. 2001;37(Suppl):S137–81.
50. Either JH, Lindsay RM, Barre PE, et al. Clinical practice guidelines for vascular access. Canadian Society of Nephrology. J Am Soc Nephrol. 1999;10 Suppl 13:S297–305.

Chapter 23
Puncture Site Management

Timothy I. Clark and Dheeraj K. Rajan

Regardless of what intervention is performed, unless the access thromboses, hemostasis remains the final post procedural access issue to deal with. Management partially is dependent on sedation status, puncture hole size, and if thrombolytics and/or heparin were used during interventions. Also, if high flow sheaths have been used for intervention, the patient may be transferred to the dialysis unit and dialysis commenced through these sheaths.

The simplest way to obtain hemostasis is to apply finger pressure to the site(s) of puncture to prevent bleeding. Enough pressure should be applied to promote hemostasis without occluding or impeding flow through the access. Hemostasis is often obtained in under 15 min for uncomplicated interventions with no heparin onboard. However, in cases where a large puncture hole exists e.g., 10 Fr with concurrent anticoagulants on board, hemostasis times can exceed an hour.

Other options beyond digital compression and clamps used within dialysis units include variations on suture techniques which include a tied purse string knot, a figure of eight suture, the Woggle technique,

T.I. Clark (✉)
Associate Professor of Radiology, Director,
Interventional Radiology, Department of Radiology,
Penn Presbyterian Medical Center, Philadelphia, Pennsylvania, USA
e-mail: timothy.clark@uphs.upenn.edu

D.K. Rajan (ed.), *Essentials of Percutaneous Dialysis Interventions*,
DOI 10.1007/978-1-4419-5657-6_23,
© Springer Science+Business Media, LLC 2011

and a suture tourniquet technique. Also, compression buttons and adhesive prothrombotic pads exist. All of these maneuvers allow for the interventionalist to be freed from time to obtain hemostasis and subsequently proceed with other tasks.

For puncture holes 4 Fr or smaller, digital compression is sufficient. For 5 Fr up to 12 Fr one of the suture techniques can be used. Each has its own advantages and disadvantages. Either a 2–0 or a 3–0 monofilament suture should be used as braided sutures have a greater risk of becoming infected and forming granulation tissue. These techniques should be reserved only for well incorporated grafts or along sites of fistula use where perivascular scar tissue has formed.

Pursestring Suture

The suture is placed subcutaneously with 2–4 bites circumferentially around the puncture site. The bites extend in to the perigraft or perivascular tissue, with care taken to not extend into the access itself. After the sheath or intervention device is removed, the suture is tied thereby closing off the hole. The following day or within days the suture can be removed. Advantages include immediate hemostasis and no need to observe the patient. Disadvantages include the need to remove the suture at a later time, difficulty in removing the suture, and if the suture is not removed within a few days it can act as a source of infection or become incorporated within the skin making removal even more difficult [1–3].

A variation of the pursestring suture is to place a small cut piece of catheter or dilator (see Fig. 23.1). A 1 cm length will suffice and tie the pursestring suture down onto the cut piece. To tighten the suture and obtain hemostasis, the cut dilator/catheter is rotated or screwed around to tighten the suture (without over rotating and tearing the skin) and then fixed in place with a steristrip. This maneuver allows for easier removal of the suture at a later time as the dilator/catheter piece is removed which now leaves a small gap between the skin and the suture facilitating passage of the scissors under the knot.

These are available through a variety of manufacturers. A technical note [6] describes use of a compression dressing that consists of 1–2 folded 4×4 in. gauzes held in place by a Tegaderm stretched tightly over it. This takes the physician a little longer to apply than a suture but since hemostasis is immediate after successful placement, the patient does not have to return for suture removal and there is no risk of infection.

For arterial punctures, direct pressure is advised until hemostasis is obtained (usually 15 min if the patient is not anticoagulated). For radial artery punctures, compression devices are available and often used by cardiologists.

References

1. Vorwerk D, Konner K, Schurmann K, Gunther RW. A simple trick to facilitate bleeding control after percutaneous hemodialysis fistula and graft interventions. Cardiovasc Intervent Radiol. 1997;20(2):159–60.
2. Vesely TM. Use of a purse string suture to close a percutaneous access site after hemodialysis graft interventions. J Vasc Interv Radiol. 1998;9(3):447–50.
3. Zaleski GX, Funaki B, Gentile L, Garofalo RS. Purse-string sutures and miniature tourniquet to achieve immediate hemostasis of percutaneous grafts and fistulas: a simple trick with a twist. AJR Am J Roentgenol. 2000;175(6):1643–5.
4. Simons ME, Rajan DK, Clark TW. The woggle technique for suture closure of hemodialysis access catheterization sites. J Vasc Interv Radiol. 2003;14(4):485–8.
5. Clark TW, Haji-Momenian S, Kwak A, et al. Angiographic changes following the use of a purse-string suture hemostasis device in hemodialysis access interventions. J Vasc Interv Radiol. 2009;20(1):61–5.
6. Barzel E. Use of a simple compression dressing to obtain hemostasis after pharmacologic thrombolysis of dialysis grafts. J Vasc Interv Radiol. 1999;10(8):1039–42.

Chapter 24
No Remaining Venous Access

Dheeraj K. Rajan and Dirk S. Baumann

When traditional sites of access have been exhausted, there are some percutaneous and surgical options remaining. These are salvage procedures and often have limited durability. The patient is now on a rapidly descending slope towards mortality, and discussions with the patient and their family should ensue. Options can be divided into catheter, AVG/AVF options and other options. Most catheter options are exotic, and associated with a high morbidity or mortality. Routes for catheter placement include translumbar, transhepatic, and via collaterals in the neck, chest or abdomen. AVG/AVF options are primarily surgical options discussed below. However, one can also attempt to salvage former accesses.

D.K. Rajan (✉)
Head and Associate Professor, Division of Vascular & Interventional Radiology, Department of Medical Imaging, University of Toronto, Toronto, Ontario, Canada
e-mail: Dheeraj.Rajan@uhn.on.ca

D.K. Rajan (ed.), *Essentials of Percutaneous Dialysis Interventions*,
DOI 10.1007/978-1-4419-5657-6_24,
© Springer Science+Business Media, LLC 2011

Translumbar Catheter Insertion

Translumbar catheter insertion requires a patent inferior vena cava. This can be assessed from prior CT examinations of the abdomen and pelvis. After appropriate consent is obtained, the patient is placed in the prone position. A puncture site is chosen just cephalic to the right iliac crest and approximately 8–10 cm (four finger breadths) to the right of midline. The skin is prepped and draped in the usual sterile fashion. Local anesthetic is infiltrated into the skin and subcutaneous tissues, and then a small skin incision is made. Under fluoroscopic guidance, a 21G, 15-cm-long needle is advanced cephalad and slightly medial to the anterolateral margin of the vertebral bodies so as to puncture the IVC at the level of L2–L3, below the renal veins. An intraluminal position is confirmed by free aspiration of blood through the needle; injection of contrast material is then performed to exclude entry into the renal vein and thereby avoid the potential complications of renal vein thrombosis, retroperitoneal hematoma, and catheter malfunction. If entry into the renal vein occurs, another entry site is chosen. Although we prefer to enter the IVC below the renal veins, entry at or above these veins is not considered a contraindication. Another option for localization, if possible, is to advance a pigtail catheter to the level of puncture within the IVC, either through femoral, collateral or upper body veins, and use the pigtail as a target for needle puncture. Finally, one can often opacify the IVC with contrast via a catheter placed into a lower extremity vein. A 0.018-in.-diameter guide wire is then advanced, and the cannula is exchanged for a 6-F coaxial introducer (Neff Set -Cook, Bloomington, MD) or Accustick II (Boston Scientific, Natick, MA). A 0.035-in.-diameter stiff Glidewire (Terumo Medical, Somerset, NJ) or Amplatz stiff guide wire (Boston Scientific or Cook) is advanced into the right atrium or preferably into the superior vena cava (SVC). The tract is then progressively dilated, and a 14 or 15 Fr, 30-cm-long Peel-Away sheath is inserted. Before insertion, the sheath is curved, which appears to facilitate passage into the IVC. Any catheter can be placed and the peel-away sheath within the set can be used. The most common length of catheter placed is a 27 cm tip to cuff length. Given near end of venous access, we prefer to use a split tip catheter, as there is evidence demonstrating longer patency than step tip catheters [1, 2].

The subcutaneous tunnel is extended laterally, approximately 8–10 cm from the initial puncture site. The tunnel length should be such that the catheter tip is positioned at the IVC-right atrial junction and the Dacron cuff remains within the tunnel. The catheter is then advanced through the tunnel and into the IVC through the sheath, which is subsequently removed. Each lumen of the catheter is aspirated and injected to verify functionality and then heparinized or citrated, and the catheter is sutured in place. The initial puncture site is closed with interrupted subcutaneous dissolvable sutures and covered with steristrips. The exit site is closed with a purse string 2–0 monofilament stitch, and after the first knot is tied, a second hanging knot is formed with both ends of the suture, then advanced through one of the securing bracket suture eyes and tied to secure the catheter in place (see Fig. 24.1).

The most common complications with this procedure/access site are common to catheter placement, regardless of the access site chosen and include catheter thrombosis, fibrin sheath formation, infection, and migration of the catheter tip. Outward migration of the catheter into the retroperitoneal soft tissues may result in a hematoma, but bleeding from this complication is generally minor and, except for the loss of access, of little clinical consequence. The catheter can also migrate to the iliac veins. Repositioning the catheter can be performed using endovascular retrieval techniques. Eventually, patients will also develop IVC stenosis with potential occlusion.

Transhepatic Catheter Insertion

Transhepatic dialysis catheter insertion techniques are similar to routine dialysis catheter insertions via the right internal jugular vein, with the exception that the access site is the middle or right hepatic vein through the hepatic parenchyma. Prior imaging of the liver should be performed to verify patency of the hepatic veins and to exclude ANY underlying liver pathology. Provided liver enzymes and the coagulation parameters are normal and the patient has a normal appearing liver with no ascites, then this option can be considered.

The right upper lateral abdominal quadrant is prepped and draped in a sterile fashion. Under ultrasound guidance, via a preferred subcostal approach with the aid of fluoroscopy, a 15 cm 21G needle is used to puncture the middle or right hepatic vein in the midportion of the vein more peripherally than centrally. Alternatively, an intercostal approach at the 10th or 11th interspace along the midaxillary line

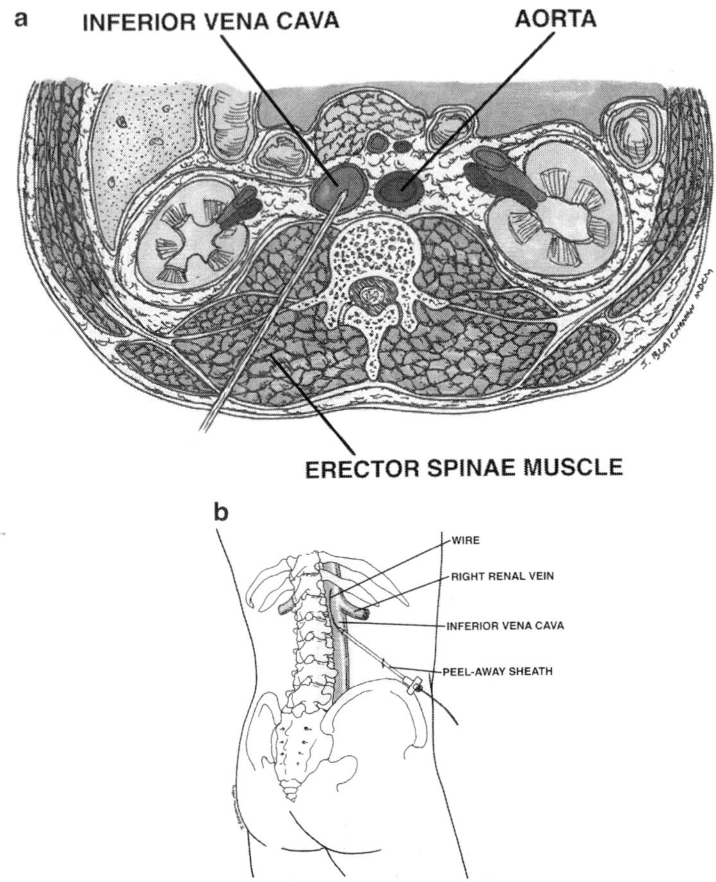

Fig. 24.1 Translumbar catheter insertion

may be used. The level of pleural reflection should be ascertained with respiratory motion observed under fluoroscopy to ensure the puncture will not cross it. A longer intravascular tract may reduce the risk of catheter migration. Puncture close to the confluence of the hepatic veins should be avoided. Contrast material is then injected to verify venous location. Contrast should flow towards the heart. If it flows towards the peripheral portions of the liver, the portal vein has been accessed and should not be cannulated. Once the middle hepatic vein is accessed, a 0.018 in. wire is advanced to the right atrium. Over this wire, a 4–6-F coaxial system (Accustick II Introducer System or

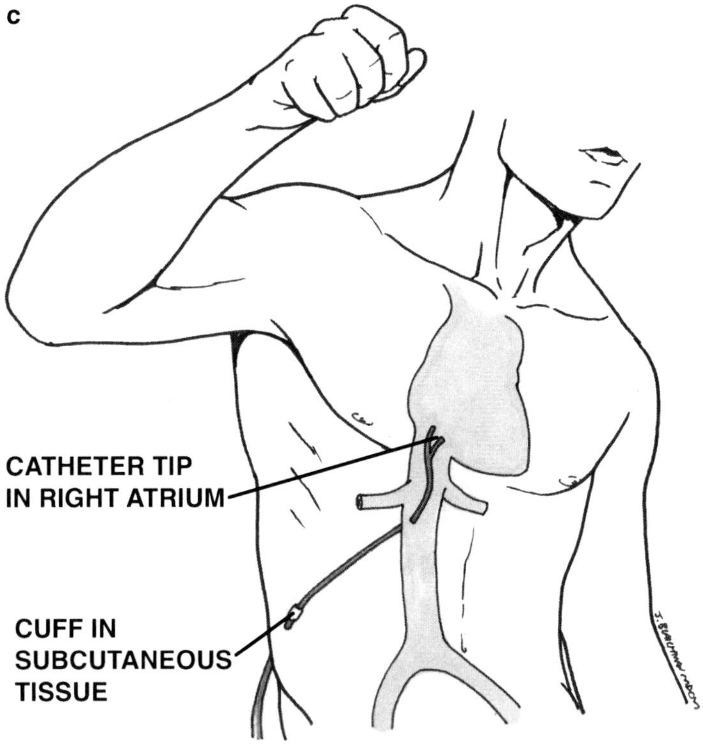

Fig. 24.1 (continued)

Neph Set) is advanced into the hepatic vein to allow placement of the 0.035-in. (0.89-mm) guide wire into the right atrium. Sequential tract dilation is performed, and a subcutaneous tunnel is created inferiorly for placement of the dual-lumen dialysis catheter. As with translumbar catheters, a split tip catheter should be used, typically with a 19 cm tip to cuff distance when possible with the tip positioned at the atrial/IVC junction (see Fig. 24.2). If removal is planned, the liver parenchymal tract requires embolization to prevent bleeding into the peritoneal space.

It is recommended that patients be kept overnight for observation and for complications of catheter placement. Complications, other than standard complications associated with dialysis catheters are significantly higher than with traditional access sites, particularly bleeding from the liver which can be fatal. Complications include

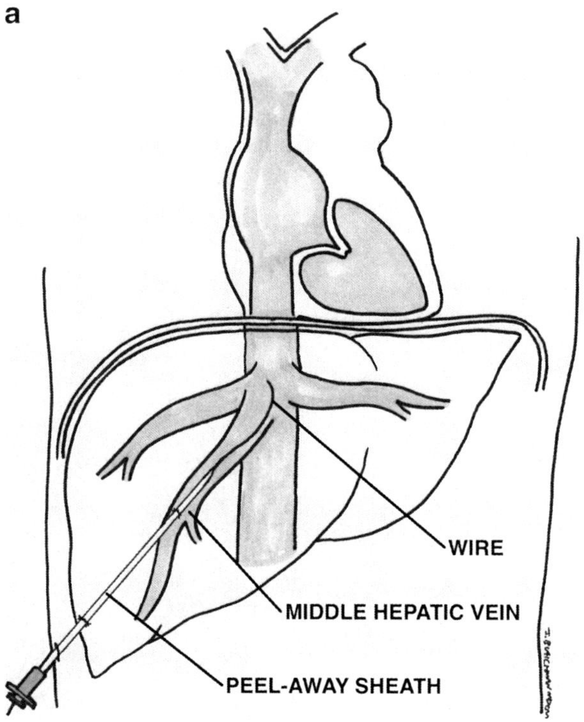

Fig. 24.2 Transhepatic catheter insertion

acute Budd–Chiari syndrome and biliary communication with the hepatic tract. In addition, there is a higher rate of catheter kinking. One study found a complication rate of 29% of the catheter placements. Primary patency also tend to be much lower than traditional sites with observed patency of 24 days although they can exceed 120 days [3, 4].

Other Pathways

Other options include searching for collateral veins in neck and chest. These collaterals can be punctured under ultrasound guidance with a micropuncture set, and using the inner dilator of the set, contrast can be

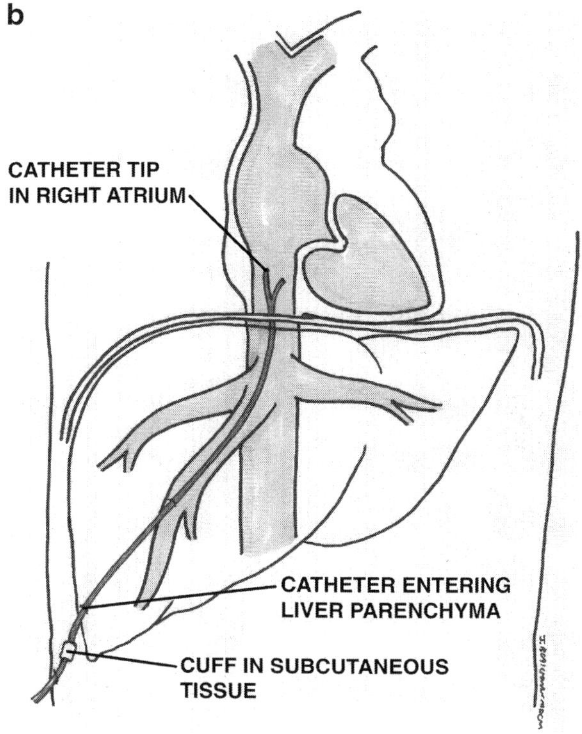

Fig. 24.2 (continued)

injected to determine the size, course, and endpoint of the collateral. If the vein collateral is close to 3–4 mm in size and has a relatively non-tortuous course, and terminates in the SVC, IVC or azygous vein, a dialysis catheter may be placed into this. Using a glidewire, if the tortuosity can be negotiated, a small 4 of 5 Fr hydrophilic or standard catheter can be advanced over the wire and the wire can then be substituted for a stiff wire to facilitate passage of a peel away sheath. The catheter can then be advanced over the wire, through the peel-away sheath. In some cases, the SVC is occluded, and the azygous vein becomes enlarged. Positioning the tip within an enlarged azygous vein has resulted in functioning catheters in selected case reports.

Novel Pathways Include

1. The external jugular vein
2. Direct puncture of the brachiocephalic veins
3. Supraclavicular puncture of the subclavian vein/brachiocephalic veins
4. Mediastinal venous collaterals (see Fig. 24.3)
5. Dilated intercostal veins
6. Transrenal puncture with entry into the renal vein to the IVC/azygous vein

These are advanced techniques with potentially life threatening hemorrhagic complications. It is recommended that these procedures be performed at tertiary care centers where emergency surgical support services exist [5, 6].

AVG/AVF Options

A novel consideration is to image abandoned fistulas and/or non thrombosed grafts with occluded outflow veins. Complete venous imaging adjacent to the access may reveal a matured collateral vein or normal adjacent outflow vein. One can then use a directional cannula and 21G needle and puncture from the occluded access to the adjacent outflow vein or collateral. When the needle enters the venous segment, location can be confirmed with contrast. If position is satisfactory, a wire can be then passed into the vein, and the subcutaneous tract dilated sequentially with balloon catheters with subsequent stenting or stent grafting of the bridging tract if required (see Fig. 24.4). Contrast should be injected at various steps to determine if the tract is sufficiently bridged and there is no extravasation. Another consideration is that one should not pass through nerves, tendons/ligaments or muscle tissue as this may cause significant morbidity for the patient. No published studies have determined the durability of this technique. Other techniques for salvage include sequential dilation of communicating or collateral veins with increasing balloon sizes over one session or multiple sessions over a couple of weeks (see Fig. 24.5) [7]. Also, ulnar basilic fistulas can be created near the wrist and transposed radiobasilic fistulas within the mid to distal third of the forearm are possible.

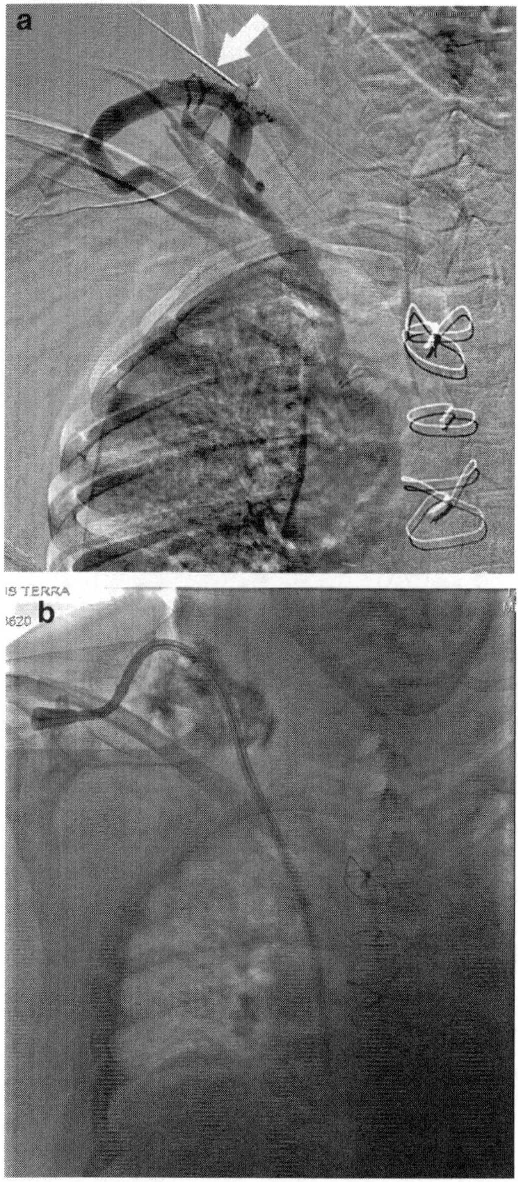

Fig. 24.3 Patient with chronic occlusion of the right SCV and jugular veins. (**a**) Puncture of scapular vein with 21G needle (*arrow*) demonstrates venous emptying to the SVC. (**b**) Tunneled catheter placed via the venous collateral pathway.

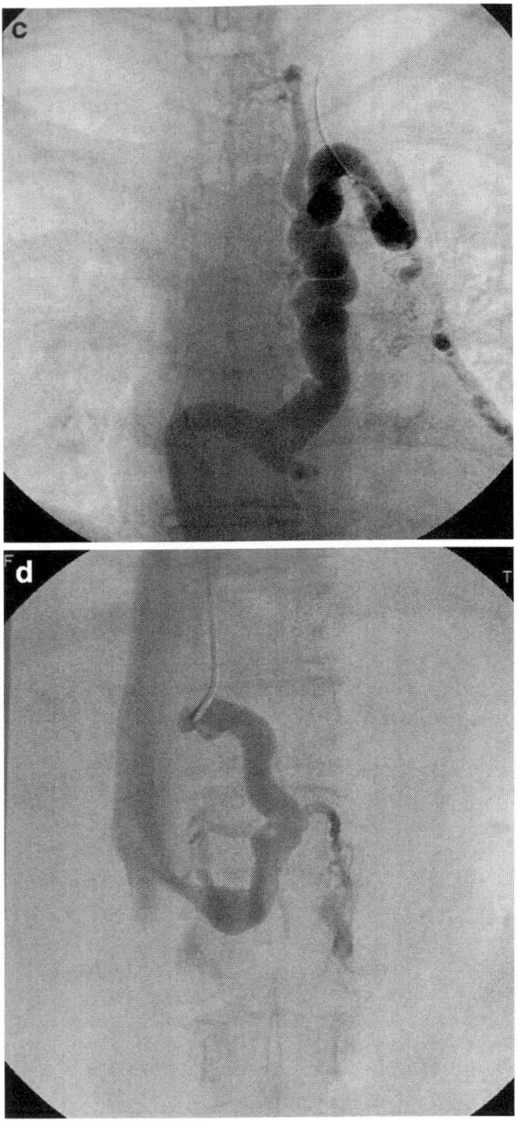

Fig. 24.3 (continued) (**c**) Cancer patient requiring chemotherapy delivered centrally. Via a neck collateral vein, contrast is injected demonstrating mediastinal collaterals emptying below the diaphragm into the (**d**) hemiazygous system which then empties back into the IVC. (**e**, **f**) Over a stiff glidewire, a Hickman catheter is inserted from the neck collateral to the right atrium

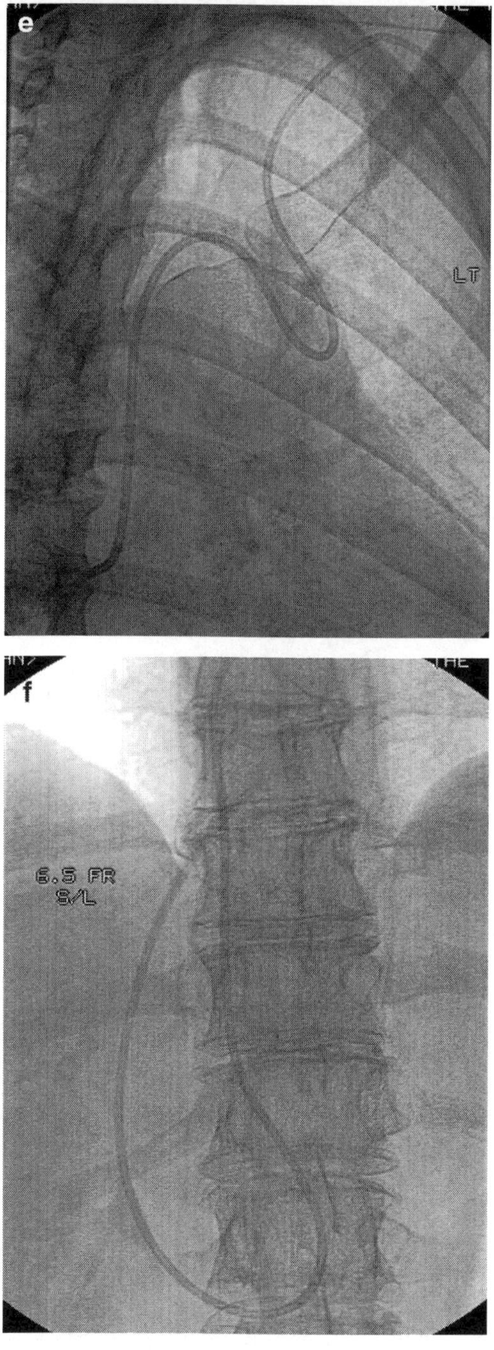

Fig. 24.3 (continued)

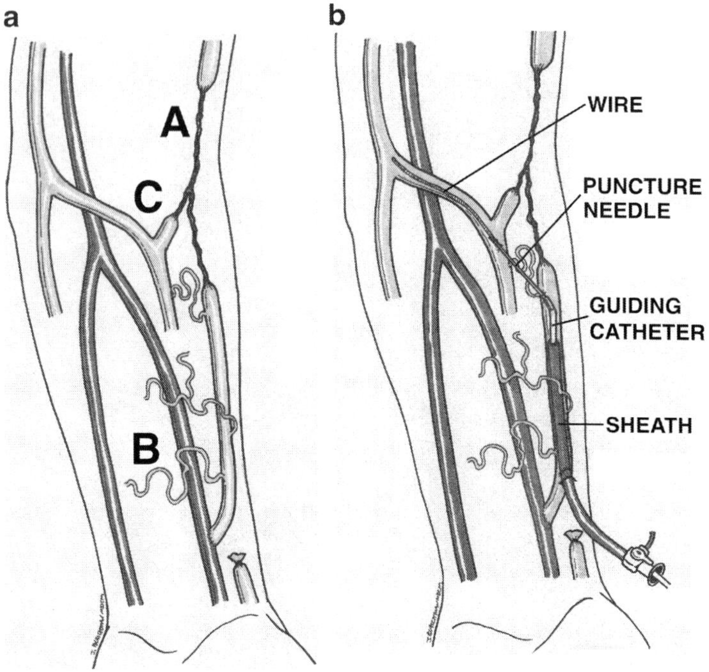

Fig. 24.4 (1) Collateral vein puncture for salvage of AV access ((**a**) occluded venous outflow, (**b**) collateral vessels filling, (**c**) larger collateral or adjacent normal vein). (2) Using a guiding catheter and needle, the adjacent vein is punctured and a wire is passed into it. (3) The needle and guiding catheter are removed and over the wire, the tract is sequentially dilated. (4) If required, a bridging stent or stent graft is placed from the access to the adjacent vessel

A hybrid percutaneous and surgical procedure with the Hemodialysis Reliable Outflow (HeRO) device (Hemosphere, Inc.) is effective for patients with central venous stenosis and/or occlusion and is approved for use within the United States (see Fig. 24.6). It is used in the upper extremities of patients who would otherwise be catheter dependent. Arterial blood is shunted from the donor artery into the central venous system without having to create a formal venous anastomosis. The device is a completely subcutaneously implanted device that can bypass central venous stenosis and/or occlusion by traversing the lesion endovascularly and terminating in the right atrium or any available large outflow target vein. This device consists of two components: a conventional ePTFE graft and

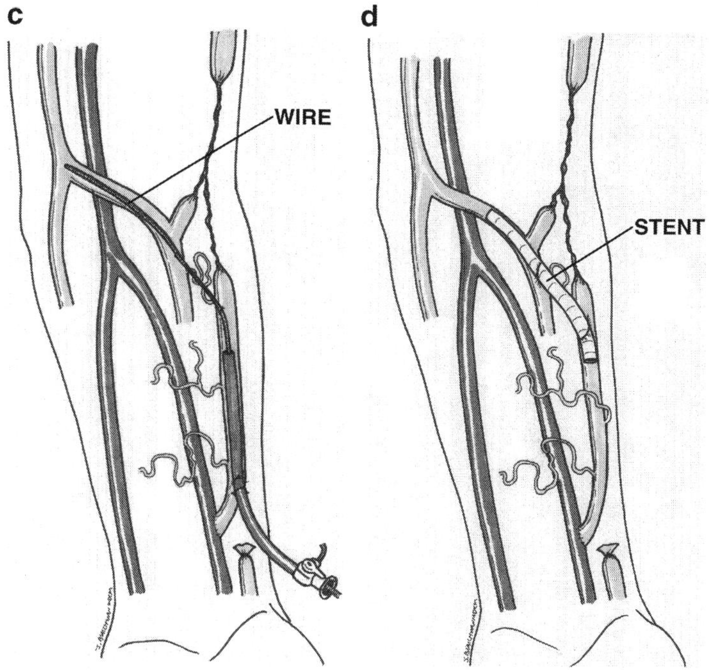

Fig. 24.4 (continued)

an endoluminal, large-bore, single-lumen, nitinol-reinforced, silicone outflow component. The silicone outflow component is inserted into the internal jugular, subclavian, femoral vein or sufficiently large collateral utilizing the Seldinger technique or via TDC exchange and then coupled with an ePTFE graft, which is tunneled subcutaneously in the standard surgical fashion and anastomosed to an upper extremity artery or inflow conduit of choice. Primary patency rates of the HeRO device are less than grafts, therefore requiring more interventions than grafts but with similar secondary patency [8].

Surgical Options

When evaluating patients for complex and potentially morbid access alternatives, it is critical to extensively review and exhaust all potential and more conventional access options. Consideration should be

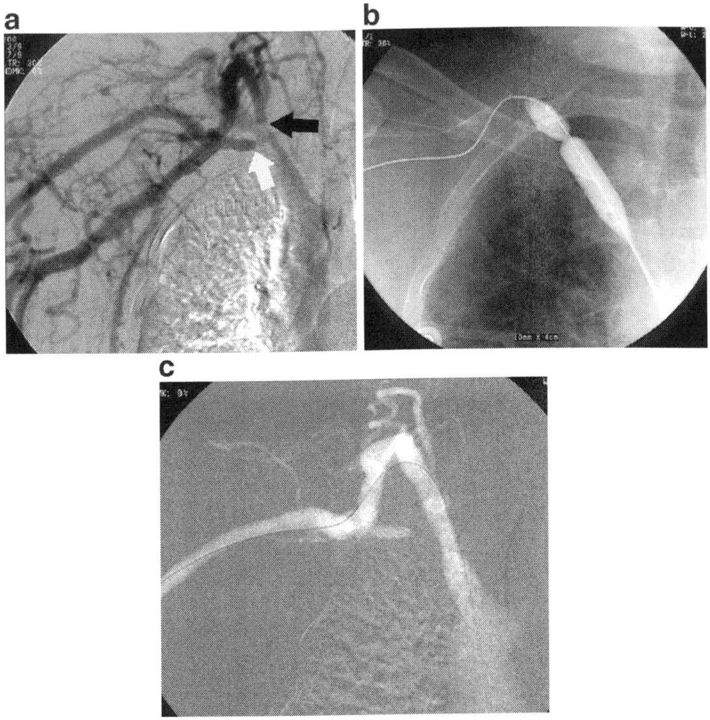

Fig. 24.5 Sixty-nine-year-old female with right forearm graft with arm swelling. (**a**) Right forearm graft fistulogram demonstrating total occlusion at the subclavian vein (*white arrow*) and a high-grade stenosis at a collateral vessel (*black arrow*). (**b**) After failed attempts at recanalization, the collateral vessel was dilated with a 10×40 mm balloon. (**c**) Post-PTA fistulogram demonstrated an excellent result with subsequent resolution of arm swelling. (Case courtesy of Dr. Goo, Soonchunhyang University Hospital, South Korea)

given to use of peritoneal dialysis. All extremities should be rescanned with ultrasound and/or venography to confirm previous evaluations. Often, thorough re-review will uncover choices which can be exploited prior to more aggressive techniques. In addition to the percutaneous approaches described above, surgical approaches to either the abdominal or thoracic central veins can be employed. Specifically, laparoscopy can be used to guide percutaneous access to the iliac veins or inferior vena cava and to allow catheter placement into these veins. Thoracoscopy alternatively allows for minimally invasive placement of a catheter into the innominate vein, azygos vein, hemiazygos

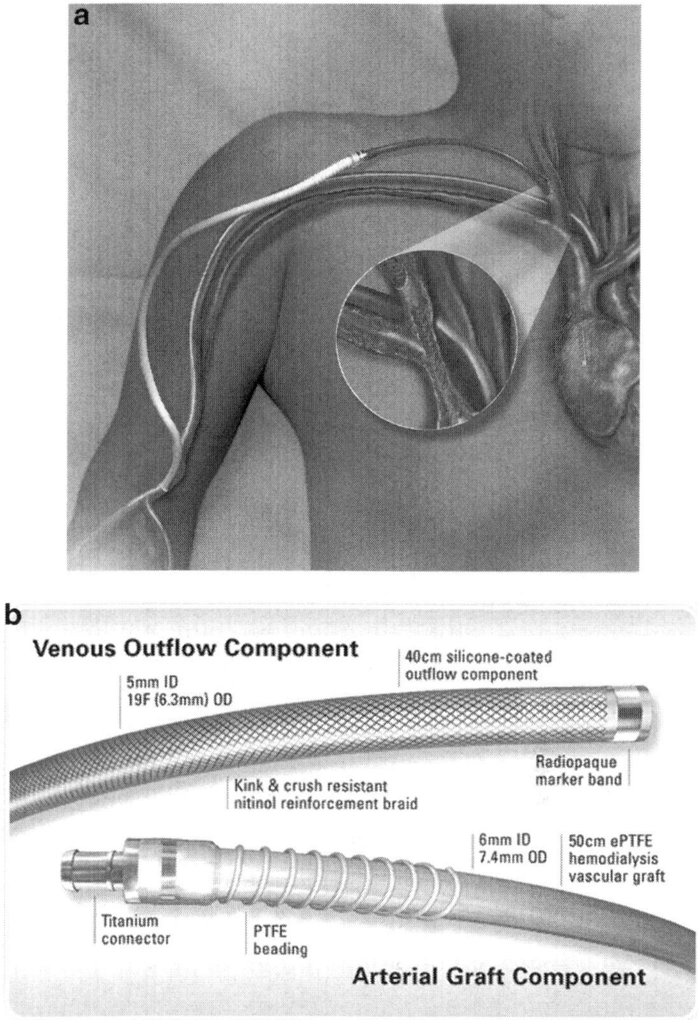

Fig. 24.6 HeRO device (Reprinted with permission and courtesy of Hemosphere, Inc., Eden Prairie, MN)

vein or right atrium. To decrease the risk of catheter infection in patients with limited access, AV grafts may be placed into these larger central veins, such as the iliac veins. These larger caliber veins tend to develop anastomotic intimal hyperplasia at a slower rate than smaller diameter veins, improving graft patency. Venous anastomotic stenoses can be treated endovascularly in the future if needed. Finally, when in-line flow is not available for patent peripheral veins, these veins can be transposed/translocated to a site with a patent central venous outflow. Preoperative evaluation and planning is critical in these patients to design ways to maximize access longevity. Close postoperative monitoring is geared toward anticipating and preventing failure and complications.

Conclusion

All the aforementioned techniques are relatively demanding and not without serious potential complications. One should have advanced knowledge of catheter, wire, and stenting techniques as well as ultrasound abilities. Surgical alternatives exist for accesses and consultation with access surgeons prior to embarking on risky interventions is recommended.

Key Points

- A CT chest venogram may demonstrate patent central veins or collaterals that can be used for access insertion.
- When novel insertion sites are required, it is time to advise the patient of their prognosis.
- Consider revising or reviving previous accesses/access sites.
- Venograms via collateral veins may expose viable routes for access insertion.

References

1. Rajan DK, Croteau DL, Sturza SG, Harvill ML, Mehall CJ. Translumbar placement of inferior vena caval catheters: a solution for challenging hemodialysis access. Radiographics. 1998;18(5):1155–67; discussion 1167–1170.
2. Trerotola SO, Kraus M, Shah H, et al. Randomized comparison of split tip versus step tip high-flow hemodialysis catheters. Kidney Int. 2002;62(1):282–9.

3. Smith TP, Ryan JM, Reddan DN. Transhepatic catheter access for hemodialysis. Radiology. 2004;232(1):246–51.
4. Stavropoulos SW, Pan JJ, Clark TW, et al. Percutaneous transhepatic venous access for hemodialysis. J Vasc Interv Radiol. 2003;14(9 Pt 1):1187–90.
5. Forauer AR, Brenner B, Haddad LF, Bocchini TP. Placement of hemodialysis catheters through dilated external jugular and collateral veins in patients with internal jugular vein occlusions. AJR Am J Roentgenol. 2000;174(2):361–2.
6. Murthy R, Arbabzadeh M, Lund G, Richard III H, Levitin A, Stainken B. Percutaneous transrenal hemodialysis catheter insertion. J Vasc Interv Radiol. 2002;13(10):1043–6.
7. Ahmad I. Salvage of arteriovenous fistula by angioplasty of collateral veins establishing a new channel. J Vasc Access. 2007;8(2):123–5.
8. Katzman HE, McLafferty RB, Ross JR, Glickman MH, Peden EK, Lawson JH. Initial experience and outcome of a new hemodialysis access device for catheter-dependent patients. J Vasc Surg. 2009;50(3):600–7. 607 e601.

Chapter 25
Radiologic Peritoneal Dialysis Catheter Insertion and Troubleshooting

Robyn A. Pugash

Peritoneal dialysis is well established as being an efficient and effective form of renal replacement therapy. It is less expensive than hemodialysis, carries lower rates of access-related morbidity and mortality, is associated with greater preservation of residual renal function, and in permitting self-therapy promotes independence and improves quality of life. Indeed, patient satisfaction with peritoneal dialysis is in general higher than it is with hemodialysis.

As is true for hemodialysis, the cornerstone of successful peritoneal dialysis is access; an ideal access will be safe, well tolerated, easy to use, durable, and as complication-free as possible while providing reliable flow rates with minimal outflow failure.

Numerous catheter designs have been tested over the years. Variations include (but are not limited to) number of cuffs (one or two), shape of the catheter tip (straight or coiled), and shape of the subcutaneous segment (straight or bent, also called "swan neck"). While no single design is conclusively superior to others with respect to catheter survival or complication rates, the available evidence

---

R.A. Pugash (✉)
Assistant Professor, University of Toronto, Sunnybrook Health Sciences Centre, Toronto, Ontario, Canada
e-mail: robyn.pugash@sunnybrook.ca

D.K. Rajan (ed.), *Essentials of Percutaneous Dialysis Interventions*, DOI 10.1007/978-1-4419-5657-6_25,
© Springer Science+Business Media, LLC 2011

favors the double cuff, coiled tip, swan neck catheter as being an excellent configuration for most patients.

Various insertion methods exist and include open surgical insertion, laparoscopic insertion, peritoneoscopic insertion, "blind" percutaneous insertion, and radiologic insertion, each having advantages and disadvantages, supporters and detractors.

While catheter type and insertion method are undoubtedly very important, the experience, expertise and level of engagement of the access team (not to mention a host of center characteristics) are at least of equal (if not greater) importance in determining outcomes, accounting for the considerable variation that exists among centers, even when comparing similar methods and catheter types.

It is beyond the scope of this discussion to address indications for peritoneal dialysis as a form of renal replacement therapy. Once peritoneal dialysis has been chosen, two contraindications exist to the specific method of radiologic insertion of peritoneal dialysis catheters, and these are surgical scars over all available entry sites (risk of underlying adhesions that can lead to gut injury) or the need for additional procedures that cannot be performed radiologically, such as hernia repairs.

Catheter Insertion

Catheter insertion is performed as a day procedure, with no need for hospital admission. Warfarin, clopidogrel and full-dose ASA are discontinued 5 days before the procedure. Patients on therapeutic doses of low molecular weight heparin are asked to hold one dose before the procedure. Prophylactic doses of LMWH are not withheld.

Patients who are not diabetic remain NPO after midnight, apart from any regular medications that are taken with sips of water. Diabetic patients are instructed to have a light breakfast early in the morning and to take their medications as usual. A full bowel prep is taken.

The following supplies are needed (in addition to those commonly available in IR suites):

- *Peritoneal catheter*. If purchased as a kit for insertion by Seldinger technique, the catheter will be accompanied by an appropriately sized peel-away sheath (Fig. 25.1).

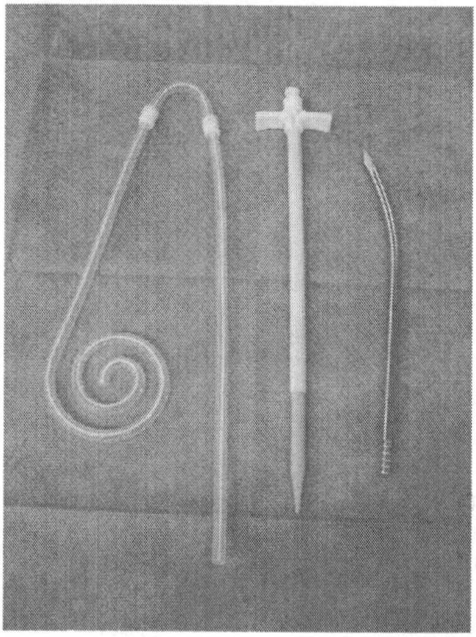

Fig. 25.1 From left to right: double cuff, coiled tip, swan neck catheter; peel-away introducer sheath; Faller stylet

- *PD stylet*, which is a malleable "coat-hanger" type of wire with a loop at one end (a catheter mounted on a PD stylet is shown in Fig. 25.8).
- *Faller stylet*, which is a stainless steel tunneling device with a cutting edge at one end and ridges at the other end (Fig. 25.1). The stylet pulls the catheter through the tunnel and creates the skin exit site in one pass, in exactly the same way as a needle pulls a suture through skin. Because the Faller stylet has the same outer diameter as the peritoneal catheter, it creates a snug exit site that requires no suturing which minimizes exit site complications.

The steps for placing a double cuff peritoneal dialysis catheter are as follows:

1. It is important to plan the exit site beforehand to ensure it is away from the belt line, deep skin creases, and bony prominences while remaining easily visible to the patient, bearing in mind that ideal catheter tip position is deep in the pelvis (to keep it away from the omentum and minimize the likelihood of outflow obstruction caused by omental wrapping), and that the tunnel/exit site should be directed inferiorly or laterally (never superiorly) to reduce the likelihood of exit site or tunnel infections. The belt line and deep

skin creases are marked with the patient dressed, sitting and leaning slightly forward; the lines are re-inked with a sterile marker if they wash off while the patient is being prepped.

2. Good catheter position is difficult to obtain in the presence of a full bladder; because few patients are anuric, routine placement of a Foley catheter for the duration of the procedure is essential.
3. Antibiotic prophylaxis (1 g cefazolin or 600 mg clindamycin if allergic) is used routinely.
4. IV sedation and analgesia are used; usually 50 μg fentanyl and 1 mg midazolam to start and repeated if needed during the procedure. Standard physiologic monitoring is used.
5. It is unclear if placement side affects catheter function. One view is that left-sided insertion leads to less tip migration on the theory that peristaltic activity of the descending colon will tend to encourage the catheter tip to stay in the pelvis. Since tip migration does not correlate well with catheter malfunction (outflow obstruction more commonly being caused by omental wrapping of the catheter than by nondependent tip position) and since left-sided catheters do not lie particularly close to the descending colon, this is probably more myth than fact but having said that, our practice is to nonetheless default to left-sided insertion, opting for the right side only if a left-sided catheter has previously failed, or if there is a contraindication to left-sided insertion, such as a surgical scar at the planned entry site.
6. Meticulous sterile technique is essential. The prep solution (2% chlorhexidine gluconate in 70% isopropyl alcohol) should be allowed to dry on the patient.
7. Once the patient has been prepped and draped, the catheter is laid over the abdomen, and positioned so that the coiled segment is superimposed on the pubic symphysis, and the uppermost end of the straight intraperitoneal segment is roughly 3 cm lateral to the midline (Fig. 25.2). While some operators place catheters through the linea alba, we prefer to place catheters through the medial border of the rectus muscle; this may improve deep cuff fixation (more robust tissue ingrowth) and lead to fewer leaks.
8. A horizontal incision will be made; if using a swan neck catheter, this is positioned slightly inferior to the swan neck itself (Fig. 25.3). 2% lidocaine with epinephrine is used to anesthetize the skin. The incision should be about 5–6 cm long; efforts to minimize cosmetic impact by using a shorter incision are not

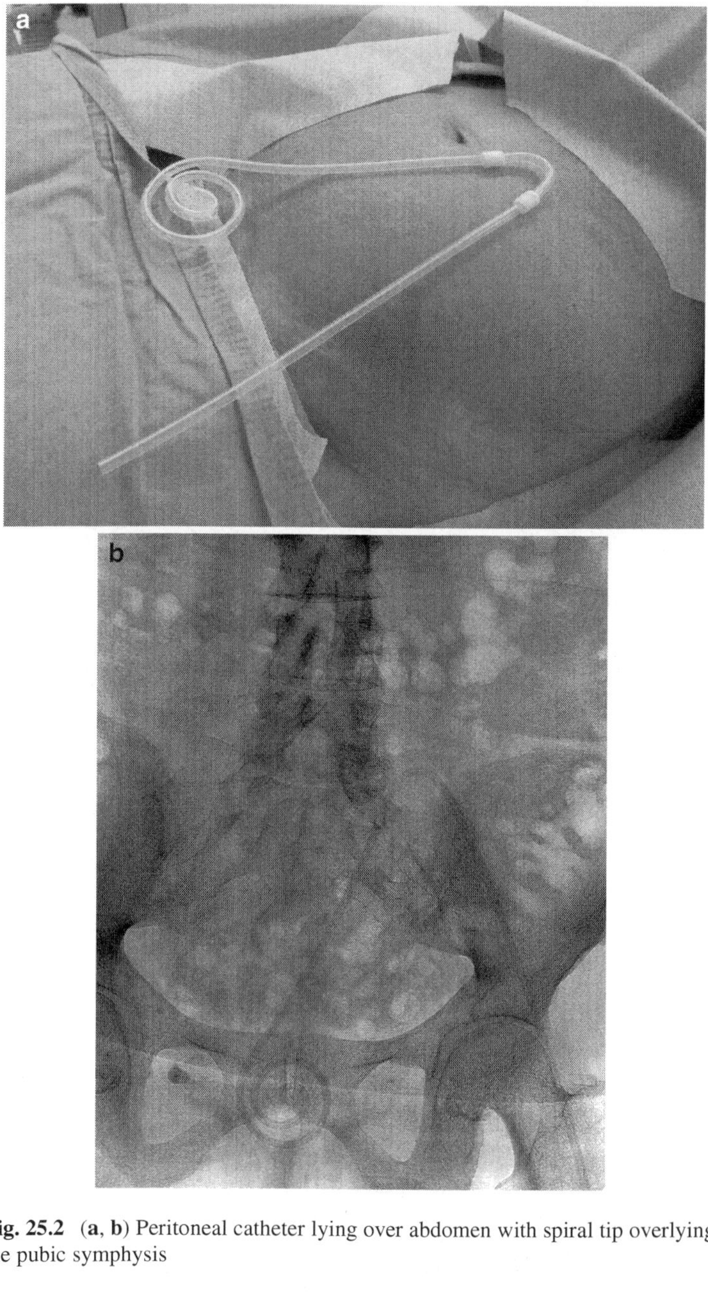

Fig. 25.2 (**a**, **b**) Peritoneal catheter lying over abdomen with spiral tip overlying the pubic symphysis

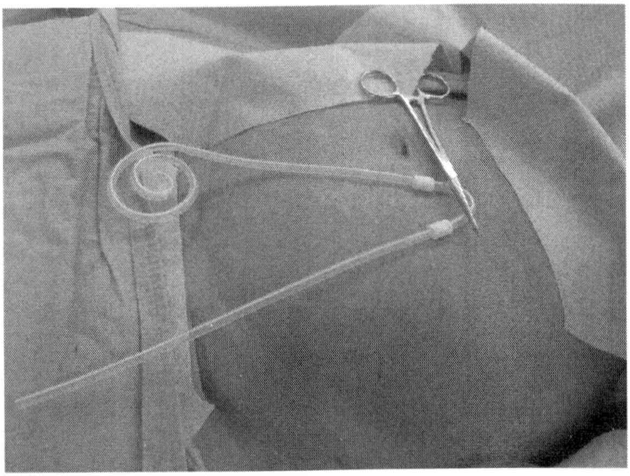

Fig. 25.3 Position of skin incision is indicated by the hemostat

recommended (can lead to difficulty in obtaining the necessary position of the deep cuff).

9. The anterior rectus sheath is exposed using blunt dissection with hemostats.
10. Needle trajectory is planned with fluoroscopy. The tip of a 22-gauge Chiba needle is placed on the anterior rectus sheath in the medial third of the incision over the medial edge of the rectus muscle. The needle is held at about a 60° angle to the abdominal wall in the parasagittal plane and under frontal fluoroscopy is aimed toward the pubic symphysis (Fig. 25.4).
11. Once trajectory has been planned, the Chiba needle is advanced through the rectus under ultrasound guidance using a linear probe. Loops of bowel will be visible moving with respiration just deep in the abdominal wall, marking the transition to the peritoneal space. Patients often wince slightly as the needle pierces the peritoneum.
12. After the puncture has been made, needle tip position is confirmed by injecting a small quantity of contrast material. If the tip is intraperitoneal, contrast will flow away from the needle and outline loops of bowel (Fig. 25.5a). If the tip is not correctly placed (either too superficial in the abdominal wall or too deep in the greater omentum), contrast will collect in a "blob" around the needle tip (Fig. 5b).

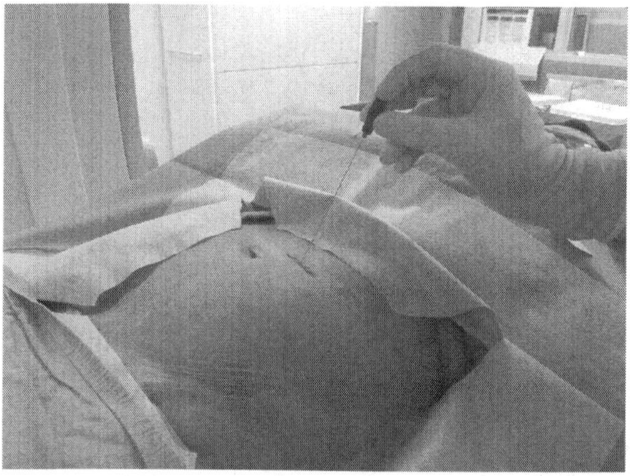

Fig. 25.4 Position of Chiba needle prior to US guided puncture. The needle is held at roughly a 60° angle to the abdominal wall in the parasagittal plane and is aimed toward the pubic symphysis

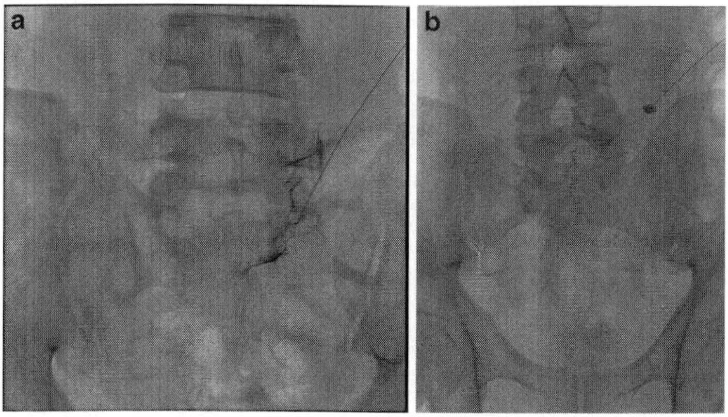

Fig. 25.5 (**a**) Contrast flowing away from the needle tip outlining bowel loops confirms intraperitoneal tip position. (**b**) Contrast collecting in a "blob" around the needle tip indicates that it is not in the peritoneal space

Will I hit the gut?: Any interventional radiologist who has ever tried to place a jejunostomy percutaneously will know just how elusive a target a normal small bowel loop can be. In the absence of adhesions that tether gut loops to the anterior abdominal wall, the likelihood of injuring highly mobile small bowel loops with

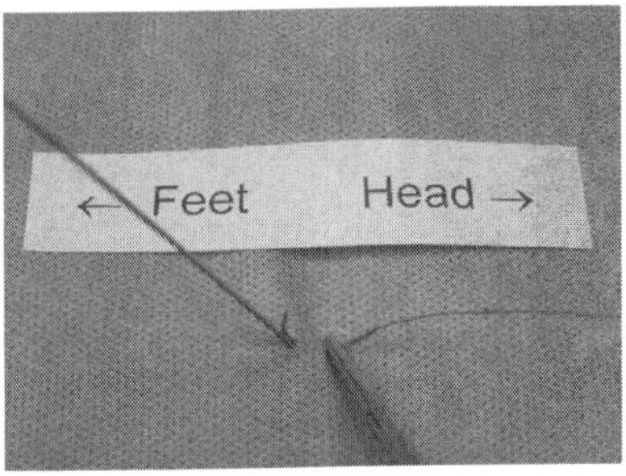

Fig. 25.6 Demonstration of correct suture placement for deep cuff. The gray background represents the anterior rectus sheath. The puncture has been performed and a wire has been placed.. The suture is placed through the anterior rectus sheath starting about 5 mm cranial to the puncture then exiting as close to the wire as possible

an ultrasound guided puncture that extends just a few millimeters into the peritoneal space is remote.

Should I try to find out if I hit the gut? Some operators routinely perform pull-back injections using an introducer, a 0.018 in. wire and a side-arm adapter. This will presumably detect any through-and-through punctures by opacifying the gut lumen. If the puncture has been performed correctly, though, through-and-through transgression of the gut is so remote a possibility as to be of no concern. If a small tag of gut wall were snagged by the Chiba needle without traversing the lumen, a pull-back injection would not pick it up (if this has occurred in our practice, it has not become clinically apparent in over 220 insertions). If the insertion site is free of surgical scars, and if the puncture is performed carefully, ensuring that needle excursion into the peritoneal space is as minimal as possible, maneuvers to assess for gut injury are not necessary.

13. After advancing a 0.018 in. wire through the Chiba needle into the peritoneal space, the access is upsized and a 0.038 in. wire is placed. An absorbable suture such as 3-0 Vicryl is used to take a bite of the anterior rectus sheath immediately adjacent to the cranial side of the wire's entry into the rectus sheath (Fig. 25.6). This suture is set aside for later use. At this point an absorbable purse-string suture can be placed in the surrounding anterior rectus sheath; this has not been our routine practice, but it is advocated by some operators as a way to minimize early leaks. If used, the purse-string suture should be tied after the catheter has been inserted.

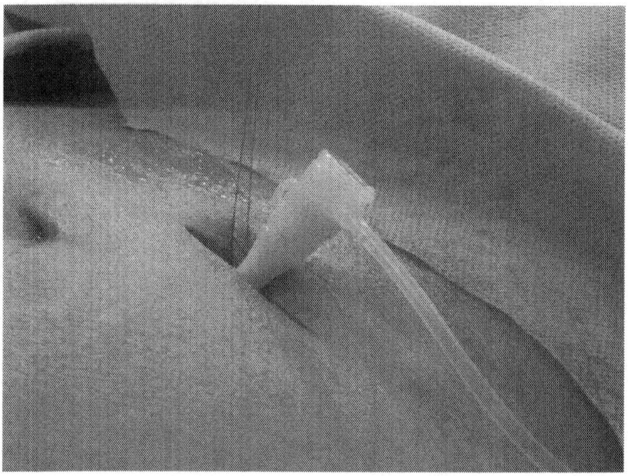

Fig. 25.7 Close-up of incision after introducer sheath has been placed. The Vicryl suture that was placed in the anterior rectus sheath is visible as well

14. A large vascular introducer sheath (11 Fr works well) is then placed over the wire (Fig. 25.7). Room temperature saline (1–1.5 L) is infused through the side-arm into the peritoneal space. The saline displaces bowel loops out of the pelvis, thereby facilitating deep pelvic catheter tip placement. Contrast is intermittently injected through the side arm during the saline infusion to get a sense of whether or not enough "room" has been created in the pelvis.
15. Once the saline has been infused (a pressure bag helps speed up the process), the vascular introducer sheath is exchanged for the peel-away sheath.
16. The peritoneal catheter is loaded on the PD stylet (Fig. 25.8), making sure the stylet does not protrude beyond the tip of the catheter. Once loaded, it is important to ensure that the opaque stripe on the catheter is straight, not spiraling (Fig. 25.9).
17. Swan neck catheters are available for left-sided and right-sided insertion; the only difference between the two is where the longitudinal opaque stripe is placed on the catheter. It is not necessary to stock both types of catheters – if inserted correctly, left-sided catheters can be placed on the right side (and vice versa) as follows:
    - When inserting a left-sided catheter on the left side of the abdomen, as the catheter/stylet is passed through the

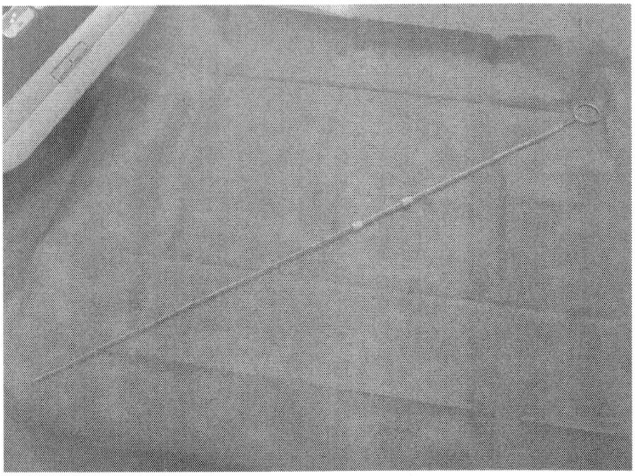

Fig. 25.8 Peritoneal catheter mounted on a PD stylet

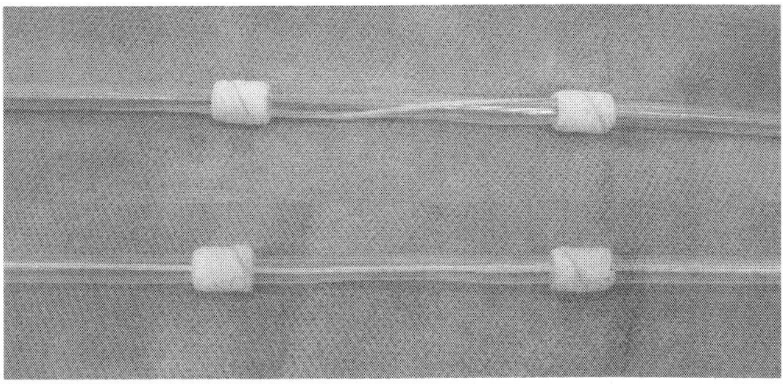

Fig. 25.9 Two catheters loaded on PD stylets. The top catheter has been incorrectly loaded (longitudinal stripe spirals around the stylet). The bottom catheter has been correctly loaded

peel-away sheath, it must be rotated so that the longitudinal stripe faces away from the patient (Fig. 25.10).

- When inserting a left-sided catheter on the right side of the abdomen, the longitudinal stripe must be turned to face the patient.
- Ensuring correct orientation of the catheter along its long axis is important when using swan neck catheters in order to prevent twisting of the swan neck in the subcutaneous tissues.

18. The catheter/stylet is advanced through the sheath and directed inferiorly toward the midline of the pelvis. Frontal fluoroscopy

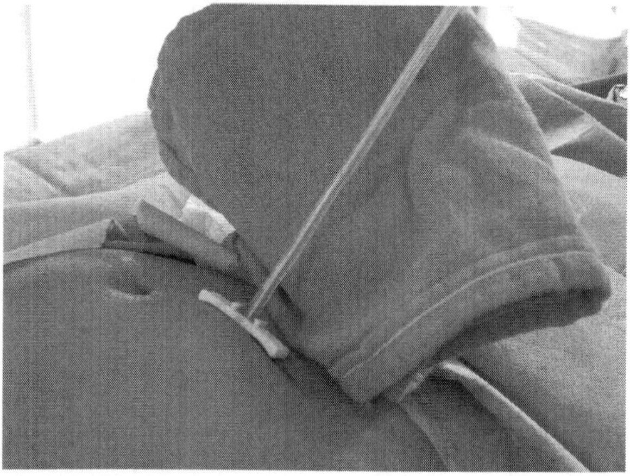

Fig. 25.10 Correct orientation of a left-sided swan neck catheter being placed on the left side of the abdomen. The catheter has been loaded on a stylet, advanced into the peel-away introducer sheath and rotated so that the stripe is facing away from the patient (the patient's head is beyond the right side of the photograph)

is used to ensure midline position of the catheter/stylet combination. The catheter/stylet is held stable in this position and the C-arm is turned to a steep oblique or lateral position.

19. With steep oblique or lateral fluoroscopy, the catheter/stylet is advanced into the rectovesical/uterine pouch. If it does not go easily, it may be necessary to inject contrast to get a sense of what might be in the way. Efforts are made to navigate past the obstacle; this often means withdrawing the catheter/stylet and peel-away sheath as far back as possible without losing access, angling anteriorly, sliding the system inferiorly along the posterior surface of the anterior abdominal wall, then once below all gut loops, angling back into the rectovesical/uterine pouch.
20. When satisfactory tip position has been obtained the sheath is peeled away while the catheter/stylet is held stable; this usually requires the help of an assistant.
21. The coiled tip of the catheter is advanced off the stylet into rectovesical/uterine pouch (Fig. 25.11). The stylet is then removed carefully under fluoroscopic observation to ensure that tip position is not disturbed in the process.
22. Using the previously placed Vicryl stitch, the deep cuff is sutured to the anterior rectus sheath; this is key in preventing catheter

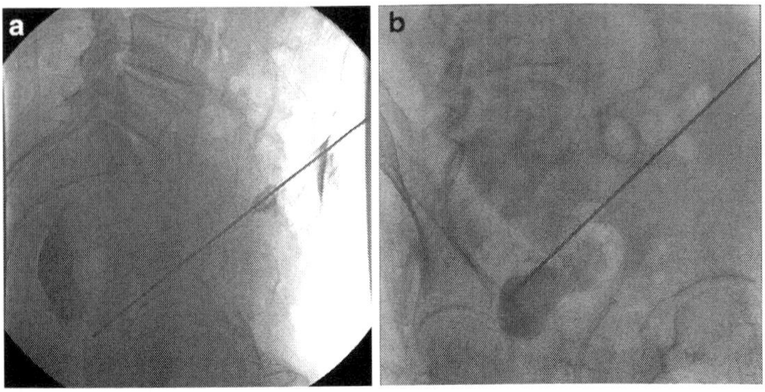

Fig. 25.11 Catheter tip being advanced off stylet into the rectovesical pouch. (**a**) Lateral view (**b**) steep oblique (different patient)

dislodgment from the abdomen until tissue ingrowth into the deep cuff has occurred. When suturing the cuff it is important to avoid piercing the catheter; it is usually fairly easy to get the needle to slide between the cuff and catheter (Fig. 25.12).

- Left-sided insertion using a left-sided catheter: The suture should be sewn through the portion of the deep cuff that is 180° away from the stripe on the catheter (Fig. 25.13).
- Right-sided insertion using a left-sided catheter: The suture should be sewn through the portion of deep cuff that is on the same side as the stripe. The suture should be in line with the stripe (Fig. 25.13b).

23. The catheter is checked for two-way flow before creating the subcutaneous tunnel; it is much easier to adjust position before the catheter has been tunneled than after. If there is outflow obstruction (failure to drain roughly the same amount of fluid that was injected), the PD stylet is used to reposition the tip.
24. The tunnel and exit site are created with the following points in mind:

- The tunnel and exit site must be either laterally or inferiorly directed to minimize infectious complications.
- Swan neck catheters must have inferiorly directed tunnels and exit sites.

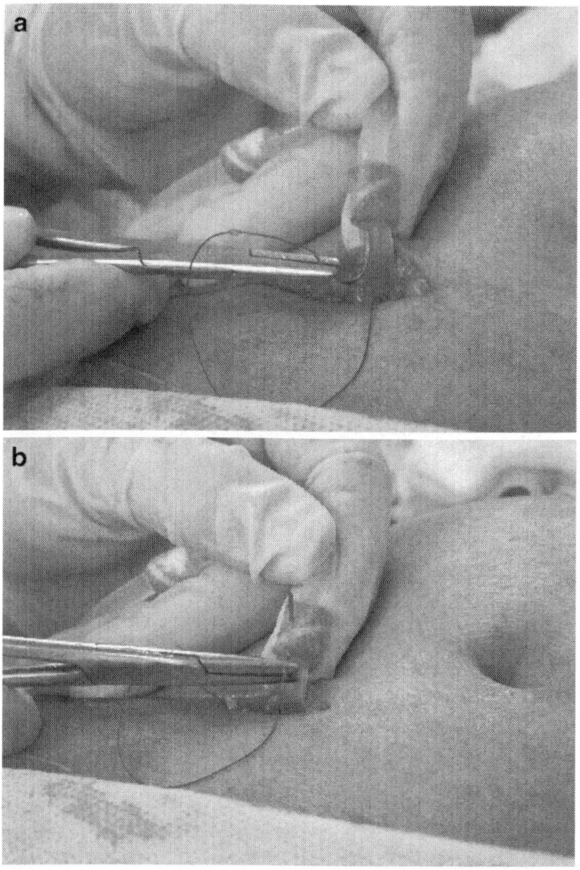

Fig. 25.12 Series of photographs showing suture placement in the deep cuff. In a, b and c the patient's feet are beyond the top right corner of the photograph. (**a**) The needle tip is slipped between the cuff and catheter. (**b**) It is usually possible to exit about mid way through the cuff. (**c**) Final suture position. (**d**) Appearance of catheter after the deep cuff has been sutured. In this photograph the patient's feet are to the left and her head is to the right. Note that the longitudinal stripe is facing away from the patient, which is the correct orientation of a left-sided catheter placed on the left side of the abdomen. If the stripe is not in correct position after the cuff has been sutured, the suture must be redone; if not, the bent segment of the catheter will be twisted in the subcutaneous tunnel. Shape memory effects of a catheter left under tension in this way can lead to tip migration or cuff extrusion

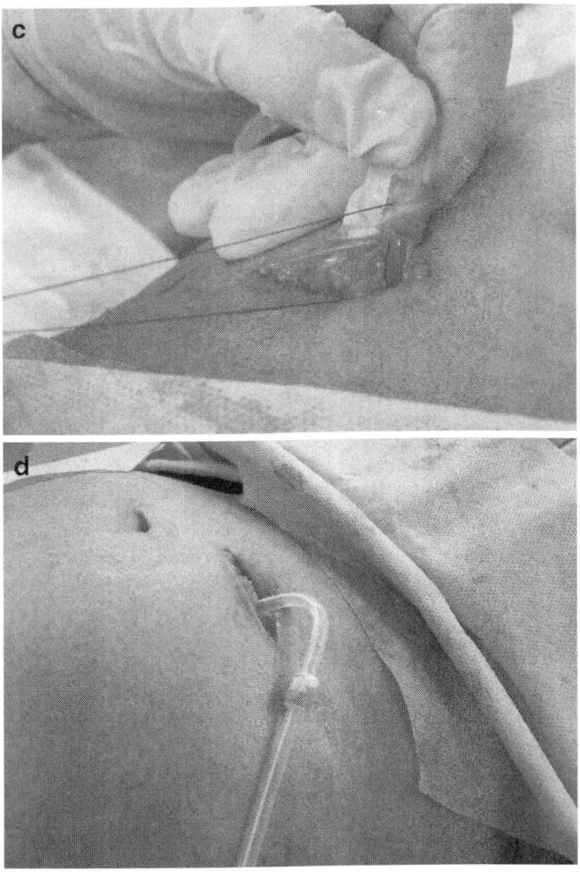

Fig. 25.12 (continued)

- Straight catheters should be given laterally directed tunnels and exit sites. If a straight catheter is bent to produce an inferiorly directed tunnel and exit site, shape memory effects can cause the tip to migrate out of the pelvis or the subcutaneous cuff to extrude from the tunnel.
- The exit site must be away from the belt line, deep skin creases and bony prominences such as the ASIS.
- The subcutaneous cuff should be placed about 4 cm from the exit site (slightly deeper than cuffs on tunneled vascular access catheters).

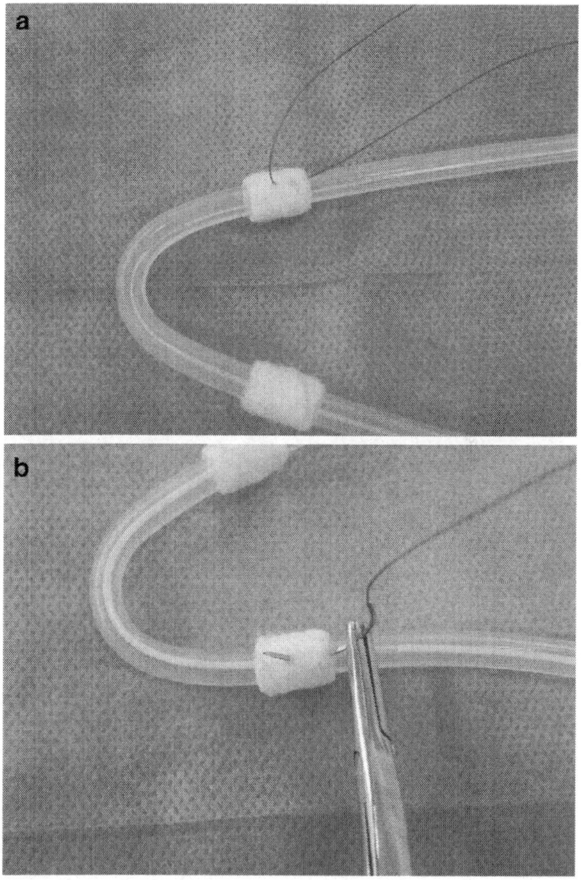

Fig. 25.13 (**a**) Position of deep cuff suture when inserting a left-sided swan neck catheter on the left side of the abdomen. The suture has been placed 180° away from the stripe (which is visible on the opposite side through the clear catheter). (**b**) Position of deep cuff suture when inserting a left-sided swan neck catheter on the right side of the abdomen. The suture has been placed through the cuff on the same side of the catheter as the stripe

25. The exit site and subcutaneous tunnel are anesthetized. The catheter is loaded onto the ridged end of the Faller stylet. The Faller stylet is carefully pushed through the subcutaneous tunnel and then out of the exit site. While traversing the subcutaneous tunnel, the Faller stylet is kept as deep as possible in the subcutaneous fat of the abdominal wall without actually penetrating the

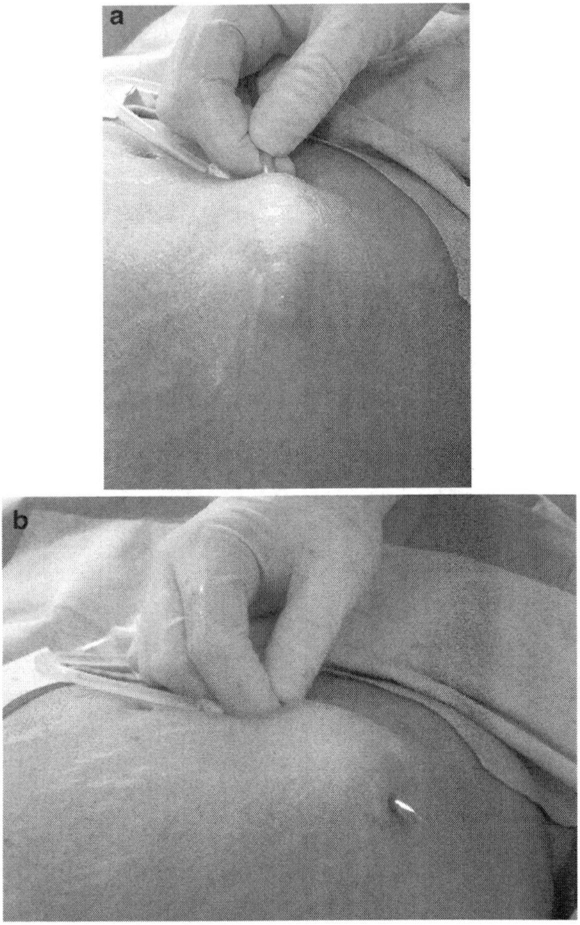

Fig. 25.14 (**a**) Tenting of the exit site over the Faller stylet as the subcutaneous tunnel is being created. (**b**) Faller stylet exiting the skin. The subcutaneous cuff is visible next to the operator's index finger; once the catheter has been pulled through the exit site, this cuff will be positioned in the subcutaneous tunnel

muscles, and is brought out superficially as it nears the exit site. The exit site is not created with a scalpel. Because the Faller stylet has the same outer diameter as the catheter, it produces a snug exit site that does not require suturing (reducing exit site complications) (Fig. 25.14).

26. The incision is closed in layers with 3-0 Monocryl. The deep layer is closed with vertical mattress sutures that are used to pull

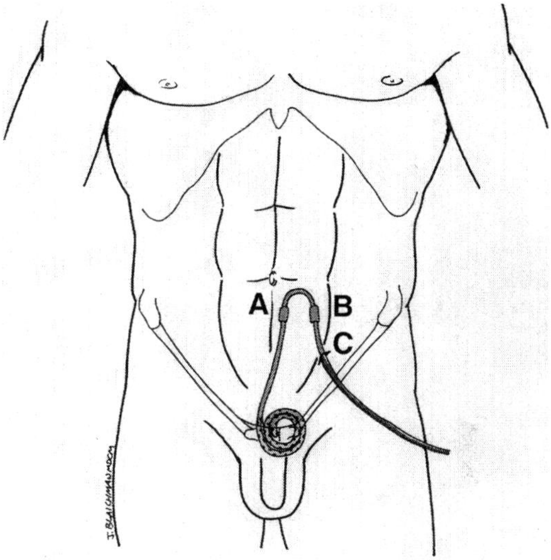

Fig. 25.15 Final position of catheter. A, deep cuff; B, subcutaneous cuff; C, exit site

the subcutaneous fat over the arc of the catheter to keep it from protruding into the incision. If done correctly, this layer will bring the skin edges together; if not done correctly, tension on the skin edges will ensue, and can lead to wound dehiscence. The skin edges are then closed with a running subcuticular suture. All knots are buried. The injected saline is allowed to drain while the incision is being closed.

27. The area is cleaned with 0.05% chlorhexidine gluconate in 4% isopropyl alcohol, gently washing away all blood from the skin and catheter.
28. After the site has dried, Steri-Strips are applied to the incision, and are followed by a gauze dressing covering both the incision and the exit site.
29. The patient is transferred to the recovery area, where a dedicated dialysis access nurse flushes the catheter.
30. The patient is discharged after a period of observation (3–4 h on average).

Final catheter position should be similar to what is illustrated in Fig. 25.15.

Peritoneal Catheter Malfunction

Catheter malfunction is very common, occurring in up to 30% of patients. Outflow obstruction (also called one way obstruction) is the most common form of catheter malfunction, and refers to the inability to consistently drain the peritoneal space completely within a reasonable amount of time, on the order of 45 min or so; it can be caused by debris (often fibrin) in the catheter lumen, as well as a variety of extraluminal factors such as constipation, omental adhesions, omental wrapping of the catheter, occlusion of sideholes by adjacent organs, tip entrapment by peritoneal adhesions, and dialysate leaks (into the pleural space or abdominal wall, for example). Inflow obstruction is caused by kinking of the catheter or intraluminal debris.

Once constipation has been ruled out as the cause of outflow obstruction, tip migration is often sought as the culprit. It is increasingly understood that tip position in and of itself does not correlate well with outflow obstruction. It is likely that much more significant are the underlying omental adhesions or omental wrapping that often the cause the tip to migrate in the first place; these produce one way obstructions to flow.

Shape memory effects can also cause tips to migrate; for example, the tip of a straight catheter given a curved subcutaneous course may have a tendency to rise up out of the pelvis; in this setting, if there are no omental adhesions or wrapping, the catheter may continue to work properly.

It is for these reasons that the position of a catheter tip on plain films does not correlate well with catheter function. Catheters in less than optimal position may work well, and catheters in seemingly perfect position may be obstructed to outflow.

In the setting of one way obstruction that is not due to constipation, catheter manipulation may be undertaken. Antibiotic coverage and IV sedation and analgesia are used. Meticulous sterile technique is mandatory. The existing titanium adapter and the transfer set are discarded and are replaced with new components after manipulation. In most cases the peritoneal space is filled with about a liter of room temperature saline. The aim of the procedure is to optimize tip position, but more importantly, to strip the catheter away from anything

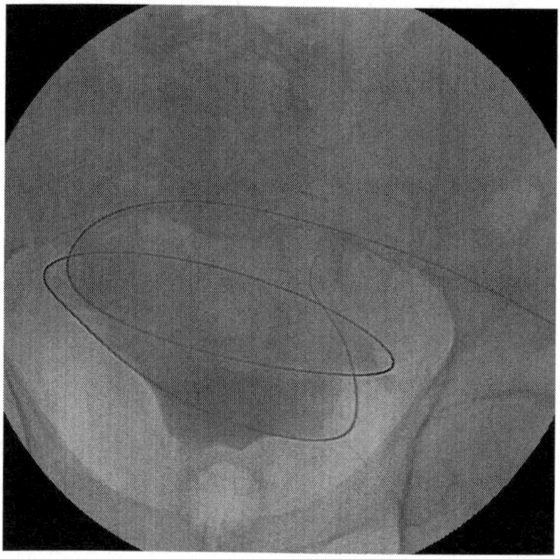

Fig. 25.16 A stiff hydrophilic wire has been passed through a malfunctioning PD catheter. It has exited from a side hole and is forming several loops in the peritoneal space. This will often produce enough tension to strip a catheter away from adhesions (c through g)

that may be adhering to it, often the omentum. Many techniques have been described for manipulating malpositioned peritoneal dialysis catheters. Among the most useful and commonly used devices are stiff hydrophilic wires and malleable PD stylets. A stiff hydrophilic wire advanced out the end of a peritoneal dialysis catheter (usually making numerous loops in the peritoneal space (Fig. 25.16) will often create enough tension to strip the catheter away from adhesions and move it to a new position. A PD stylet that has been bent into a gentle curve can be very helpful in moving the catheter back into the pelvis. It can be difficult to advance a curved stylet through the segment of catheter that traverses the abdominal wall; this can usually be accomplished by oscillating the tip of the stylet while massaging this segment of the catheter through the abdominal wall. This must be done cautiously to avoid perforating the catheter with the stylet. It is often

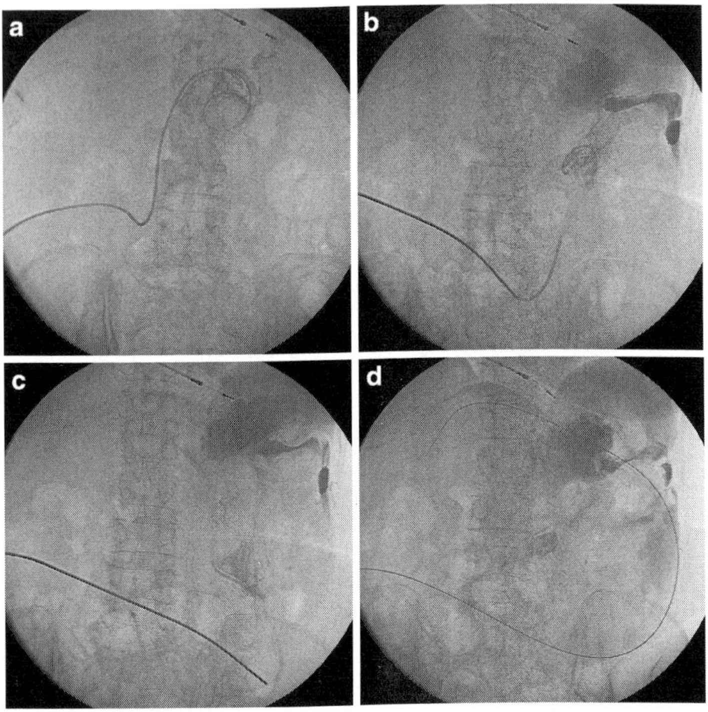

Fig. 25.17 In addition to outflow obstruction, this patient had started to experience epigastric pain when dialysate was being infused into her PD catheter. Plain films showed the tip over the epigastric region. This series of spot images was taken during manipulation of the catheter with a stiff wire and a curved stylet. The catheter was stuck to omentum; this is shown in (**b**) as mottled contrast collecting around the catheter rather than flowing away from it. As the stylet was being used to exert traction on the catheter the patient complained of epigastric pain. It was eventually possible to strip the catheter away from the omentum and reposition it in the pelvis (c through g)

necessary to alternate between the stiff wire and stylet, revising the curve on the stylet as needed; PD catheter manipulations can require considerable patience and perseverance (Figs. 25.17 and 25.18). Even in the most experienced hands, though, there will be a subset that simply cannot be corrected transluminally; these catheters are

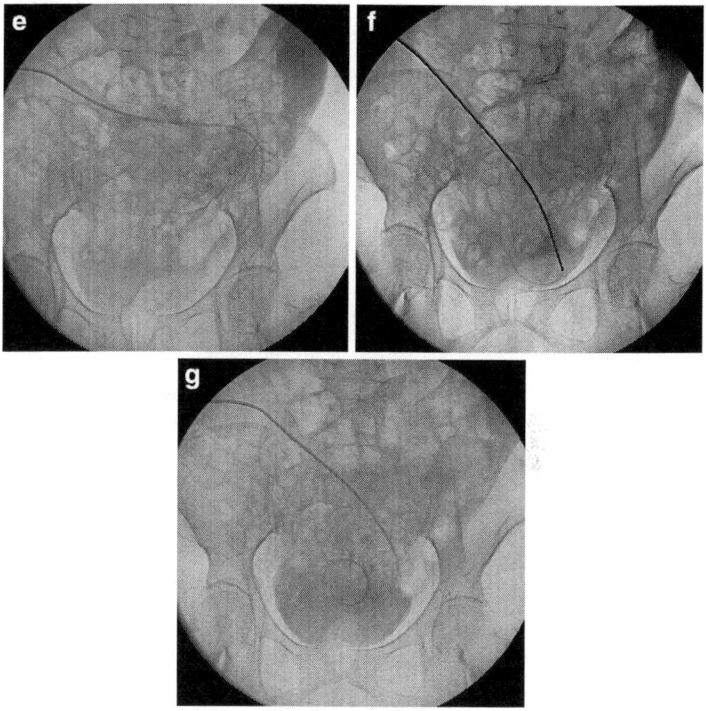

Fig. 25.17 (continued)

typically extensively wrapped in omentum or tethered by strong adhesions that cannot be disrupted using radiologic techniques.

While manipulation is relatively successful at restoring catheter function in the short term, the result is not always durable; this depends in part on the underlying cause of malfunction. CT peritoneography may be helpful in cases where manipulation fails or malfunction recurs. It can document leaks, hernias and tip entrapment by peritoneal adhesions; it can also suggest omental adhesions/wrapping. If radiologic techniques cannot correct the underlying cause of malfunction, laparoscopic techniques should be considered before the catheter is abandoned.

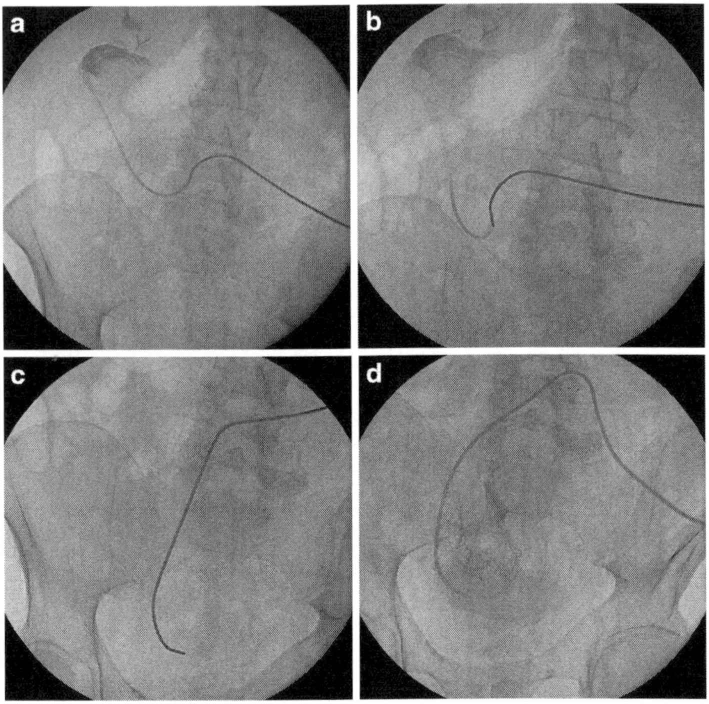

Fig. 25.18 This man had been experiencing outflow obstruction for about 2 months; he could only get full drainage when lying in a right decubitus position. The catheter tip had migrated into the right upper quadrant. It was possible to reposition it into the pelvis with a curved stylet. The catheter continued to work well over the next 4 years with no need for further intervention

Peritoneal Catheter Removal

Indications for removal

- Uncorrectable catheter malfunction.
- Complications, such as persistent exit site infection, peritonitis secondary to a tunnel infection, tunnel infection with abscess formation, bowel perforation, refractory peritonitis, fungal or mycobacterial peritonitis, cuff extrusion.
- Catheter no longer needed.

Steps for removal of a well-established double cuff peritoneal access catheter are as follows:

1. The original incision is anesthetized and re-opened with a scalpel.
2. Blunt dissection is performed through the subcutaneous fat to the fibrous tunnel.
3. A portion of the fibrous tunnel is dissected free of the surrounding tissues and is elevated with a hemostat placed under the freed segment, straddling the incision.
4. The fibrous tunnel is lifted with forceps and opened with scissors to expose the catheter.
5. The catheter is clamped with two hemostats and the intervening segment is cut with scissors.
6. With traction on the deep portion of the catheter, the fibrous tunnel is cut longitudinally with scissors until the deep cuff is reached.
7. The surrounding anterior rectus sheath is anesthetized and an 0-Maxon purse-string suture is placed and set aside.
8. With traction on the deep portion of the catheter, scissors held parallel and as close as possible to the deep cuff are used to cut the adherent fibrous tissue from the cuff.
9. Once the deep portion of the catheter has been freed, it is removed and the purse-string suture is tied.
10. Traction is then placed on the subcutaneous portion of the catheter. The fibrous tunnel is cut longitudinally with scissors until the subcutaneous cuff is reached. This cuff is dissected free and the remaining segment of the catheter is removed.
11. The incision is closed in layers in the same fashion at the time of initial insertion. The exit site is not closed; it is simply covered with a gauze dressing.

Key Points

- Interventional Radiology can play an important role in the success of peritoneal dialysis programs.
- Radiologic techniques are effective in gaining stable and durable peritoneal access.
- Absolute contraindications to radiologic insertion are rare.

- Main objectives for catheter insertion are to obtain stable tip position deep in the pelvis and to create an exit site that heals well, is comfortable, is visible to the patient and is directed either laterally or inferiorly.
- Manipulation can be helpful in salvaging some malfunctioning peritoneal dialysis catheters.

References

1. Rubin HR, Fink NE, Plantinga LC, Sadler JH, Kliger AS, Powe NR. Patient ratings of dialysis care with peritoneal dialysis vs hemodialysis. JAMA. 2004;291(6):697–703.
2. Moist LM, Port FK, Orzol SM, et al. Predictors of loss of residual renal function among new dialysis patients. J Am Soc Nephrol. 2000;11(3):556–64.
3. Tokgoz B. Clinical advantages of peritoneal dialysis. Perit Dial Int. 2009;29 Suppl 2:S59–61.
4. Mujais S, Holmes C. Modern peritoneal dialysis: concepts and approaches. Kidney Int Suppl. 2006;103:S1–2.
5. Dell'Aquila R, Chiaramonte S, Rodighiero MP, et al. Rational choice of peritoneal dialysis catheter. Perit Dial Int. 2007;27 Suppl 2:S119–25.
6. Eklund B, Honkanen E, Kyllonen L, Salmela K, Kala AR. Peritoneal dialysis access: prospective randomized comparison of single-cuff and double-cuff straight Tenckhoff catheters. Nephrol Dial Transplant. 1997;12(12):2664–6.
7. Nessim SJ, Bargman JM, Jassal SV. Relationship between double-cuff versus single-cuff peritoneal dialysis catheters and risk of peritonitis. Nephrol Dial Transplant. 2010;25(7):2310–4.
8. Eklund BH, Honkanen EO, Kala AR, Kyllonen LE. Peritoneal dialysis access: prospective randomized comparison of the Swan neck and Tenckhoff catheters. Perit Dial Int. 1995;15(8):353–6.
9. Nielsen PK, Hemmingsen C, Friis SU, Ladefoged J, Olgaard K. Comparison of straight and curled Tenckhoff peritoneal dialysis catheters implanted by percutaneous technique: a prospective randomized study. Perit Dial Int. 1995;15(1):18–21.
10. Gadallah MF, Mignone J, Torres C, Ramdeen G, Pervez A. The role of peritoneal dialysis catheter configuration in preventing catheter tip migration. Adv Perit Dial. 2000;16:47–50.
11. Jacobs IG, Gray RR, Elliott DS, Grosman H. Radiologic placement of peritoneal dialysis catheters: preliminary experience. Radiology. 1992;182(1):251–5.
12. Savader SJ. Percutaneous radiologic placement of peritoneal dialysis catheters. J Vasc Interv Radiol. 1999;10(3):249–56.

13. Savader SJ, Geschwind JF, Lund GB, Scheel PJ. Percutaneous radiologic placement of peritoneal dialysis catheters: long-term results. J Vasc Interv Radiol. 2000;11(8):965–70.
14. Rosenthal M, Yang P, Liu In-Lu. Comparison of outcomes of peritoneal dialysis catheters placed by the fluoroscopically guided percutaneous method versus directly visualized surgical method. J Vasc Interv Radiol. 2008;19(8):1202–7.
15. Vaux EC, Torrie PH, Barker LC, Naik RB, Gibson MR. Percutaneous fluoroscopically guided placement of peritoneal dialysis catheters – a 10-year experience. Semin Dial. 2008;21(5):459–65.
16. Maya ID. Ultrasound/fluoroscopy-assisted placement of peritoneal dialysis catheters. Semin Dial. 2007;20(6):611–5.
17. Moon JY, Song S, Jung KH, et al. Fluoroscopically guided peritoneal dialysis catheter placement: long-term results from a single center. Perit Dial Int. 2008;28(2):163–9.
18. Brunier G, Hiller J, Drayton S, Pugash RA, Tobe SW. A change to radiological peritoneal dialysis catheter insertion: three-month outcomes. Perit Dial Int. 2010;30:528–33.
19. Crabtree JH, Fishman A. A laparoscopic method for optimal peritoneal dialysis access. Am Surg. 2005;71(2):135–43.
20. Veys N, Biesen WV, Vanholder R, Lameire N. Peritoneal dialysis catheters: the beauty of simplicity or the glamour of technicality? Percutaneous vs surgical placement. Nephrol Dial Transplant. 2002;17(2):210–2.
21. Crabtree JH. Fluoroscopic placement of peritoneal dialysis catheters: a harvest of the low-hanging fruits. Perit Dial Int. 2008;28(2):134–7.
22. Perakis KE, Stylianou KG, Kyriazis JP, et al. Long-term complication rates and survival of peritoneal dialysis catheters: the role of percutaneous versus surgical placement. Semin Dial. 2009;22(5):569–75.
23. Dombros N, Dratwa M, Feriani M, et al. European best practice guidelines for peritoneal dialysis. 3 Peritoneal access. Nephrol Dial Transplant. 2005;20 Suppl 9:ix8–12.
24. Gokal R, Ash SR, Helfrich GB, et al. Peritoneal catheters and exit-site practices: toward optimum peritoneal access. Perit Dial Int. 1993;13(1):29–39.
25. Gokal R, Alexander S, Ash S, et al. Peritoneal catheters and exit-site practices toward optimum peritoneal access: 1998 update. (Official report from the International Society for Peritoneal Dialysis). Perit Dial Int. 1998;18(1):11–33.
26. Flanigan M, Gokal R. Peritoneal catheters and exit-site practices toward optimum peritoneal access: a review of current developments. Perit Dial Int. 2005;25(2):132–9.
27. Crabtree JH. Selected best demonstrated practices in peritoneal dialysis access. Kidney Int Suppl. 2006;103:S27–37.
28. Ash SR. Chronic peritoneal dialysis catheters: overview of design, placement, and removal procedures. Semin Dial. 2003;16(4):323–34.
29. Crabtree JH, Burchette RJ. Prospective comparison of downward and lateral peritoneal dialysis catheter tunnel-tract and exit-site directions. Perit Dial Int. 2006;26(6):677–83.

30. Crabtree JH, Burchette RJ, Siddiqi NA. Optimal peritoneal dialysis catheter type and exit site location: an anthropometric analysis. ASAIO J. 2005;51(6):743–7.
31. Kappel JE, Ferguson GM, Kudel RM, Kudel TA, Lawlor BJ, Pylypchuk GB. Stiff wire manipulation of peritoneal dialysis catheters. Adv Perit Dial. 1995;11:202–7.
32. Simons ME, Pron G, Voros M, Vanderburgh LC, Rao PS, Oreopoulos DG. Fluoroscopically-guided manipulation of malfunctioning peritoneal dialysis catheters. Perit Dial Int. 1999;19(6):544–9.
33. Diaz-Buxo JA, Turner MW, Nelms M. Fluoroscopic manipulation of Tenckhoff catheters: outcome analysis. Clin Nephrol. 1997;47(6):384–8.
34. Moss JS, Minda SA, Newman GE, Dunnick NR, Vernon WB, Schwab SJ. Malpositioned peritoneal dialysis catheters: a critical reappraisal of correction by stiff-wire manipulation. Am J Kidney Dis. 1990;15(4):305–8.
35. Dobrashian RD, Conway B, Hutchison A, Gokal R, Taylor PM. The repositioning of migrated Tenckhoff continuous ambulatory peritoneal dialysis catheters under fluoroscopic control. Br J Radiol. 1999;72(857):452–6.
36. Gadallah MF, Arora N, Arumugam R, Moles K. Role of Fogarty catheter manipulation in management of migrated, nonfunctional peritoneal dialysis catheters. Am J Kidney Dis. 2000;35(2):301–5.
37. Yilmazlar T, Yavuz M, Ceylan H. Laparoscopic management of malfunctioning peritoneal dialysis catheters. Surg Endosc. 2001;15(8):820–2.
38. Yilmazlar T, Kirdak T, Bilgin S, Yavuz M, Yurtkuran M. Laparoscopic findings of peritoneal dialysis catheter malfunction and management outcomes. Perit Dial Int. 2006;26(3):374–9.

Chapter 26
Complications and Possible Solutions

Dheeraj K. Rajan

One should not assume that percutaneous interventions within hemodialysis accesses are routine and simple. While a dominant majority of interventions are low risk, complications are inevitable when one has performed a sufficient number of cases. While many of the potential complications can be managed with endovascular techniques, others are true surgical emergencies and should be recognized as such rather than persevering to avoid having to call the surgeon or transport the patient to tertiary care center. While the following represents a majority of complications one may encounter, this list is not exhaustive and the methods discussed are not "the only way" to manage these complications. There are many ways to solve a problem/complication. Knowing your limitations and options are paramount. Secondly, ignoring complications does not mean that they magically disappear.

D.K. Rajan (✉)
Head and Associate Professor, Division of Vascular & Interventional Radiology, Department of Medical Imaging, University of Toronto, Toronto, Ontario, Canada
e-mail: Dheeraj.Rajan@uhn.on.ca

D.K. Rajan (ed.), *Essentials of Percutaneous Dialysis Interventions*,
DOI 10.1007/978-1-4419-5657-6_26,
© Springer Science+Business Media, LLC 2011

The Lost or Migrated Stent/Stent Graft

Management of this scenario depends on many factors, including the type of stent versus stent graft, what area was being stented, and the location the device has migrated to. Although a basic concept, veins get bigger as you progress more centrally. When a stent or stent graft migrates, there is real risk of migration all the way out to the pulmonary arteries. Given that most devices have points to them, if the stent/stent graft is left in the pulmonary artery, erosion through the artery may occur leading to risk of delayed fatal pulmonary hemorrhage. If devices become lodged in the heart, arrhythmias and cardiac perforation are possibilities.

If the stent/stent graft has migrated a short distance forward, the device may be pulled back by inflating a balloon within it, and capturing the device and pulling it back. For example, if the stent/stent graft is 8 mm in diameter, inflating an 8 or 9 mm balloon within it will grab it from the inside possibly allowing repositioning across the lesion or to another location. Considerations include that a stent may crumble against the lesion when being pulled back, and stent graft material has relatively little friction and may pull off the balloon when pulling back across the lesion (see Fig. 26.1).

If this is unsuccessful or not possible, one can try and "trap" the stent or stent graft with another stent/stent graft. The concept is to stent within the stent back to the lesion. A stent or stent graft 1–2 mm larger than the migrated stent is deployed partially within the migrated stent with a minimum of 1 cm overlap (see Fig. 26.2). This traps the migrated stent, and this method is effective if the stent/stent graft has migrated only a short distance. In the event that the device has migrated more centrally, but short of the SVC, one can also trap the stent by placing a much larger diameter self expanding stent through the migrated device, thereby fixing it within the vein segment (see Fig. 26.3).

Prior to considering this option, or if the stent or stent graft has migrated into the heart, one can attempt to retrieve the device. Retrieval techniques are partially dependent on if the device is a stent or stent graft. For stents, most have open cell structures and snares will catch within the interstices of the stent. For covered stents, the covering prevents snares from holding the device securely.

To retrieve a stent, a loop snare or a tulip loop snare (see Fig. 26.4) can be used to engage the stent at one end. The edge of the stent

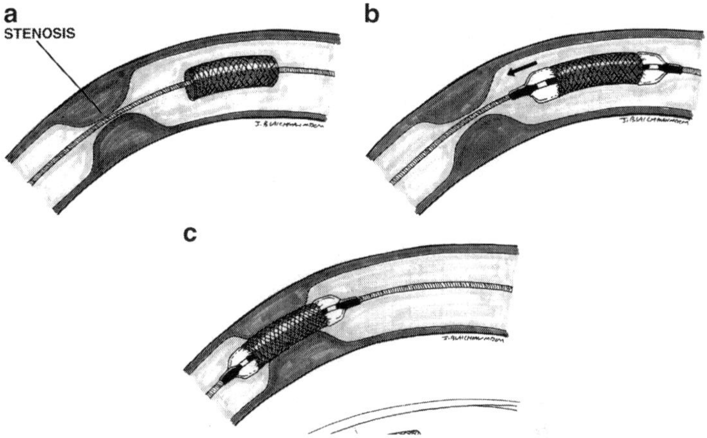

Fig. 26.1 Balloon retrieval of migrated stent

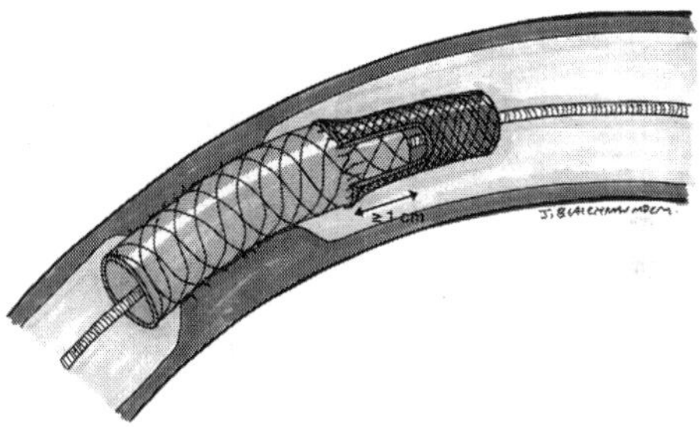

Fig. 26.2 Trapping or securing of migrated stent with another stent

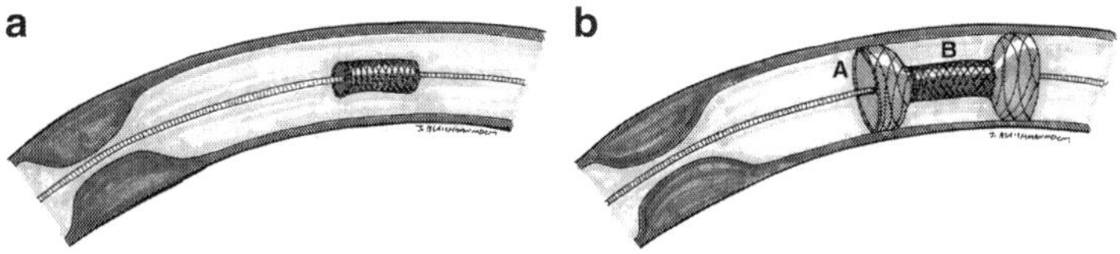

Fig. 26.3 Trapping of migrated stent (**b**) with larger stent (**a**) within a more central vessel

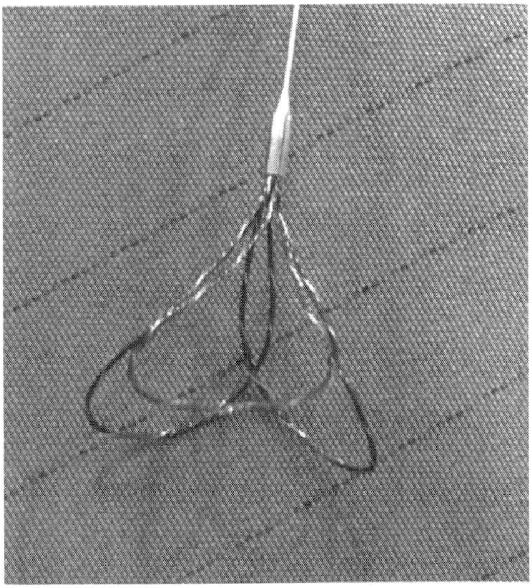

Fig. 26.4 The EN Snare (Merit Medical) or tulip snare composed of three nitinol loops allowing for more circumferential snaring of foreign bodies

should be engaged to allow the captured end to be compressed or funnelled down to allow the stent to be pulled into the sheath, rather than catching on the edge of the sheath. Once snared, the device can be pulled into a large sheath and the snare, and sheath with the stent within it are pulled out (see Fig. 26.5). Prior to attempting this, a large sheath has to be placed to allow a stent to be pulled into it. The sheath size should be large enough for the stent to relatively easily pass into it and is often 14 Fr or higher. Given the large size, the retrieval is often performed from the femoral vein although one can pass the sheath through the access if it is an upper arm access and later purse string the hole shut. Most self expanding stents have an open cell structure and are actually very fragile. As one attempts to pull the stent into the sheath, the struts of the open structure may catch on the lip of the sheath (see Fig. 26.6). There are two percutaneous options. One is simply to pull harder and hope the stent pulls into the sheath, or to grab the stent with another snare from the other end through another access point. When the stent has been snared from both ends, one can put traction on both snares and stretch the stent to a lower profile (see Fig. 26.7). If the stent fractures, individual pieces will have to be retrieved, but given poor visibility of nitinol with fluoroscopy, fragments may be missed [1].

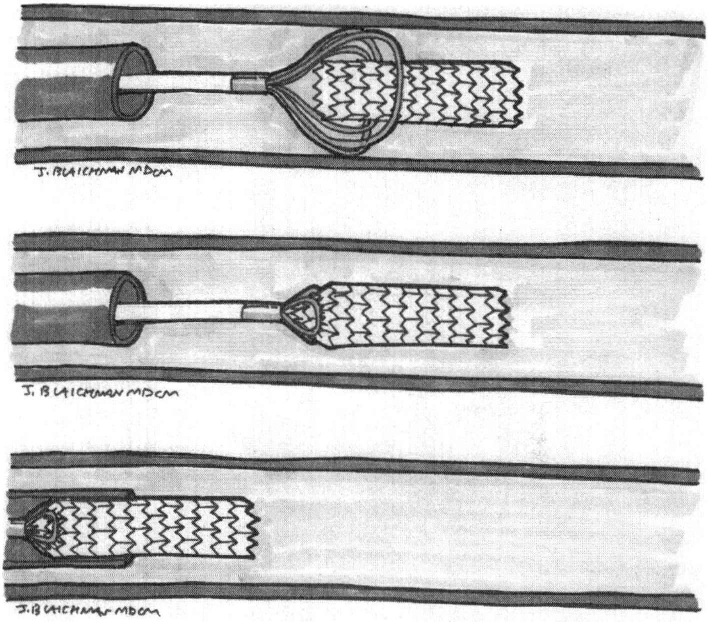

Fig. 26.5 Snare retrieval of migrated stent or stent graft

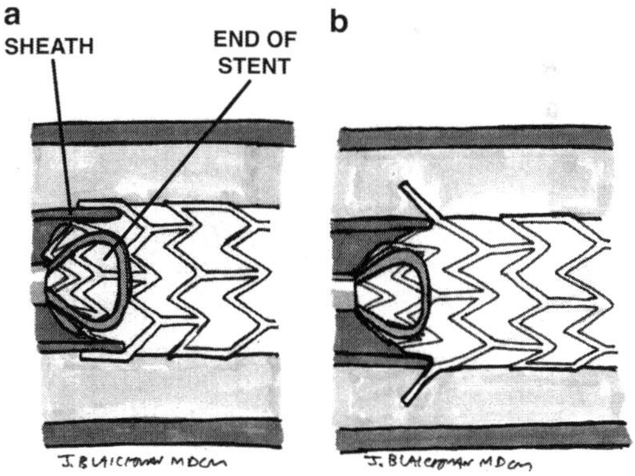

Fig. 26.6 Insufficient sheath size results in end of stent/stent graft catching on the tip of the sheath

For stent grafts, if the snare does not successfully hold onto the migrated device, one can advance a glidewire up beside the stent graft and with a hooked guiding catheter, pass the wire back through the stent graft, thereby going around over and back through the stent

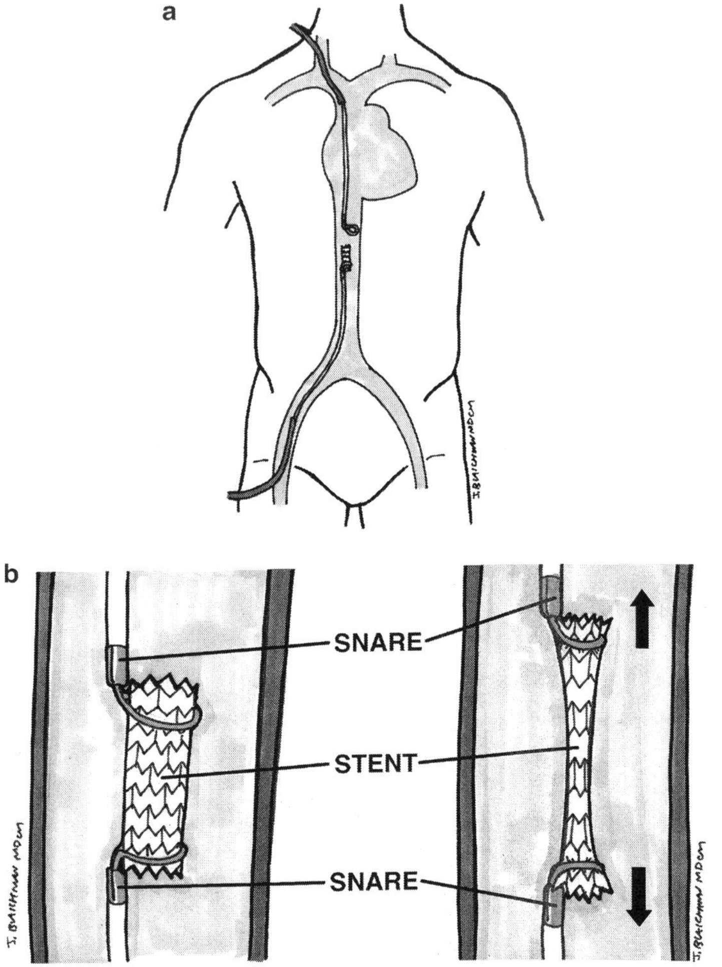

Fig. 26.7 (**a**) Access from upper central veins and femoral vein obtained and snares advanced from both directions. (**b**) The migrated stent/stent graft is captured from both ends and with traction from both directions the device is stretched to a lower profile for retrieval

graft allows the device to be captured. The end of the wire is then snared and pulled through the sheath thereby capturing the stent graft (see Fig. 26.8). One can also use biopsy forceps to grab onto the stent graft. Such devices include myocardial biopsy forceps and an alligator biopsy forceps. The Bard Recovery cone (used for Bard IVC filter

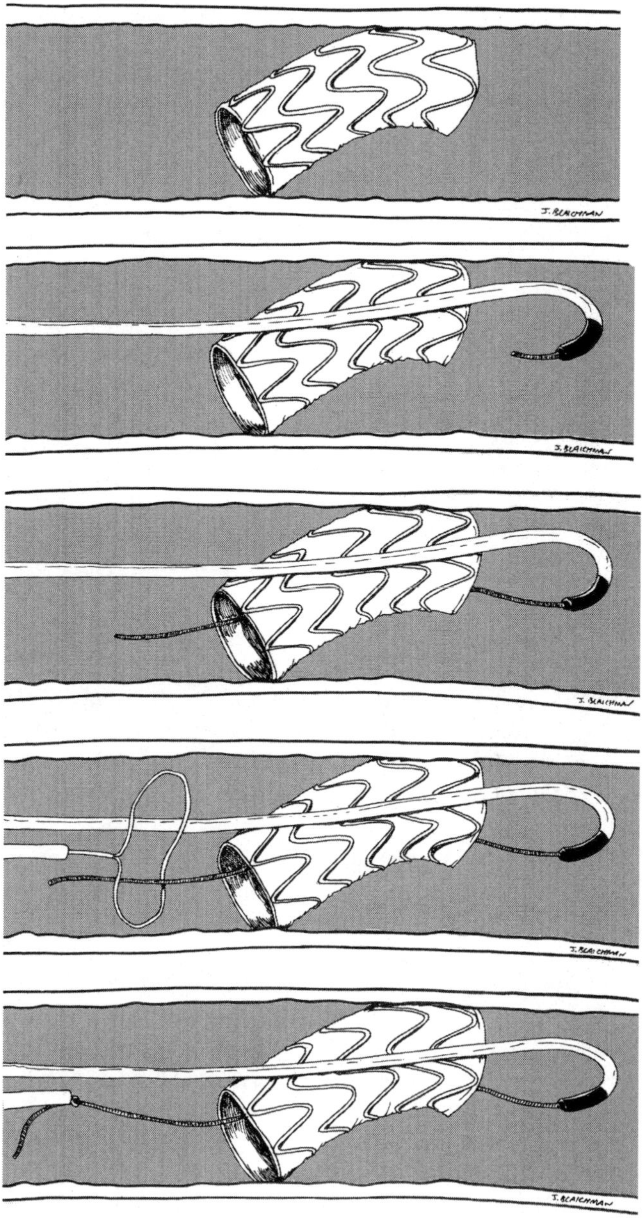

Fig. 26.8 Retrieval of stent graft

removals) is a collapsible umbrella with a large diameter opening that allows capture of most smaller (<8–10 mm) diameter stents/stent grafts. The device also allows a wire through it which can be directed through the stent and then the cone is directed over end of stent. The cone is then collapsed thereby capturing and securing the end of the stent/stent graft.

Once the device is pulled into the sheath, the sheath is simply pulled out of the patient while maintaining a grasp on the stent/stent graft. These deployed devices do not pass through the diaphragm of access sheaths. If the device to be retrieved as migrated beyond the tricuspid valve, when removing the device, one must ensure that the tricuspid valve leaflets are not caught or will get torn when pulling out the device. This will precipitate right heart failure and the need for surgical intervention.

Rupture of Dialysis Graft/Fistula/Vein

During balloon dilation, one can sometimes tell when rupture has occurred, before deflating the balloon and doing a contrast fistulogram. When rupture of the vessel occurs, one feels a "popping" or sudden split second snapping sensation through the shaft of the balloon catheter. As dilation should always be performed under active fluoroscopic monitoring, one may see a waist in the balloon suddenly disappear, instead of gradually dilating with a drop in pressure with the balloon inflator.

If conservative measures fail for management of rupture, these alternatives may be considered. Conservative measures include reversal of heparin, external compression, and balloon tamponade. Compression and balloon tamponade should be attempted for at least 10 min and up to three times if possible. For venous segment ruptures at sites of previous stenosis, uncovered stents can be placed. Sizing is based on the diameter of the next adjacent normal vein segment. Uncovered stents have been found to have a similar patency as balloon angioplasty [2]. Although a rare occurrence, during angioplasty of an intragraft stenosis, the graft may rupture. Although perigraft scar tissue often contains the rupture, rarely, a perforation or tear through the skin may occur. When this happens, the graft has now been exposed to the skin surface and is now considered infected. Options for treatment include blowing up a balloon across the site of rupture and transferring the patient to the operating room emergently or sacrificing the graft by occluding it with either coils, an Amplatzer device or suture ligation. For the latter scenario, one has to occlude both the inflow and outflow of the graft. Lastly, a stent graft can be placed across the rupture site. This is a temporizing measure as the graft is still considered infected, but this option allows for more time to manage the patient and allow for possible surgical revision of the graft (see Fig. 26.9).

When fistulas rupture through the skin, they are often at sites of aneurysms where the skin is thinned to the point of appearing shiny with a blood scab, eschar, or blister at the shiny portion. A simple physical test mentioned in Chap. 17 is to pinch the overlying skin. If the skin cannot be pinched, there is a high risk of rupture. When one sees this appearance, there is a relatively high risk of spontaneous rupture and life threatening hemorrhage. When such an appearance is seen, surgical revision should be considered. Another option is to place a stent graft across this location, thereby excluding the aneurysm. If this is to be done, careful attention should be made to make sure the device is long enough to provide a proper seal on either end to exclude the aneurysm. Gram positive antibiotics should be administered as clot within the aneurysm is often colonized with gram positive bacteria. Lastly, the aneurysm should be aspirated after stent graft placement to prevent future seroma formation.

Embolization of Clot into the Artery

During AVG/AVF procedures if proper care is not taken and volume of any sort is introduced into the thrombosed access, the arterial plug or clot may be forced into the feeding artery and travel distally. Although most emboli are asymptomatic within the arm and do not require intervention [3], some events do lead to acute hand or arm ischemia followed by permanent deficits. If the clot burden is minimal and the patient has no symptoms, one may consider no intervention at all although long term implications have not yet been determined. An attempt at treatment/removal of visualized emboli should be made. Depending on the clot burden, and configuration of the access, a variety of techniques may be attempted.

1. Bleed back technique [4]. With this technique, if embolization occurs down the radial or ulnar artery, the artery affected is compressed before the access origin. Blood flow through the palmar

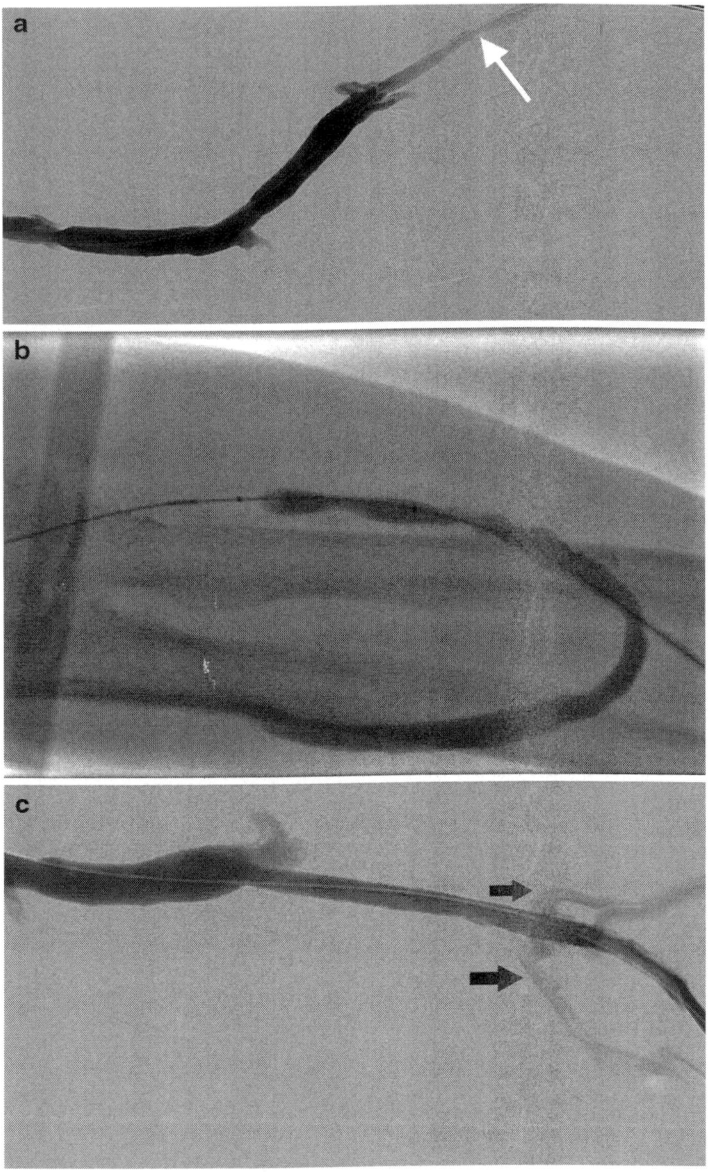

Fig. 26.9 Patient with forearm loop graft with decreased flows and skin ulceration at site of arterial needle insertion. (**a**) Fistulogram demonstrates arterial limb intragraft stenosis (*arrow*). (**b**) A clear waist to the balloon is seen during inflation verifying location of stenosis. (**c**) Completion fistulogram demonstrates frank

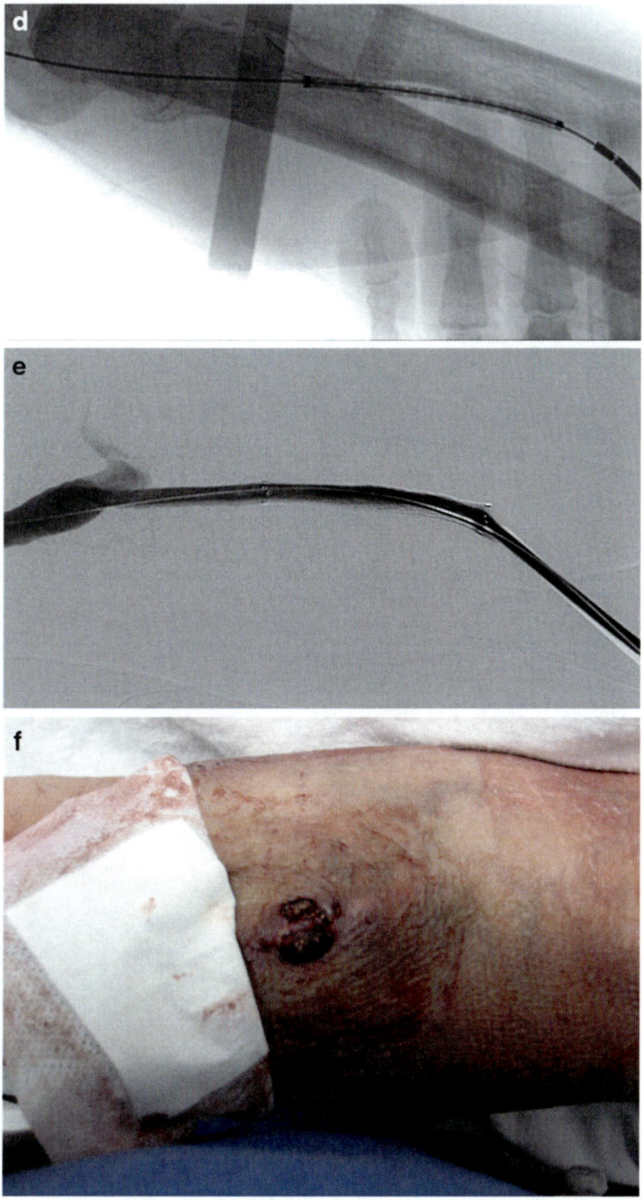

Fig. 26.9 (continued) extravasation (*arrows*) out of the graft and examination of the site revealed the ulceration had ruptured open with blood pouring out over the skin. (**d**) With direct compression of the bleeding site (fingers), a Fluency 7 × 40 mm

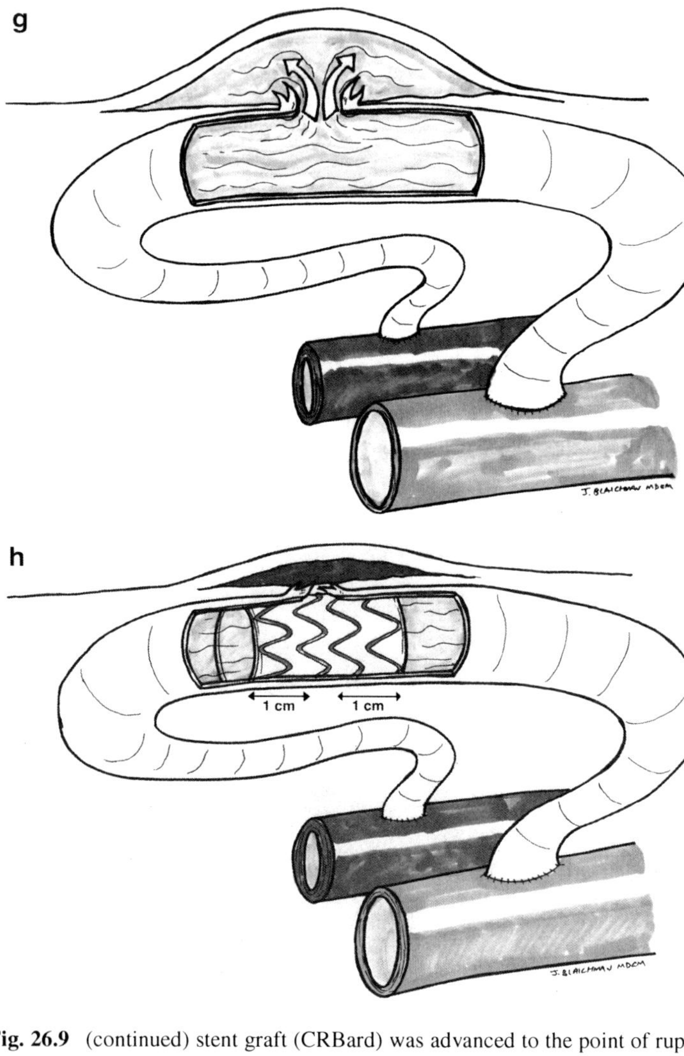

Fig. 26.9 (continued) stent graft (CRBard) was advanced to the point of rupture and deployed. (**e**) Post deployment fistulogram with no continued extravation. (**f**) Ulceration of the skin at point of rupture. The patient subsequently had elective replacement of the arterial limb of the graft (open rupture by surgical literature is considered an infected access) thereby preserving the access. (**g**) Illustration of graft rupture. (**h**) A minimum of 1 cm margins beyond the rupture is recommended to prevent migration and ensure an adequate seal for hemostasis

arches of the hand then fill the affected artery retrograde and backwash the embolism into the dialysis access (see Fig. 26.10). The backbleeding technique relies on the principle of backbleeding via collateral arteries to float an embolus retrograde into the graft or fistula. For this procedure to work, the graft or fistula must be patent. A Fogarty balloon or other occlusion type balloon is placed in the brachial artery just above the anastomosis and the patient exercises their hand for approximately one minute. The balloon is then deflated and repeat fistulography is performed. A variant of this method is placement of a 4–5 Fr catheter distal to the embolus, and administering forceful injections in an attempt to dislodge the embolus retrograde by volume displacement, into the patent graft or fistula. Care must be exercised not to displace or fragment the embolus into smaller emboli that occlude end vessel arteries.

2. Fogarty embolectomy. The Fogarty balloon is advanced beyond the embolism and inflated. The inflated balloon is then pulled back slowly to the arterial anastomosis and the embolism is allowed to wash up into the access (see Fig. 26.11).
3. Thrombolysis. An endhole catheter is advanced up to the embolism, and tissue plasminogen activator (tPA) or urokinase is injected in tiny forced aliquots to dissolve the clot. The aliquots are administered as 2–3 cc injections using a 3–10 cc syringe to generate more injection pressure to force the thrombolytic into the clot (figure). If the clot burden is over a long segment of artery, a multi-sidehole infusion catheter can be inserted to pulse spray the thrombolytic into the clot. For tPA, 2–10 mg may be injected over a few minutes in 2 mg aliquots until or if the clot dissolves. For urokinase, the dose ranges from 250,000–1,000,000 units.
4. Suction embolectomy (see Fig. 26.12). A large endhole catheter or guiding catheter is advanced up to and touching the clot. A large syringe is then attached to the catheter ≥20 cc and suction is applied and the catheter is pulled back. With this method the clot may become lodged within the entry sheath within the access after the suction catheter is pulled out. In such an event, the clot typically lodges at the diaphragm of the sheath and may be pulled out by grabbing it with forceps advanced through the diaphragm. Otherwise, the sheath can be removed over a wire and flushed clean or the clot can be aspirated out the sidearm or flushed into the access.

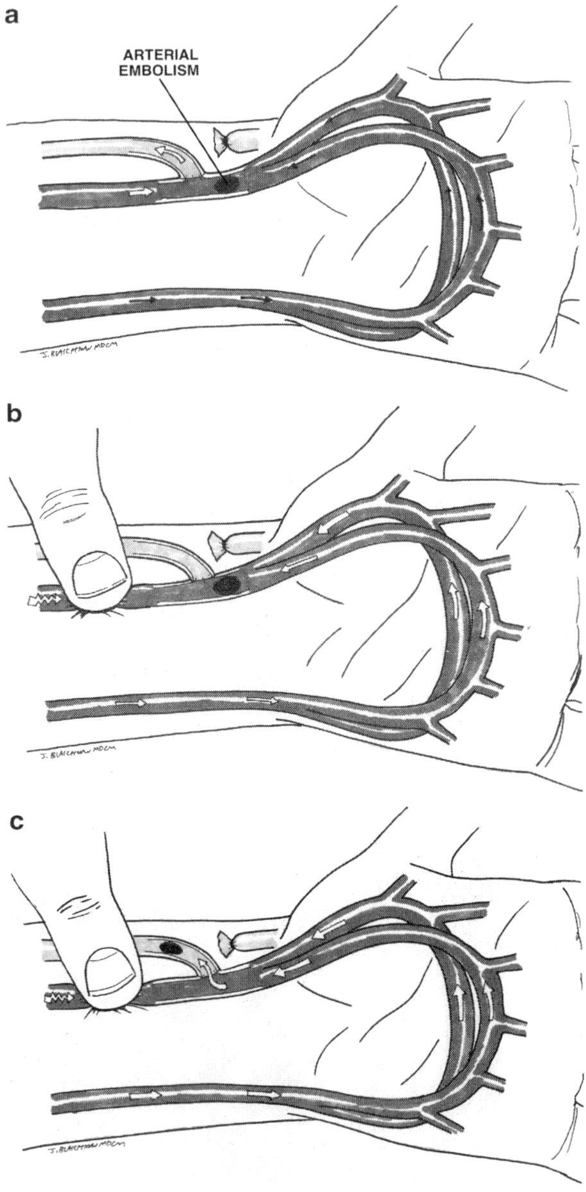

Fig. 26.10 Compression of the feeding artery to the dialysis access leads to preferential backflow through collateral arterial pathways to the access pushing the embolism back into the access

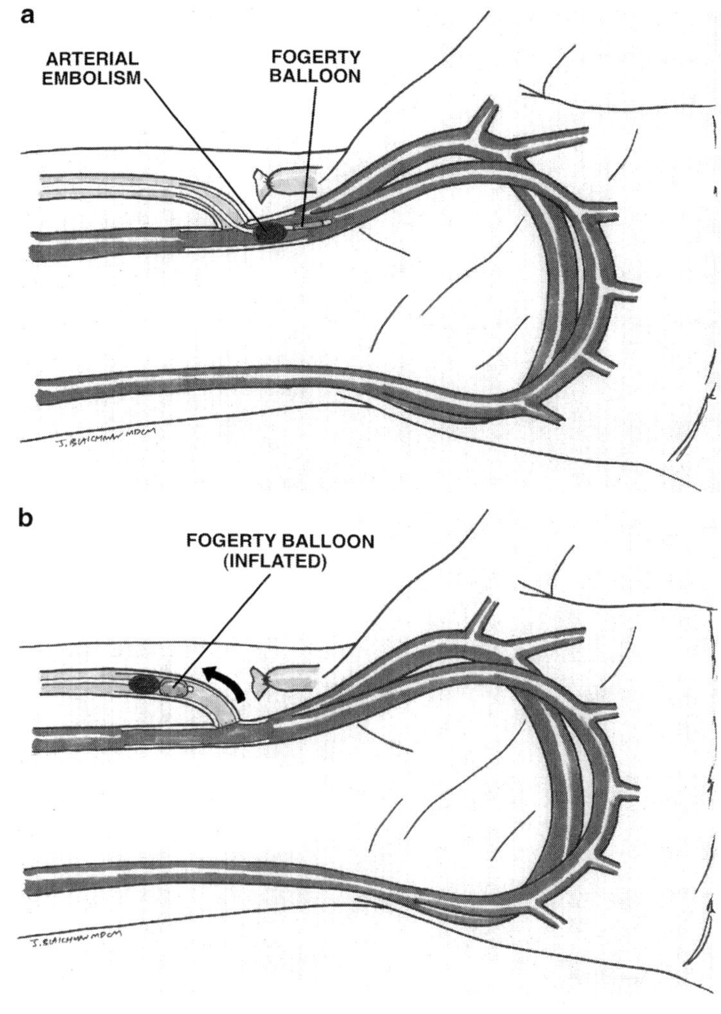

Fig. 26.11 (**a**) Distal arterial embolism. Deflated Fogarty embolectomy catheter is advanced across the clot. (**b**) Catheter is inflated and clot is dragged back into the access

5. Call a surgeon. If the clinical situation warrants intervention, a surgical exploration and thrombectomy may be required. In this event, the patient should be appropriately systemically anticoagulated to prevent propagation of clot.

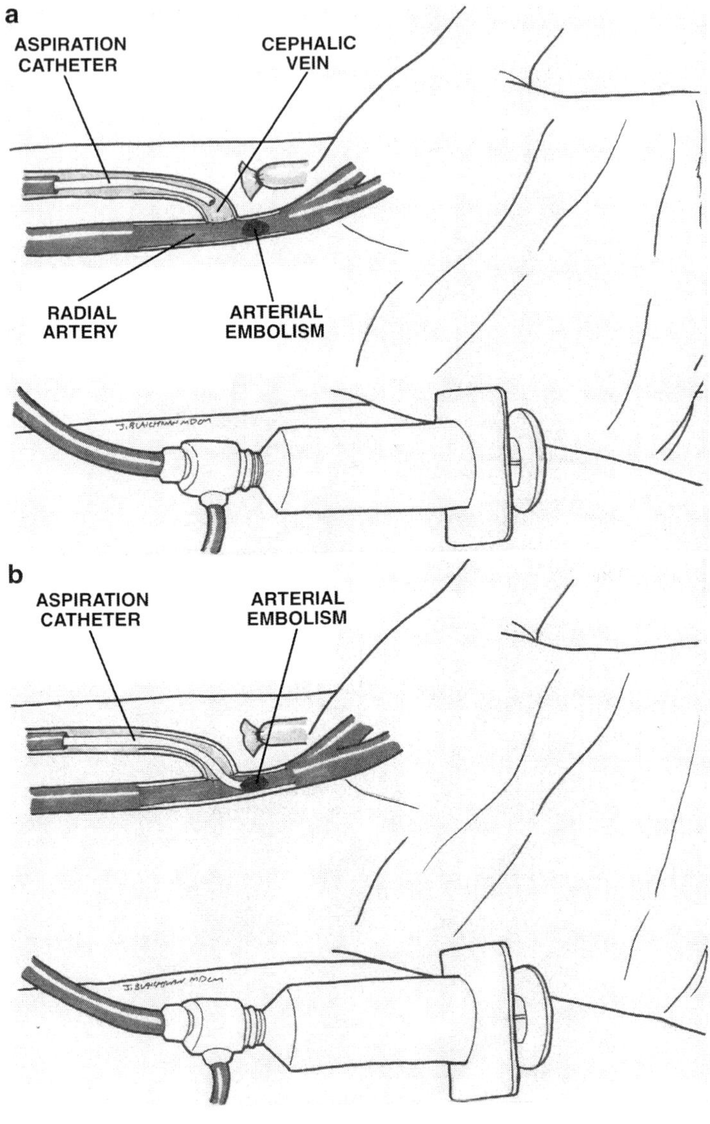

Fig. 26.12 (**a**) Embolism in distal radial artery. (**b**) Large end hole catheter or guiding sheath advanced up to clot. (**c**) Suction is applied with a 20 or 50 cc syringe and the catheter/sheath is withdrawn. (**d**) During declotting of upper arm BC AVF, clot embolized down the brachial artery causing the hand to go numb and cold. Embolisms commonly catch at points of vessel bifurcation (*arrow*) and

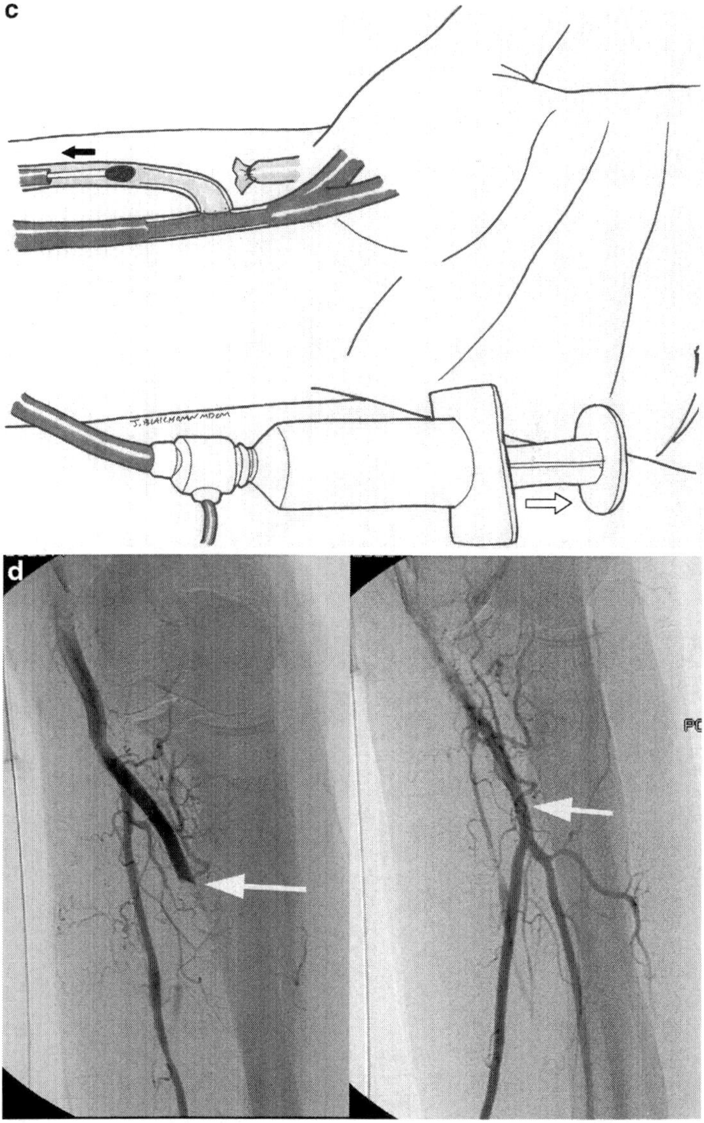

Fig. 26.12 (continued) in this case, where the brachial artery bifurcates into the radial and ulnar arteries. With suction aspiration using a 6 Fr. guiding catheter, the clot was removed restoring flow to the brachial artery. The radial and ulnar arteries are now seen

Lost Balloon Fragments

Although balloon catheters are designed so that in instances of rupture, they tear longitudinally allowing for full retrieval of the device, occasionally components may detach. One can usually tell when the balloon has ruptured, as there is a sudden release of pressure and the balloon deflates rapidly. This can happen if the balloon catches on the struts of a fractured stent, the ends of a stent or in the case of Fogarty balloons, if the balloon is inflated to a size bigger than the area the balloon is being pulled back across, and one pulls with a large amount of force, the balloon and tip can shear off.

Reasonable attempts should be made to retrieve the fragments, as they are potential sources of thrombus formation, can migrate to the lungs, and can be sources of infection. As fragments are often not radiopaque, injections of contrast with DSA are often needed to identify where the fragments are as they will show up as flow voids, or flow defects (see Fig. 26.13). One should examine the balloon catheter itself to determine how much of the device is missing. For fragments, the Ensnare device is perhaps best at retrieving fragments as the multiple petal design allows to a greater chance of grasping. Loop snares and biopsy forceps can also be used. If using a snare, the device size chosen should correspond to the vessel size the fragments lie in.

If retrieval attempts fail, the fragments can be stented down along the vessel wall to trap them and create laminar flow (see Fig. 26.14). Nitinol stents are recommended and post dilation angioplasty should be performed to push the fragments up against the wall thereby reducing flow disruption and potential clot formation.

Balloon will not Deflate

Rarely, an angioplasty balloon or a Fogarty balloon will not deflate completely. This occurs due to either of the following or a combination of both. If the balloon is inflated with undiluted contrast, the viscosity of the contrast may prevent deflation of the balloon by jamming the inflation fluid port. Another possibility is the balloon is pulled back when not fully deflated causing the shaft of the balloon catheter to stretch out, narrow down, and therefore occlude the

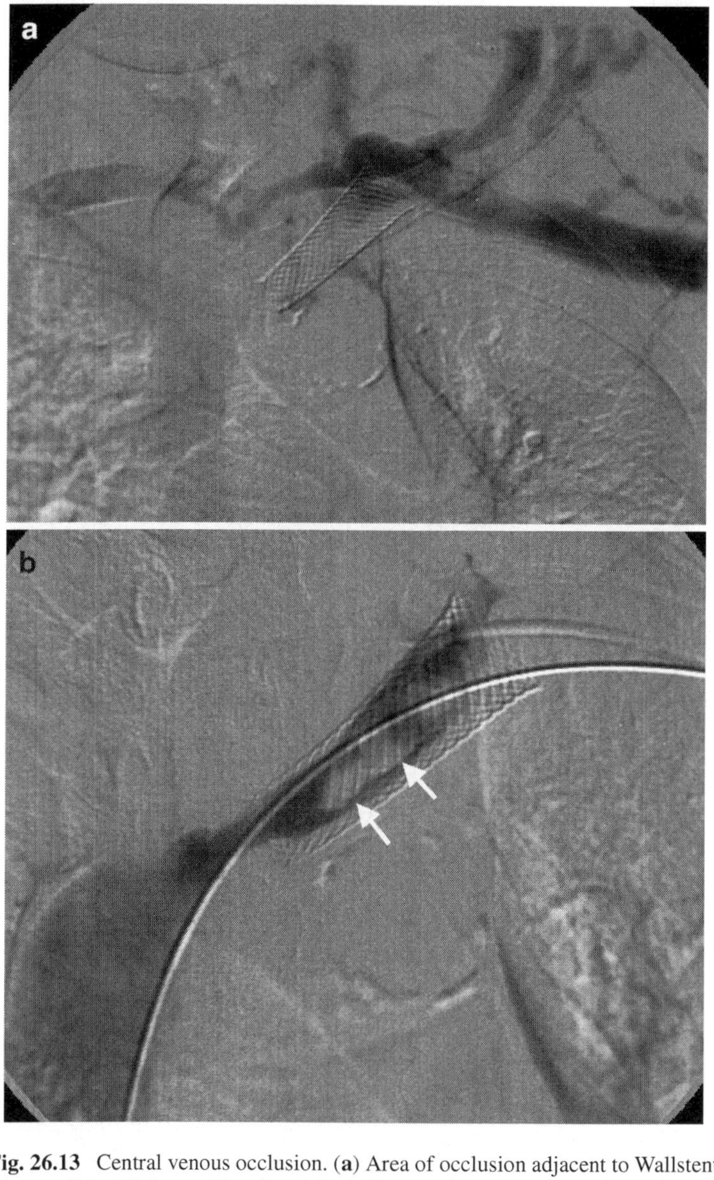

Fig. 26.13 Central venous occlusion. (**a**) Area of occlusion adjacent to Wallstent (Boston Scientific) was dilated and the balloon catheter caught on the end wires of the stent and tore off. (**b–d**) The balloon fragment was visualized as a filling defect (*arrows*) with contrast injection and successfully retrieved with a nitinol loop snare. (**e**) During declotting procedure when arterial plug was pulled, the

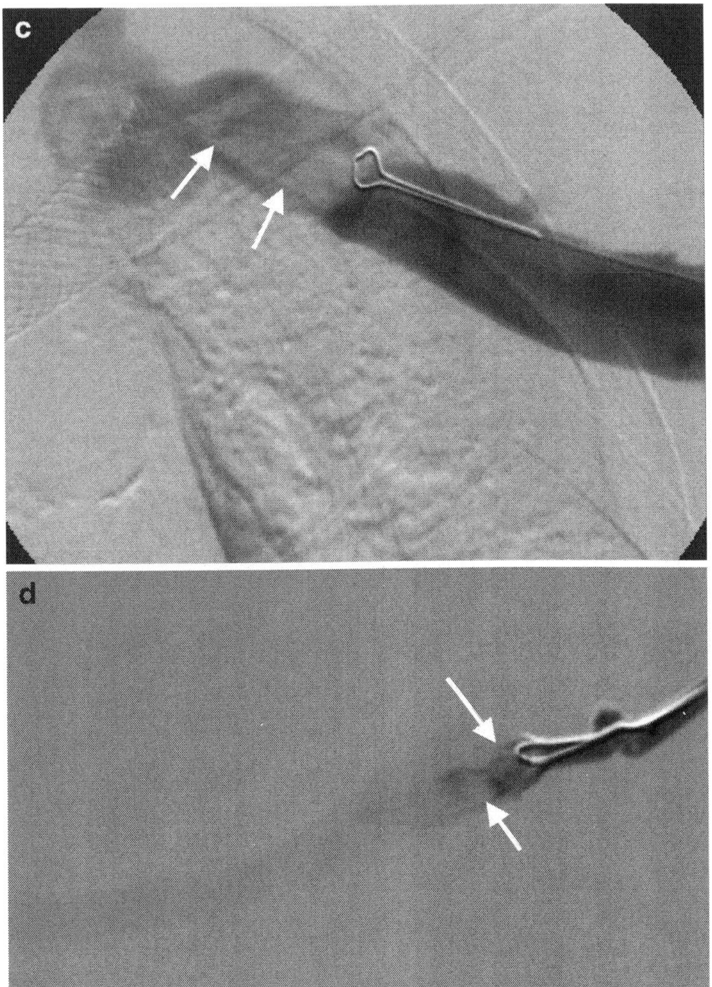

Fig. 26.13 (continued) balloon tip of the Fogarty catheter broke off with retained contrast within it (*arrow*). The PTA balloon was kept inflated to prevent embolization to the lungs and a 5-mm loop snare was used to retrieve the fragment

outflow/inflow tract of the balloon. To overcome this problem, peripherally, one can simply take a small gauge needle (e.g., 25 gauge) and under fluoroscopic guidance, percutaneously puncture the balloon allowing it to deflate (see Fig. 26.15). Within the central

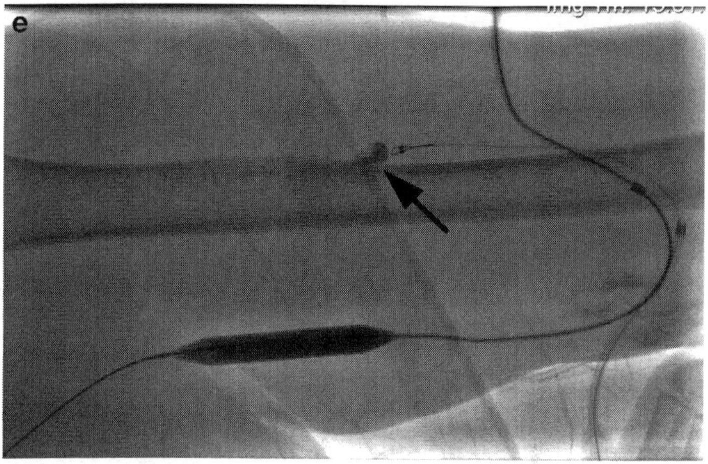

Fig. 26.13 (continued)

system, a second puncture and sheath are required. The puncture may be performed within the access more central to the puncture site. A directional catheter is then advanced up to the balloon and using the back end of a wire, advanced through the catheter, the balloon can be punctured (see Fig. 26.15).

Lost Wire

A lost wire is often the result of simply not paying enough attention to making sure the end of the wire is always visible. Secondly, it can result when a device that is longer than the portion of the wire outside the patient is advanced.

It is important to ascertain which portion of the wire is floppy and which end is the stiff end. This can be done based on the site of entry and verified fluoroscopically. The floppy end (provided one has followed normal convention of advancing the floppy end of the wire first) should lie more centrally with the stiff end lying more peripherally. This can be verified with fluoroscopically as the J or shaped portion of the wire should be visible and in the case of a straight

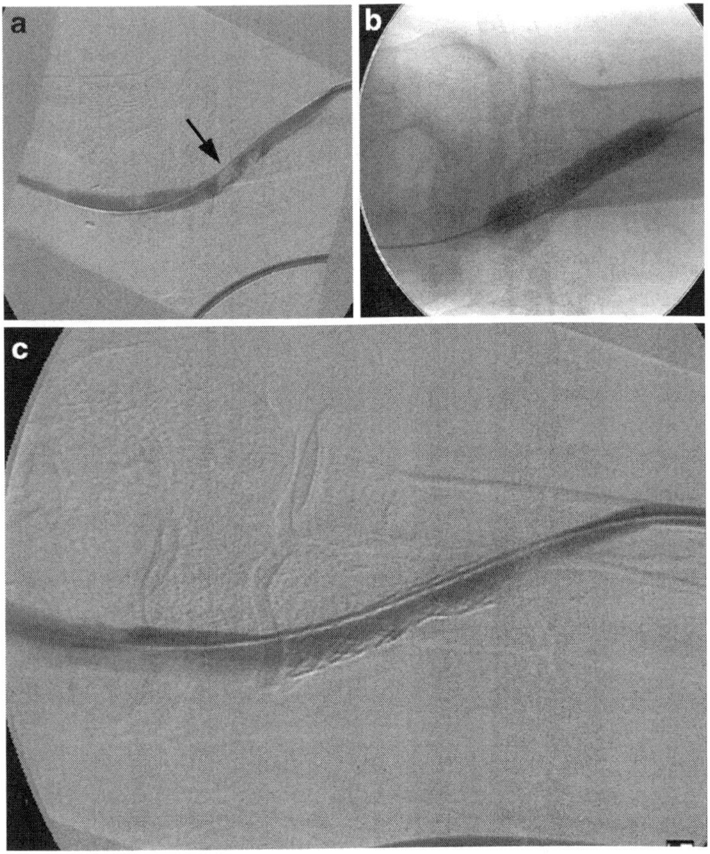

Fig. 26.14 (**a**) Ruptured balloon fragment (*arrow*). (**b**) A self expanding stent was deployed across the balloon fragment thereby pinning it against the vessel wall. (**c**) Balloon fragment is now excluded from the vascular access outflow vein. (**d**) Illustration of balloon fragment stented against vessel wall

wire, the floppy portion is often not completely linear. When retrieval is attempted, the floppy end should be retrieved first. Retrieving the stiff end may lead to vessel perforation and/or laceration which may cause life threatening bleeding. In addition, the stiff end may catch outside the sheath whereas the floppy end will pull into it (see Fig. 26.16).

After the location of the wire has been ascertained and the floppy end determined, access should be obtained that allows easiest and the

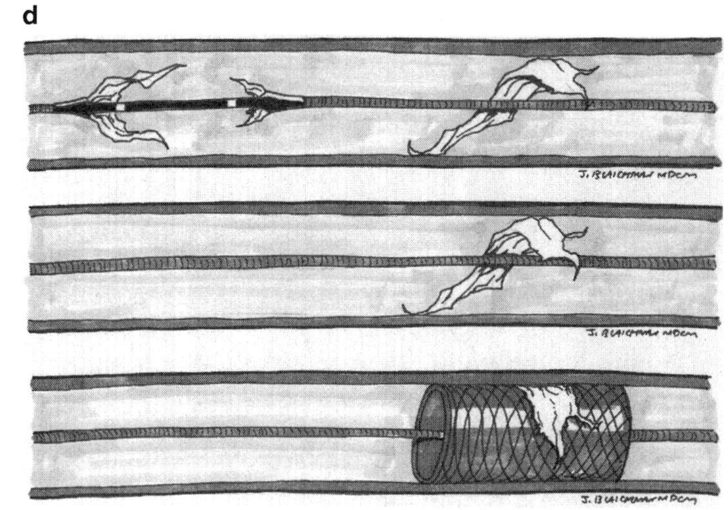

Fig. 26.14 (continued)

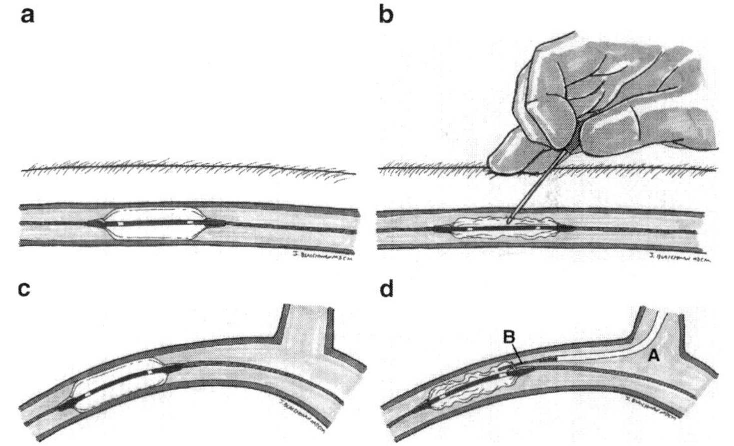

Fig. 26.15 Balloon deflation techniques when balloon will not deflate normally

most direct access to the floppy portion of the wire. This is often from the femoral vein. An appropriately sized sheath should be placed to allow for the retrieval device and the wire. Usually a sheath size 2 Fr bigger than the sheath size required for the retrieval device is

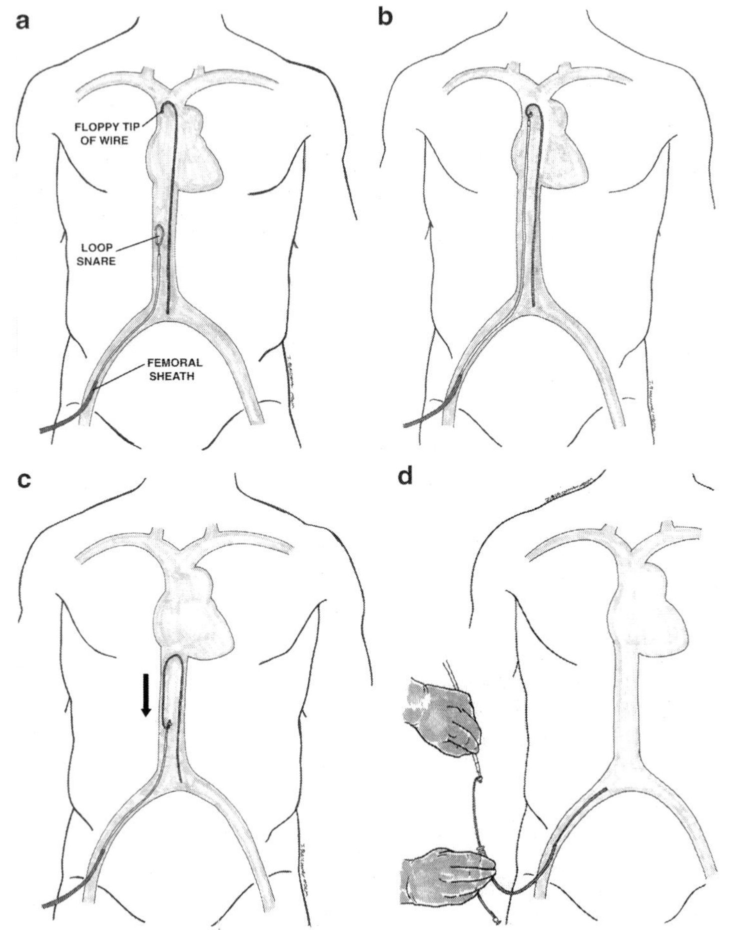

Fig. 26.16 (**a–d**) Illustration of basic steps to lost wire retrieval ensuring access sheath large enough to accommodate retrieval device and the wire. (**e**) Directional catheter (C2) is advanced to the soft tip portion of the guidewire. (**f**) Soft tip or J portion of guidewire is snared with a 10 mm nitinol loop snare. (**g**, **h**) Guidewire removed via an arm vein

sufficient. Using either an Ensnare or a loop snare, the floppy end of the wire should be captured near the tip to allow it to be retrieved. If the wire is engaged farther down its length, it may buckle on itself and not fit into the sheath.

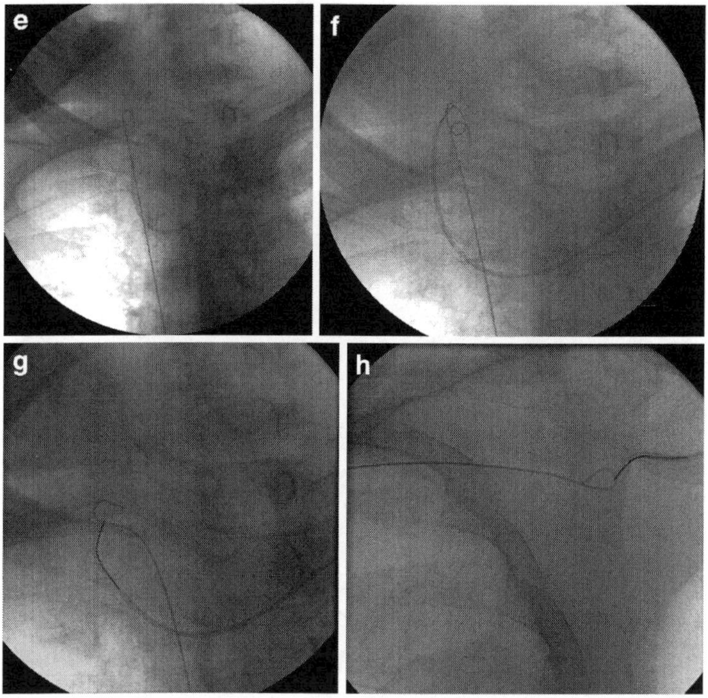

Fig. 26.16 (continued)

Vessel Dissection

Vessel dissection is not necessarily a negative event and in fact all angioplasty events cause limited dissection. A dissection is considered a problem that requires intervention when the dissection flap compromises the vessel lumen and limits flow. Prolonged repeat balloon inflations across the flap with the same diameter balloon should be attempted for at least 45 s to attempt to "tack up" the dissection flap. If this does not correct the flow limitation after a few attempts, a self expanding stent can be placed across the flap. However, this should be avoided as a first step as there is limited patency of stents in the venous system. Within the arterial system, patency is somewhat better. The stent should be sized according to the diameter of the normal adjacent vein or artery segment.

Thrombosis of Vein Catheter Resides in

It is important to ascertain if thrombosis is the result of infection or not. If thrombosis is the result of infection, the catheter should be removed. If there is no evidence of infection, removal of the catheter will result in loss of the access site. Removal of the catheter will not aid in resolution of the clot either. In this situation, the access site should be maintained and the catheter exchanged when needed.

Air Embolization

Despite common thought, 5–10 cc of air within the venous system is not of concern in the absence of a right to left shunt or patent foramen ovale. Air embolism is a concern when volumes exceeding 150 cc as a bolus enter the venous system and enter the heart and becomes lodged in the main pulmonary artery blocking blood entry or "air lock." One might consider that >150 cc is a lot of air. However, the tidal volume in an average patient with a single inspiration is >400–500 cc. Hence, air embolism is particularly of concern during dialysis catheter insertions in the upper body. The air will be visible with appropriate fluoroscopic equipment.

There are basically three immediate treatments which can be used in isolation or in combination:

1. Turn the patient into the left lateral decubitus position. This will trap the air in the right atrium and prevent migration to the pulmonary artery. The patient should be maintained in this position until the air resolves.
2. Place the patient on 100% oxygen. As room air is composed of >70% nitrogen, 100% oxygen assists in dissolving the air embolism.
3. Place a catheter into the air embolism and suck it out. As most cases happen during dialysis catheter insertion, the dialysis catheter itself can be advanced into the air bubble and used to aspirate the air.
4. Although rarely considered, a semi acute treatment option is hyperbaric therapy which is available at most tertiary care centers.

Pulmonary Embolism

Although it is rare to have a potentially fatal pulmonary embolism from declotting procedures, it is possible if outflow veins are also thrombosed and/or dealing with a clotted megafistula. Management is equivalent to standard care which includes conservative supportive care, systemic thrombolysis and regional thrombolytic/mechanical treatment of the pulmonary embolism. Appropriate referral services should be contacted for admission and management. Percutaneous management requires advanced endovascular skills, and is associated with high mortality and morbidity.

Pneumothorax

With ultrasound guidance, this complication should be rare. In most cases, the pneumothorax is small and can be managed conservatively with supplemental oxygen, observation for an additional 4–6 h with chest x-rays obtained at 2-h intervals to document no change or reduction of the pneumothorax. If the pneumothorax is large or expanding, a small bore chest tube with a Heimlich valve can be inserted most commonly through the second interspace of the chest wall anteriorly. There are prefabricated insertion kits available for this purpose.

Pericardial Tamponade

This condition represents a surgical emergency, and the best treatment for this complication is recognizing that this event is occurring. Common causes include wire or dilator perforation of the SVC or the heart, perforation of the SVC related to catheter or dilator insertion, angioplasty induced tear and perforation of metallic stents. Attempts at opening occluded central venous segments can also lead to this complication. The superior pericardial recess can extend up into the supraclavicular area [5]. This list is not exhaustive. Some clinical signs include patient agitation, tachycardia, hypotension, breathlessness, jugular distension, and muffled heart sounds. On ECG, one may see low voltage QRS complexes and ST segment changes.

One should be aware of this potential complication whenever working in the central upper venous system and maintain a high level of suspicion. If suspected, one can use an ultrasound to examine the pericardium to determine if there is accumulating fluid or blood within the pericardial space. Blood will have varying densities on ultrasound.

Treatment is emergent and dependent on the patent's clinical condition but often requires placement of a catheter into the pericardial space or a surgical pericardial window to relieve the pressure on the heart. Call for surgical assistance immediately.

Contrast/Allergic Reaction

Despite to prior reactions to intravenous dye, a patient may at a later time develop an acute hypersensitivity to contrast leading to an allergic or anaphylactic reaction. The allergic reaction can be delayed by greater than 24 h. Mild reactions including pruritus and/or urticaria are often self limiting and can be treated with diphenylhydramine, 25–50 mg PO or IV. For anaphylactic reactions, symptoms often develop within 30 min of injection of contrast. Treatment is based on severity of the reaction. If the patient develops an anaphylactic reaction, aggressive interventions including intubation may be needed.

Anaphylaxis is likely to occur if the patient develops rapid onset and progression of symptoms including:

1. Airway/breathing/circulation problems
2. Skin changes including flushing, angioedema and/or urticaria

Vague symptoms such as restlessness, vomiting, and/or abdominal pain may be present. For minor reactions limited to skin changes and skin irritation, diphenylhydramine in doses of 25–50 mg may be given IV every 4 h. Ranitidine (Zantac) 50 mg IV can also be given for mild reactions. For severe reactions including anaphylaxis, IV or IM adrenaline is the most important drug. The IM route is preferred as this reduces risk of inappropriate dosage or misdiagnosis. IV dosing should be reserved to practitioners familiar with vasopressor use in their practice.

Doses are:

Adult patient

0.3–0.5 mL 1:1,000 solution SC or IM q15 min
0.5–1 mL 1:10,000 solution IV; slow administration; repeat prn
IV infusion: 0.1–1 μg/kg/min

Pediatric patient

0.01 mL/kg (minimum 0.1 mL) 1:1,000 solution IM (preferred) or SC q15 min
0.1 mL/kg 1:10,000 solution IV prn slow administration; repeat prn
IV infusion: 0.1–1 μg/kg/min

Cardiovascular and/or respiratory collapses are very possible complications and acute supportive care should be provided within an acute care setting. This includes high concentration of oxygen usually greater than 10 L/min and large volumes of fluid (500–1,000 mL for adults, 20 mL/kg for children, and monitor response). In addition, administration of epinephrine has risks as well. One has to be aware of the dose administered, as an overdose (particularly when the wrong concentration is used) can cause cardiac arrhythmias, cardiovascular collapse, and cerebrovascular hemorrhage.

Key Points

- Don't be a hero. If the situation is beyond you, ask for help.
- Don't ignore the problem. Devices and mistakes don't dissolve.
- Leaving something alone may lead to bigger problems in the future.
- Surgical options exist. Enquire about them if you fail or you are beyond your level of comfort.
- For interventions or catheter placements in the central veins, always be aware of pericardial tamponade as a potential complication.
- Overall risks for complications are <1% for routine interventions. However, this risk increases with increasing complexity of interventions.

References

1. Taneja M, Rajan DK. Percutaneous removal of migrated nitinol stents from the right ventricle. J Vasc Interv Radiol. 2006;17(7):1213–5.
2. Rajan DK, Clark TW. Patency of wallstents placed at the venous anastomosis of dialysis grafts for salvage of angioplasty-induced rupture. Cardiovasc Intervent Radiol. 2003;26(3):242–5.
3. Trerotola SO, Johnson MS, Shah H, Namyslowski J, Filo RS. Incidence and management of arterial emboli from hemodialysis graft surgical thrombectomy. J Vasc Interv Radiol. 1997;8(4):557–62.
4. Trerotola SO, Johnson MS, Shah H, Namyslowski J. Backbleeding technique for treatment of arterial emboli resulting from dialysis graft thrombolysis. J Vasc Interv Radiol. 1998;9(1 Pt 1):141–3.
5. Choi YW, McAdams HP, Jeon SC, Seo HS, Hahm CK. The "high-riding" superior pericardial recess: CT findings. AJR Am J Roentgenol. 2000;175(4):1025–8.

Chapter 27
On-Label, Off-Label, Misconceptions and Devices that Do not Work

Dheeraj K. Rajan

Within North America, devices used for on-label indications represent that the corresponding government health authorities recognize the device as designed and tested for the indications on the label or indications for use (IFU). For stents indicated for vascular use, the stent would have been tested for fatigability, crush resistance, and flexibility. For example, most stents are tested for a minimum of 60 million pulsations to simulate arterial pulsations and to verify resistance to fatigue. Furthermore, appropriate clinical studies have been performed to validate use for the indications on the label. These factors all add up to a device that is safer for the patient. As physicians seeking the optimal welfare of our patients, it is important that we collectively insist that on label devices be utilized and companies seek on-label approval of their devices.

Off-label use simply indicates that the device has not been tested for the indication for which the device is being used. Device companies are incentivised to avoid on-label indications as this is costly both time wise and fiscally. Such practice also allows them to market similar devices without incurring the costs of other companies who

D.K. Rajan (✉)
Head and Associate Professor, Division of Vascular & Interventional Radiology, Department of Medical Imaging, University of Toronto, Toronto, ON, Canada
e-mail: Dheeraj.Rajan@uhn.on.ca

D.K. Rajan (ed.), *Essentials of Percutaneous Dialysis Interventions*,
DOI 10.1007/978-1-4419-5657-6_27,
© Springer Science+Business Media, LLC 2011

seek on-label indication. This is mostly a pure profit motive. Since many interventionists do not insist on on-label indications and most devices used are not available on-label, current practice of off-label use continues and is indirectly supported. The caveat to this practice is devices are being used for indications for which they have not been properly investigated or tested. This should be kept in mind when treating patients.

Misconceptions

Lesion dilation is performed to the point at which effacement of the "waist" occurs. This may require pressures near the rated burst pressure of the balloon. Some operators will deliberately exceed the rated burst pressure of a balloon, although this risks balloon rupture and constitutes off-label use of the device. Some even deliberately rupture angioplasty balloons thinking that this action causes an extra stretch to the vessel wall. In the face of no evidence of this action improving angioplasty patency, one introduces the risk of vessel rupture from a sudden release of force and the risk of having fragments of the balloon embolizing or dislodging in the patient.

An adequate angioplasty result, according to the guidelines published by the Society of Interventional Radiology, is less than 30% residual stenosis measured angiographically [1, 2]. One should keep in mind that <30% residual stenosis after treatment has not been a validated treatment success endpoint and there is no evidence that reaching this endpoint translates into improved patency from intervention.

Acute elastic recoil of the vein following PTA causing >50% is considered an indication for stenting by K/DOQI guidelines. However, elastic recoil is a poorly defined entity that has neither been qualified nor quantified. Is a permanently implanted device insertion justified by such a vaguely defined pathological event?

What Likely Does not Work

Given that over 120,000 POBA's are performed in the United States alone and that POBA is recognized as the gold standard with relatively poor patency and not infrequent technical failures, a number of devices have been introduced and continue to be introduced to improve on POBA. Highlighted below are brief descriptions of limitations of some of these devices.

Ultra High-Pressure Inflation Balloons

For venous stenoses that are refractory to dilation with conventional angioplasty balloons, dilation with high-pressure balloons may allow successful treatment of the stenosis. These devices include the Blue Max 20 (Boston Scientific, Natick, MA) and the Powerflex Extreme (Cordis, Nutley, NJ). These devices are capable of dilation to 20 atm of rated burst pressure, although some interventionalists will routinely exceed this limit by several atmospheres. More recently, ultra-high-pressure balloons have become available, such as the Conquest balloon (C. R. Bard, Covington, GA). This balloon is constructed of Kevlar but maintains a low profile, and the 8-mm balloon can be inserted through a conventional 6-Fr vascular sheath. The rated burst pressure is 27 atm, although in our practice we have routinely inflated it to 35 atm without balloon disruption, and a recent study supports this practice [3]. This can result in successful treatment of lesions that do not respond to conventional or other high-pressure angioplasty balloons. However, clear patency advantage in fistulas or grafts has not been demonstrated [4]. Furthermore, there is no evidence to indicate that a technically successful angioplasty translates into improved patency.

Stenting

The results of stent placement for venous stenoses in dialysis access have been disappointing, and no prospective randomized trials exist to support their routine use [5, 6]. Furthermore, retrospective studies indicate no advantage of stents over POBA for improved patency outcomes with one study. One retrospective study actually found worse outcomes with stents compared to angioplasty [7]. Within the United States, reimbursement rather than good evidence and good clinical practice has driven increased usage of these devices from 0% in 1991 to >12% in 2008 (www.usrds.org).

The adage that "a stent is only as good as your first angioplasty" should be borne in mind when considering stent placement. At present, stent placement should be reserved for circumstances in strict accordance with the K/DOQI guidelines [8]. It should also be recognized that a stent will not provide any additional radial force to a lesion that cannot be effaced with an angioplasty balloon, so there is little rationale to stent a lesion that has a persistent waist on an angioplasty balloon. Lesions with extensive elastic recoil, those, which recur within a short period (2–3 months following successful angioplasty), or those that occur in association with flow-limiting dissections of the vein wall may be appropriate candidates for stent placement [9].

Stent Grafts

The rationale for the use of stents with a synthetic covering is that they may provide a relatively inert matrix for the ingrowth of normal endothelial cells without a hyperplastic response leading to intimal thickening. There is also evidence that stent grafts may help to prevent or reduce migration of adventitial macrophages and smooth muscle cells to the intima-media level, thereby also reducing the hyperplastic host response. A recently completed randomized comparing conventional balloon angioplasty with angioplasty plus placement of an encapsulated PTFE-covered nitinol stent for the treatment of stenosis at the venous anastomosis of synthetic grafts demonstrated superior and significant improvement in 6 month primary patency of 50–23% [10]. This randomized, multicenter trial population consisted of grafts only and only at the venous anastomosis. *Efficacy in other locations of grafts, fistulas, and central stenosis cannot be extrapolated from this study and should not be.* However, one small randomized study and two retrospective studies are demonstrating initial promise within fistulas [11–13]. Until better evidence exists, routine stent graft use has only been proven efficacious at the venous anastomosis in dialysis grafts compared with POBA.

Cutting Balloons

These balloon catheters have tiny, longitudinally mounted atherotomes (microsurgical blades) embedded within the balloon material which, when inflated, “score” the intima to create controlled trauma to the vessel wall. The scored vessel is then dilated with a standard angioplasty balloon. Results of the prospective randomized "Cutting Edge" trial in patients with dialysis grafts, demonstrated no significant difference in primary patency at 6 months compared to angioplasty [14]. Within fistulas, no clear patency advantage was demonstrated as well [15]. No good scientific evidence exists for routine use of cutting balloons in any dialysis intervention.

Cryoplasty

The most significant study to date consisted primarily of dysfunctional dialysis grafts. The authors found a poor technical success of 35% with a primary lesion patency of 25% at 6 months. Outcomes were far below K/DOQI guidelines and traditionally observed outcomes with angioplasty [16]. Again, there is no evidence to support use of this device for dialysis interventions.

Hemodialysis Ports

While the concept was good, these devices are still prone to fibrin sheath formation and a failure mode similar to dialysis catheters yet with higher resource utilization and a significantly higher cost for the device itself compared to a catheter. Revisions are more difficult and time consuming. Also, one study examining outcomes demonstrated a very high rate of jugular vein thrombosis after insertion (100%) and also suggested similar infection rates to traditional catheters. In patients with limited venous capital, vein thrombosis is a serious negative outcome [17, 18].

Other

There are no sufficient studies to date to suggest any improved outcomes to angioplasty for fistula stenosis with brachytherapy, directional atherectomy catheters, drug eluding stents (DES), and drug eluding balloons or perivascular drug delivery. This is likely to change within the near future. The use of intravascular ultrasound for dialysis interventions is subject to debate. Although the device allows for accurate vessel sizing, this is rarely needed with access interventions. There is a potential role for aiding in central and peripheral venous occlusion interventions where it may assist in directing puncture across to open vein segments.

Conclusion

Despite multiple new devices in existence that may be applied to treat stenosis in hemodialysis fistulas and grafts, none has clearly demonstrated patency advantage over POBA and routine use of these devices cannot be justified. Stent grafts have been proven to be superior to POBA only at the venous anastomosis in dialysis grafts. However, these devices appear to hold initial promise of improved outcomes in fistulas as well but further study is required prior to change in practice.

Key Points

- Insist on using on-label devices when the option is available. They have been properly investigated for the indications on package labeling.
- There are many "fun" devices available for dialysis interventions but does the "pretty" picture translate into a better outcome?

References

1. Aruny JE, Lewis CA, Cardella JF, et al. Quality improvement guidelines for percutaneous management of the thrombosed or dysfunctional dialysis access. Standards of Practice Committee of the Society of Cardiovascular and Interventional Radiology. J Vasc Interv Radiol. 1999;10(4):491–8.
2. Gray RJ, Sacks D, Martin LG, Trerotola SO. Reporting standards for percutaneous interventions in dialysis access. Technology Assessment Committee [see comments]. J Vasc Interv Radiol. 1999;10(10):1405–15.
3. Trerotola SO, Stavropoulos SW, Shlansky-Goldberg R, Tuite CM, Kobrin S, Rudnick MR. Hemodialysis-related venous stenosis: treatment with ultra-high-pressure angioplasty balloons. Radiology. 2004;231(1):259–62.

4. Rajan D, Platzker T, Lok CE, et al. Ultrahigh-pressure versus high-pressure angioplasty for treatment of venous anastomotic stenosis in hemodialysis grafts: is there a difference in patency? J Vasc Interv Radiol. 2007;18(6):709–14.
5. Patel RI, Peck SH, Cooper SG, et al. Patency of Wallstents placed across the venous anastomosis of hemodialysis grafts after percutaneous recanalization [see comments]. Radiology. 1998;209(2):365–70.
6. Rajan D, Clark TW. Patency of Wallstents placed at the venous anastomosis of dialysis grafts for salvage of angioplasty-induced rupture. Cardiovasc Intervent Radiol. 2003;26(3):242–5.
7. Kariya S, Tanigawa N, Kojima H, et al. Peripheral stent placement in hemodialysis grafts. Cardiovasc Intervent Radiol. 2009;32(5):960–6.
8. Eknoyan G, Levin NW, Eschbach JW, et al. Continuous quality improvement: DOQI becomes K/DOQI and is updated. National Kidney Foundation's Dialysis Outcomes Quality Initiative. Am J Kidney Dis. 2001;37(1):179–94.
9. Gray RJ, Horton KM, Dolmatch BL, et al. Use of Wallstents for hemodialysis access-related venous stenoses and occlusions untreatable with balloon angioplasty. Radiology. 1995;195(2):479–84.
10. Haskal ZJ, Trerotola S, Dolmatch B, et al. Stent graft versus balloon angioplasty for failing dialysis-access grafts. N Engl J Med. 2010;362(6):494–503.
11. Shemesh D, Goldin I, Zaghal I, Berlowitz D, Raveh D, Olsha O. Angioplasty with stent graft versus bare stent for recurrent cephalic arch stenosis in autogenous arteriovenous access for hemodialysis: a prospective randomized clinical trial. J Vasc Surg. 2008;48(6):1524–31, 1531.e1–2.
12. Bent CL, Rajan D, Tan K, et al. Effectiveness of stent-graft placement for salvage of dysfunctional arteriovenous hemodialysis fistulas. J Vasc Interv Radiol. 2010;21(4):496–502.
13. Gupta M, Rajan D, Tan KT, Sniderman KW, Simons ME. Use of expanded polytetrafluoroethylene-covered nitinol stents for the salvage of dysfunctional autogenous hemodialysis fistulas. J Vasc Interv Radiol. 2008;19(6):950–4.
14. Vesely TM, Siegel JB. Use of the peripheral cutting balloon to treat hemodialysis-related stenoses. J Vasc Interv Radiol. 2005;16(12):1593–603.
15. Bhat R, McBride K, Chakraverty S, Vikram R, Severn A. Primary cutting balloon angioplasty for treatment of venous stenoses in native hemodialysis fistulas: long-term results from three centers. Cardiovasc Intervent Radiol. 2007;30(6):1166–70; discussion 1171–1162.
16. Gray RJ, Varma JD, Cho SS, Brown LC. Pilot study of cryoplasty with use of PolarCath peripheral balloon catheter system for dialysis access. J Vasc Interv Radiol. 2008;19(10):1460–6.
17. Rosenblatt M, Caridi JG, Hakki FZ, et al. Efficacy and safety results with the LifeSite hemodialysis access system versus the Tesio-Cath hemodialysis catheter at 12 months. J Vasc Interv Radiol. 2006;17(3):497–504.
18. Trerotola SO. Hemodialysis catheter placement and management. Radiology. 2000;215(3):651–8.

Chapter 28
Publications of Hemodialysis Interventions: What Is Relevant?

Dheeraj K. Rajan

Evidence-based medicine represents the foundation for which the clinical practices are based. Unfortunately within the field of percutaneous analysis interventions, not many well-constructed and scientific studies exist. The strongest evidence that can be relied upon is a review of multiple prospective randomized studies whereas the weakest evidence that exists is a retrospective case publication.

For percutaneous dialysis interventions, most of the published studies represent larger retrospective series with little published randomized prospective data (see Fig. 28.1). In addition, some current practices are based on anecdotal data or personal experiences. Since interventionalists and patients are relying on published data to guide interventions and therefore outcomes, it is important to insist on proper research. In addition, it is up to the responsible physician who is treating patients to understand literature that exists regarding interventions they wish to perform.

D.K. Rajan (✉)
Head and Associate Professor, Division of Vascular & Interventional Radiology, Department of Medical Imaging, University of Toronto, Toronto, Ontario, Canada
e-mail: Dheeraj.Rajan@uhn.on.ca

D.K. Rajan (ed.), *Essentials of Percutaneous Dialysis Interventions*,
DOI 10.1007/978-1-4419-5657-6_28,

© Springer Science+Business Media, LLC 2011

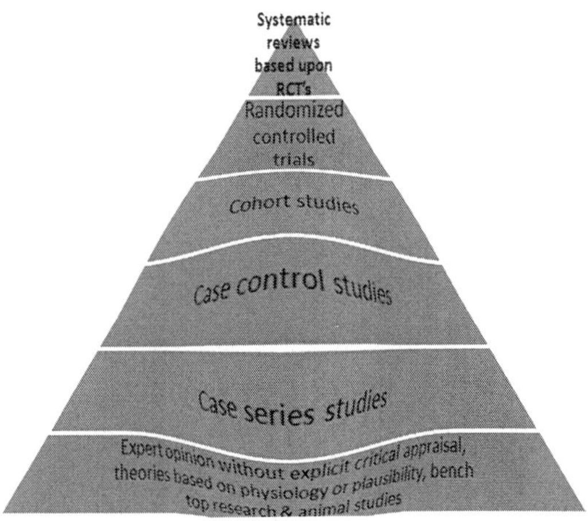

Fig. 28.1 Literature evidence pyramid

As such, it is important to understand the literature that is published. Understanding begins with understanding the quality of the published study itself. Is the publication a randomized prospective blinded study or is it a case report or series? Is the journal within which the article appears peer reviewed or not? What is the impact factor of the journal or is it a well-respected journal? Is the patient population a reflection of your practice? What are definitions of failure, success, complications, and how are outcomes designed? These are some of the basic questions we should all ask ourselves when reading published outcomes before adopting new technologies or methods. For example, primary patency can be defined in multiple ways. Primary patency for surgically created accesses is from the time of creation to time of revision or intervention whereas for percutaneous interventions, it is the time from intervention to failure of that intervention. Furthermore, results can be misstated simply based on if an "intent to treat" analysis is performed. For example, if one has ten patients and there are five technical failures of intervention, patency cannot exceed 50%. However, if one ignores the "intent to treat" methodology and excludes failures, patency up to 100% can be observed. It is important to remember the saying, "There is truth, there are lies and then there are statistics."

First, the best level of evidence that exists is randomized multicenter prospective studies. The main reasons are that patient selection bias is removed and there is an unbiased comparison to another form of therapy. The next major level is a meta-analysis of multiple retrospective studies. Meta-analysis overcome some of the deficiencies of single retrospective studies which include selection and population biases [1].

The most common published type of study within the field of percutaneous hemodialysis interventions is the retrospective single center study. Limitations of such studies include the following:

1. Retrospective – there is selection bias and this study only represents the experiences of a single institution and their study population which may not translate into similar outcomes at other sites.
2. No randomization of the comparison group if there is any which again introduces bias. There may be certain patient characteristics that influence outcome but are not recognized. Randomization reduces or eliminates influence of variables not considered.
3. Preprocedure, periprocedure, and postprocedure methods are not standardized thereby making the findings more subjective to interpretation.
4. The statistical findings are subject to interpretation as a statistical power to a study cannot be determined due to the retrospective nature of the study.
5. Quoted significance is often a comparison of a single variable without considering or controlling for or considering confounding variables.

Case series or case reports represent the lowest level of evidence-based medicine as they represent single events and therefore outcomes are subject to chance. One should not change their clinical practice based on this evidence alone although such reports may be instructional for isolated or rare events.

Why are published outcomes so important? Many physicians are now presenting or discussing their outcomes with new techniques and/or devices without publishing their findings. Without proper peer review, there is no independent assessment of methodology and outcomes. Any physician should at least expect publication in a reputable peer reviewed journal or an independent review by an unbiased expert of findings prior to adopting change in practice.

Within percutaneous dialysis interventions, there are only limited published randomized prospective studies with proper study statistical design [2–4]. The first is related to the type of dialysis catheter used and impact on survival functionality. The last two relate to two different types of treatments for venous anastomotic stenosis in patients with upper arm dialysis grafts compared to angioplasty. Randomized outcomes are more representative of true outcomes. This is highlighted by the findings of the two studies examining grafts. Within the K/DOQI guidelines, minimum POBA recommended primary outcomes are 50% at 6 months. This threshold was determined based on retrospective studies. In randomized prospective studies, POBA patency was 23–40% at 6 months indicating that POBA is not as effective in dialysis grafts as once thought (and suspected) and falls below the published standard within the K/DOQI guidelines.

An area of controversy continues to be the use of stents in dialysis grafts and fistulas. One study published by Vogel and Parise examined the use of nitinol stents versus POBA, the mean primary patency was significantly better with stenting than POBA. However, no standardized continuous or invasive monitoring of patency was performed. There was no accounting of possible interventions performed at other centers. At a mean angiographic follow-up of 348 days, 86% of patients with follow-up angiograms had a mean 55% in-stent stenosis. Given no current approved therapies for in-stent stenosis, a majority of the patients at follow-up had significant stenoses with no defined future treatment. What is highlighted by this study is: (1) one should know how patency was assessed and (2) reading the full publication rather than the abstract sometimes highlights findings with implications to clinical practice one might otherwise not observe. In this case, a 100% intimal hyperplasia rate was observed at 1 year with nitinol stents [5].

In another study examining use of a percutaneous declotting device in dialysis fistulas, a 100% technical success rate was observed. However, if one reads the materials and methods section, patients with large pseudoaneurysms and central occlusions were excluded. Hence, the study was not based on "intent to treat" and excluded a subset of patients one would normally see in daily practice [6].

In a recently published study by Haskal et al., this randomized, multicenter prospective study required 2 and 6 month mandatory angiographic follow-up. It should be noted that since most studies are retrospective, they are observational and do not allow for such uniform objective follow-up of patients. This is one of the advantages of prospective study designs [3].

Basic common definitions for percutaneous dialysis interventions are as follows [7]:

Anatomic or technical success is defined as less than 30% residual diameter stenosis postdilation. For treatment of thrombosed accesses, restoration of flow combined with a less than 30% maximal residual diameter stenosis for any significant underlying stenosis.

Procedural success is defined as anatomic success and at least one indicator of either hemodynamic or clinical success.

Clinical success: After treatment of a thrombosed access, resumption of normal dialysis for at least one session constitutes clinical success. After treatment of a stenosis, reduction of recirculation below threshold values constitutes clinical success.

Primary patency: Interval following intervention until the next access thrombosis or repeated intervention. It ends with treatment of a lesion anywhere within the access circuit, from the arterial inflow to the superior vena cava-right atrial junction.

Assisted primary patency: Interval after intervention until access thrombosis or a surgical intervention that excludes the treated lesion from the access circuit.

Secondary patency: Interval after intervention until the access is surgically declotted, revised, or abandoned because of inability to treat the original lesion, choice of surgeon, transplant, or loss to follow-up.

Outcomes are based on "intent to treat" inclusion criteria and when comparing studies, these definitions should be kept in mind.

In summary, it is up to the practicing interventionalist to interpret the literature mentioned at conferences and published within medical journals. There is value for the physician and particularly patients if one exercises a bit of pessimism when confronted with new findings that may alter practice. I advise that one should discount hearsay and accept findings when published in peer-reviewed journals. However, this alone is perhaps not enough. Reading the published article personally and understanding the study design, the patient population, and results are invaluable. Patients deserve this effort from their physicians.

Key Points

- Small retrospective cases series should be interpreted with some skepticism if results seem overly positive.
- Read beyond the abstract.

References

1. Guyatt G. Users' guides to the medical literature: essentials of evidence-based clinical practice. 2nd ed. New York: McGraw-Hill Medical; 2008.
2. Trerotola SO, Kraus M, Shah H, et al. Randomized comparison of split tip versus step tip high-flow hemodialysis catheters. Kidney Int. 2002;62(1):282–9.
3. Haskal ZJ, Trerotola S, Dolmatch B, et al. Stent graft versus balloon angioplasty for failing dialysis-access grafts. N Engl J Med. 2010;362(6):494–503.
4. Vesely TM, Siegel JB. Use of the peripheral cutting balloon to treat hemodialysis-related stenoses. J Vasc Interv Radiol. 2005;16(12):1593–603.
5. Vogel PM, Parise C. SMART stent for salvage of hemodialysis access grafts. J Vasc Interv Radiol. 2004;15(10):1051–60.
6. Rocek M, Peregrin JH, Lasovickova J, Krajickova D, Slaviokova M. Mechanical thrombolysis of thrombosed hemodialysis native fistulas with use of the Arrow-Trerotola percutaneous thrombolytic device: our preliminary experience. J Vasc Interv Radiol. 2000;11(9):1153–8.
7. Gray RJ, Sacks D, Martin LG, Trerotola SO. Reporting standards for percutaneous interventions in dialysis access. Technology Assessment Committee [see comments]. J Vasc Interv Radiol. 1999;10(10):1405–15.

Chapter 29
Interesting Cases

D.K. Rajan (ed.), *Essentials of Percutaneous Dialysis Interventions*,
DOI 10.1007/978-1-4419-5657-6_29,
© Springer Science+Business Media, LLC 2011

Case 1
Sharp Needle Recanalization for Salvaging AV Accesses with Chronically Occluded Outflow

Naveen Goel

Introduction

There is a subset of patients in which the fistula upper body and/or outflow veins are chronically occluded. These peripherally occluded (Fig. 29.1), blind-ended AV accesses drain through multiple accessory veins ultimately into the central circulation. An AV access becomes dysfunctional due to lack of straight line outflow which can manifest as, or be associated with prolonged bleeding, high venous pressures, poor clearances due to recirculation, swelling of the extremity, and even thrombosis of the access. When conventional recanalization techniques fail, the definitive treatment has been surgery to salvage these accesses, which has its own associated morbidity and mortality. The technique described here percutaneously creates a new anastomosis of the occluded outflow to a patent adjacent outflow vein. This percutaneous technique is feasible, safe, and easily done in the outpatient setting. It is an excellent option to salvage these dying accesses.

Procedure

The procedure is performed using local anesthesia and moderate sedation. A detailed duplex ultrasound exam is performed to search for an adjacent patent outflow vein. An area is then identified where

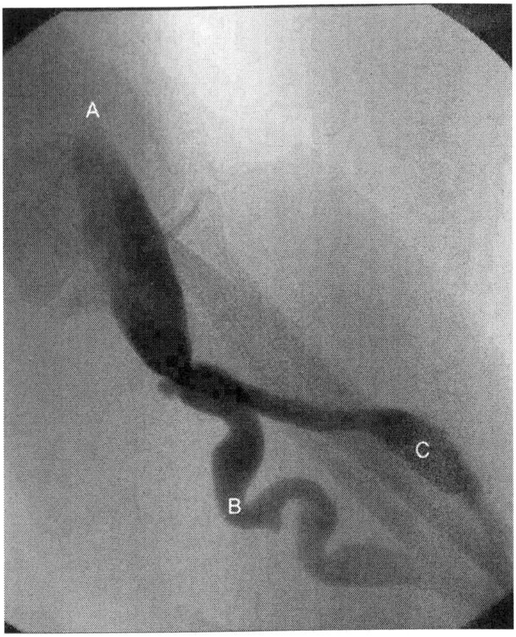

Fig. 29.1 A, Occluded outflow; B, retrograde emptying; C, main body of the access

the main body of the AV access and the selected outflow vein were superficial and closest to each other.

Access is gained into the main body of the fistula or graft in an antegrade manner (Access A, Fig. 29.2) and a 7 Fr sheath is inserted. We choose a 7 Fr sheath in anticipation of the predicted maximum balloon size and stent if required. Multiple fistulogram are obtained and in majority of cases, the selected outflow vein can be accessed in the retrograde manner (Access C, Fig. 29.2) with an angled 4 Fr catheter with or without placement of a sheath. Patency of the outflow vein is again confirmed with contrast injections. The catheter or inflated angioplasty balloon can be used as target in this selected outflow vein for the needle advancement under fluoroscopic guidance (Fig. 29.3). Under direct visualization using ultrasound guidance (Fig. 29.2) or fluoroscopic guidance (Fig. 29.3) a 21 gauge needle (Micro-puncture Introducer; Cook, Bloomington, IN) is advanced

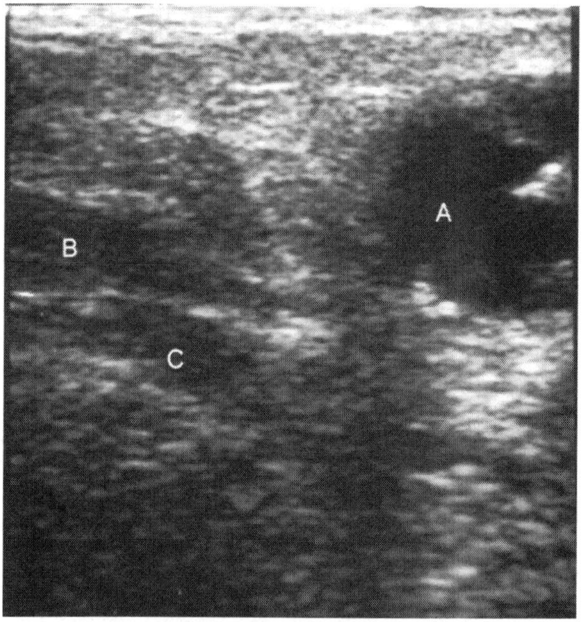

Fig. 29.2 Sharp needle advancing from occluded outflow towards patent outflow vein under ultrasound guidance. A, Occluded outflow with needle; B, targeted patent outflow vein; C, artery in close proximity to the vein

from the patent portion of the outflow fistula body or vein, distal to the occluded site to an adjacent patent vein. The direction of the needle advancement through the subcutaneous tract should be as parallel to the access and the targeted outflow vein as possible. Direction of the puncture decision is based on ease of maneuverability during the procedure. It usually takes two to three needle passes to gain access to the collateral vein. A 0.018-in. wire is advanced and needle is exchanged for 5 Fr coaxial dilator sheath (Micro-puncture Introducer; Cook, Bloomington, IN). The inner dilator was removed and test bolus of contrast is injected to confirm the position in the selected patent outflow vein. This 5 Fr dilator is then exchanged for a 6 or 7 Fr sheath (Access B, Fig. 29.2) over a hydrophilic wire (Terumo). Sequential balloon dilatation is performed of this newly created tract and the outflow vein to accommodate the increased blood flowing through this channel. A hydrophilic wire and angled

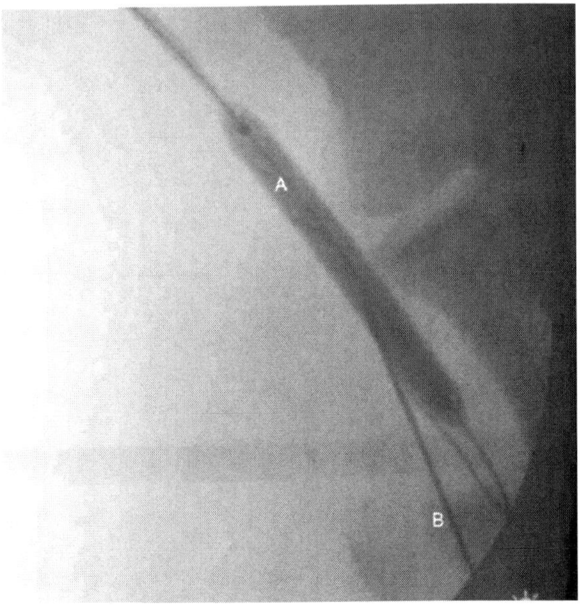

Fig. 29.3 Angioplasty balloon is used as target under fluoroscopy guidance. A, Inflated angioplasty balloon; B, 21 gauge needle

catheter are then traversed from antegrade access A and manipulated across the tract into the new outflow vein and this newly created tract is further dilated. The starting size of the balloon depends upon the outflow vein diameter. Usually, we start with a 4–6 mm diameter balloon and progress to an 8×40 mm diameter balloon. The goal is to achieve most of blood flowing through this new outflow with diminished collateral veins and establishment of a good thrill. Uncovered stents are required in a majority of cases. Reasons for using uncovered stents instead of stent grafts are twofold. First, based on our experience, uncovered stents work as good as stent grafts for venous perforations and second stent grafts were twice the cost of the uncovered stents and nonreimbursable for this indication in outpatient settings. Stent grafts are an option for continued extravasation or pseudoaneurysm formation and potentially longer durability. If the tract is 1–2 mm and the previous mentioned goals are achieved, one does not necessarily need a stent placed.

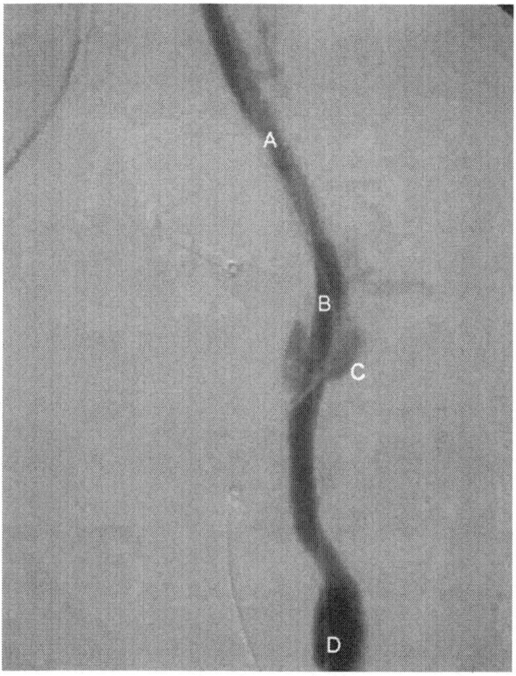

Fig. 29.4 After stent placement flow through the newly created tract. A, Outflow vein; B, occluded outflow; C, stent in newly created tract; D, main body of the access

The stent size recommended is approximately 20–30% bigger than the diameter of the AV access and the outflow vein. The stents are usually inserted from the antegrade access A, but could also be placed from the retrograde access C. It is not recommended to deploy the stents from access point B. Immediate follow-up fistulogram shows brisk flow through the AV access into the new outflow vein (Fig. 29.4). The patient is followed at intervals of 1 week, 1 month, and every 3 months thereafter. Postprocedure, the patient receives aspirin 81 mg orally and then daily indefinitely. Also Plavix 150 mg is administered orally as a bolus and then 75 mg daily for at least 3 months. The procedure is considered successful if the patient's symptoms are resolved and the patient is able to be dialyzed for more than one time.

Outcomes

In an unpublished series, our immediate technical success was achieved in 100% (16/16) of the patients and 93.75% (15/16) of the patients had clinical success with full restoration of normal fistulae function with complete reversal of symptoms. The distance traversed using sharp needle ranged from 2 to 10 mm. 12/16 patients required 8–10 mm diameter stents (uncovered). One patient required a stent graft after 9 weeks to treat a large pseudoaneurysm that occurred in the subcutaneous tract even though an uncovered stent was placed initially. Mean follow-up of 22.7 weeks demonstrated 94% (15/16) of the accesses remaining functioning well during follow-up.

Educational Points

1. Percutaneous salvage of occluded accesses is possible by creation of a new anastomosis to an appropriately selected adjacent outflow vein.
2. If doing so, uncovered stents are often required.

Case 2
Pain After Bare Metal Stent Placement

Shuji Kariya

CASE 2.1

Introduction

A 60-year-old woman with right radiocephalic fistula presented with chronic occlusion of the outflow cephalic vein in the forearm. Venous outflow was maintained by a collateral vein. Stenosis of the collateral vein was impeding access flow. Balloon angioplasty was performed to treat the stenosis, but blood flow was not sufficiently improved due to recoil (see Fig. 29.5a). Two Wallstents (Easy Wallstent; Boston Scientific, Natick, MA) were therefore placed to oppose the recoil (see Fig. 29.5b). Access flow improved as a result.

Issue/Complication

Two months after placement, pain resembling "a needle piercing the skin" developed at the stent placement site. Fistulography revealed that the stent had shortened and the distal edge of the stent had moved into the area of stenosis (see Fig. 29.5c). This had caused the distal edge to deform, resulting in several struts buckling outward toward the skin (see Fig. 29.5d). Although the strut tips remained subcutaneous, every time the skin at the site was touched the patient felt sharp, stabbing pain.

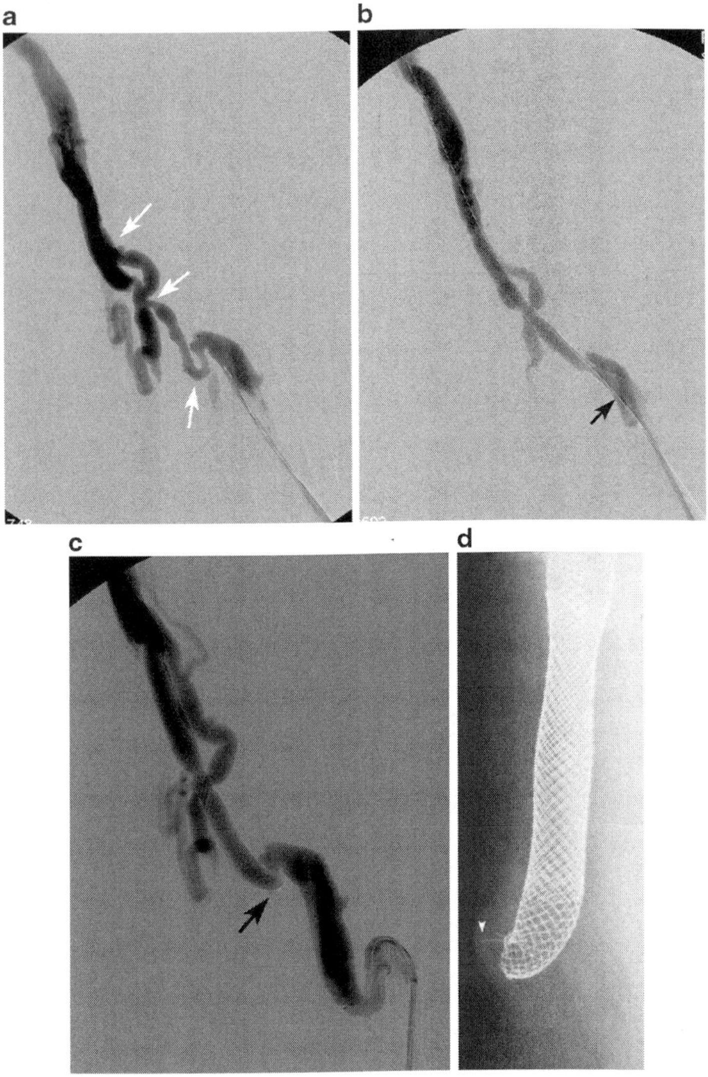

Fig. 29.5 A 60-year-old woman with right radiocephalic fistula in which outflow was maintained by a collateral vein. (**a**) Balloon angioplasty was performed to treat the stenosed collateral vein, but blood flow did not improve due to recoil (*white arrow*). (**b**) Two Wallstents were placed. The *black arrow* shows the distal edge of the stent. (**c**) Pain resembling a needle piercing the skin developed 2 months after stent placement. Shortening of the stent had caused the stent edge to move into the area of stenosis, where deformation occurred. (**d**) Plain radiography, showing struts buckling outward toward the skin at the deformed stent edge (*white arrowhead*)

Management

The stent was surgically removed, and the stenosis was bypassed with a graft.

CASE 2.2

Introduction

A 66-year-old man with right radiocephalic fistula underwent balloon angioplasty twice to treat stenosis in the brachiocephalic vein. The patency period was less than 2 months after each procedure. A third balloon angioplasty was performed at the same site with simultaneous implantation of a Wallstent (Easy Wallstent; Boston Scientific).

Issue/Complication

Sharp needle-like pain developed at the stent placement site during deployment. Fluoroscopy revealed that some struts had buckled at the stent edge during deployment (see Fig. 29.6a).

Management

Pain resolved when the stent was retracted back into the delivery system. The stent was then redeployed. The redeployment was completed without strut buckling or pain (see Fig. 29.6b).

Educational Points

Both patients experienced buckling of stent struts and sharp pain resembling the feeling of a needle piercing the skin. Wallstents are known to be associated with complications of stent migration and lesion uncovering resulting from shortening [1, 2]. In Case 1, these

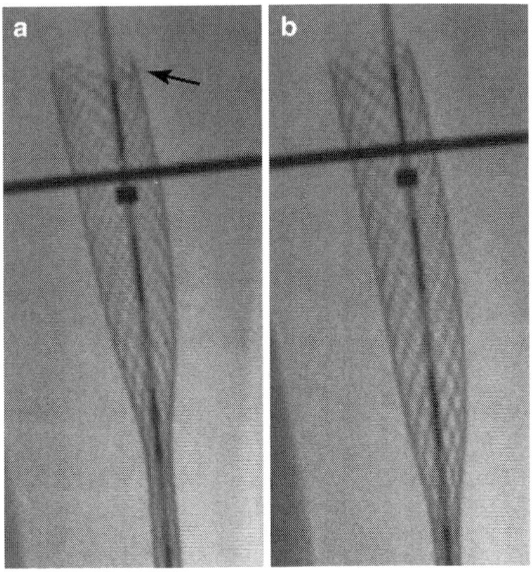

Fig. 29.6 A 66-year-old man developed pain during deployment of a Wallstent into the stenotic region of the brachiocephalic vein. (**a**) Struts at the stent edge had buckled (*arrow*). (**b**) The stent was retracted and redeployed. Redeployment was completed without strut buckling or pain

complications were conjectured to be accompanied by fracture of the stent edge, causing the struts to bend toward the skin. In Case 2, pain developed after struts buckled outward toward the skin during stent deployment. When pain develops after stent placement, stents must be examined for buckling of struts toward the skin. Patients must also be asked if they are experiencing pain during stent deployment. The complications in these two cases may be specific to Wallstents, as adjacent struts are not joined at the stent edge in the Wallstent. Nitinol stents are also widely known to be susceptible to fracture, which may result in separated struts becoming oriented in the direction of the skin [3]. The complication of pain experienced by these patients can be considered specific to vascular access, which involves vessels just underneath the skin.

Case 3
External Jugular Tunneled Catheter Placement as an Alternative Access

Micah Chan

Introduction

Currently, up to 60% of incident dialysis patients and nearly 30% of prevalent patients are using a CVC for hemodialysis [4, 5]. The right internal jugular vein is widely accepted as the vessel of choice for placement of long-term central venous catheters (CVC) for hemodialysis. The most common second choice for central venous catheter placement is the left internal jugular vein, but use of this vessel potentially puts the left arm's vasculature at risk and is associated with poor blood flow rates (Qb) and high rates of subsequent vascular stenosis and thrombosis.

A 63-year-old African-American male with end-stage renal disease (ESRD) was referred to interventional nephrology for placement of a hemodialysis catheter. Physical and ultrasound exam of the neck revealed absence of the right internal jugular (RIJ) vein but presence of the right external jugular (REJ) vein (see Fig. 29.7). Contrast venogram of the left internal jugular (LIJ) vein showed 100% stenosis and multiple collaterals (see Fig. 29.8).

Issue/Complication

The issue arises when hemodialysis patients do not have right or left internal jugular access and often times are relegated to a tunneled femoral catheter.

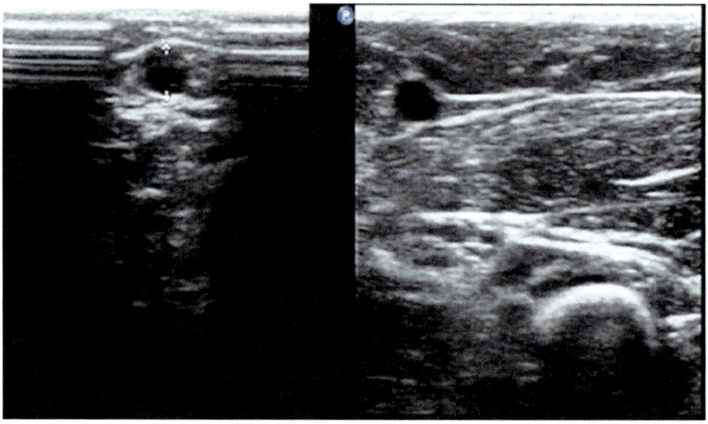

Fig. 29.7 Ultrasound guidance showed patent right external jugular vein and absence of right internal jugular vein

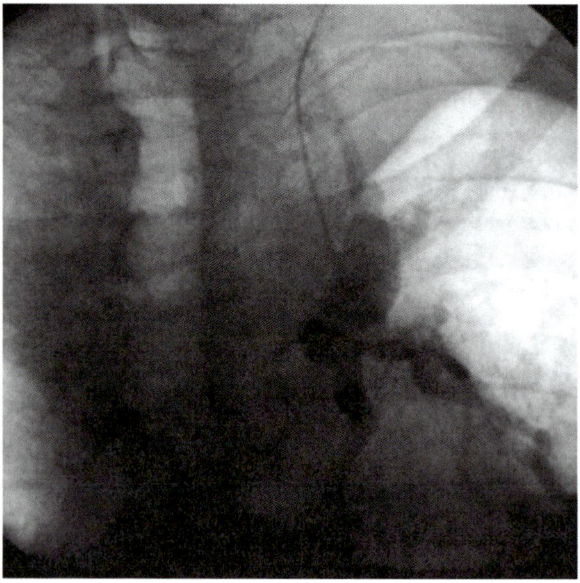

Fig. 29.8 Venogram of left internal jugular vein showing collateral vessels and 100% stenosis

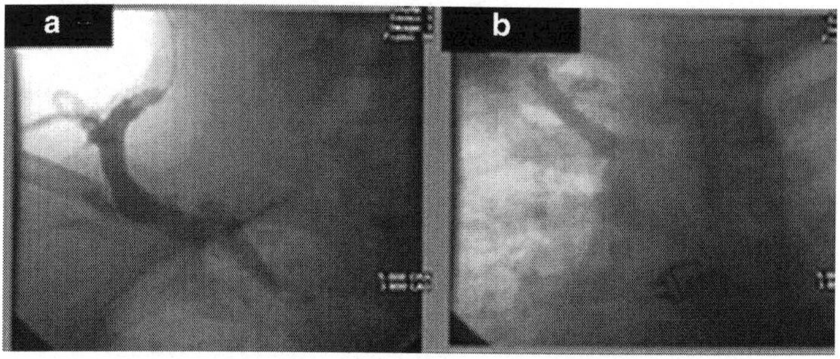

Fig. 29.9 Venogram of right external jugular vein shows patent vessel and flow to right side of heart

Management

Given the complications and infectious risks of a long-term tunneled femoral catheter, the REJ vein was used as an access for placement of a tunneled catheter [6]. A 4 Fr micropuncture was used to cannulate the REJ vein. A venogram was performed to define the EJ vein anatomy and blood flow to right heart (see Fig. 29.9). A 23-cm Tal-Palindrome tunneled catheter was prepared and inserted under standard technique in the EJ vein (see Fig. 29.10). Blood flows on dialysis and dialysis adequacy for the next 3-months were excellent.

Educational Points

1. Interventionalists should consider the external jugular veins as alternate access choice if the internal jugular veins are unavailable.
2. Placement of an external jugular vein tunneled catheter is a relatively simple and safe procedure if ultrasound and angiography is utilized.

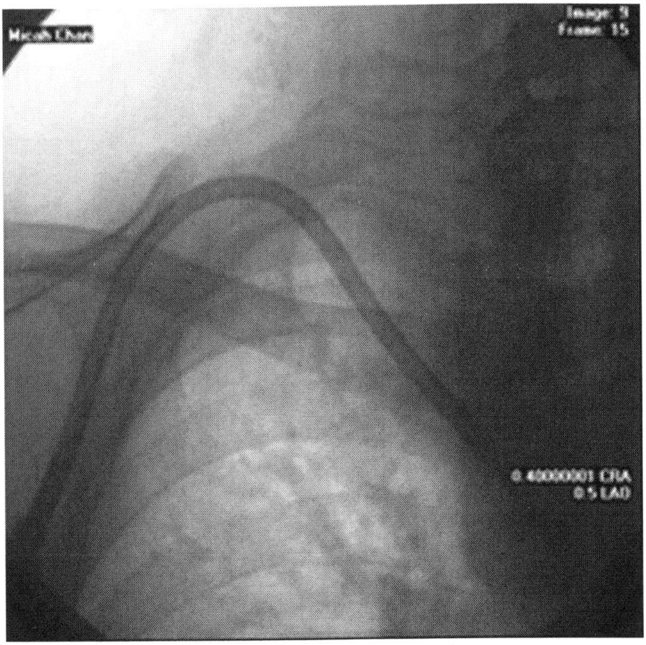

Fig. 29.10 Right external jugular tunneled catheter successfully placed

Case 4
Placement of PTFE Stent Graft Using CO_2 Angiography

Micah Chan

Introduction

The epidemic of end-stage renal disease (ESRD) in the United States is growing each year with an estimated 450,000 persons in need of renal replacement therapy in 2003 and projected 650,000 persons by 2010 [7]. The successes of kidney transplantation over the last 50 years have dramatically altered the quality of life and lifespan of many patients who were otherwise relegated to chronic renal replacement therapy. Even though allograft survival has improved based on the most recent UNOS transplant registry, chronic allograft nephropathy continues to be the most prevalent cause of late transplant graft failure [8].

A 44-year-old white female with a living unrelated kidney transplant was referred for evaluation of gradual swelling and pain over her previously placed right femoral polytetrafluoroethylene (PTFE) arteriovenous graft (AVG). The patient was on immunosuppression with mycophenolate mofetil and prednisone. The patient had biopsy proven chronic allograft nephropathy and calcineurin inhibitor toxicity with a baseline creatinine of 2.2 mg/dL and estimated glomerular filtration rate (eGFR) of 24 mL/min/1.73 m^2.

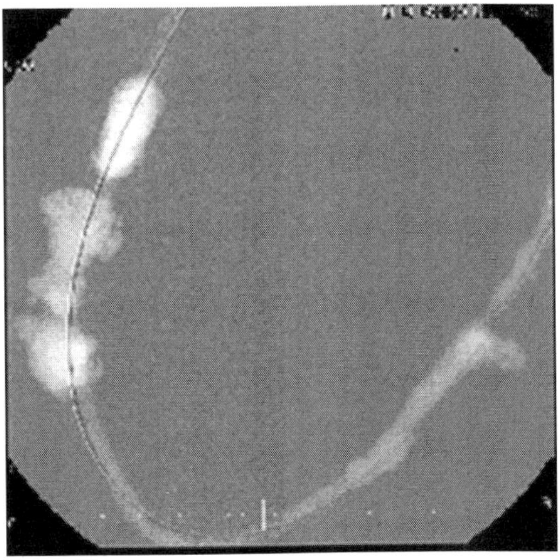

Fig. 29.11 CO_2 AVG fistulagram showing expanding pseudoaneurysms

Issue/Complication

The issue arises when chronic kidney disease (CKD) and transplant patients with abnormal eGFR need evaluation of arteriovenous access with contrast.

Management

Given the risk of contrast induced nephropathy in this renal transplant patient, CO_2 angiography was utilized to study the AVG. A 4 Fr micropuncture was used to cannulate the AVG. A 6 Fr 5-cm introducer was then exchanged over a wire and CO_2 AVG fistulagraphy was performed showing an 8-cm segment of pseudoaneurysms (see Fig. 29.11). These pseudoaneurysms were pulsatile and extended close to the skin surface. The 6 Fr introducer was then exchanged over a wire for a 9 Fr 12-cm introducer. Then an 8 × 40 and 8 × 60 mm BARD Fluency® PTFE stent graft was deployed over a 0.035 in.

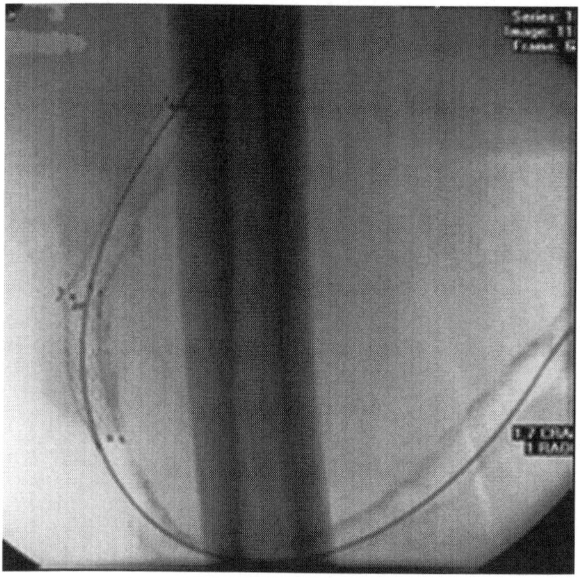

Fig. 29.12 CO_2 AVG fistulagram after deployment of two stent grafts showing resolution of pseudoaneurysms

angled glidewire sequentially. Repeat fistulography after stent graft deployment showed resolution of the pseudoaneuryms and leakage (Fig. 29.12). The patient returned 1-month for follow-up and stent graft was patent without residual pseudoaneurysm.

Educational Points

1. Interventionalists should consider CO_2 angiography in patients who are at high risk for contrast nephropathy.
2. Placement of stent grafts are commonly used for expanding pseudoaneurysms which avoids complicated surgery [9].

Case 5
May-Thurner Physiology Complicating Left Femoral Dialysis Graft

Ahmad I. Alomari, Brian J. Dillon, and Horacio M. Padua

History

This is a 24-year-old female patient with Goldenhar syndrome and end-stage renal disease secondary to reflux nephropathy into a solitary kidney. History of scoliosis corrected with spinal fusion. She is on hemodialysis via a revised left femoral PTFE graft. The graft flow measured with a transit-time ultrasonic blood flow meter (Transonic System, Ithaca, NY) has been steadily decreasing over the last few months from 1,200–1,300 to 850 mL/min. Contrast study demonstrated a marked stenosis of the left common iliac vein with extensive network of pelvic collaterals, which has worsened compared to a venogram obtained 2 years earlier (see Fig. 29.13a, b). There was a mild stenosis of the venous anastomosis (see Fig. 29.13c).

Intervention

Under anesthesia, the right common femoral vein was accessed with sonographic guidance and a 7 Fr sheath was placed. Initial venogram confirmed the presence of severe stenosis of the left common iliac vein with a pressure gradient of 6 mmHg across the lesion. There was a moderate stenosis of the venous anastomosis. Over a guide wire, angioplasty of the lesion was performed with a 12 mm×4 cm and

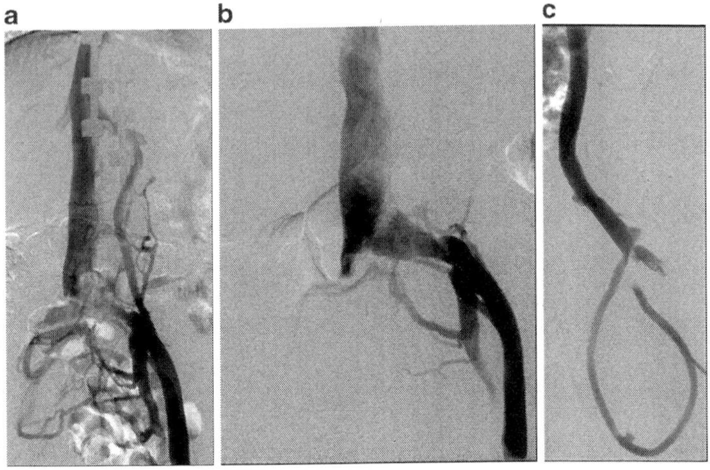

Fig. 29.13 (**a**) Marked stenosis of common iliac vein. (**b**) Venogram 2 years earlier demonstrated mild stenosis. (**c**) Moderate stenosis of venous anastomosis of the thigh PTFE graft

14 mm×4 cm Atlas balloon catheters, respectively. Post-angioplasty venography demonstrated markedly improved caliber of the stenotic segment, though residual stenosis and filling of collateral veins were significant (see Fig. 29.14a). As the etiology of this stenosis is related to external compression, the stenotic segment of the iliac vein was stented with a 14 mm×4 cm Protegé stent. The stent was then dilated. Venography demonstrated excellent reduction of the diameter of the stenosis with minimal residual stenosis in the lower peripheral portion of the stent (see Fig. 29.14b). Filling of collateral veins was markedly diminished and pressure gradient dropped to 0 mmHg. The venous anastomosis was dilated with a 6 mm×4 cm Profiler balloon catheter with improvement of the caliber of the stenosis.

Following the procedure, the graft flow improved to 1,200–1,300 mL/min level. However, over the next 6 months the flow gradually deteriorated to ~800 mL/min. Contrast study showed narrowing of the lower portion of the stent (see Fig. 29.15a). Balloon angioplasty reduced the gradient from 4 to 0 mmHg and restored the flow >1,200 mL/min (see Fig. 29.15b).

The flow dropped again 3 months later and contrast study showed restenosis of the lower segment of the common iliac stent. Currently, the plan is to extend the stent caudally over the ostium of the internal iliac vein and into the cranial portion of the external iliac vein.

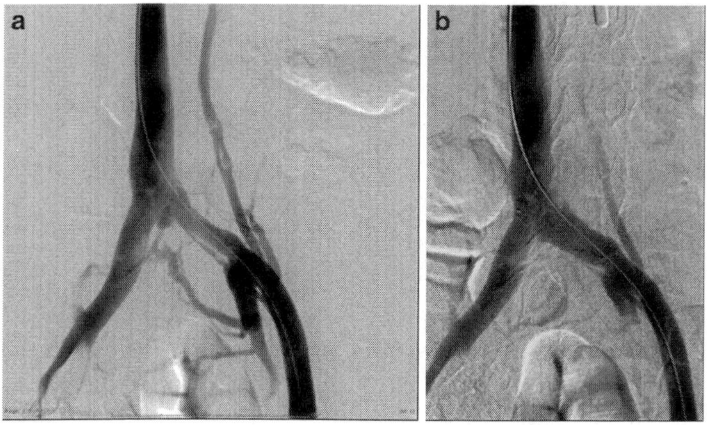

Fig. 29.14 (**a**) Postballoon dilation demonstrates luminal improvement; however, collaterals persist. (**b**) Following stent deployment, luminal caliber is further improved with resolution of collaterals

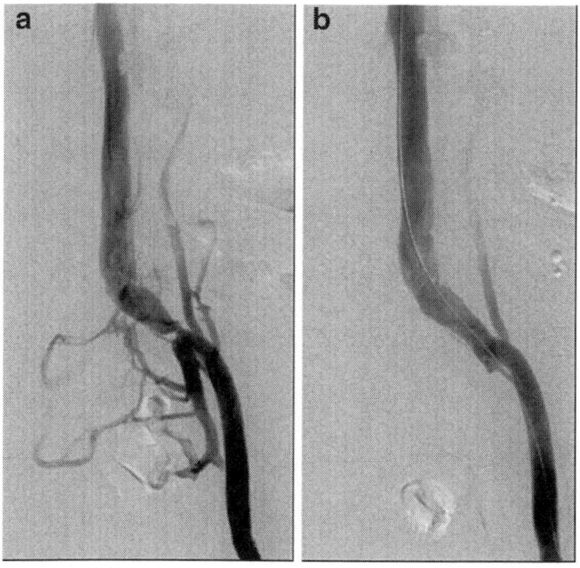

Fig. 29.15 (**a**) New area of stenosis has formed immediately below prior placed stent consistent with stent induced edge stenosis. (**b**) Following PTA, the stenosis has resolved

Educational Points

1. One should be aware of the etiology and treatment of vascular pathology outside of common hemodialysis problems that may adversely affect access function.
2. Edge stenosis or intimal hyperplasia at the edge of stents or along the length of the stents is a common problem eventually requiring intervention in many cases.

Case 6
Morbid Complication of Dialysis Graft Thrombolysis

Ahmad I. Alomari, Brian J. Dillon, and Horacio M. Padua

History

Seventeen-year-old female patient on hemodialysis for end-stage renal disease secondary to cloacal abnormality was referred for with clotted right femoral PTFE graft. The past surgical history is significant for failed cadaveric renal transplant, steroid-induced insulin-dependent diabetes mellitus, right hip replacement secondary to avascular necrosis of the femoral head, cholecystectomy, and bladder augmentation. The patient was thrombophilic (factor V Leiden deficiency and prothrombin gene mutation (G20210A) on long-term Warfarin treatment.

Intervention

Thrombolysis and angioplasty of the dialysis graft was performed under general anesthesia. The clot was initially lysed with an AngioJet thrombolysis catheter, pulse spray thrombolysis with heparin, balloon angioplasty of the venous anastomosis, and pullback thrombectomy through the arterial anastomosis with a Fogarty balloon.

The venous anastomosis showed moderate stenosis which was successfully treated with balloon angioplasty. The common femoral and iliac veins and the IVC were completely and chronically occluded

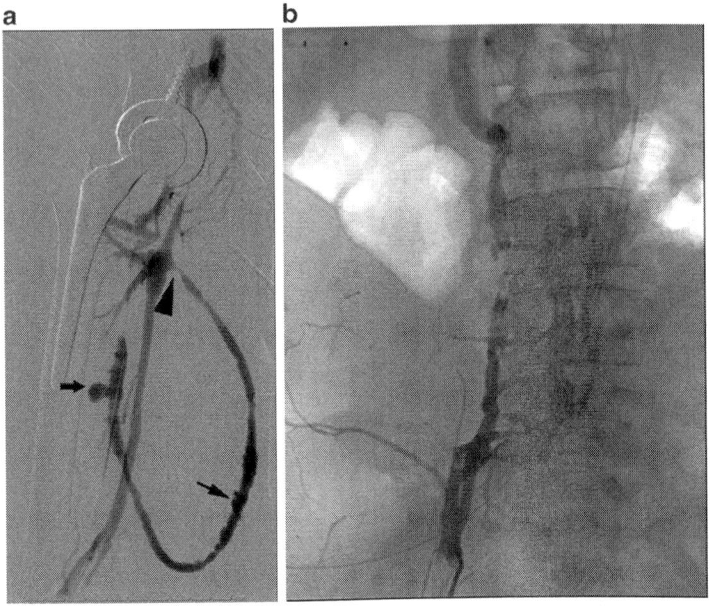

Fig. 29.16 (**a**) Thigh graft with pseudoaneurysms (*arrows*) and venous anastomotic stenosis (*arrowhead*). (**b**) Chronically occluded venous outflow

with retrograde drainage into the thigh femoral vein and via a large collateral vein cranially. The graft had a couple of small pseudoaneurysms from repeated needle punctures (see Fig. 29.16).

Complication

In the recovery room, the patient developed pain and decreased pulses in the right foot. The physical exam was difficult as the patient was not fully awake and the pulse was difficult to palpate prior to the exam. As it was late in the evening, the patient was admitted for dialysis and observation. However, pain worsened over night. The procedure was reviewed and, in retrospect, clots were noticed in the femoral artery in one of the fluoroscopic images (see Fig. 29.17).

The patient was brought back to the angiography suite for urgent thrombolysis. Initial angiographic images showed multiple clots in

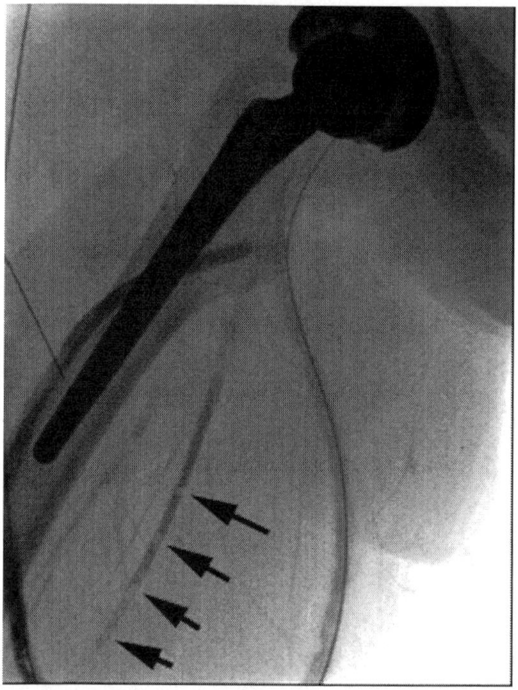

Fig. 29.17 Reflux of contrast to assess arterial anastomosis after completion of declotting procedure. In retrospect, multiple filling defects are seen within the superficial femoral artery (*arrows*) consistent with clot emboli

the popliteal artery with near complete occlusion of the popliteal bifurcation and tibioperoneal trunk. The femoral artery was patent (see Fig. 29.18).

Mechanical and pharmacologic thrombolysis using tissue plasminogen activator, heparin, and AngioJet thrombolysis catheter was performed. Though flow was restored into these two vessels, spasm developed which was not responsive to intra-arterial nitroglycerin. In addition, the flow into the tibial and peroneal arteries was tenuous and no significant flow was restored into the anterior tibial artery (see Fig. 29.19). The posterior tibial artery had a small proximal clot and filled distally via peroneal collaterals. The plantar arch and the dorsalis pedis artery were patent but markedly attenuated.

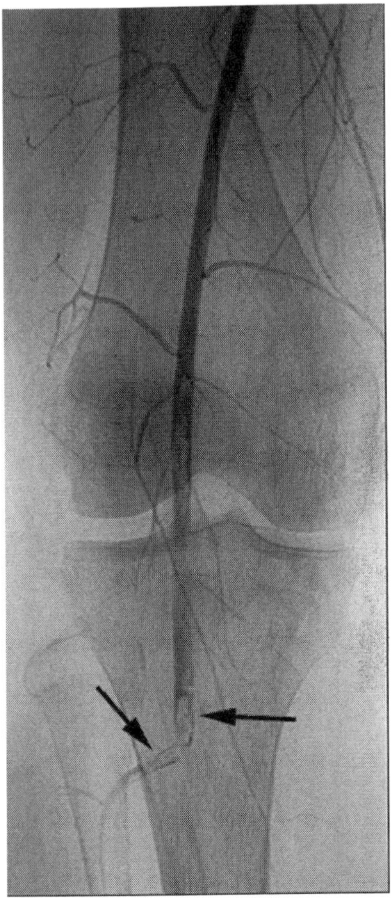

Fig. 29.18 Angiogram of the distal SFA and popliteal artery demonstrates emboli within the distal popliteal artery and origin of the anterior tibial artery (*arrows*) with almost no flow into leg arteries beyond this point

Following the procedure, therapeutic anticoagulation was initiated. Overnight, perfusion and swelling of the leg worsened. The clinical diagnosis was concerning for compartment syndrome. This was confirmed elevated compartment pressures measured in the operating room where urgent fasciotomy was performed. This unfortunate cascade of events resulted in right foot drop and sensory loss. Physical therapy was then started and the wound was eventually closed with a skin graft.

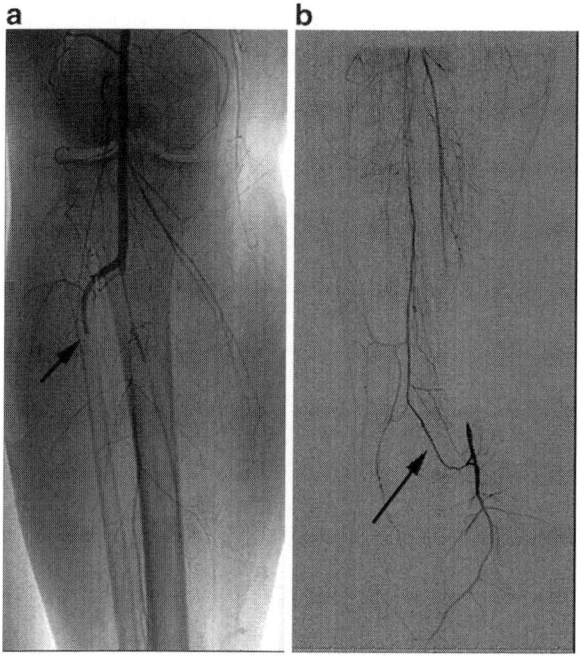

Fig. 29.19 After thrombolysis and mechanical thrombectomy. (**a**) The anterior tibial artery remains occluded (*arrow*) and (**b**) there is minimal flow to the foot via a patent peroneal artery with collateral supply (*arrow*) to the distal posterior tibial artery

Educational Points

1. The arterial anastomosis should be assessed after flow is reestablished within the access.
2. When assessing the arterial anastomosis, postthrombolysis/thrombectomy, gently inject contrast in the event that there is retained clot within the access.
3. Arterial embolization, although asymptomatic in most patients, can be a very serious complication and immediate measures to deal with the complication, including appropriate consultations with a surgeon when indicated, should be undertaken.

Case 7
Extra-Anatomic Use of Stent Grafts to Treat Central Venous Obstruction

Bart Dolmatch

Introduction

Central venous obstruction with associated arm swelling has become ever more common in the dialysis patient population largely related to use of large-bore indwelling dialysis catheters [10, 11]. Current therapy has largely been directed at direct angioplasty of the occlusion, with or without stents, to achieve patency [12]. However, some occlusions cannot be treated by direct intervention, and alternative therapy may be needed to preserve the ipsilateral AV access and treat swelling of the extremity.

This 48-year-old black woman had dysfunction of her left upper arm arteriovenous graft, and the venous anstomosis of her AV graft had been treated with declotting and stent grafts on prior occasions. Stent grafts were placed up to the axillary vein, and two subsequent episodes of thrombosis of the access were not associated with any evidence of stenosis. CT scan (Fig. 29.20) demonstrated that the stent grafts were kinked due to 90° angulation at the venous anastomosis, and the AV graft was abandoned. The surgeon placed a new AV graft adjacent to the abandoned one, suturing the venous anastomosis to a residual patent portion of left axillary vein, and the patient developed marked swelling of her left shoulder, upper arm, forearm, wrist, and hand.

Fistulogram (Fig. 29.21) demonstrated a patent AV graft and the occluded "old" stent grafts within the central portion of the axillary vein.

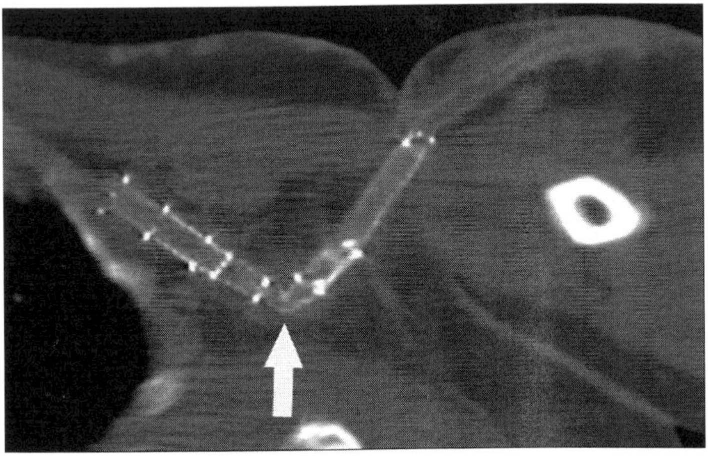

Fig. 29.20 Curved planar reformation CT through the "old" stent grafts reveal a kink (*arrow*) due to excessive angulation at the venous anastomosis of the arterio-venous graft, causing recurrent thrombosis with no obvious stenosis seen on frontal angiography. Kinking of the stent grafts may have been exaggerated during CT scanning because the patient's arms were raised. However, subsequent attempts to demonstrate kinking of the stent grafts during angiography did not show appreciable deformation

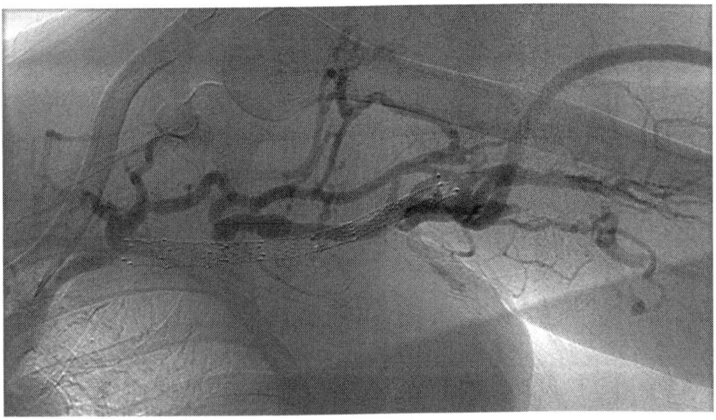

Fig. 29.21 A new AV graft has been placed adjacent to the old one at the left upper arm, with the venous end of the graft anastomosed to a short segment of axillary vein. Central to this portion of axillary vein, the "old" stent grafts cause venous occlusion, and there are many collaterals seen in the left upper arm and shoulder, as well as marked swelling that was seen, clinically

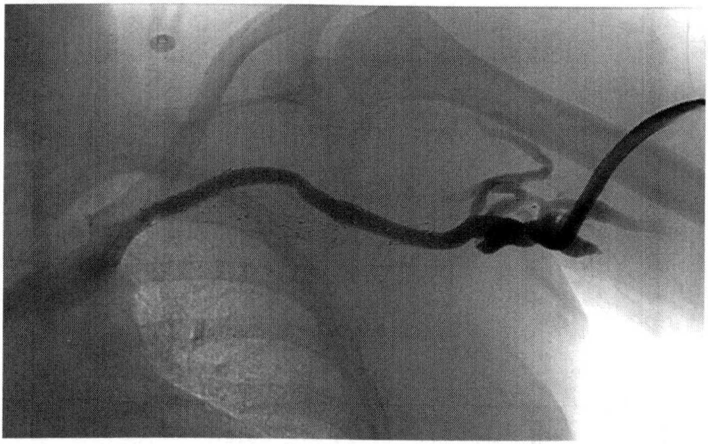

Fig. 29.22 Using the dominant collateral pathways around the occluded axillary vein stent grafts, an endoluminal bypass has been created with 8 mm diameter stent grafts. Note that after creation of this extra-anatomic endoluminal bypass, nearly all collaterals have resolved

Rather than ligate the AV graft, an attempt was made to use the existing collateral pathway around the occlusion as a channel in which overlapping stent grafts would restore sufficient flow to reduce arm swelling. A 0.035 in. hydrophilic wire was passed through the dominant collateral pathway to the left subclavian vein, the tract was balloon dilated to 8 mm, and three overlapping 8 mm diameter Fluency stent grafts (Bard Peripheral Vascular, Inc.) were placed within the dilated collateral pathway, restoring inline flow around the occluded axillary vein, with resolution of the collateral veins at the left arm and shoulder (Fig. 29.22).

Though hemodynamics were improved within the venous system, the patient developed immediate severe left shoulder pain and an isolated sensory deficit involving only her radial nerve, with numbness of her thumb, second, and third fingers. ACT scan was performed to look for a hematoma, but there was none. Neurology consult confirmed the suspicion that the stent grafts were compressing a portion of the left brachial plexus related to the radial nerve. The patient was treated with Neurontin and analgesics. After several weeks, her shoulder pain had mostly resolved. After 6 months, her radial neuropathy had resolved. At 14 months, she developed recurrent swelling, though it was milder than on initial presentation. A focal central stent graft stenosis (Figs. 29.23 and 29.24) was treated with one

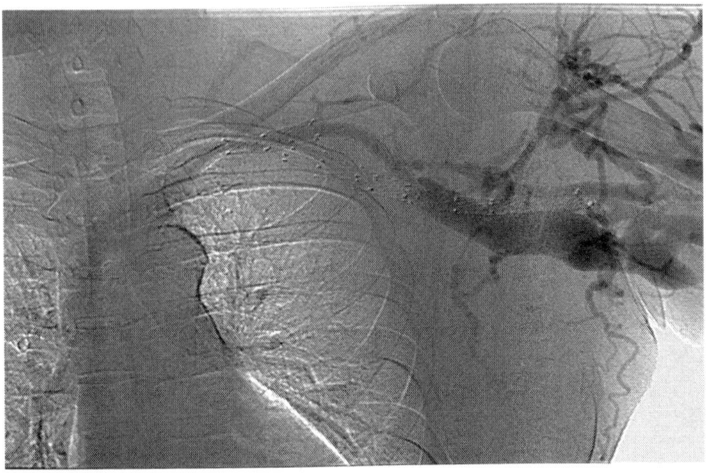

Fig. 29.23 At 14 months, this patient has recurrent swelling. Fistulogram shows that the collateral veins are returned, though the endoluminal stent graft bypass appears to be patent

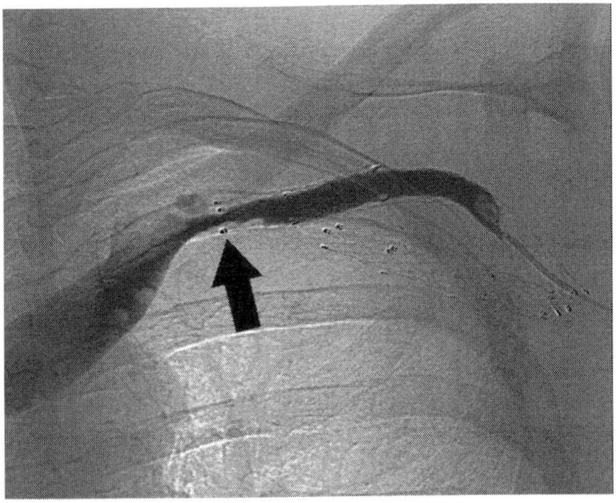

Fig. 29.24 Upon closer evaluation, a focal edge stenosis (*arrow*) is seen at the central end of the stent grafts

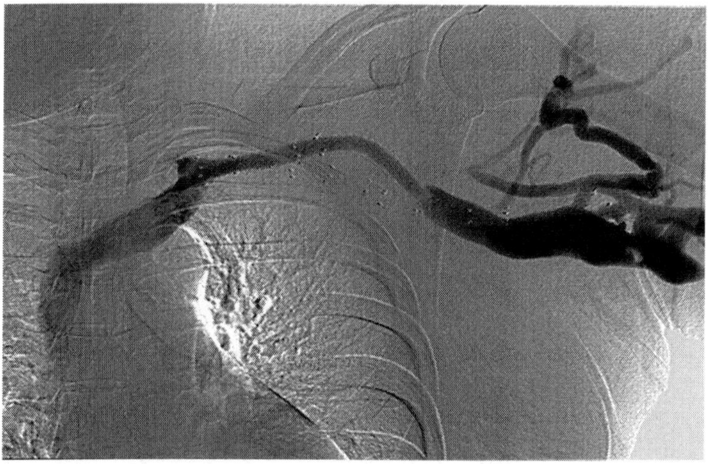

Fig. 29.25 Angioplasty and placement of an additional stent graft was sufficient to restore patency to the stent grafts, affording clinical resolution of swelling until the AV graft was ligated after successful kidney transplantion. The cumulative patency of this extra-anatomic endoluminal stent graft bypass was nearly 2 years

additional Fluency stent graft (Fig. 29.25), and this patient did will until she received a kidney transplant within the next several months. A second episode of recurrent mild left arm swelling following kidney transplantion was treated by ligation of the AV Graft, since her renal transplant was working well.

Issue/Complication

Significant arm swelling due to central venous occlusion is usually treated by direct intervention, but when the occlusion cannot be treated, aggressive surgical bypass options, flow-reducing procedures, or ligation of the AV access are usually all that remains. In this case, an extra-anatomic stent graft bypass was created through collateral channels. It treated the patient's swelling. However, the course of the extra-anatomic pathway involved the distal brachial plexus and radial nerve consideration of structures that are not seen during fistulography (e.g. nerves, arteries) must be considered before proceeding with novel interventions.

Management

Direct recanalization of the axillary vein was not possible due to the old stent grafts. Ligation of the left arm AV graft was only considered as a last option. Creation of an "endoluminal bypass" by placing stent grafts within existing collaterals was a novel solution, and it worked very well to treat arm swelling. However, the extra-anatomic path of these stent grafts caused neurologic deficits that, fortunately, reversed over time.

Educational Points

1. Stent grafts can be used effectively to maintain dialysis access patency and may have a role in treating central venous obstruction.
2. Stent grafts, like all vascular structures, reside in 3-D space. The "old" stent grafts. failed due to angular anatomy that caused them to kink, though this was not obvious on 2-D angiography. The "new" endoluminal bypass created with stent grafts placed in a collateral pathway compressed nerves. Always think about what 3-D space you are working within, and be aware of nonvisualized structures and anatomy.

Case 8
Salvage of an Unsalvageable AV Fistula with Stent Grafts

Bart Dolmatch

Introduction

This 47-year-old systems engineer developed end-stage renal disease due to long-standing hypertension (biopsy proven). He started hemodialysis with a right IJ tunneled catheter, and underwent vascular mapping for ultimate creation of a left brachiocephalic AV Fistula in the spring of 2007. By August 2007, the fistula had not been used successfully for dialysis and a fistulogram was performed (Fig. 29.26). The patient continued on hemodialysis through his right IJ tunneled catheter for another year awaiting "maturation" of his AV fistula, but in August 2008 the fistula was still not being used for dialysis. A fistulogram at another center (not shown) led to the decision that this AVF should be abandoned, and the patient was referred to our access surgeon for consideration of a new AV access.

I saw this patient with our access surgeon in clinic. The fistula was extremely pulsatile with a marginal flow volume of 660 mL/min. We decided to repeat an AV fistulogram with the intent to reconsider salvage of the fistula. A long cephalic vein stensosis was seen (Fig. 29.27) and angioplastied to 7 mm with extensive perivenous extravasation and pre-occlusive stenosis (Fig. 29.28). Bailout was achieved with an 8 × 150 mm Viabahn stent graft (WL Gore and Associates) on the central side, and two overlapping Fluency stent grafts (8 × 80 and 9 × 80 mm; Bard Peripheral Vascular, Inc.) distally

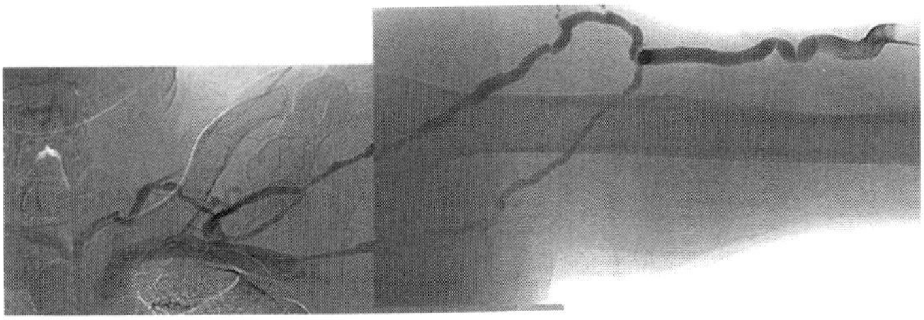

Fig. 29.26 Fistulogram of immature left brachiocephalic AVF several months postoperatively

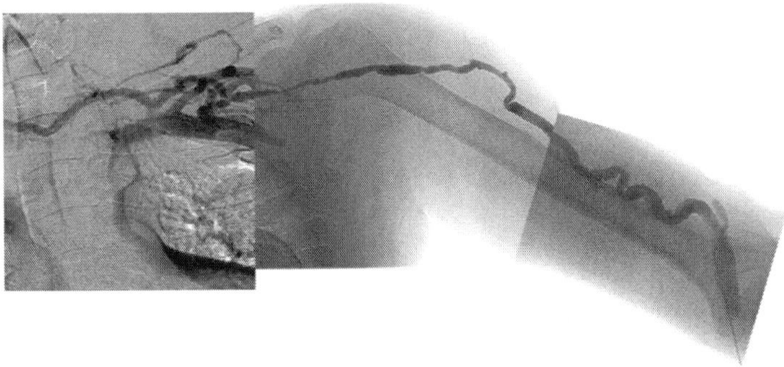

Fig. 29.27 Fistulogram of immature left brachiocephalic AVF more than a year after it was created. There is a diffuse stenosis of the cephalic vein over a long segment, centrally

(Fig. 29.29). Thereafter, the catheter was removed and the AVF was used successfully for hemodialysis with flow of 1.6 L/min 1 month after intervention.

Six months after intervention, increased pressures were noted in the AVF, and repeat duplex was performed with deterioration of flow volume to around 800 mL/min and stenosis within the Viabahn stent grafts (Fig. 29.30). Repeat AV fistulogram confirmed the duplex findings (Fig. 29.31), and in-covered-stent stenosis within the Viabahn was treated with overlapping 8 mm diameter Fluency stent grafts (Fig. 29.32), as well as distal extension of the sent grafts segment with one more Fluency sent grafts. Postprocedure flow volume improved to 1.8 L/min and dialysis continued uneventfully for another 7 months when the AVF again became pulsatile and flow volume dropped to 1.0 L/min. Repeat fistulogram shows a widely

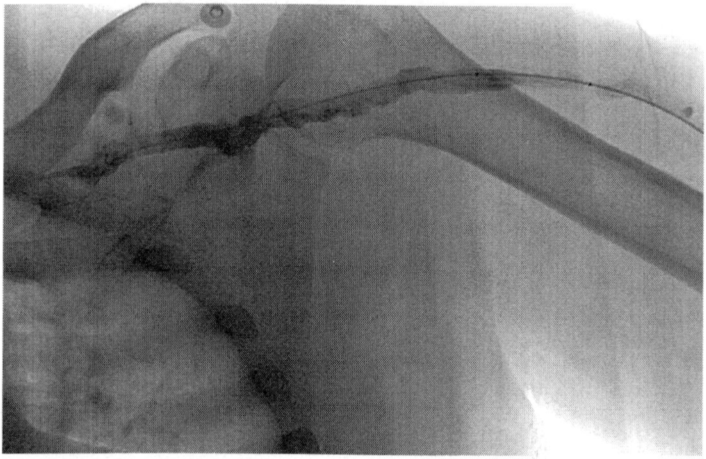

Fig. 29.28 Post-angioplasty to 7 mm. Contrast stains the perivenous PTA sites, and residual stenosis caused impairment to flow that was considered to be pre-thrombotic

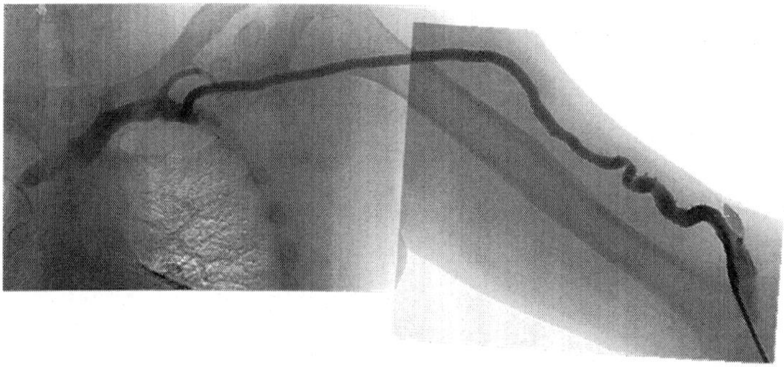

Fig. 29.29 Salvage of the AVF with a central 8 × 150 mm Viabahn and two overlapping Fluency stent grafts (8 × 80 mm and 9 × 80 mm), distally

patent series of stent grafts except for a focal edge stenosis of the central-most Fluency (Fig. 29.33) related to the terminus of the cephalic arch. This was dilated and an 8 × 40 mm Flair sent grafts was deployed at the site, covering the area of restenosis (Fig. 29.34).

Hemodialysis was performed without further difficulty until the patient received a renal transplant 21 months after the first intervention. He volunteered to undergo a "no-charge" duplex of his AVF at 25 months, and the access flow volume was 1.9 L/min (Fig. 29.35).

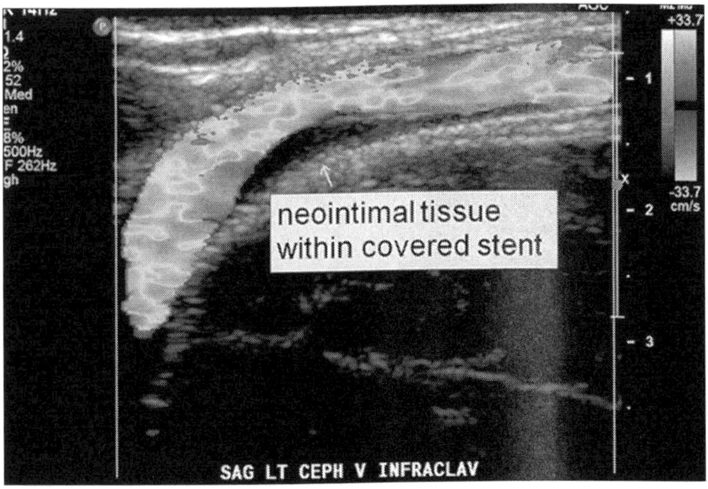

Fig. 29.30 At 6 months, the access flow had deteriorated to around 800 cc/min and restenotic neointimal tissue has formed only within the Viabahn stent graft in the region of the cephalic arch

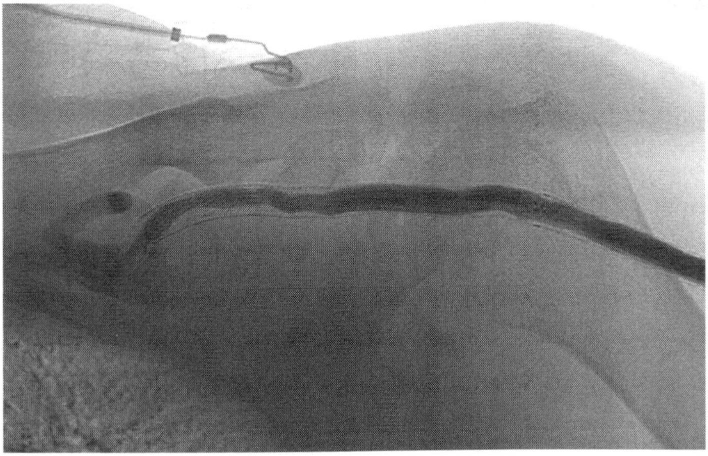

Fig. 29.31 Fistulogram following the 6-month duplex confirms in-covered-stent restenosis within the Viabahn, only. The Fluency stent grafts are widely patent

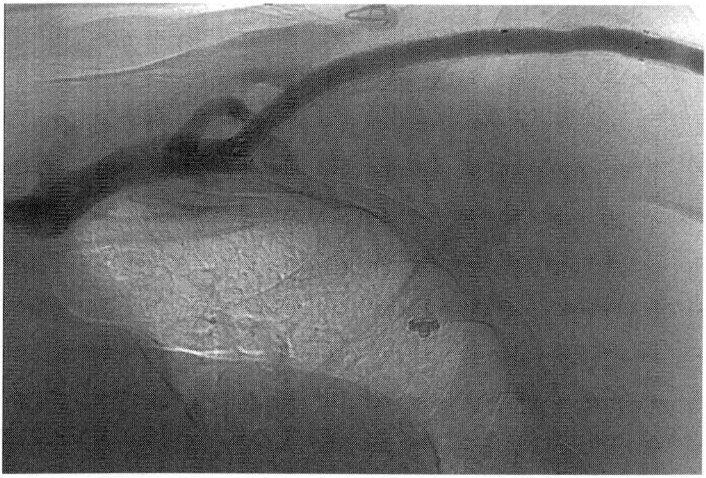

Fig. 29.32 In-covered-stent restenosis within the Viabahn has been treated with 8 mm angioplasty and placement of an 8×80 mm Fluency stent graft within the lumen of the Viabahn

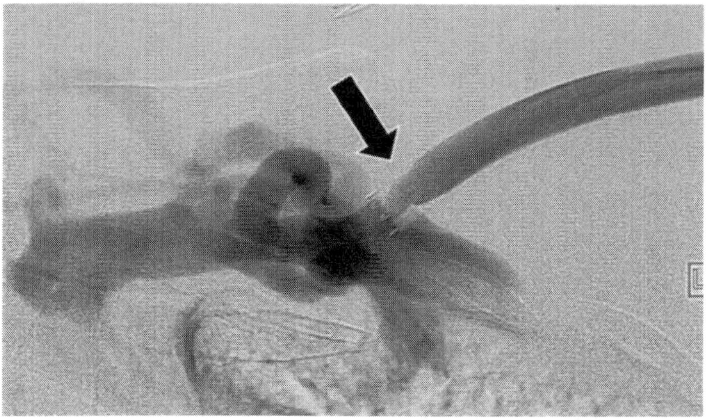

Fig. 29.33 Seven months later, the entire AVF is widely patent except for one focal 50–60% edge stenosis at the central end of the Fluency within the terminus of the cephalic arch (*arrow*)

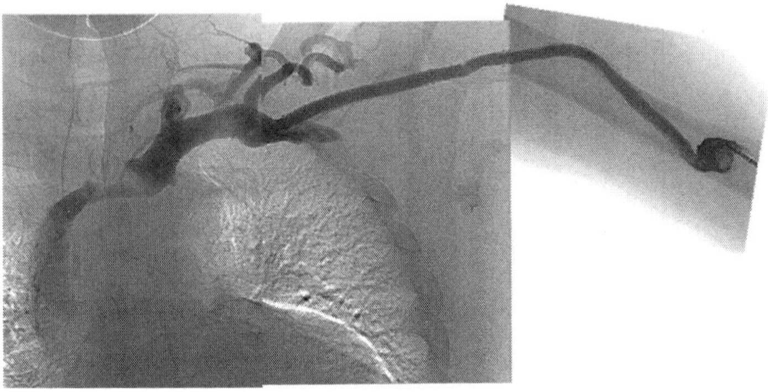

Fig. 29.34 The edge stenosis shown in Fig 29.33 has been balloon dilated and treated with a final 8 mm diameter Flair stent graft across the terminus of the cephalic arch

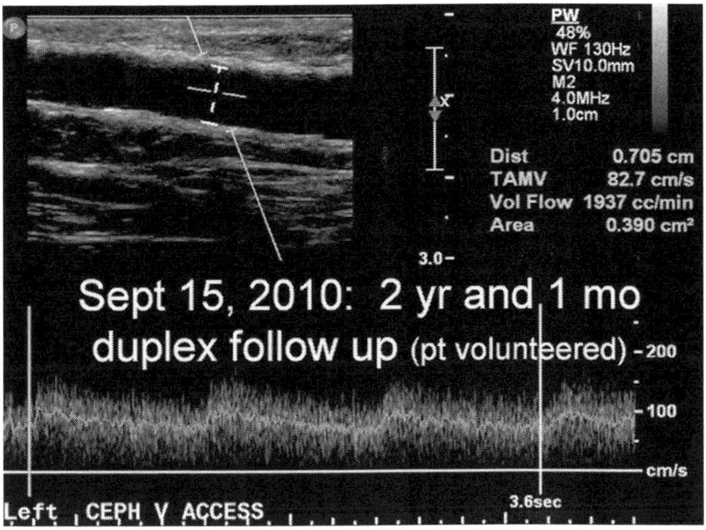

Fig. 29.35 Duplex of the AV fistula 25 months after the initial intervention (and several months after the patient received a successful renal transplant) showing excellent flow volume of 1.9 L/min

He may undergo elective ligation of his left brachiocephalic AVF now that it is no longer being used.

Issue/Complication

The issue of AVF immaturity has been of great concern, particularly in light of data from a recent multicenter study where AVF immaturity in the US was 60% within the first 5 postoperative months [13]. In that study, half of the immature or unuseable AVF's were abandoned. Use of stent grafts to salvage AV fistulae is relatively new [14], and use of these devices is not approved for this indication in the US. However, in select cases like this one they can salvage the unsalvageable AV fistula.

Management

In this case, the heroics of salvage must be balanced with the risk/benefit/cost of intervention versus abandonment after creation of a new AV access. Those calculations are complex, and we are never sure if creation of a new AV access will afford a durable solution or if it will also be fraught with early failure and need for repeated treatments.

Here, use of stent grafts successfully rescued and maintained this AVF, though this treatment pathway required several visits and use of expensive therapy. Curiously, there was initial restenosis only within the Viabahn over a relatively diffuse length while the Fluency stent grafts showed no restenosis. This raises the question of whether all stent grafts are really interchangeable. Perhaps some are more prone to specific problems. The second restenosis was related to the central uncovered end of the Fluency at the terminus of the cephalic vein, a site that is particularly vulnerable to restenosis. Through close monitoring and aggressive intervention, this AVF has been kept patent for over 2 years.

Educational Points

1. AVF immaturity is a frequent problem in the US.
2. Stent grafts can be used to mature AV fistulae, but there may be differences in durability and restenosis patterns for different devices. Use of these devices, while "off-label," can afford remarkable results.
3. Close monitoring of patients can help detect problems in AV access before the circuit clots. It also affords the opportunity for the interventionalist to develop a relationship with the patient.

Case 9
Salvage of Occluded Aneurysmal Arteriovenous Fistula by Incision for Direct Thrombus Extraction: Adjunct to Failed Percutaneous Thrombectomy

Theodore F. Saad

Introduction

A 61-year-old African-American male presented with thrombosis of his left forearm radial artery to cephalic vein fistula. This had been constructed 22 months earlier and had undergone three prior percutaneous interventions for maturation and maintenance of function, including percutaneous thrombectomy 2 months prior to this presentation. It was being used successfully for the past 6 months but developed large needle puncture site aneurysms which were firm and noncompressible; there was no ulceration, eschar formation, or other sign of local infection (Fig. 29.36). Percutaneous thrombectomy was attempted but unsuccessful due to the large amount of residual organized thrombus (Fig. 29.37) that resisted mechanical manuevers including catheter aspiration [15] and balloon maceration. No thrombolytic agent was used. Due to the large volume and organized nature of thrombus, it was not deemed amenable to local thrombolytic therapy [16] and the risks of central thrombo-embolism were significant.

Issue/Complication

Organized thrombus in large fistula needle-site aneurysms resistant to conventional percutaneous thrombectomy.

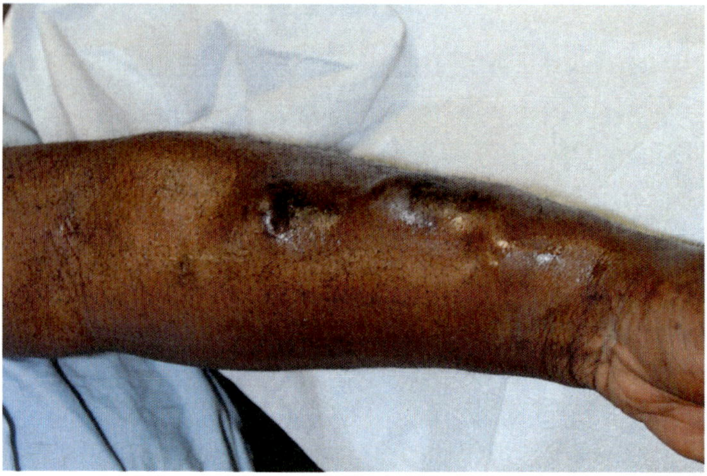

Fig. 29.36 Thrombosed radiocephalic fistula with two large venous aneurysms

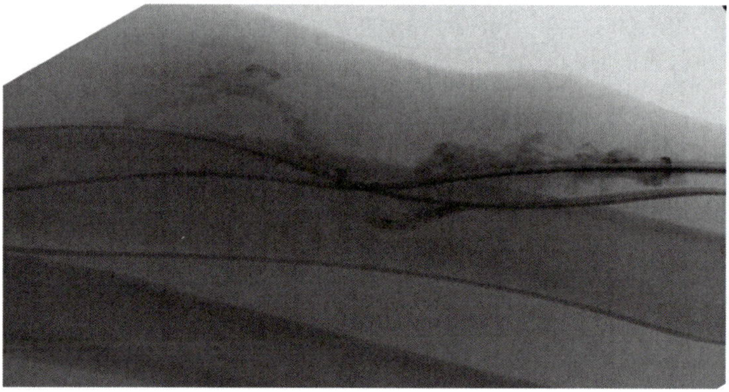

Fig. 29.37

Management

Consideration was given placing a venous hemodialysis catheter, and either abandoning the fistula or referring the patient for attempted open surgical thrombectomy. In this case, in order to achieve immediate fistula salvage we performed direct thrombectomy via a small incision

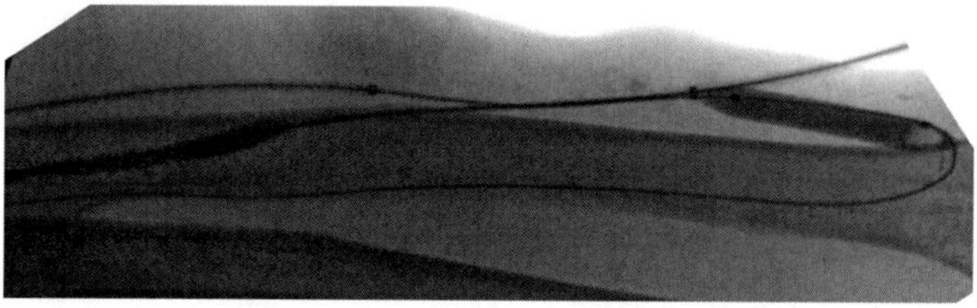

Fig. 29.38

with balloon occlusion of the fistula inflow and outflow. Guide wires were placed via two sheaths, peripherally across the arterial anastomosis and centrally through the venous outflow. An 8 by 80 mm angioplasty balloon was advanced across the venous outflow stenosis and a 7 by 40 mm balloon advanced into the arterial inflow segment of the fistula; both were inflated to achieve proximal and distal occlusion (Fig. 29.38). A site was selected for incision where there was thick healthy skin and vessel wall, along the lateral aspect of the venous aneurysm, avoiding recent needle puncture areas. After local lidocaine anesthesia, a 1–1.5 cm incision was made through the skin and vein using a number 11 scalpel; there was no discernable plane of separation between vein and skin. Thrombus was then extracted by manually squeezing the fistula, "milking" thrombus from both ends toward the incision, and grasping thrombus with a curved haemostat yielding abundant thrombus (Fig. 29.39). Serial imaging was performed until no significant residual thrombus could be seen. The incision was closed securely with a layered interrupted subcutaneous 3-0 Vicryl and a running superficial 3-0 Nylon suture. The outflow lesion was then angioplastied fully to 8 mm; the arterial segment occlusion balloon was deflated and inflow restored with brisk angiographic flow of contrast and a strong palpable thrill. Completion imaging showed no residual thrombus or stenosis (Fig. 29.40). The fistula has remained patent and functional without requirement for repeat intervention 6 months post-thrombectomy.

Educational Points

Thrombosed fistulae with large aneurysms are challenging to treat using conventional percutaneous methods due to the large volume of

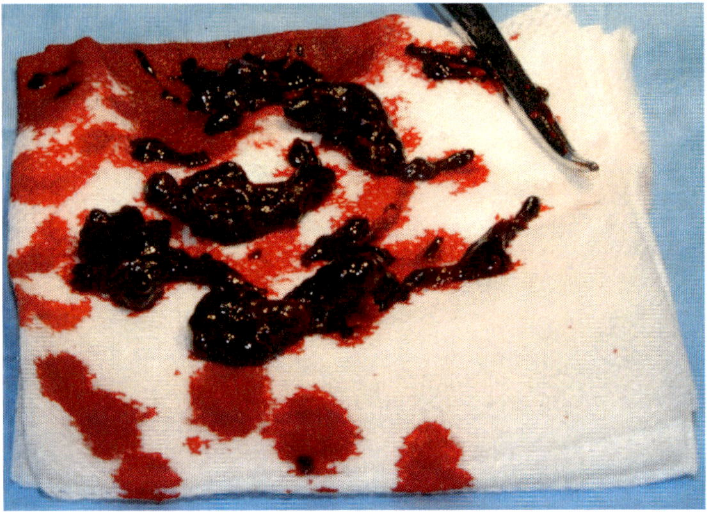

Fig. 29.39 Extracted clots

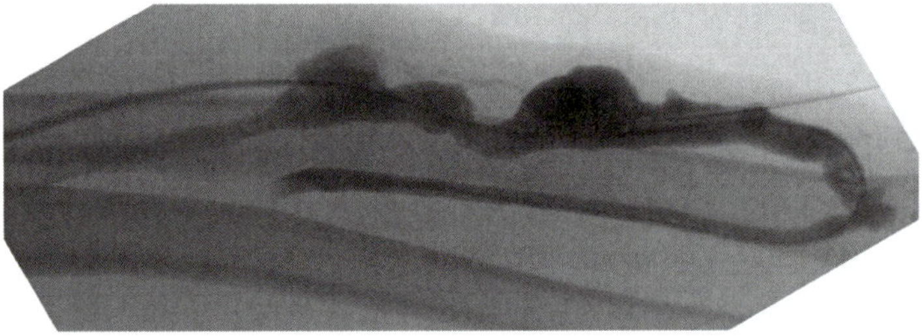

Fig. 29.40

organized thrombus. When aspiration, maceration, or pharmacologic thrombolysis are ineffective in removing thrombus, the fistula may be lost and there may be increased risk for clinically significant thrombo-embolism. Direct thrombus extraction via a small incision utilizing balloon occlusion of the fistula inflow and outflow provides an effective alternative for such cases and may avoid the morbidity of venous catheter access and new access surgery.

Case 10
Clotted Left Upper Arm Graft with Pseudoaneurysms: Salvage with Stent Grafts

Martin E. Simons

Introduction

A 66-year-old woman with a 13-year-old left upper arm prosthetic graft presents to the hemodialysis clinic, with her graft clotted. This is the first episode of thrombosis. She has had previous venous anastomotic angioplasty, 8 months earlier.

Issue/Complication

The graft was declotted using a crossed catheter technique. Two 6 Fr sheaths (Performer, Cook), were placed. The patient was given heparin 3,000 IU, intravenously, and the graft was laced with 6 mg of rt-PA. Using a 5 Fr over-the-wire Fogarty balloon (Edwards Life Science), the platelet plug was dislodged from the arterial anastomosis (Fig. 29.41), and the remainder of the graft was angioplastied with an 8 mm × 4 cm low compliance balloon (Dorado, Bard) (Fig. 29.42). At this point there was significant clot burden retained in two pseudoaneurysms at previous needle puncture sites (Fig. 29.43).

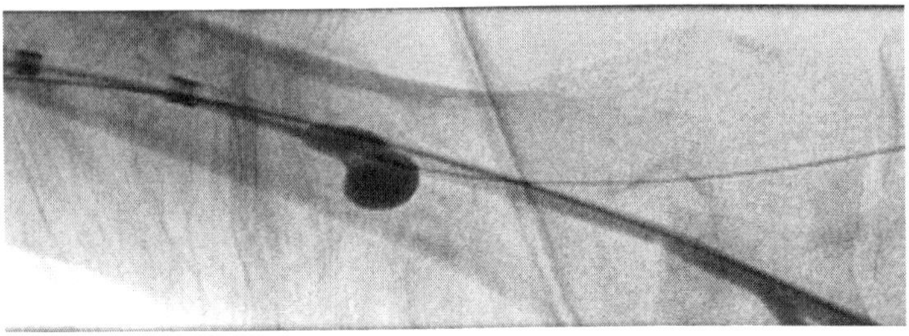

Fig. 29.41

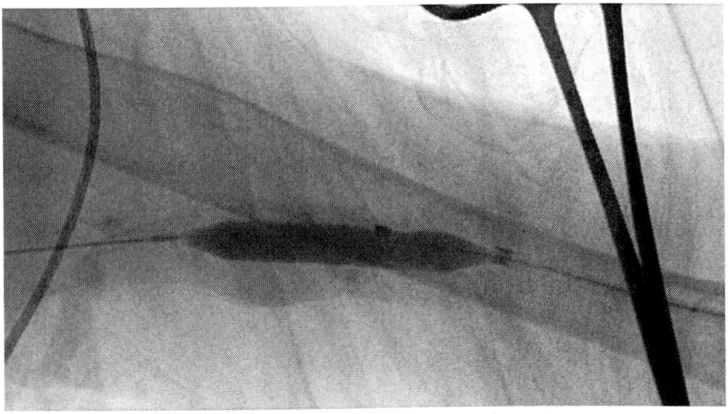

Fig. 29.42

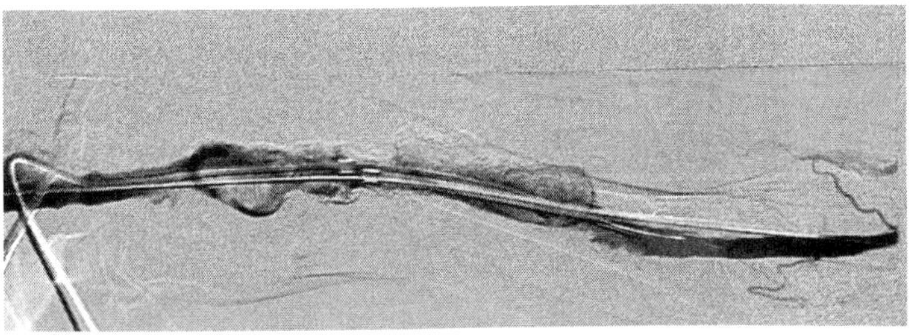

Fig. 29.43

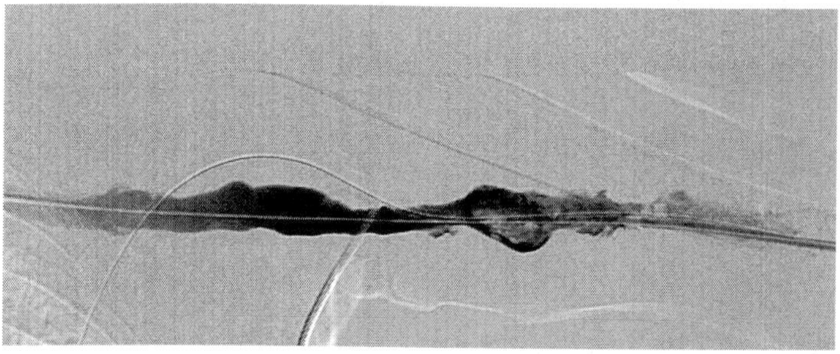

Fig. 29.44

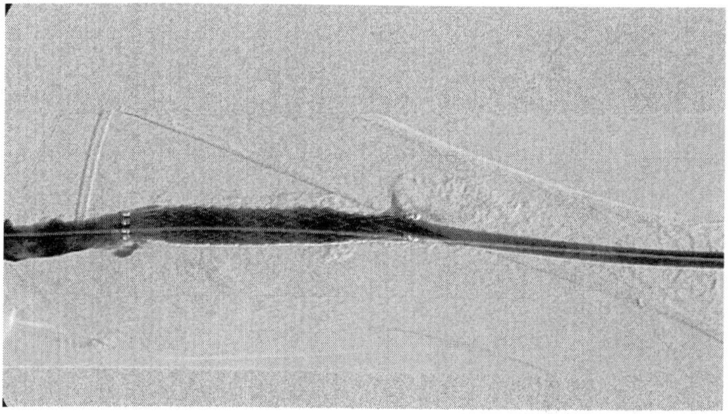

Fig. 29.45

Management

Initially, the angioplasty balloon was used to try free up the clot in the pseudoaneurysms using external pressure with fingers and subsequently the barrel of a 10 cc syringe. Figure 29.44 shows that this technique worked to clear out the venous puncture site aneurysm but failed to clear out the thrombus in the arterial puncture site pseudoaneurysm. We then deployed a stent graft (Fluency, 8 × 60 mm, CR Bard), to isolate the pseudoaneurysm and the clot within it from the circuit. Any residual clot exposed to blood in the graft, will tend to propagate and cause early thrombosis and there was concern of this happening in this case. The final angiogram (Fig. 29.45), shows brisk flow and no evidence of endoleak. We considered, but did not aspirate the blood out of the pseudoaneurysms as most of it was clotted. The graft was used the next day, and the hemodialysis needles were placed easily through the sent graft without complication. At 3-month follow-up, the graft was working well. There were no issues with needle placement through the Fluency stent graft.

Educational Points

When declotting a graft, it is mandatory, to remove all visible thrombus, and to have brisk flow in the graft. Any residual clot can lead to early rethrombosis, within a few hours. After failing to clear the pseudoaneurysms of thrombus using pharmacokinetic techniques (rt-PA, balloon maceration and external massage), stent grafts are a viable option in excluding the thrombus from the graft and returning brisk antegrade flow to the circuit.

Case 11
Duplication of SVC with Placement of a Dialysis Catheter on the Left Side

John R. Ross

Introduction

The patient underwent a first stage basilic vein transposition on the left with a right side IJ catheter in place. The right catheter became infected. Upon removal of the right catheter, insertion of a left sided catheter revealed duplication of SVC (see Fig. 29.46).

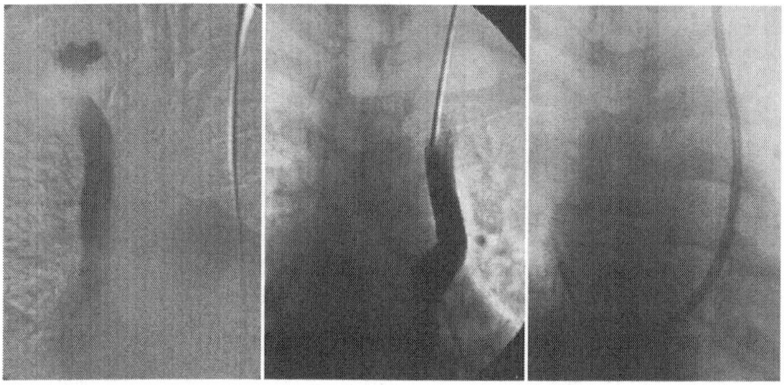

Fig. 29.46 Venogram done on the right side demonstrates a normal right sided SVC. A venogram from the left demonstrates a persistent left SVC with no left brachiocephalic vein. The new dialysis catheter was inserted with the tip passing into the coronary sinus

Issue/Complication

The patient will require a central catheter for 8 weeks for second stage basilic vein transposition and maturation. Will hemodialysis with this catheter configuration result in a patient safety issue?

Management

A left sided dialysis catheter in a patient with SVC duplication may be left in place without any safety issues. A peristent or duplicated SVC is present in 0.5% of the population and the left brachiocephalic vein is absent. The left SVC almost always drains to the coronary sinus [17].

Educational Points

Although somewhat rare, this central venous variation does occur.

Case 12
Rupture of SVC during PTA with Massive Hemothorax and Shock

John R. Ross

Introduction

The patient had been classified as catheter dependent for 2 years. The plan was to place a percutaneous sutureless anastomosis graft placement on the right side (Case 15). An initial venogram revealed a high-grade stenosis in brachiocephalic/SVC vein junction (see Fig. 29.47).

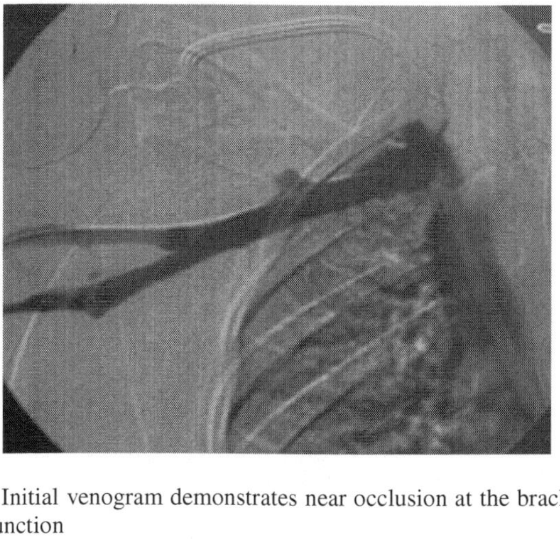

Fig. 29.47 Initial venogram demonstrates near occlusion at the brachiocephalic vein/SVC junction

A 10 mm×4 cm balloon was inflated to 16 atm to treat the stenosis. The post-angioplasty imaging revealed no obvious extravasation.

Issue/Complication

The patient developed hemothorax and shock within a couple hours of the dilation.

Management

The patient was admitted and required fluid and blood product resuscitation. An initial chest X-ray demonstrated complete opacification of the right hemithorax and a chest tube was placed returning blood (see Fig. 29.48). A repeat angiogram revealed no contrast beyond previous stricture with no obvious extravasation. A 10×100 mm Viabahn stent graft placed across the area of previous angioplasty with excellent results (see Fig. 29.49). The patient's bleeding and shock resolved and they were subsequently discharged three days later without complications.

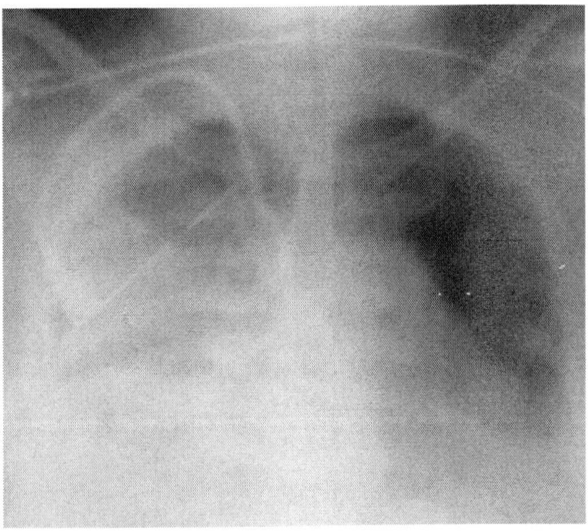

Fig. 29.48 Chest X-ray with near complete opacification of the right hemothorax. A chest tube has been placed

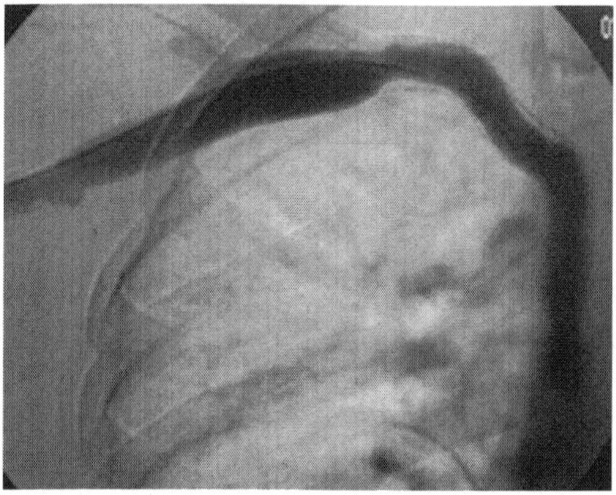

Fig. 29.49 Venogram after placement of Viabahn stent graft showing good flow and no extravasation of contrast

Educational Points

Central venous PTA ruptures are rare but can be quite lethal. A rule of thumb is if PTA is performed on the central veins, the appropriate size stent graft can be life saving.

Case 13
Ischemic Foot with Thigh PTFE Loop Groin Graft

John R. Ross

Introduction

The patient had 6 mm PTFE graft in place for 3 years without problems. Foot ischemia developed over a 2 month time frame (see Fig. 29.50). Significantly, prior to ischemia developing, the patient experienced a myocardial infarction (MI) and beta blockers were initiated. Prior to the MI the systolic blood pressures were 160–180. Following treatment initiation with beta blockers the systolic blood pressures were 100–110.

Issue/Complication

Could the leg and thigh graft be salvaged?

Management

An aortogram with runoff was performed and essentially negative for significant peripheral vascular disease. Severe steal syndrome was present. Central graft banding was performed with a 7 × 50 mm Viabahn stent graft and a 3 mm PTA balloon.

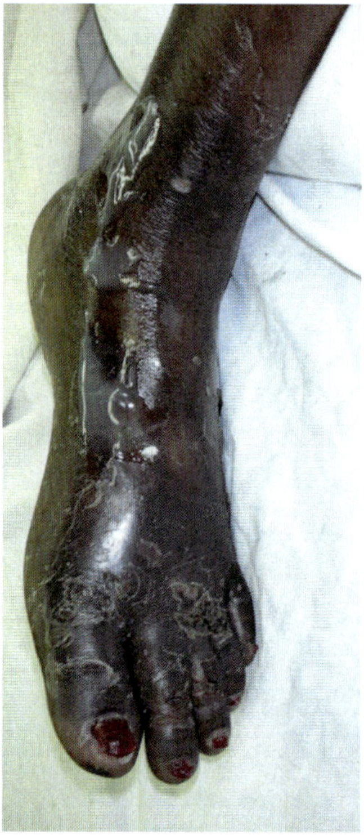

Fig. 29.50 Ischemic changes of the foot

Technique

The 7×50 mm stent graft was placed in the central portion of the graft. A 3 mm PTA balloon is placed in the center of the stent graft (see Fig. 29.51). With the balloon inflated to burst pressure a 2-0 monofilament tie is placed around the stent graft onto the balloon resulting in a 3 mm stricture (see Fig. 29.52). The graft rarely clots with this technique but will frequently clot without the stent graft (see Fig. 29.53).

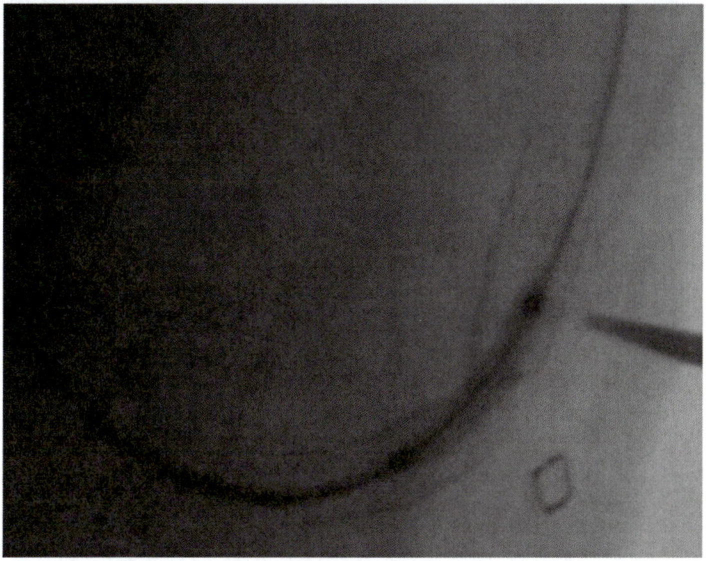

Fig. 29.51 Viabahn stent graft within the thigh graft with 3 mm balloon inflated within it. A 2-0 monofilament suture has been placed around the graft and tied narrowing the graft and intraluminal stent graft to a luminal diameter of 3 mm

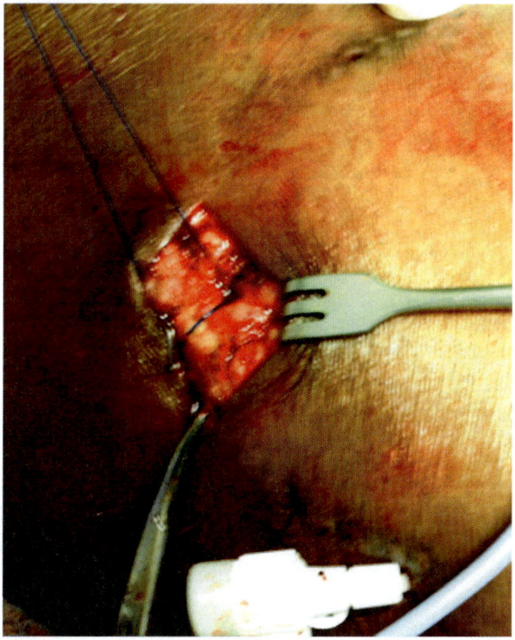

Fig. 29.52 The suture has been placed with a small incision in the skin over the midpoint of the stent graft visualized with fluoroscopy

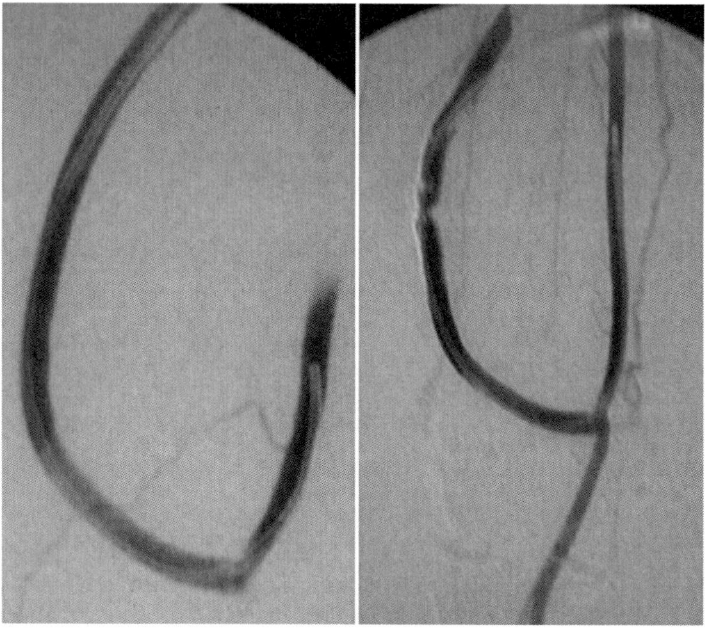

Fig. 29.53 Pre- and postfistulograms with flow reduced from 1,000 to 200 mL/min. Arterial needle is placed in graft before the banded area and venous needle is placed into the graft beyond the banded area

Educational Points

Thigh graft ischemia is very difficult to manage. The central banding technique drops blood flow substantially. The arterial needle is placed on the inflow part of the graft proximal to banding with the venous needle distal to the banding. This allows for good dialysis with low flow in the graft. The parallel circuit will flow at the prescribed blood flow rate on the dialysis machine.

Case 14
Rapidly Expanding Fistula Aneurysm with Thin Skin

John R. Ross

Introduction

A patient presented with a 6-year-old brachiocephalic fistula with rapid increase in size of an aneurysm. The patient had a previous history of cephalic arch stenosis requiring repeated PTAs and placement of a 8×100 mm stent graft. The most recent angiogram revealed a stenosis only at the outflow of the aneurysm.

Issue/Complication

Surgical or percutaneous repair of a true aneurysm with thin skin.

Management

Surgical resection of the anterior portion of the aneurysm with the skin to section off the stricture area (see Figs. 29.54–29.57).

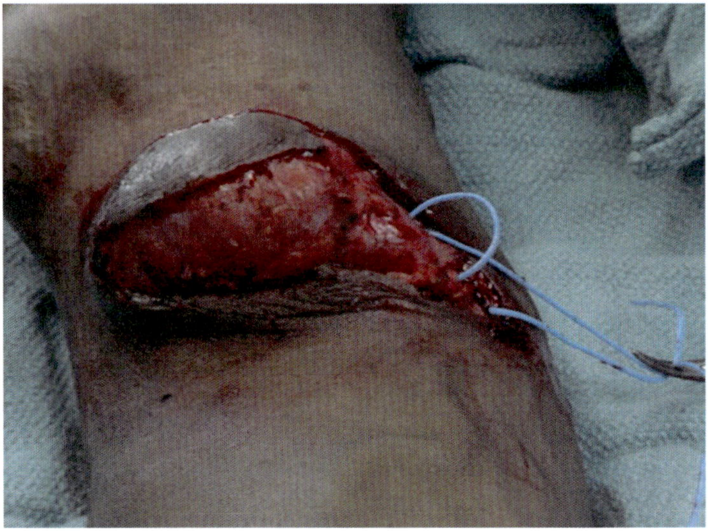

Fig. 29.54 Large aneurysm dissected out from surrounding skin

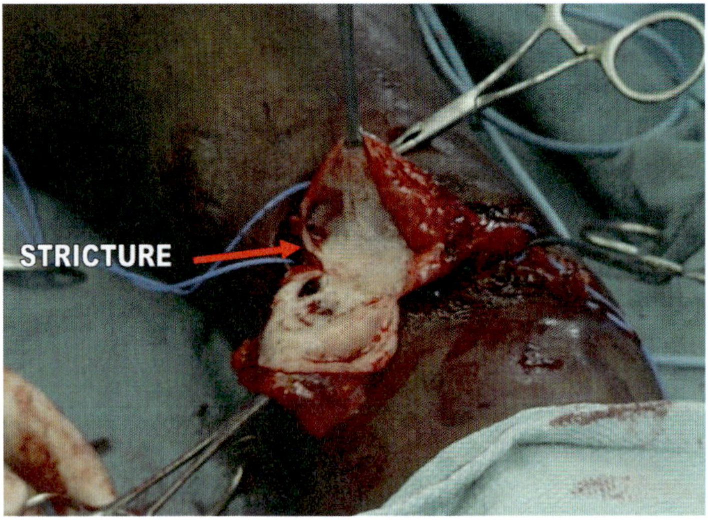

Fig. 29.55 Inflow and outflow control is obtained with lateral resection of aneurysm wall

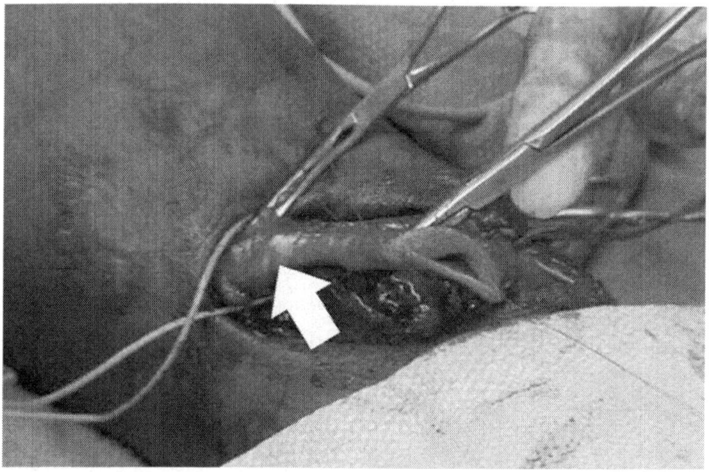

Fig. 29.56 Reconstruction of vessel with patch repair of outflow stenosis (*arrow*) at the end of the aneurysm

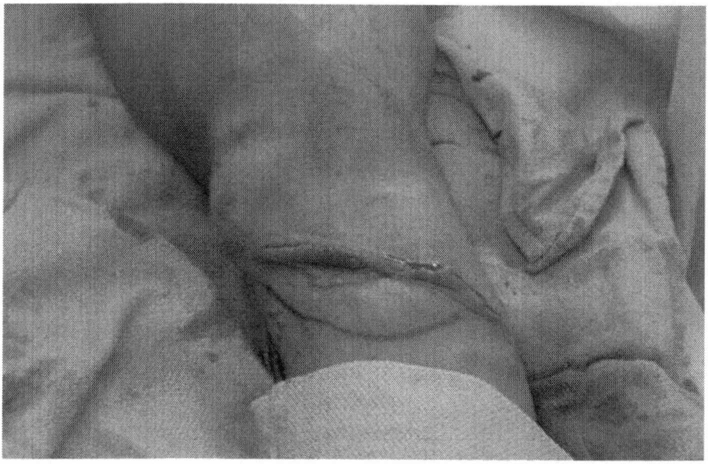

Fig. 29.57 The repaired fistula is tucked under skin flap and the skin is closed

Educational Points

Most aneurysms of fistulae are TRUE aneurysms. A simple anterior resection with a lateral repair and "tucking" of the repair under the skin resolves the problem providing a more durable and safer solution than percutaneous exclusion.

Case 15
Hybrid Surgical/Percutaneous Access Placement

John R. Ross

Introduction

The patient was presented for new access placement The prior access history included three axillary access procedures on the left, a prior basilic vein transposition, cephalic fistula with drop down to axilla, and a prior exploration of axilla for graft placement all on the left (see Fig. 29.58).

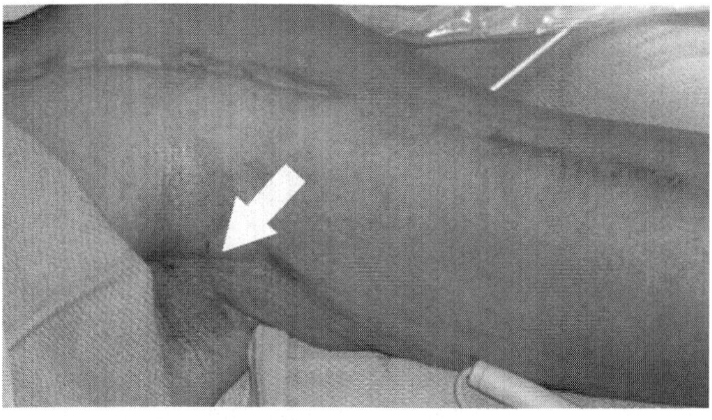

Fig. 29.58 Basilic vein transposition failure and cephalic drop down failure (*arrow*)

Issue/Complication

Abandon thoughts of left access placement?

Management

Creation of a percutaneous sutureless venous anastomosis graft placement on the left. Using ultrasound, the left axillary vein is easily identified. The axillary vein was punctured in an antegrade direction and over-a-wire, a peel-away vascular sheath was placed following a venogram confirming patency of the vein. The brachial artery was then exposed near the elbow with subcutaneous tunneling of 6 mm PTFE graft to the percutaneous axillary puncture where a small subcutaneous pocket was created. The 0.035 in. wire was backloaded through the tunneled graft (see Fig. 29.59). A 8×150 mm Viabahn stent graft (W.L. Gore, Flagstaff, AZ) was then threaded over the wire through the graft and then through the peel-away sheath to an adequate outflow vein. The peel-away sheath was then removed (see Fig. 29.60)

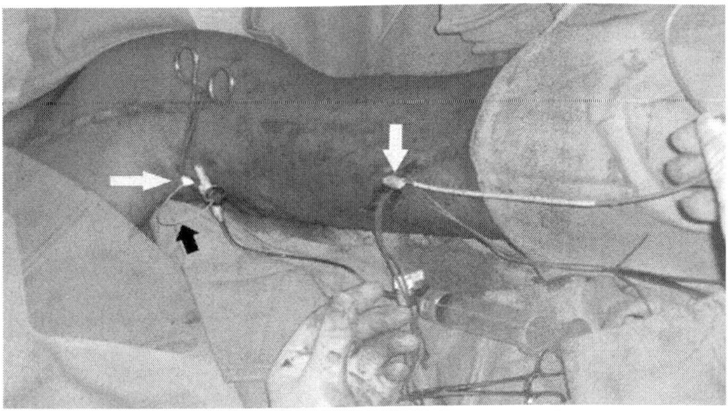

Fig. 29.59 Graft has been tunneled subcutaneously from brachial site to the percutaneous axillary puncture site (*white arrows*). The wire passing through the axillary peel-away sheath was backloaded (*black arrow*) through the graft

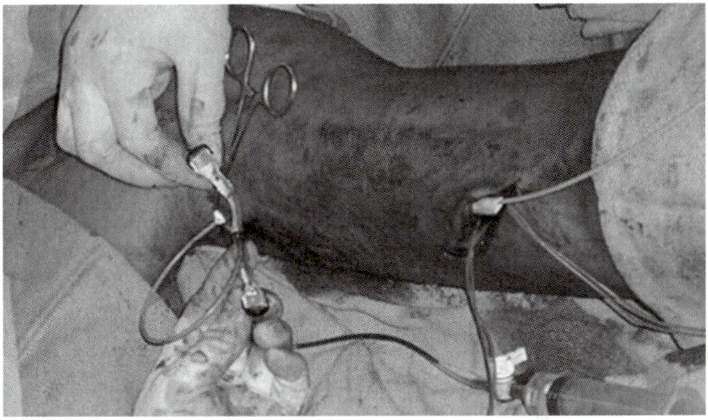

Fig. 29.60 After the stent graft is passed through the graft and through the peel-away sheath, the peel-away sheath is removed

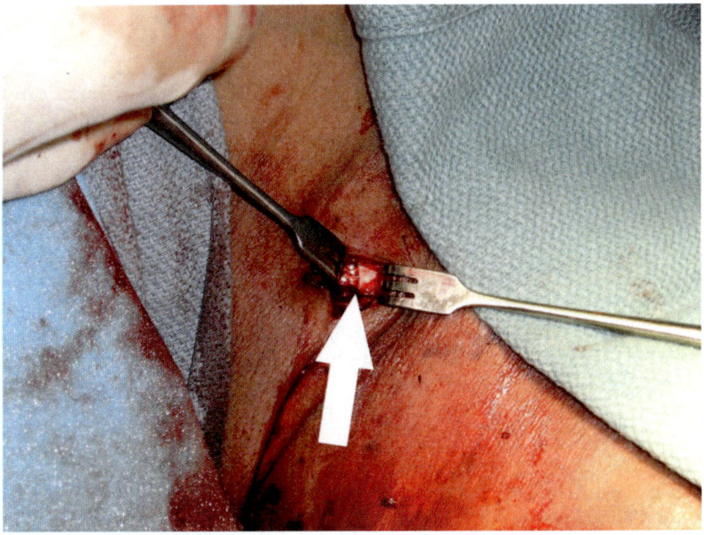

Fig. 29.61 The sutureless "stengraftomosis" (*arrow*) at the axillary puncture site

and the Viabahn was then deployed from the vein with 4 cm of the Viabahn extending into the graft creating a sutureless anastomosis (see Fig. 29.61). A standard arterial anastomosis is then performed with the tunneled graft to the brachial artery.

Educational Points

1. Novel combinations of surgery and percutaneous techniques can be used to create accesses previously not considered or possible.
2. A sutureless venous anastomosis potentially avoids later formation of venous anastomotic stenosis.

References

1. Kariya S, Tanigawa N, Kojima H, Komemushi A, Shomura Y, Shiraishi T, et al. Peripheral stent placement in hemodialysis grafts. Cardiovasc Intervent Radiol. 2009;32(5):960–6.
2. Haage P, Vorwerk D, Piroth W, Schuermann K, Guenther RW. Treatment of hemodialysis-related central venous stenosis or occlusion: results of primary Wallstent placement and follow-up in 50 patients. Radiology. 1999;212(1): 175–80.
3. Kapoor B, Lockhart M, Sharma D, Maya ID. Brachiocephalic vein stent fracture: case series and literature review. Semin Dial. 2010;23(1):110–3.
4. Lee T, Barker J, Allon M. Tunneled catheters in hemodialysis patients: reasons and subsequent outcomes. Am J Kidney Dis. 2005;46:501–8.
5. Rayner HC, Besarab A, Brown WW, Disney A, Saito A, Pisoni RL. Vascular access results from the dialysis outcomes and practice patterns study (DOPPS): Performance against kidney disease outcomes quality initiative (K/DOQI) clinical practice guidelines. Am J Kidney Dis. 2004;44:22–6.
6. Maya ID, Allon M. Outcomes of tunneled femoral hemodialysis catheters: comparison with internal jugular vein catheters. Kidney Int. 2005;68: 2886–9.
7. Chan MR, Dall AT, Fletcher KE, Lu N, Trivedi H. Outcomes in patients with chronic kidney disease referred late to nephrologists: a meta-analysis. Am J Med. 2007;120:1063–70.
8. Cecka JM. The OPTN/UNOS Renal Transplant Registry. Clin Transpl. 2005;1–16.
9. Barshes NR, Annambhotla S, Bechara C, Kougias P, Huynh TT, Dardik A, et al. Endovascular repair of hemodialysis graft-related pseudoaneurysm: an alternative treatment strategy in salvaging failing dialysis access. Vasc Endovascular Surg. 2008;42(3):228–34.
10. Barrett N, Spencer S, McIvor J, et al. "Subclavian stenosis": a major complication of subclavian dialysis catheters. Nephrol Dial Transplant. 1988;3: 423–5.
11. Agarwal AK, Patel BM, Farhan NJ. Central venous stenosis in hemodialysis patients is a common complication of ipsilateral central vein catheterization. J Am Soc Nephrol. 2004;15:368A–9.
12. Kundu S. Central venous disease in hemodialysis patients: prevalence, etiology and treatment. J Vasc Access. 2010;11:1–7.

13. Dember LM, Beck GJ, Allon M, et al. Effect of clopidogrel on early failure of arteriovenous fistulas for hemodialysis: a randomized controlled trial. JAMA. 2008;299:2164–71.
14. Bent CL, Rajan DK, Tan K, Simons ME, et al. Effectiveness of stent-graft placement for salvage of dysfunctional arteriovenous hemodialysis fistulas. J Vasc Interv Radiol. 2010;21:496–502.
15. Turmel-Rodriguez L, Pengloan J, Rodrigue H, et al. Treatment of failed native arteriovenous fistulae for hemodialysis by interventional radiology. Kidney Int. 2000;57:1124–40.
16. Schon D, Mishler R. Pharmacomechanical thrombolysis of natural vein fistulas: Reduced dose of TPA and long-term follow-up. Semin Dialysis. 2003;16: 272–5.
17. Demos TC, Posniak HV, Pierce KL, Olson MC, Muscato M. Venous anomalies of the thorax. AJR Am J Roentgenol. 2004;182(5):1139–50.

Abbreviations

abN	abnormal
ASA	Acetylsalicylic acid
Atm	atmospheres
AVF	arteriovenous fistula
AVG	arteriovenous graft
Avg	average
BAM	balloon assisted maturation
BB	brachiobasilic
BBT	brachiobasilic transposed
BC	brachiocephalic
bFGF	basic fibroblast growth factor
BFR	blood flow rate
BMS	bare metal stent
BP	blood pressure
CBA	cutting balloon angioplasty
CDC	Centers for disease control and prevention
CKD	chronic kidney disease
CMS	Centers of medicare and medicaid services
CO	cardiac output
CO2	carbon dioxide
CPR	cardiopulmonary resuscitation/recirculation
CQI	continuous quality improvement
CR	crude rates
CVC	central venous catheter
CVI-Q	quantitative color velocity index
CVP	central venous pressure
DDAVP	desmopressin
DES	drug eluding stent
DOPPS	dialysis outcomes and practice plans study
DOQI	dialysis outcomes quality initiative
DRIL	distal revascularization with interval ligation
DSA	digital subtraction angiography
DVP	Dynamic venous pressure
ECG	electrocardiogram
ESRD	end stage renal disease
FDA	Food and drug administration
FFBI	Fistula first breakthrough initiative
Fr	French
Gd	gadolinium
GFR	glomerular filtration rate
HD	hemodialysis
HIF-1	hypoxia inducible factor-1
ICC	intraclass correlation coefficients
IFU	Indications for use
II	image intensifier
IJV	internal jugular vein
INR	international normalized ratio
IR	interventional radiology
IV	intravenous

D.K. Rajan (ed.), *Essentials of Percutaneous Dialysis Interventions*,
DOI 10.1007/978-1-4419-5657-6,

© Springer Science+Business Media, LLC 2011

IVC	inferior vena cava
JAS	juxtaanastomotic segment
K/DOQI	kidney disease outcomes quality initiative
Kt/V	quantification of hemodialysis adequacy (K-dialyzer clearance of urea, t-time, V-volume of distribution of urea)
kVp	peak kilovoltage
MAP	mean arterial pressure
Min	minute
mm	millimeter
MMP	matrix metalloproteinases
MRA	magnetic resonance angiography
MRI	magnetic resonance imaging
NCRR	National center for research resources
NIH	National institutes of health
NPO	nil per os (nothing by mouth)
NSF	nephrogenic systemic fibrosis
OP	outpatient
OTW	over the wire
PAI	proximalization of arterial inflow
PD	peritoneal dialysis
PDGF	platelet derived growth factor
PDSA	plan-do-study-act
PICC	peripherally inserted central catheter
Pmp	per million population
PO	per oral
POBA	plain old balloon angioplasty
PT	prothrombin time
PSV	Peak systolic velocity
PTA	percutaneous transluminal (balloon) angioplasty
PTD	percutaneous thrombectomy device
PTFE	polytetrafluoroethylene
PTT	partial thromboplastin time
Q	blood flow
Qa	access blood flow
Qb	blood pump flow
QA	Quality assurance
QI	Quality initiative
R	resistance or recirculation
RC	radiocephalic
RCT	randomized controlled trial
ROC	receiver operating characteristic
ROS	reactive oxygen species
RUDI	revision using distal inflow
r-tPA	recombinant tissue plasminogen activator
SCV	subclavian vein
SIR	Society of interventional radiology
SVC	superior vena cava
SVP	Static venous pressure
TCC	tunneled cuffed catheter
TGF-β	transforming growth factor-beta
TIMPs	tissue inhibitors of matrix metalloproteinases
tPA	tissue plasminogen activator
UD	ultrasound dilution
UK	urokinase
US	ultrasound
VA	vascular access
VAC	vascular access coordinator
VAT	vascular access team
VEGF-A	vascular endothelial growth factor-A
VNH	venous neointimal hyperplasia
VP	venous pressure
VPF	vascular permeability factor
WSS	wall shear stress

Index

Printed by Publishers' Graphics LLC